AF556936

This small volume is dedicated to my teachers,
Dr. Harry M. Zimmerman and Dr. Robert D. Terry,
as the two individuals to whom
I owe my greatest debt for both introducing me to
the fundamentals of neuropathology and inspiring me
to enter the field and commit myself to it.

FOREWORD

The beginner in neuropathology, be he medical student or nonmorphologist in the neurosciences, will find this book invaluable. The aim obviously is to provide the background for future exploration in this field. Elementary considerations of normal neuroanatomy are provided which are basic to an understanding of morbid neuroanatomy, both macro- and microscopical. And much more is included, such as methods of removal of the human nervous system from the body for detailed study by sectioning, fixation for preservation, and staining for light and electron microscopy. This book is a veritable vade mecum, hardly needing a living mentor to supervise procedures and interpretations. It is quite practical, for it is based on methods derived from years of usage in training many generations of neuropathologists at the Montefiore Hospital and Medical Center in New York.

It is to be noted that the contents of this book are arranged in a novel fashion. There is no attempt, as is the case in the usual textbook of pathology, to group the contents according to disease entities. Rather, pathologic states are illustrated according to their topography. That is, conditions that affect the cortical gray matter are grouped in one section; those affecting the central gray in another; those in the central white matter in another; the blood vessels, glia and meninges in yet other sections. The same topographic determinant applies to the spinal cord. This method of presentation has proved to be effective in over twenty years of instruction of fellows and residents, which is the span of the author's experience in teaching neuropathology.

In an important sense this book is more than a beginner's guide. Numerous illustrations depicting known, and less well known, alterations in the neuropil, neurons, glia and blood vessels serve as reminders of morphologic change and offer quick help even to the initiated in neuropathology. A serviceable index provides aid in locating the graphic examples of these morphologic alterations.

It will be noticed that the majority of the sectional citations to the literature refer to the author's own publications. This provides a certain sense of immediacy and assurance, and cannot help but document the prodigious knowledge on which this book is based. But there is also a helpful, more inclusive bibliography at the end of the volume to satisfy the wants of the reader who may desire to delve more deeply.

H.M. Zimmerman, M.D.

PREFACE

The present volume was written with two, somewhat contradictory, purposes in mind. The first purpose was to provide a practical guide for the beginning neuropathologist. In general, the text describes the methods used at Montefiore Hospital for the training of the young neuropathologist. The student is acquainted with the requirement for careful collection of clinical data and pathologic material and is introduced to the techniques used in neuropathology. He or she is then led in a stepwise fashion to the examination of the brain beginning with gross external examination and proceeding to the investigation of sectioned gross material. The latter includes the horizontal sections so useful for correlation with the CT scanner. Eventually the student is introduced to the microscopic examination of tissue. In keeping with the overall approach, the book is organized on an anatomic basis rather than from the point of view of disease classifications as are most other texts of neuropathology.

The second purpose was to serve as a single reference for the wealth of fine structural information concerning neuropathologic alterations which has become available in the last two or three decades. While detailed reviews of selected, specialized areas such as demyelination and aging are available there is, as yet, no single volume that attempts to gather all this information and present it in a way useful to the neuropathologist.

Two areas of practical importance to the neuropathologist have been omitted. These are muscle and peripheral nerve pathology. Recently, several excellent books on these subjects have appeared and are in wide use. The reader is referred to these in the text.

The bibliography is limited to my own publications and to other selected key references and is by no means complete. The list of textbooks will serve as a point of access to the literature.

The material used for the illustrations is derived from the collection at Montefiore Hospital and from a number of referred cases. I am grateful to the numerous individuals who have allowed me to examine those cases.

ASAO HIRANO

ACKNOWLEDGEMENTS

Many individuals have participated either directly or indirectly in the preparation of this volume. Among them are some who require special thanks. Dr. Leopold G. Koss, Professor and Chairman, Department of Pathology, Albert Einstein College of Medicine at Montefiore has provided us with support and encouragement throughout this undertaking. Drs. Nitya Ghatak and Josefina F. Llena, my associates in the Division of Neuropathology, have been constant collaborators. I am grateful to Dr. Herbert M. Dembitzer who has played such a valuable role in the preparation of this manuscript.

Finally, I must express my thanks to Mrs. Pearl Parsowith for her indefatigable service as secretary, typist and editor, to Miss Ernestine Middleton and Mrs. Glenna Smith for their expert technical assistance, and to Igaku-Shoin for their patience and help throughout this undertaking.

CONTENTS

I
The First Approach

A. THE MATERIAL (Fig. 1)

Neuropathology is that part of pathology which is primarily concerned with the nervous system; both the central and peripheral. Theoretically, it should be limited to these systems but, as a practical matter, it is really concerned with any specimen of interest to the neurologist or neurosurgeon. Thus, specimens of the scalp and skull are sometimes received in the neuropathology laboratory when removed by a neurosurgeon. Similarly, not only spinal cord material but also the vertebrae and certainly intervertebral discs, as well as epidural tissue, may often be the subject of neuropathologic examination. Because of the close relationship between the musculature and nervous tissue, the study of skeletal muscle is always an important part of neuropathology. In addition, the study of skin in such conditions as dermatomyositis and even examination of rectal biopsies in certain lipidoses are all valid parts of neuropathology (Landing et al., 1972; Fidelman and Lagunoff, 1972). In certain cases, parts of the sensory organs, too, such as the retina or the orbital contents become important subjects of study for the neuropathologist.

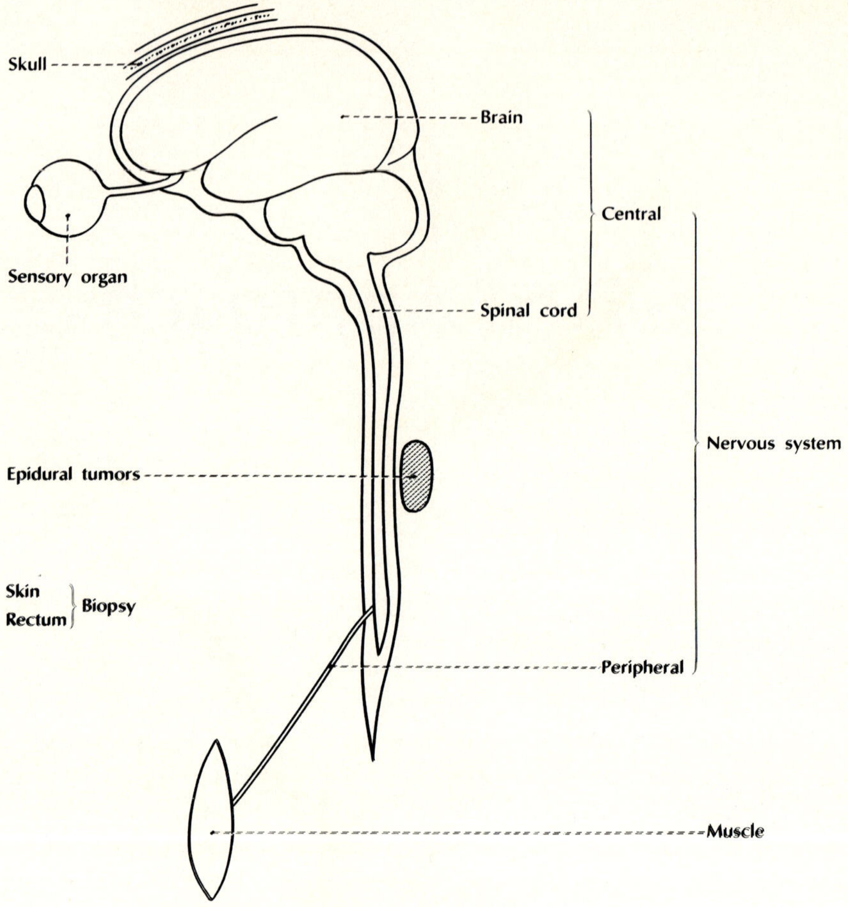

Fig. 1 Tissue for neuropathological study.

REFERENCES

Landing, B.H., Neustein, H.B., & Kamoshita, S.: Biopsy diagnosis of lipidosis: Background considerations, general concepts and practical aspects. *In* Sphingolipids, Sphingolipidoses and Allied Disorders. pp. 15-35, Volk, B.W., & Aronson, S.M. (eds.), Plenum Publishing Co., New York, 1972.

Fidelman, S., & Lagunoff, D.: The morphology of the normal human rectal biopsy. Human Pathol., 3: 389-401, 1972.

Dubowitz, V., & Brooke, M.H.: Muscle Biopsy: A Modern Approach. W.B. Saunders Co., Ltd, London, 1973.

Hughes, J.T.: Pathology of Muscle. W.B. Saunders Co., Philadelphia, 1974.

Burger, P.C., & Vogel, F.S.: Surgical Pathology of the Nervous System and its Coverings. John Wiley & Sons, New York, 1976.

B. TRAINING IN NEUROPATHOLOGY (Fig. 2)

In general, the individuals entering the training program will be derived from two sources. One is the clinician, either neurologist or neurosurgeon. The second is derived from general pathology. In most cases the career neuropathologist is derived from the department of general pathology but it is not uncommon to have neurologists or neurosurgeons enter the field on a full time basis.

The amount of time an individual spends in the department of neuropathology will depend, of course, on the future plans of the trainee. Those wishing to enter careers in neuropathology will spend at least two years in neuropathology in addition to other training requirements in order to qualify for board certification. Others may spend as little as three months in neuropathology wishing to gain only a superficial background in the field.

It is our experience that a period of less than six months is not feasible for even a minimum amount of training in the field. It is only at that time that the discipline is sufficiently understood to excite the interest of a serious student. Thus, even committed neurologists and neurosurgeons should plan on spending six months in neuropathology. As a practical matter, however, sometimes only three months are available in the busy schedules of the clinicians.

In an important sense, this mixture of clinician and pathologist is useful in a department of neuropathology. Generally, the neurologist or neurosurgeon brings with him a talent for relating the clinical symptoms and signs to the gross anatomy. He is, however, often deficient in appreciating microscopic change. The training pathologist, on the other hand, usually has a good grasp of microscopic morphology and is quick to evaluate alteration but he is often less than expert in correlating clinical data with morphological change, especially at the macroscopic level. Thus, a good department of neuropathology is a healthy mixture of clinicians and pathologists. In many ways they complement one another and each can learn from the other. When one adds the extra ingredient of an active research program, often involving basic scientists, then the neuropathology department becomes an exciting, vibrant place of academic excellence as well as a valuable service to the clinical departments.

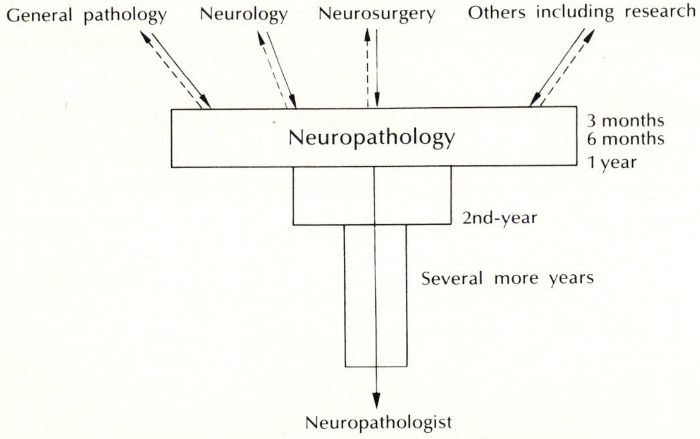

Fig. 2 Those who come to neuropathology.

C. THE IMPORTANCE OF CLINICAL DATA

When the novice neuropathologist is first informed of an impending autopsy of a patient of neurological interest, his first impulse is to immediately remove the brain and, perhaps, the spinal cord and submit them to formalin fixation. This is often not the wisest approach. Before approaching the cadaver, the neuropathologist must learn as much as he can concerning the patient from all the clinical data he can assemble. The general pathologist is, of course, at hand to help in this task and the clinician should also be available.

With the clinical data in mind, the neuropathologist can proceed with intelligence in the autopsy. The first question, of course, is which tissue is really of greatest interest? The brain is taken in almost every case. However, often other material is even more significant and should be removed for study. For example, in cases involving peripheral neuropathy, affected muscles and their associated nerves as well as the spinal cord are essential specimens. In other instances, effects on the brain or spinal cord are secondary to extradural pathologies such as metastases or abscess. In these cases the adjacent tissues are of at least equal interest and must be preserved.

When occlusion of the carotid artery is suspected then the bifurcation of the internal and external carotid arteries in the neck must be examined and removed if it is, indeed, occluded. If the bifurcation is patent, then water or saline must be injected into the internal carotid artery in the neck, after the brain is removed, to see whether the vessel is patent throughout its course. If occluded, it should be removed and preserved for the study of the siphon which is the second most common point of occlusion.

The point being made here is that an uninformed post mortem examination may be essentially useless. It is only by being forearmed with the clinical data that the neuropathologist can be sure of obtaining all the important specimens which, if lost, can never be retrieved.

D. REMOVAL AND PRESERVATION OF TISSUES (Fig. 3)

Once the decision concerning which tissues are needed has been made, the removal of these specimens must be performed promptly and with proper care. In most instances the brain and spinal cord will be removed by the morgue attendant and fixed in formalin. In some cases, however, when special studies are to be made, other means of preservation must be used. These decisions must be made before the tissue is taken.

For example, in cases of suggested viral or other infection, material must be selected from appropriate areas for culture, immunofluorescence, etc. before formalin fixation. Similarly, when other studies are indicated such as tissue culture, electron microscopy and some histochemistry, it may be necessary to preserve important areas by methods other than formalin fixation. For histochemical or neurochemical analysis of certain lipidoses and other conditions, samples of the material must be stored in the deep freeze rather than in fixative. Tissue culture requires that no fixative be used, but that sterile procedures be applied. For electron microscopy, glutaraldehyde rather than formalin is the fixative of choice.

As mentioned above, the morgue attendant usually removes the brain and spinal cord under routine conditions. Nevertheless, it is wise for the beginning neuropathologist to thoroughly familiarize himself with the procedure. Various methods have been described by a number of authors. The simple technique outlined by K.M. Earle is probably the most practical for the beginner.

Briefly, the method consists of cutting through the scalp from the mastoid over the crown. The scalp is then reflected anteriorly and posteriorly exposing the skull. After severing the temporal muscles, the skull is sawed through in a horizontal plane from a few centimeters above the upper edge of the orbit to above the external occipital protuberance. The dura mater is cut in the same plane. The falx cerebri is detached at the crista galli. The brain is lifted from the calvarium by raising the frontal lobe. The various attachments such as the optic nerves, pituitary

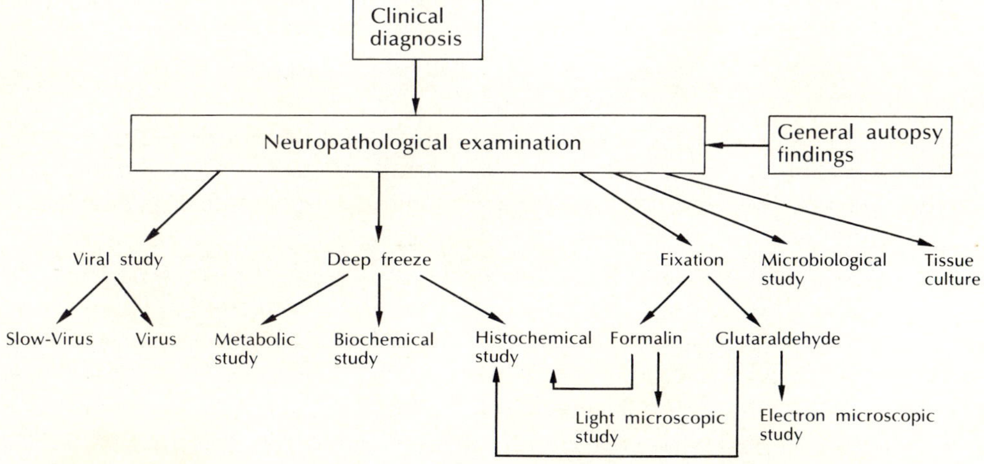

Fig. 3 Neuropathological study.

stalk, internal carotid arteries, etc. are cut as the brain is raised. As the brain is raised further, the cerebellar tentorium is cut along its edge. The cranial nerves and vertebral arteries are cut and finally the brain is detached from the spinal cord. The attached dura mater is cut and the brain is lifted free. In the adult, the dura mater separates easily from the skull. In infants, however, the dura mater is the periosteum of the skull and is, therefore, tightly adherent to the bone.

At this point the brain is weighed and, except when subarachnoid hemorrhage is present and barring any need for the special methods described above, it is fixed in 10% buffered formalin. Except for the time necessary for weighing, the unfixed brain should not be left on a hard surface. Perfusion fixation is preferred to simple immersion. About 100 ml of fixative are injected into the stump of each internal carotid artery and into the vertebral artery. The brain is then suspended in a jar of fixative by twine passed through the basilar artery and attached to the top of the jar. In those cases in which perfusion is unfeasible, such as when one or more major vessels are occluded, the brain is fixed by immersion alone.

When subarachnoid hemorrhage is seen, it is best to wash the brain in cold running water to remove as much blood as possible so as to more easily visualize the blood vessels. After washing, the brain is fixed as usual.

Once the brain is safely suspended in fixative, the base of the skull is examined for abnormalities. At this time the pituitary gland is usually removed and placed in fixative.

Removal of the spinal cord is more tedious and time consuming. There are two popular methods; the anterior and the posterior approaches. We have found the anterior approach more practical. After the thorax and abdomen are eviscerated, each vertebral arch is cut at the pedicle along with the surrounding soft tissue. The spinal cord and attached dura are lifted out and the roots are severed starting at the cervical level. Finally, the filum terminale is cut and the cord lifted free. Unless special methods are indicated, the entire cord is immersed in an elongated container of fixative.

Under routine circumstances, the brain and spinal cord are left in fixative for one or two weeks although they can be stored indefinitely. If left too long, however, the staining properties deteriorate. On the other hand, cutting fresh tissue invariably leads to distortion of the normal anatomy. By a week or two the tissue is firm and suitable for examination.

The importance of prompt fixation and gentle handling cannot be overemphasized. First, autolysis is a common artifact resulting from delayed fixation. In extreme cases this can lead to gross spongy changes as the result of gas formation in the tissue. This is the well-known "Swiss cheese-like" appearance (Fig. 4). Postmortem autolysis can also lead to the more confusing microscopic sponginess as a result of cellular disintegration. Second, rough handling of unfixed or incompletely fixed tissue can easily result in artifactual deformities in both the brain and the spinal cord. One well-known example is the so-called "tooth-paste" artifact of the spinal cord in which a portion is constricted leading to the abnormal displacement of tissue above and below the constriction (Figs. 5 and 6). Areas of interest, such as infarcts or tumors, are especially prone to these changes.

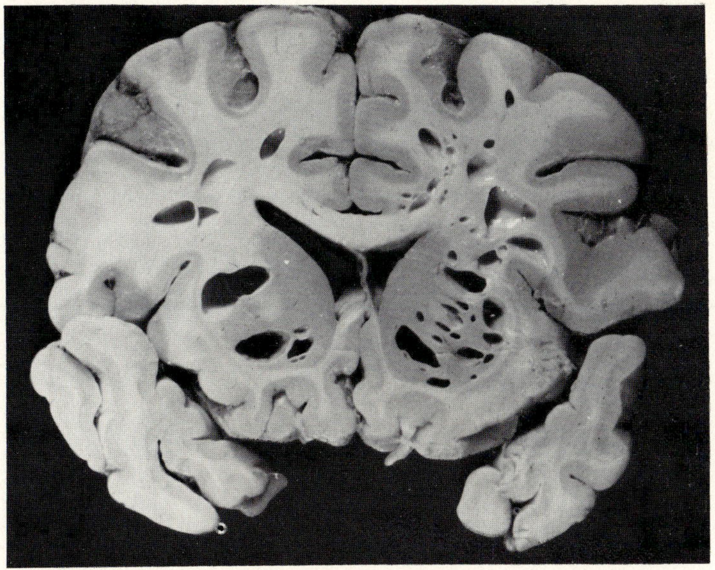

Fig. 4 "Swiss cheese" postmortem artifact.

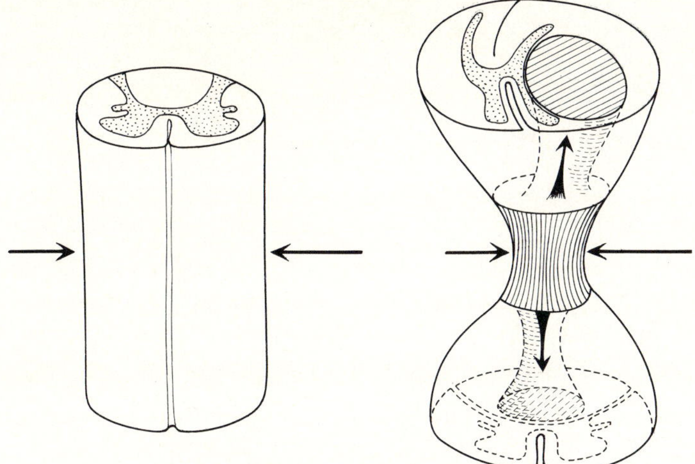

Fig. 5 "Toothpaste" artifact.

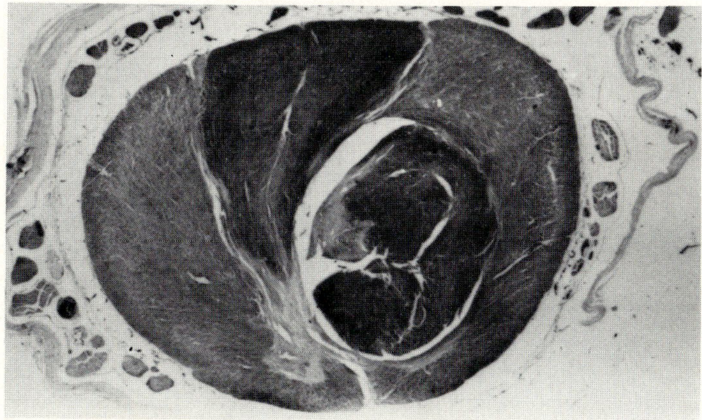

Fig. 6 "Toothpaste" artifact (myelin stain).

REFERENCES

Symposium on methods for the study of the central nervous system. *In* The Central Nervous System: International Academy of Pathology Monograph, pp. 284-347, Bailey, O.T., & Smith, P.E. (eds.), The Williams and Wilkins Company, Baltimore, 1968.

Hirano, A.: Electron microscopy in neuropathology. *In* Progress in Neuropathology. Vol. 1, pp. 1-61, Zimmerman, H.M. (ed.), Grune and Stratton, New York, 1971.

Earle, K.M.: Examination of the Brain, American Registry of Pathology, Armed Forces Institute of Pathology, Washington, D.C.

Hughes, J.T.: Pathology of the Spinal Cord. 2nd Ed., pp. 181-190, Lloyd Luke, London, 1978.

E. MACROSCOPIC EXAMINATION OF THE BRAIN AND SPINAL CORD

1. Concerning the Correlation of Clinical and Pathological Findings

Since a minimum of one or two weeks must elapse between the removal of the brain and its examination, it is a good practice to review the clinical data once more before the brain and spinal cord are cut for macroscopic examination. By this time, too, the data from the general autopsy should be available.

This is an extremely valuable review for the neuropathologist in training as well as for the diagnostic neuropathologist. It is at this time that the intellectual efforts of the diagnostician must be fully utilized. The object, of course, is to be able to predict the pathological findings as closely as possible.

In this regard, it is important to realize that the correlation between clinical and pathological findings is not always as clear cut as might be wished. First, sometimes obvious clinical features may be present with no discernible morphological alteration at either the macroscopic or microscopic levels. Functional psychoses, many paroxysmal disorders and certain infantile mental retardations are good examples of this. In other conditions, the macroscopic appearance of the brain may be essentially unremarkable whereas microscopic changes may be striking. Unless we are fully aware of the clinical features, essential parts of the brain may go unexamined and may even be discarded as normal brain. A good example of this situation is amyotrophic lateral sclerosis, where the reported obvious changes in the motor cortex are usually very hard to find with the naked eye. Some cases of Creutzfeldt-Jakob disease may also fail to reveal gross atrophic changes.

On the other hand, macroscopic examination may sometimes reveal lesions that are unexpected and missed by the clinician. Frequently, meningiomas and even acoustic neuromas may be detected during gross examination which were previously unsuspected, usually because of the prominence of other medical problems. We can expect that with increasing use of the computerized tomography method (CT Scan) these surprises will be fewer in the future. On the other hand, with the increased use of chemotherapy and steroids as well as antibiotics after, or in conjunction with organ transplants, or treatment of lymphomas and other malignancies, we can expect a greater number of occult viral and fungal infections of the brain. It is therefore wise to remove random samples of tissue for microscopic study even though gross lesions are absent. In general, it is to be remembered that once the brain is discarded it cannot be retrieved.

REFERENCE

Friedman, A.P., Carton, C.A., & Hirano, A.: Facial pain. Post-graduate Medicine., 27: 756-775, 1960.

2. Examination of the Brain

Before the brain can be conveniently examined it must be washed in cold running tap water for six to twelve hours in order to remove the excess formalin. The gross examination should be carried out in a well ventilated room because of the persistence of formalin vapors.

The brain weight was recorded before fixation and should again be noted for indication of pathology. The average adult brain weight is 1300 grams, but fairly wide variations around this average are not necessarily signs of pathology. Nevertheless, brain weight of less than 1000 grams or greater than 1500 grams in an adult suggests either atrophy or swelling, often accompanying a space-occupying lesion.

The average weight of children's brains is given in Fig. 7. Older individuals, especially after the age of 65 tend to have smaller brains. Finally, women tend to have smaller brains than men.

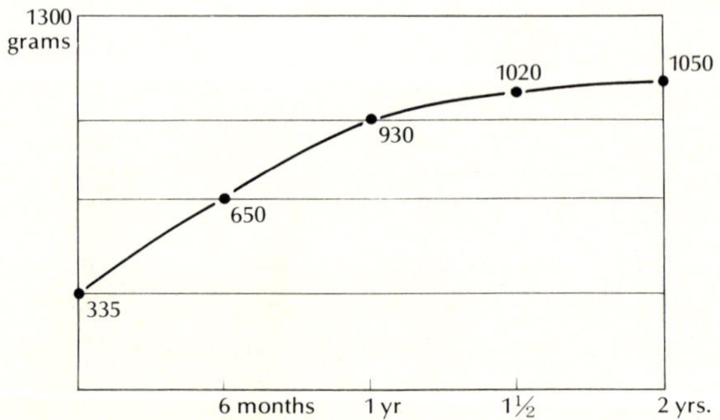

Fig. 7 Brain weight of the infant.

After fixation the brain and its meningeal coverings and attached blood vessels and cranial nerves are examined before the parenchyma itself is approached. This requires the removal of the dura mater and the careful examination of the leptomeninges, cranial nerves and the blood vessels in the subarachnoid space. Pathological changes in these structures will provide us with clues as to what may be expected in the underlying parenchyma both on external examination and after sectioning.

DURA MATER

Normally the dura mater is a thick, tough, white, smooth membrane containing venous sinuses. The most obvious change of the dura mater is the presence of either *epidural* (Fig. 8) or *subdural* (Figs. 9—12) *hematomas*. The age of the hematoma and the amount of bleeding will determine the details of its appearance.

Tumors may appear as protuberances on either the inner or the outer surface of the dura mater. Most often they are either *meningiomas* (Figs. 13, 14) or *metastatic lesions* (Figs. 15—17). Each may have either single or multiple foci.

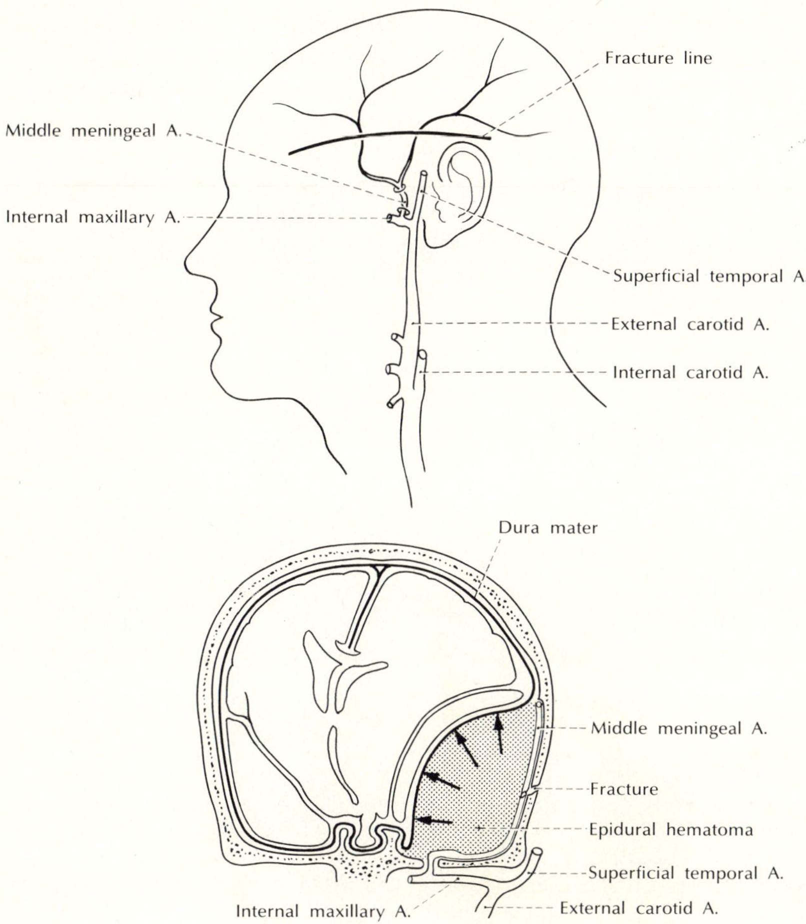

Fig. 8 Epidural hematoma.

The common carotid artery branches in the neck giving rise to the internal and external carotid arteries. The latter branches into the superficial temporal artery and the internal maxillary artery. The first branch of the internal maxillary artery is the middle meningeal artery which penetrates the skull through the foramen spinosum and appears at the base of the brain. It courses in a shallow groove between the dura mater and the skull, where it branches and supplies the temporal region of the skull. A transverse fracture such as that illustrated here may cause the rupture of the middle meningeal artery resulting in arterial bleeding between the dura and the skull and the formation of an expanding hematoma. This presses the dura against the parenchyma resulting in increased intracranial pressure and attendant serious sequelae. This phenomenon is particularly serious in adults where the dura has lost its strong adhesion to the skull. In children the dura mater is the periosteum of the still-developing skull and the strong adhesion prevents the separation of the dura from the bone. It is therefore rare to find large hematomas in newborn children. In addition, the skull itself is fairly elastic so that fracture is less likely in the first place.

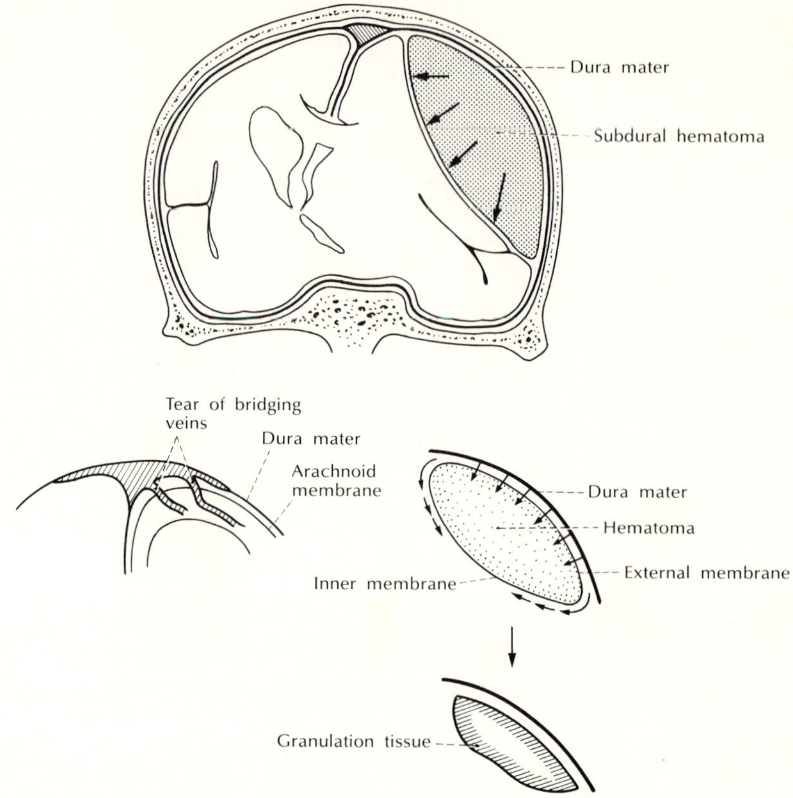

Fig. 9 Subdural hematoma.

In the event of a head injury in which the brain as a whole moves relative to the skull, a shearing force may develop across the bridging vein where the vein enters the sagittal sinus. If this force is great enough the vein will rupture and bleeding will occur into the subdural space between the dura mater and the arachnoid membrane. Unlike the epidural space the subdural space is real and permits the spread of the blood. This process represents the acute phase of the formation of a subdural hematoma.

The dura mater reacts to the presence of the extravasated blood by the formation of granulation tissue which encapsulates the hematoma. Eventually a blood-filled sac is formed often with thick membranous walls. The chronic subdural hematoma usually continues to expand slowly. The mechanism for this is obscure but it should be noted that fresh blood can often be found within a chronic subdural hematoma. When bleeding into the subdural space is minimal no encapsulation occurs. In such case the inner aspect of the dura mater presents a fine brown, friable membrane which can be easily peeled from the smooth, white dura mater. This phenomenon is often mistaken by the beginner as a stain due to post-mortem bleeding. In reality it represents a healed subdural hematoma.

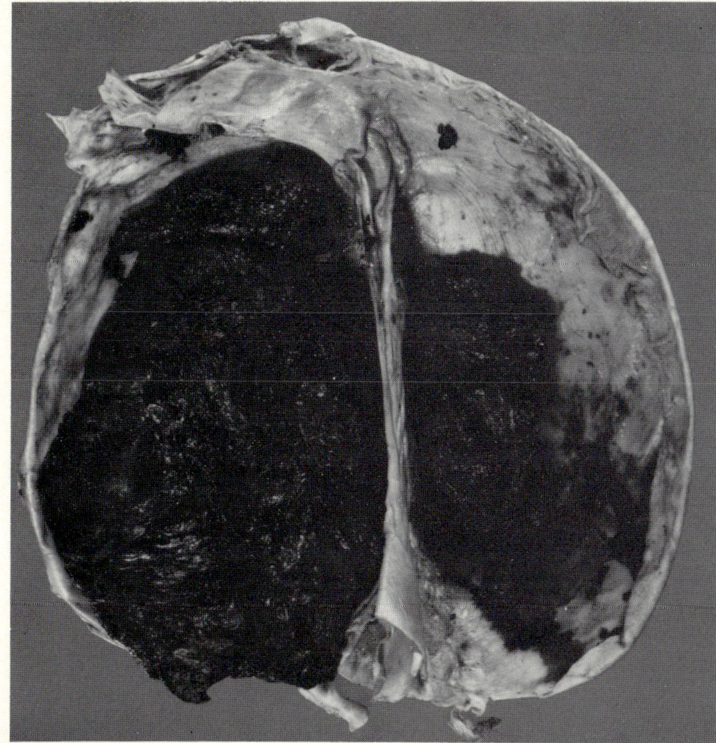

Fig. 10 Bilateral subdural hematomas.

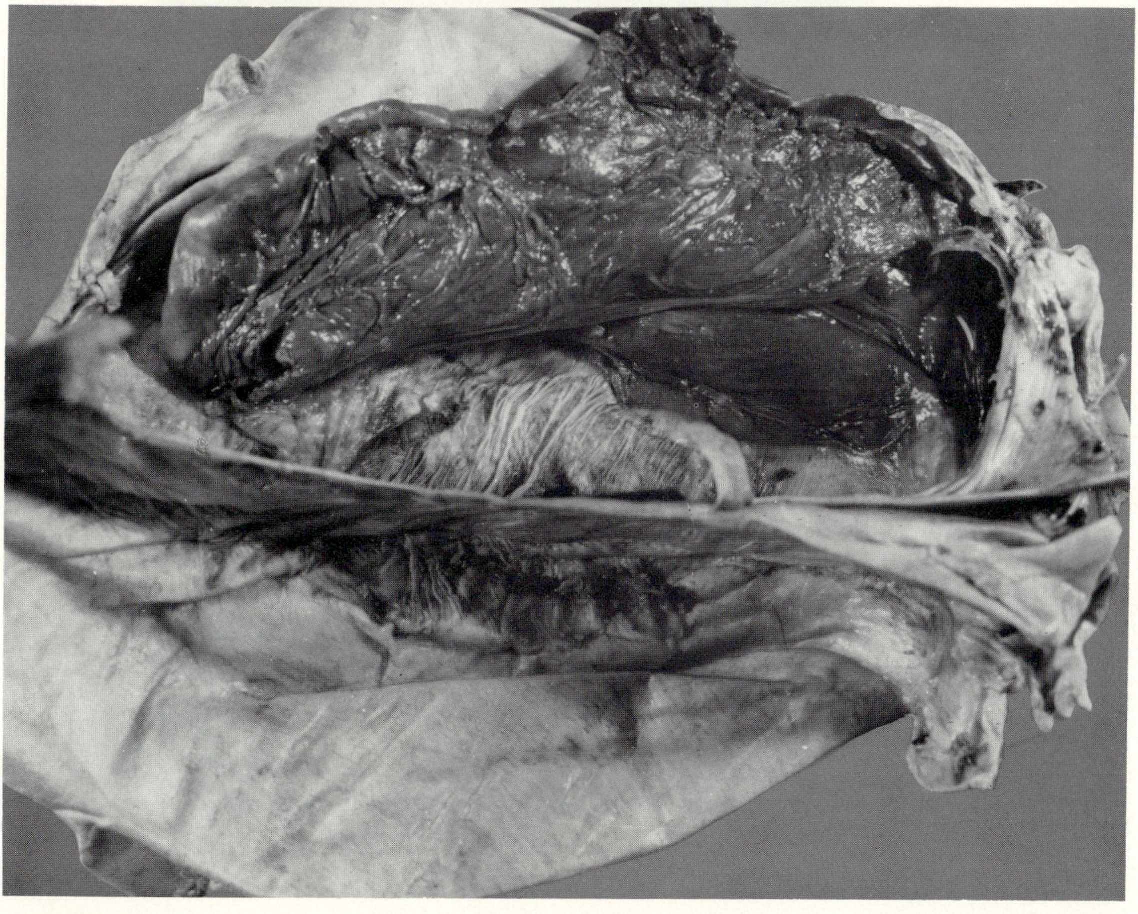

Fig. 11 Unilateral subdural hematoma.

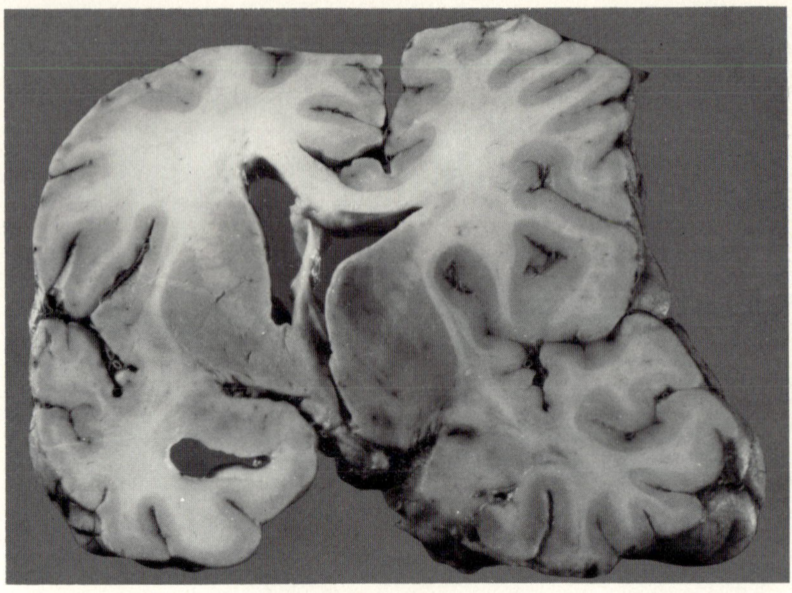

Fig. 12 Deformity of brain due to subdural hematoma.

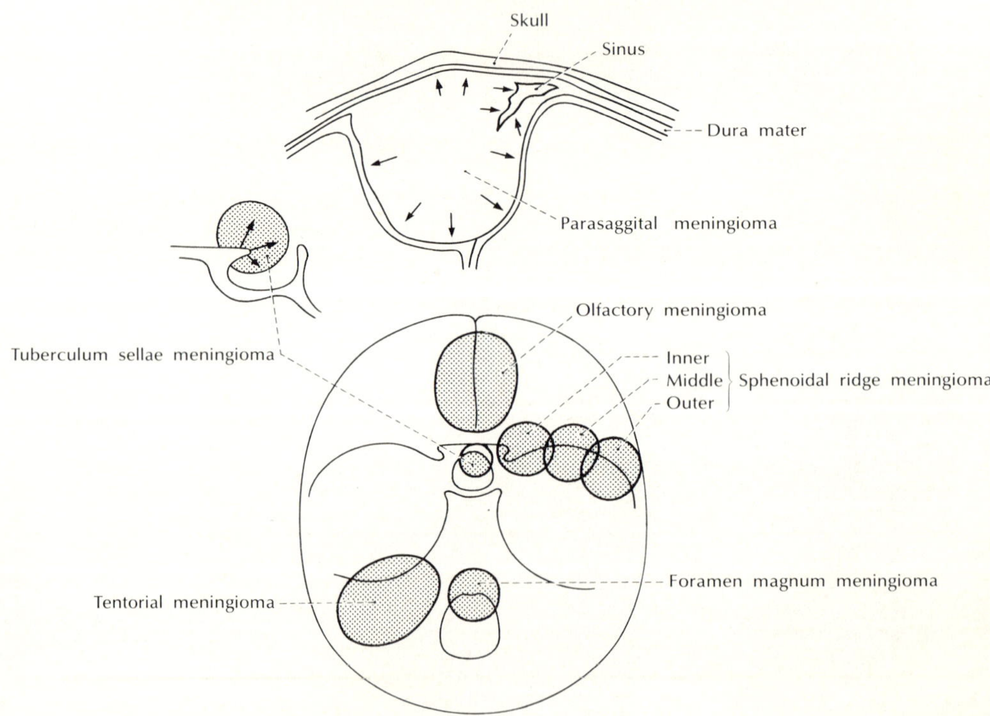

Fig. 13 Meningioma.

Meningiomas are among the most common and benign primary intracranial tumors affecting adults. They affect more women than men. They tend to occur in regions where arachnoid granulations are frequent, especially in the parasagittal area (about 50%). The sites of predilection are outlined here, and include the olfactory groove, sphenoidal ridge, tuberculum sellae, tentorial ridge and the foramen magnum. Meningiomas are well-circumscribed tumors attached to the dura mater. They may compress the underlying brain tissue but usually do not cause necrosis or hemorrhage. Most often they are single, but multiple tumors are not uncommon. Since total removal is often very difficult in the region of the superior sagittal sinus, recurrence in this area is virtually inevitable. Malignant meningiomas are exceptional.

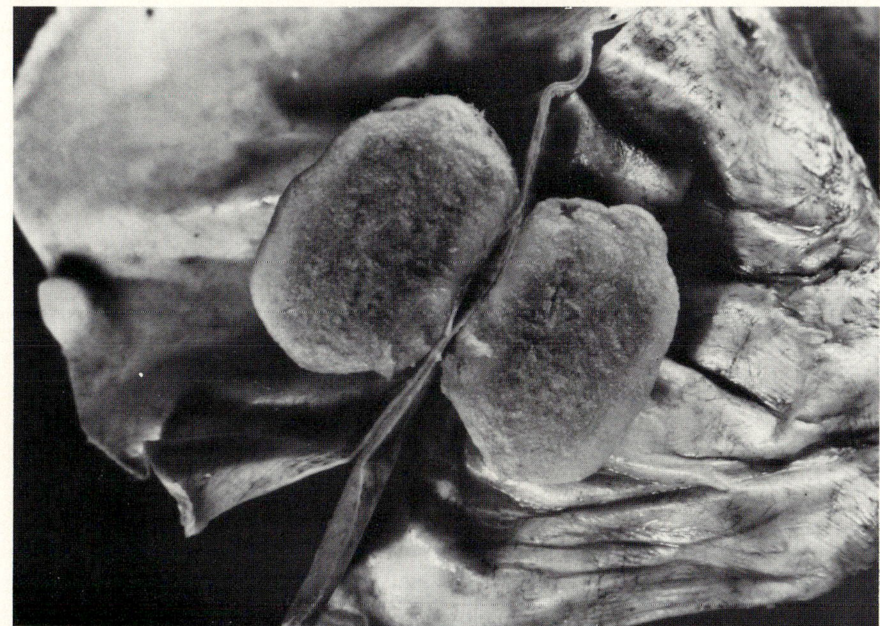

Fig. 14
Meningioma.

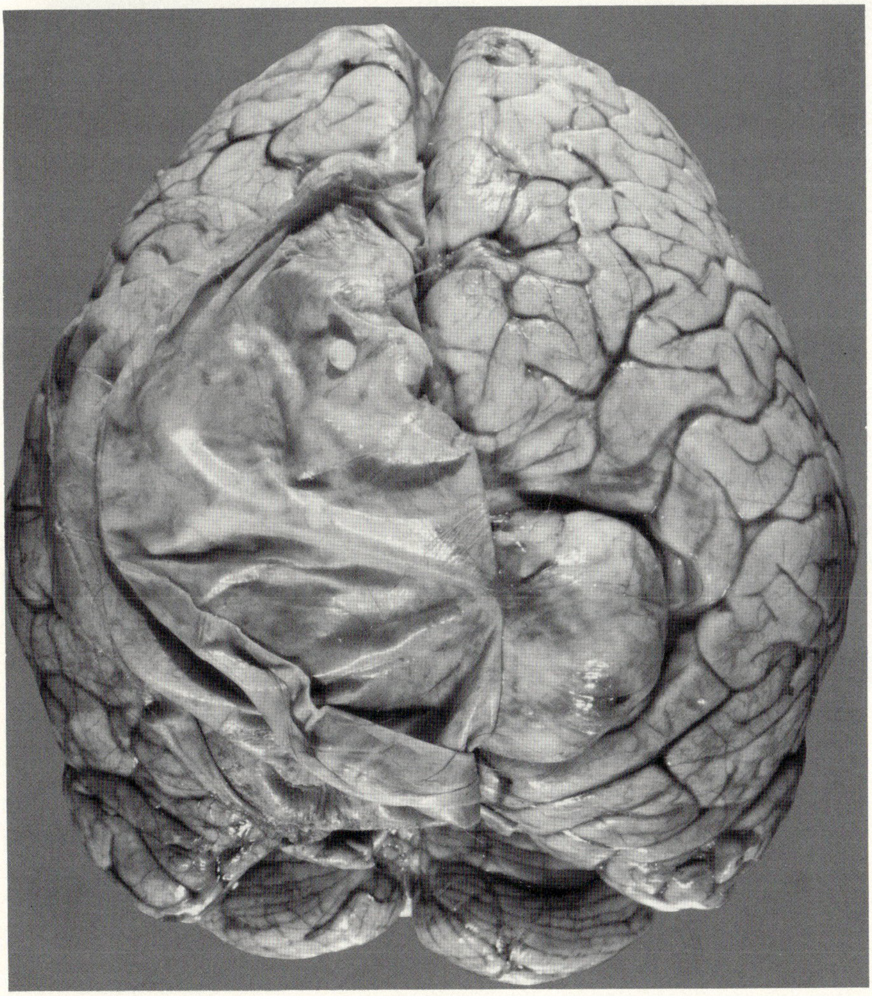

Fig. 15
Metastatic tumor resembling a meningioma.

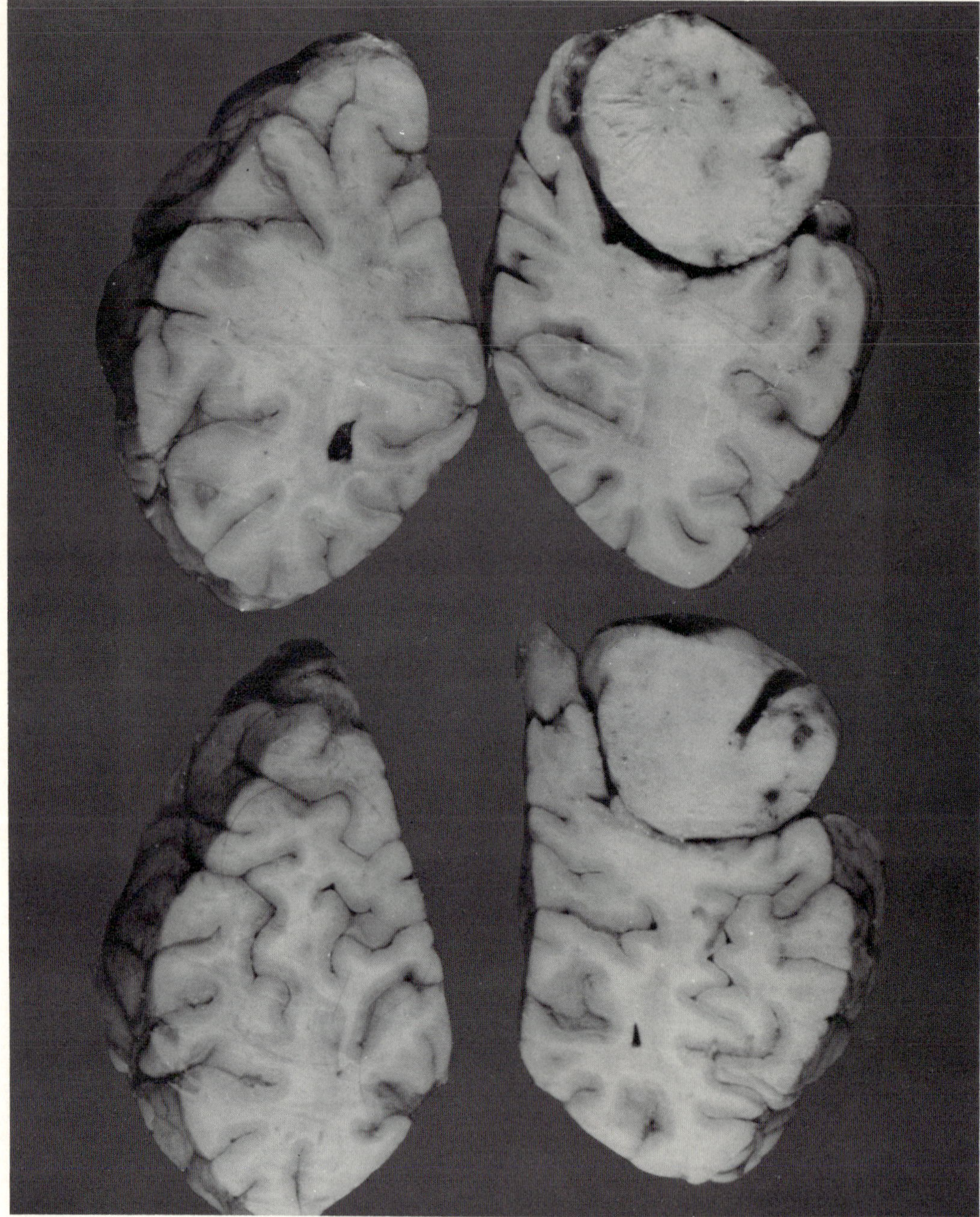

Fig. 16 Coronal sections of a brain with a metastatic tumor resembling a meningioma.

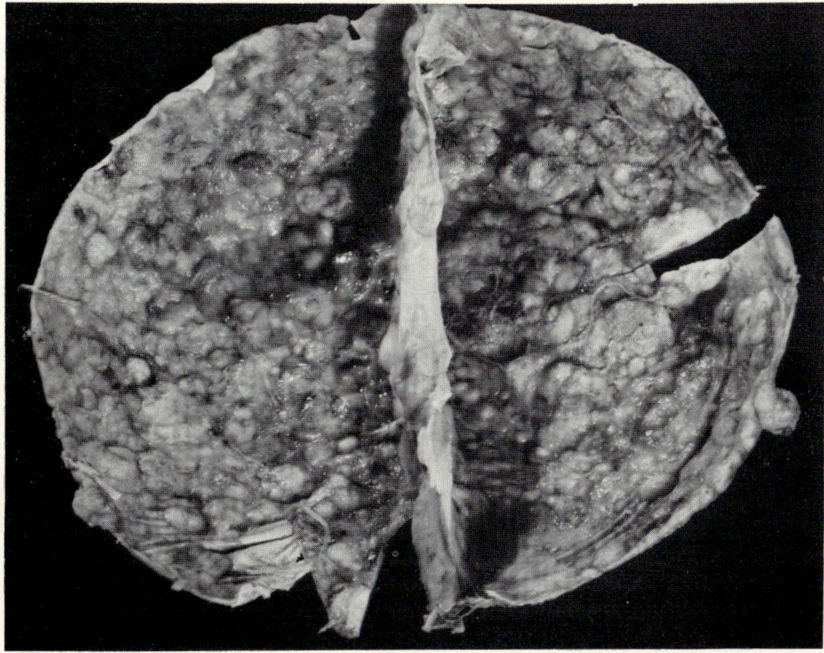

Fig. 17 Metastatic breast carcinoma to the dura mater.

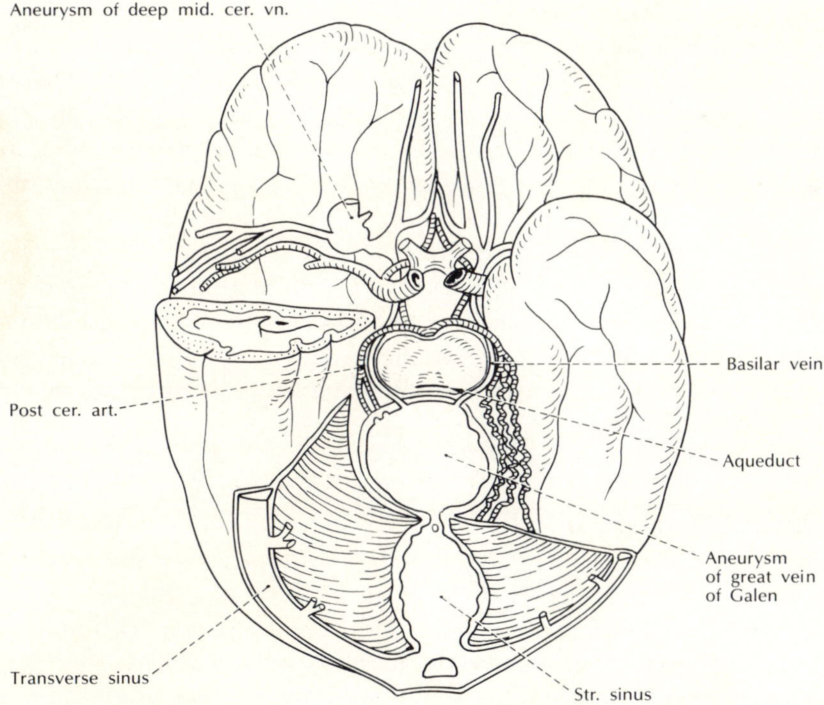

Fig. 18 Aneurysm of the vein of Galen. Dilation of the vein of Galen results from anastomoses with the posterior cerebral artery. Compression of the midbrain produces stenosis of the aqueduct. (From Hirano, A., & Terry, R.D.: Aneurysm of the vein of Galen. J. Neuropathol. Exp. Neurol. 18: 424-429, 1958.) (Hirano, A., & Solomon, S.: Arterio-venous aneurysm of the vein of Galen. Arch. Neurol., 3:589-593, 1960.)

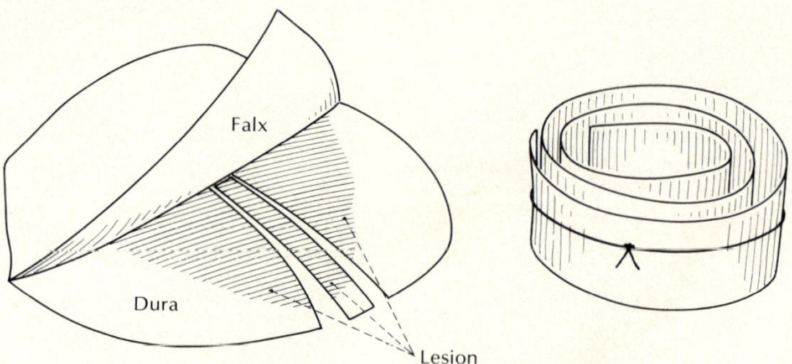

Fig. 19 Preparation of dura for embedding.

Often they will be large enough to indent the underlying brain. It is not uncommon, especially in women, to find unsuspected small meningiomas or metastatic lesions on the basis of a gross examination. Breast carcinoma is the most common metastatic tumor found in the dura mater (Fig. 17). Although it is rare, breast tumors can even metastasize into a pre-existing meningioma.

After the surfaces of the dura mater have been examined, it is lifted off the brain. At this point one inspects the surface of the underlying brain. The presence of parasagittal bilateral softening corresponding to sinus drainage territories indicates an occlusion in the sinus within the dura mater; generally a sinus thrombosis. In such cases samples of the sinus must be removed for microscopic study.

Some apparent changes may not be the result of pathology. Calcification of the falx cerebri is a common finding, especially in older individuals. These changes should not be confused with tumors.

Aneurysms of the vein of Galen (Fig. 18) are detectable on external examination. These are the result of arterio-venous malformations in which usually either the anterior or posterior cerebral arteries fuse with the vein of Galen.

In some cases, it is necessary to examine fairly large expanses of the dura mater. For the sake of convenience one can remove a strip of affected dura mater and roll it into a coil secured by a thread as illustrated in Fig. 19. Such preparations enable one to view long stretches of membrane in a single section. It is wise to note how the strip was coiled so that one can be sure which aspect of the dura mater is being examined in the microscope.

LEPTOMENINGES (Fig. 20)

As the dura mater is lifted off the surface of the brain the outer aspect of the arachnoid membrane is exposed. This membrane, along with its underlying subarachnoid space and the delicate pia mater, constitute the leptomeninx (pl. = leptomeninges). Removing the dura mater from the brain requires undercutting a number of adhesions, especially along the superior sagittal sinus, as well as at the vein of Galen. These adhesions are the numerous *arachnoid villi (arachnoid granulations* or *pacchionian corpuscles)* and emissary veins to the sinus in the dura

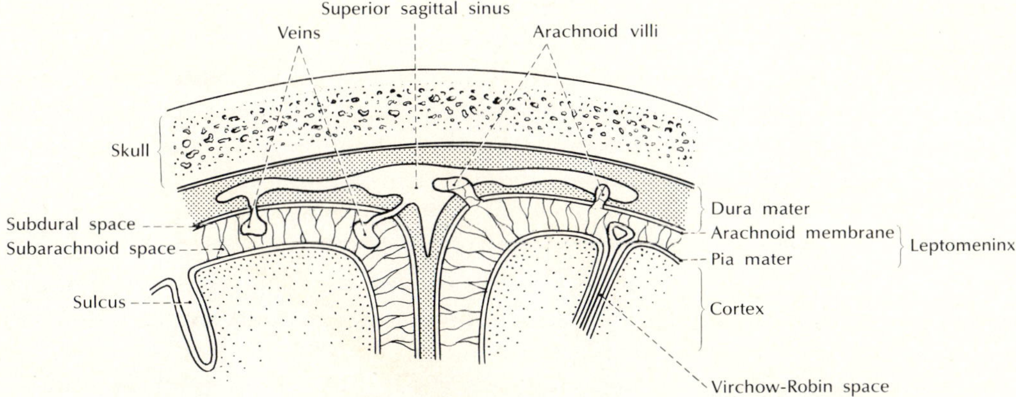

Fig. 20 Relationship between superior sagittal sinus and meninges.

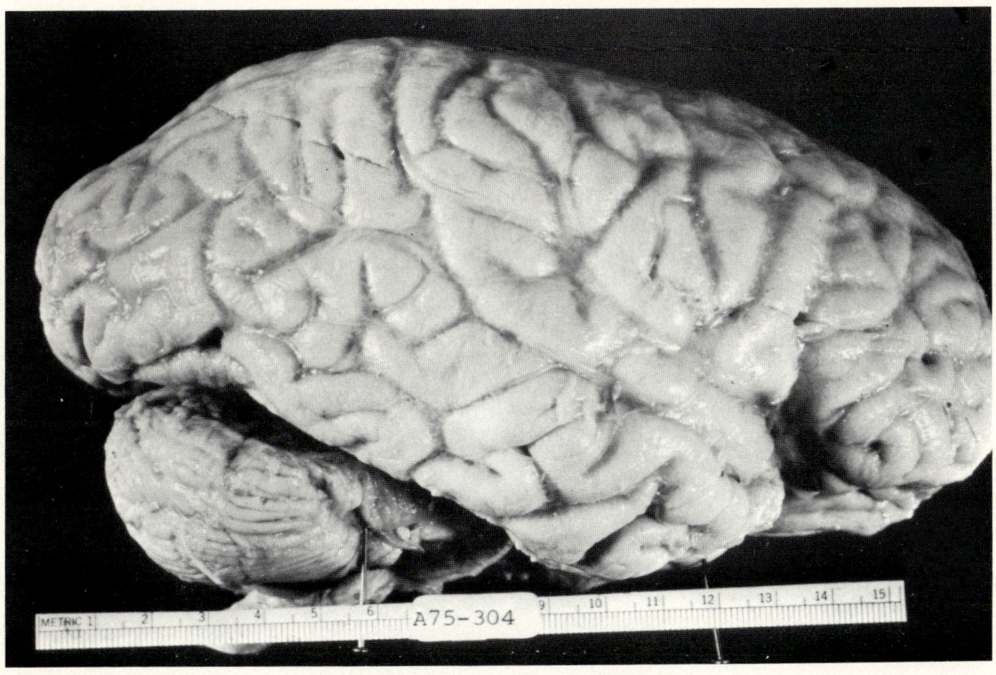

Fig. 21 Cryptococcal meningitis.

mater. The villi are sites of absorption of cerebrospinal fluid from the subarachnoid space. Histologically, these structures mimic miniature meningiomas. Interestingly, areas rich in arachnoid villi are areas of predilection for meningioma formation. Tears of the emissary veins by traumatic force are believed to be the major cause of subdural hematomas.

The *arachnoid membrane* closely covers the entire surface of the brain. It extends down into the major fissures but not into the finer sulci. The underlying *subarachnoid space* contains cerebrospinal fluid, blood vessels, and a complex network of trabeculae. *The pia mater* extends into all the sulci, covering a much greater surface than the arachnoid membrane. In infants the leptomeninges separate easily from the surface of the brain parenchyma.

The surface of the base of the brain, especially the medulla oblongata, sometimes appears dark. This is a normal phenomenon and is due to the presence of melanin-bearing cells, melanophores, in the subarachnoid spaces. It is more common in darker-skinned individuals and is absent in albinos.

Meningitis (Fig. 21) results in a clouding of the leptomeninges due to the accumulation of inflammatory cells in the subarachnoid space in addition to the reaction of the arachnoid cells and fibroblasts themselves. This is easily seen in the young patient where the leptomeninges are otherwise clear and relatively thin. In older patients, however, these changes become progressively less obvious because of the normal aging changes which result in a thicker, less transparent membrane. Unless the meningitis is quite severe, the inexperienced observer may find it

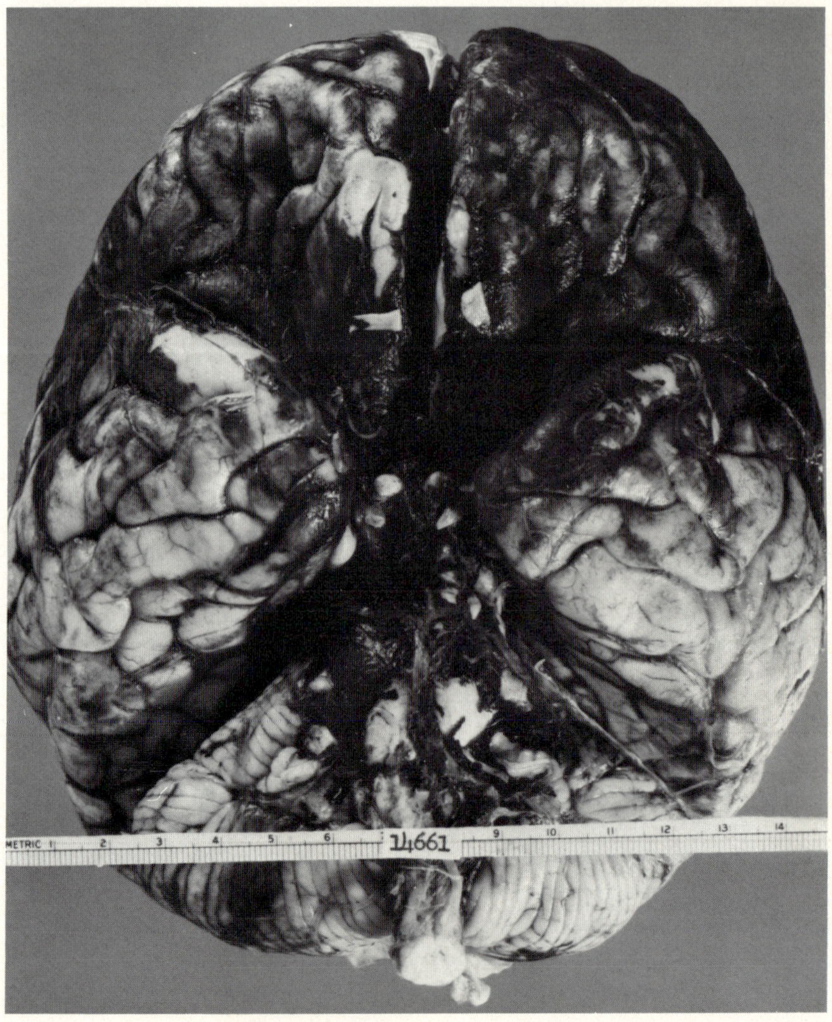

Fig. 22 Subarachnoid hemorrhage.

difficult to detect. These considerations are especially important nowadays when many patients come to autopsy after lengthy regimens of immunosuppressant drugs and antibiotics, and in which mild, occult meningitis may be present as a terminal event. Since the subarachnoid space is continuous with the ventricles, meningitis may often be accompanied by ependymitis. In chronic meningitis, thickening of the membrane may lead to obstruction of the foramen of Magendie and Luschka causing hydrocephalus.

The neuropathologist in training may mistake the normally blood-filled vessels of the arachnoid space for a sign of vascular congestion. This is especially likely in cases in which, for one reason or another, the brain was not perfused.

Subarachnoid hemorrhage is probably the most obvious alteration of the leptomeninges (Fig. 22). This is most often due to a *ruptured aneurysm* at the circle of Willis (Fig. 23). Accumulations of large amounts of blood occur within

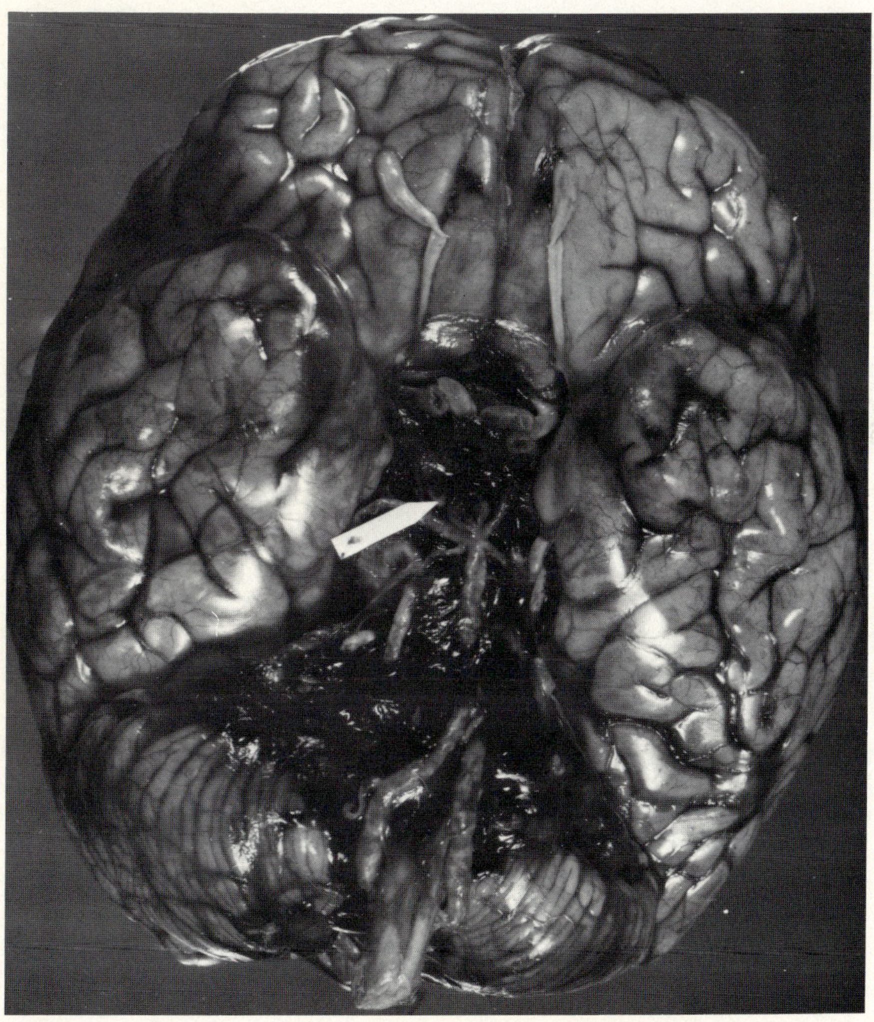

Fig. 23 Ruptured aneurysm of the basilar artery.

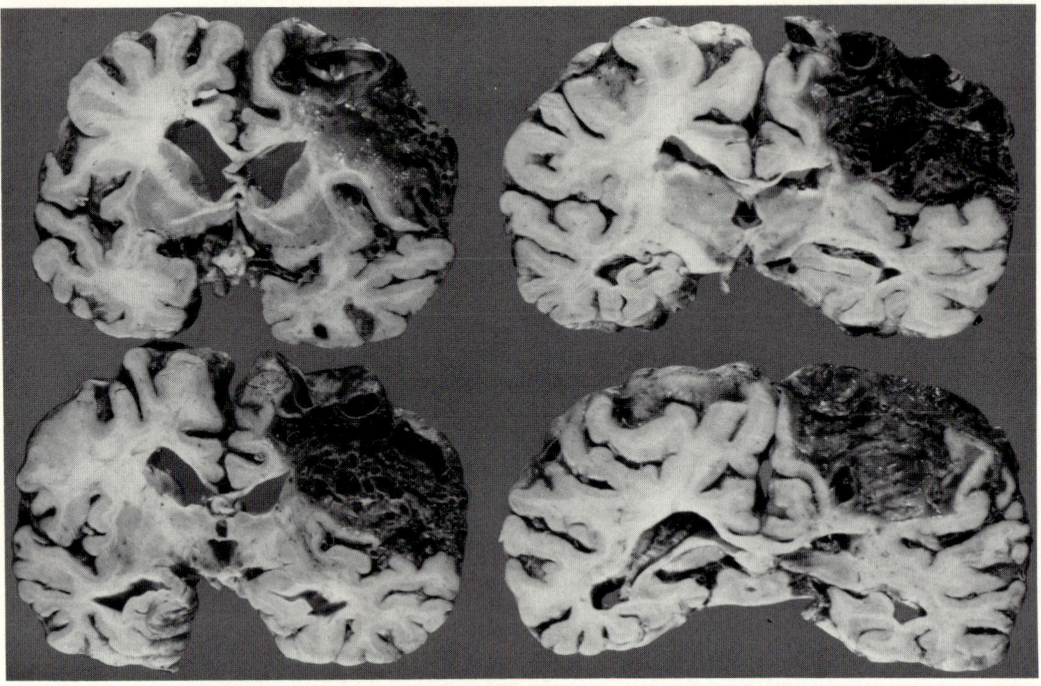

Fig. 24 Arterio-venous malformation. (AVM).
In these congenital anomalies the blood vessels develop abnormally sometimes forming large aggregates of blood vessels. Some arteries anastomose directly with veins thus subjecting the veins to unusually high pressure. This may result in distention of the vein with thickening of the vessel wall so that it is often difficult to distinguish between these veins and arteries during gross post-mortem examination. Although abnormal masses of blood vessels may compress the underlying brain tissue resulting in deformity and gliosis, AVM's are often asymptomatic. However, the abnormal pressure on the vein often leads to rupture or thrombosis and subsequent infarct. Since AVM's are usually located in the subarachnoid space the lesions take on a characteristic wedge shape.

the subarachnoid space especially at the base of the brain. Rupture of abnormal vessels in *arterio-venous malformations* is another major cause of subarachnoid hemorrhage (Fig. 24).

Old or recurrent hemorrhage at the surface of the brain results in a brownish discoloration. This pigment is hemosiderin which, on microscopic examination, is found to be localized within the subpial astrocytes and in some meningeal cells. In addition, meningeal fibrosis may occur following bleeding. If excessive, the abnormally thickened membranes may narrow the exit of the fourth ventricle at the foramina of Luschka and Magendie leading to obstructive hydrocephalus.

THE CIRCLE OF WILLIS

Normal Anatomy and Its Variations

The *circle of Willis* is at the base of the brain. The accompanying illustrations (Figs. 25, 26A) show, in diagramatic fashion, the anatomy of the normal configuration. There are two arterial inputs on each side, the internal carotid artery anteriorly, and the vertebral artery, posteriorly. The effect of the normal anatomy is to ensure collateral circulation to virtually all parts of the brain. This is in addition to the circulation provided by the meningeal vessels which anastomose with those arising from the circle of Willis. However, large degrees of variation in the size, shape and caliber of the arteries of the circle of Willis exist. Indeed, it is rather unusual to find the symmetrical, well-formed circulation diagramed in Fig.

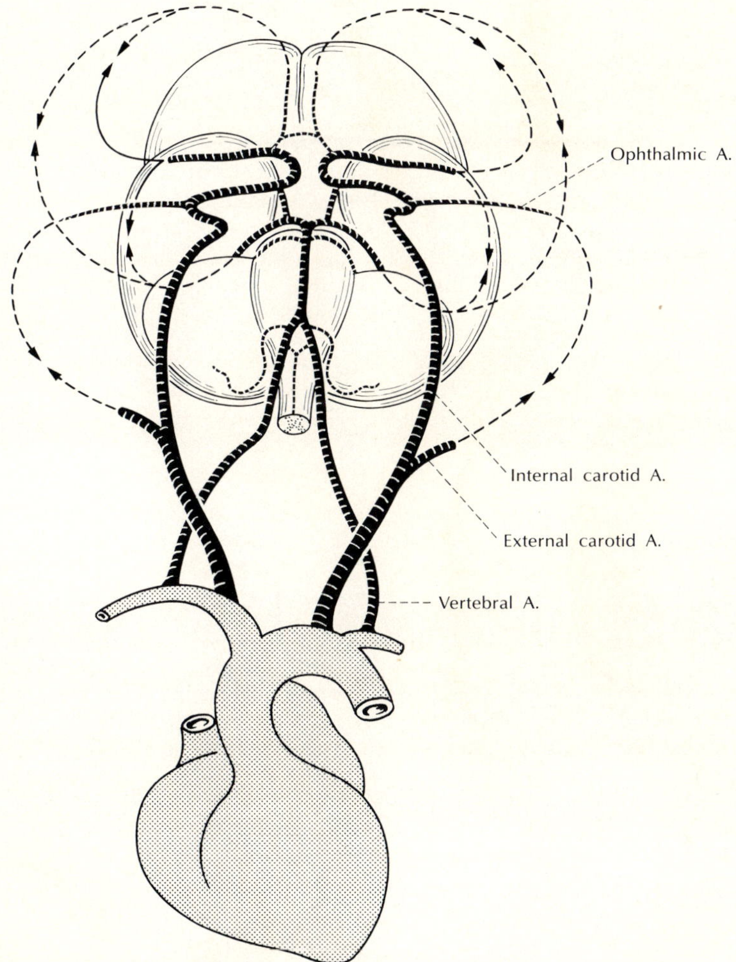

Fig. 25 Anastomoses of the intracranial arteries.

26. Many times one or more of the vessels, especially the posterior and anterior communicating arteries, may be present in only a rudimentary form. This may not lead to any pathological alteration in the otherwise normal individual. However, should occlusion occur in one of the major nearby intracranial vessels, such as the internal carotid artery, then large regions of necrosis in the area of distribution will result. Examples of this phenomenon are illustrated in Figs. 26B and C. Note that in both cases the internal carotid artery is occluded, but the area of necrosis varies depending on the developmental state of smaller vessels. The complexity of the topography of pathologic change increases dramatically when one adds variable degrees of atherosclerotic changes, increasing in severity with age, to vessels which may have had pre-existing variations in caliber. Thus, areas of necrosis resulting from interruption of the blood supply should be explored on the basis of both pathological or aging changes superimposed on the pre-existing conditions of the circle of Willis.

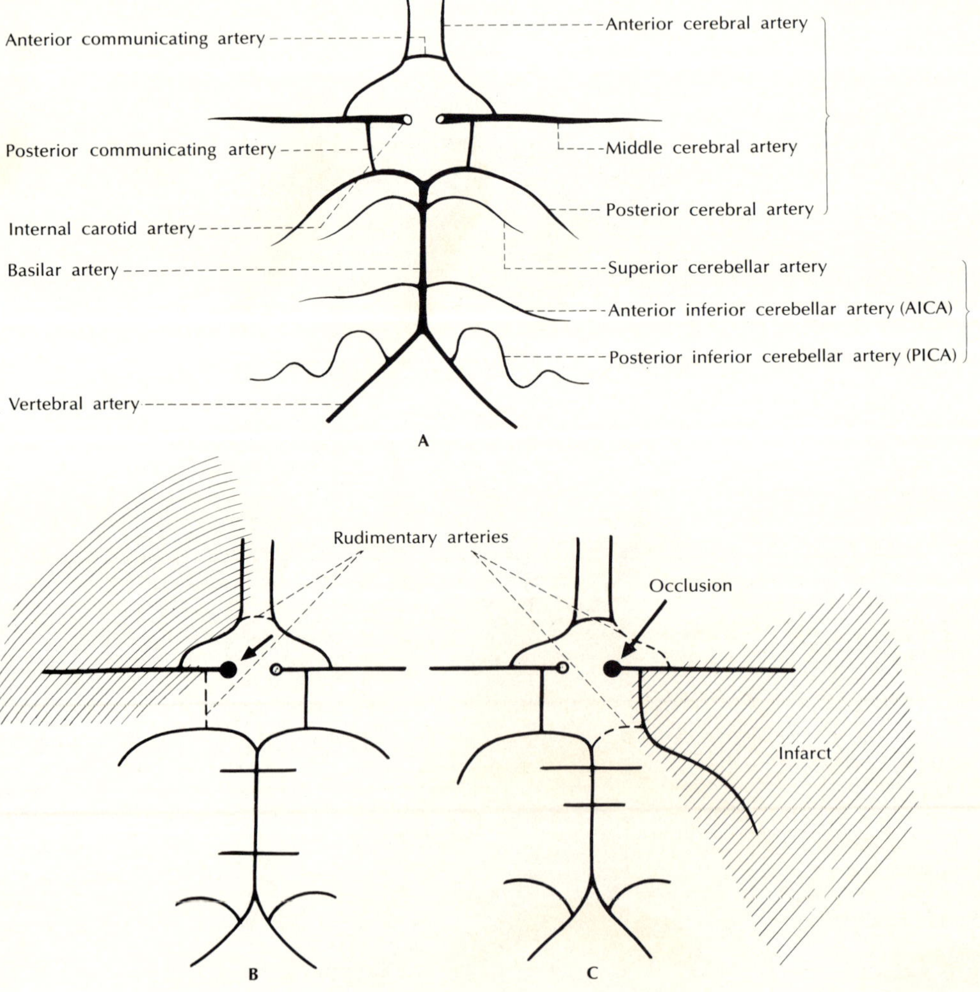

Fig. 26 Circle of Willis.

Atherosclerosis and Occlusion of the Lumen (Fig. 27)

In the adult, especially elderly individuals, atherosclerosis is one of the most conspicuous changes of the circle of Willis and its feeding vessels, the internal carotid and vertebral arteries. The sclerotic artery is thickened, tortuous and often has a yellow discoloration. Despite its apparent wide caliber the lumen is often narrowed as can be seen in sections. It is important to look for occlusion of the lumen when cerebral softening is present.

Occlusion of the arteries of the brain may also result from *emboli* derived from other parts of the body which usually result in multiple lesions. Most commonly the emboli represent detached thrombi from the heart or major proximal arteries.

Smaller vessels in the brain may be occluded by "*shower emboli*" which are microemboli consisting of detached thrombi, foreign material or fat droplets. Metastatic tumors or blood-borne infectious material may also be considered as kinds of microemboli.

When embolic occlusion is suspected, one should always look for the source of the emboli. Clinical data as well as the post mortem findings in the general organs, especially the heart, are essential for this purpose.

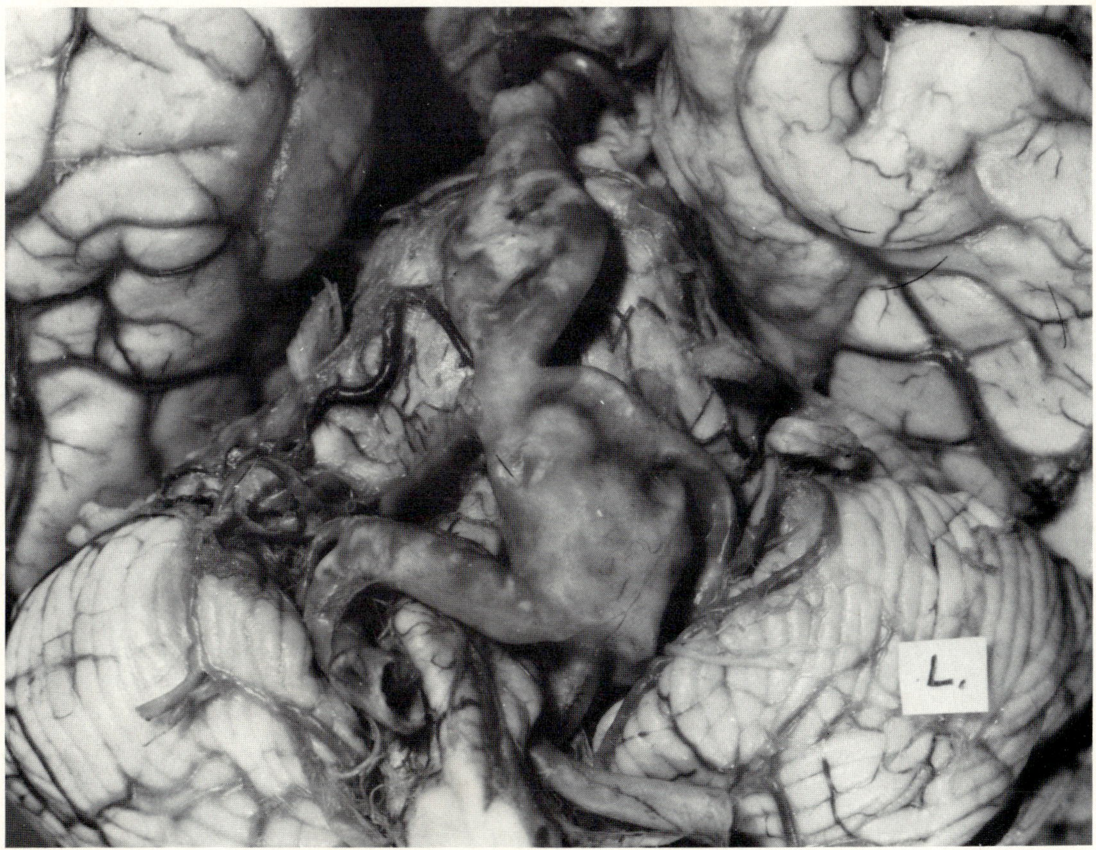

Fig. 27 Severe atherosclerosis in the base of the brain.

Aneurysms (Fig. 28)

The discovery of small unruptured aneurysms during routine examination is a rather common finding in the atheromatous circle of Willis. They usually protrude in the direction of blood flow at a site of major bifurcation. The sites of predilection

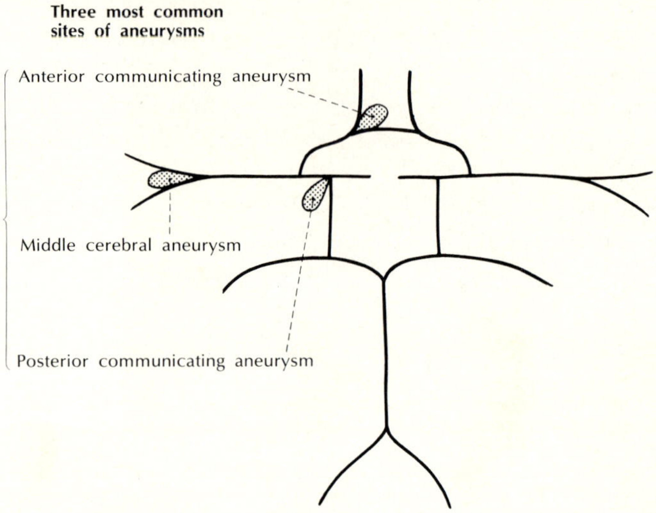

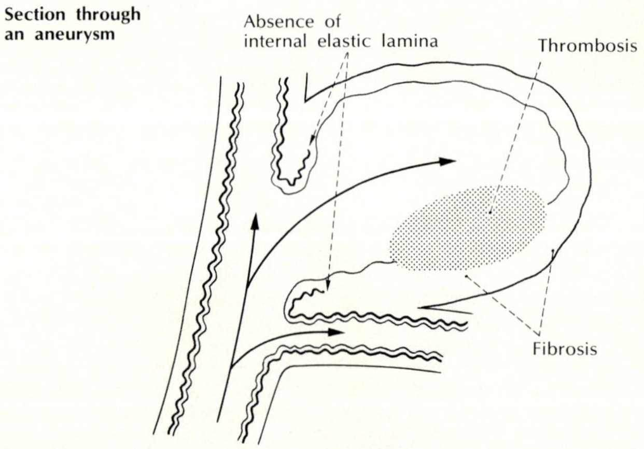

Fig. 28 Aneurysm. Discontinuity of the internal elastic lamina, atheromatous changes, as well as marked stretching of the vascular wall are the characteristic features of the protruded aneurysmal sac on microscopic examination.

Fig. 30 Ruptured anterior communicating aneurysms (from Hirano, A.: Advances in Neurological Sciences (Tokyo), 5: 480, 1961.).

Aneurysms at the junction of the anterior cerebral and the anterior communicating arteries are usually small and asymptomatic until they rupture. They may easily be overlooked unless the hemispheres are separated and the anterior commissure is exposed. After rupture the hemorrhage is usually restricted to the subarachnoid space and does not penetrate the parenchyma. On the other hand the hemorrhage may extend into the anterior horn of the lateral ventricle from below (A). Less commonly the hemorrhagic tract dissects between the corpus callosum and the cingulate gyrus forcing the elevation of the anterior cerebral arteries causing a tear of the perforating branches of the anterior cerebral arteries, resulting in necrosis of the corpus callosum. Eventually the corpus callosum ruptures allowing bleeding from above into the anterior horn and the body of the lateral ventricle (B).
(Hirano, A., Terry, R.D., and Zimmerman, H.M.: Ruptured aneurysm of the anterior communicating artery. J. Nerv. and Ment. Dis., 128: 309-322, 1959.)

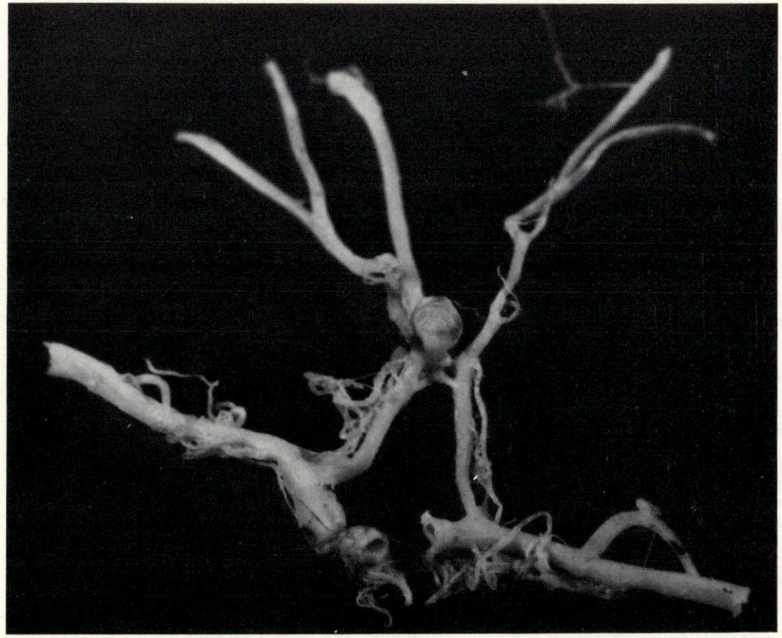

Fig. 29 Anterior communicating aneurysm.

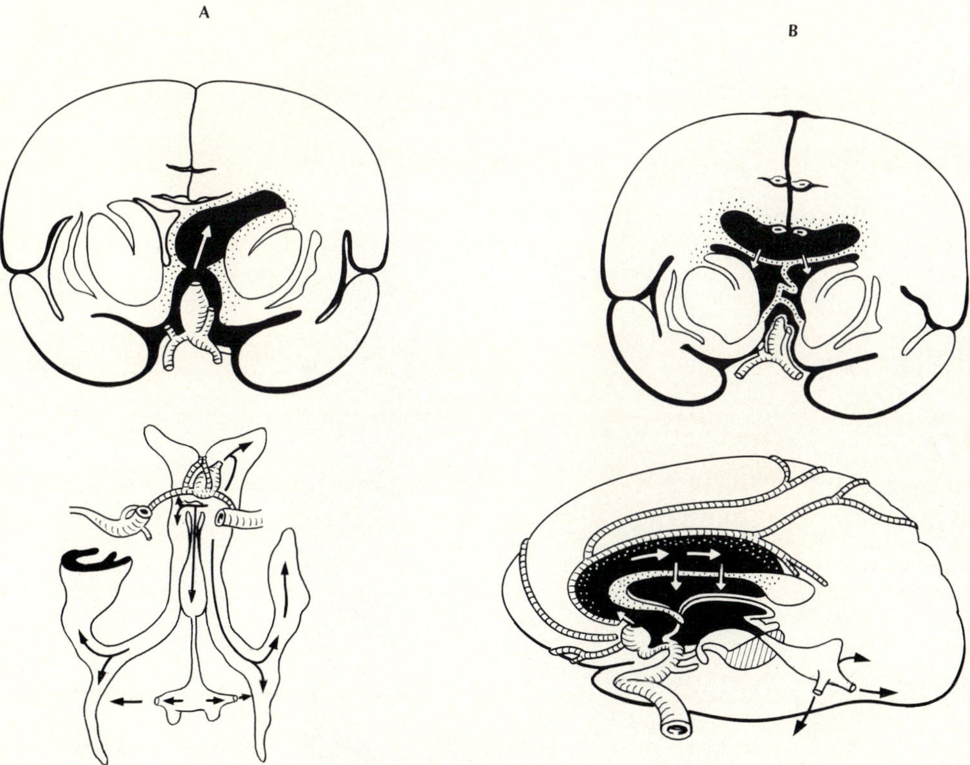

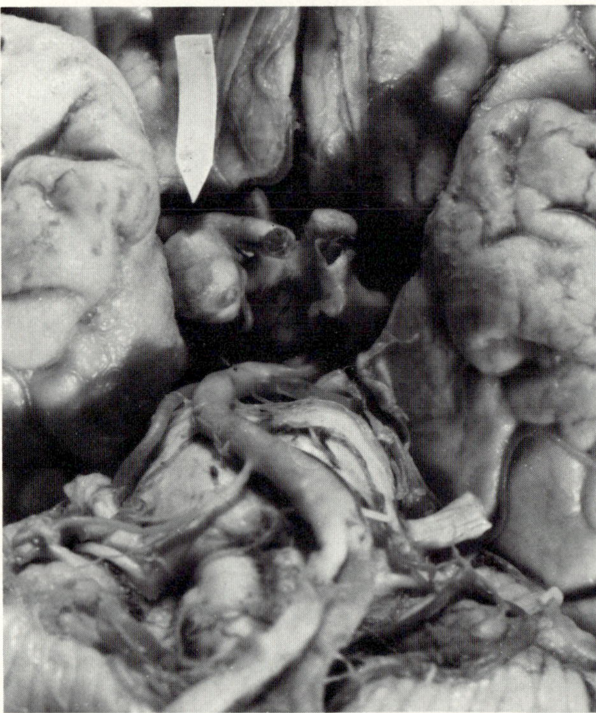

Fig. 31 Posterior communicating aneurysm.

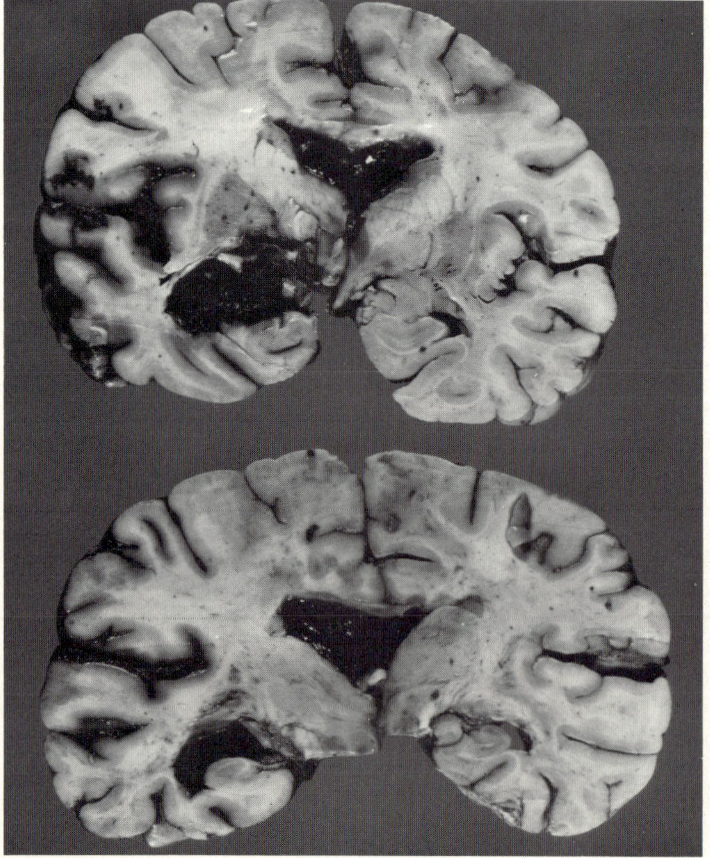

Fig. 32 Intraventricular hemorrhage due to a ruptured posterior communicating aneurysm.

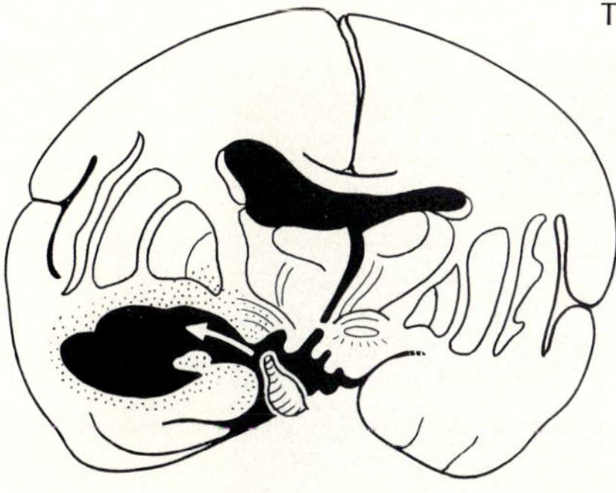

Fig. 33 Ruptured posterior communication aneurysm with a resulting hemorrhage into the ipsilateral temporal horn (from Hirano, A. Recent Advances in Research of the Nervous System (Tokyo), 5: 480, 1961).

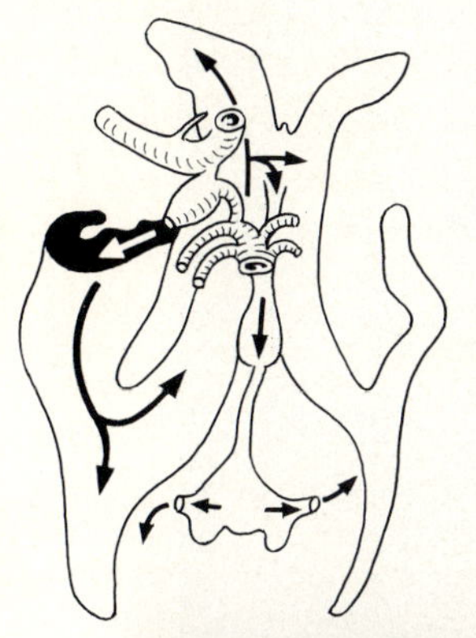

Posterior communicating aneurysms occur at the junction of the internal carotid and the posterior communicating arteries. They usually protrude in a lateral and posterior direction. The third cranial nerve courses between the uncus and this junction so that when an aneurysm occurs the nerve may be compressed by it. Thus paralysis of the third nerve may be a symptom of an expanding unruptured posterior communicating aneurysm. After rupture the hemorrhage may remain in the subarachnoid space or may extend into the temporal horn of the lateral ventricle damaging the median aspect of the temporal lobe.

(Hirano, A., Barron, K.D. and Zimmerman, H.M.: Ruptured aneurysms of the supraclinoid portion of the internal carotid and of the middle cerebral arteries. J. Nerv. and Ment. Dis., 129: 34-53, 1959.)

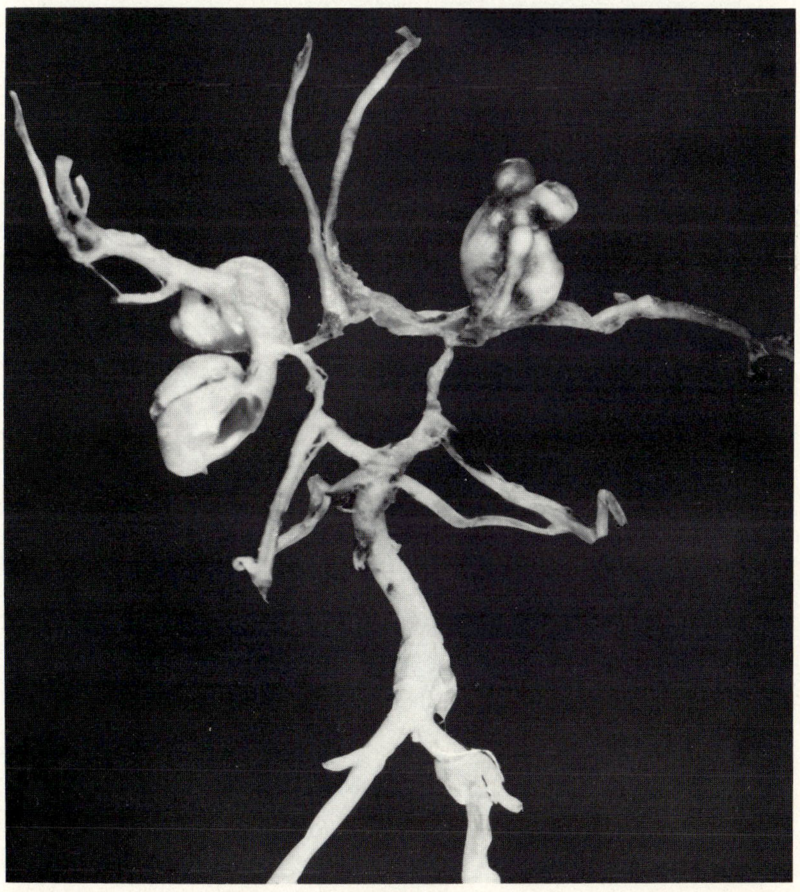

Fig. 34 Multiple aneurysms.

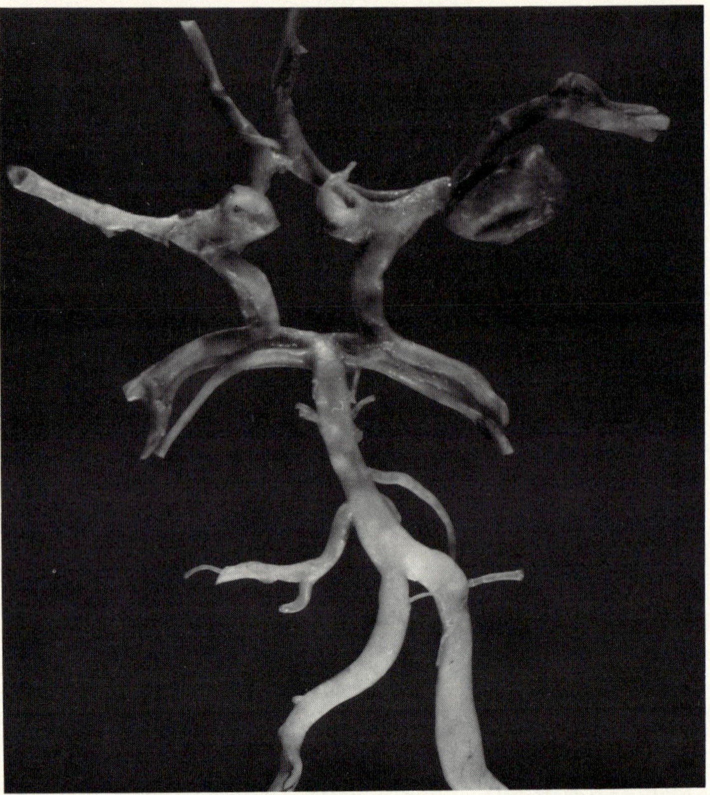

Fig. 35 Middle cerebral artery aneurysm.

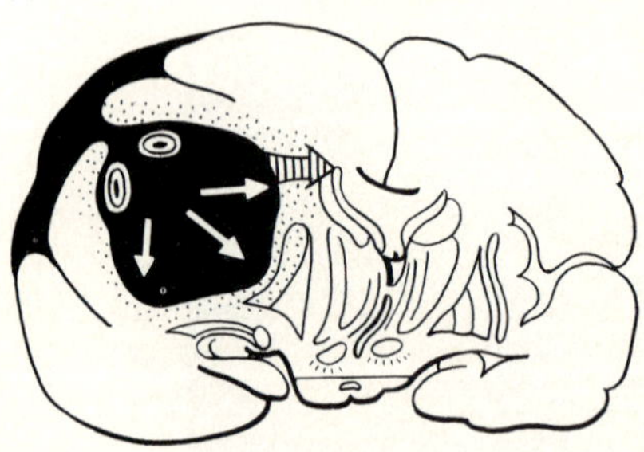

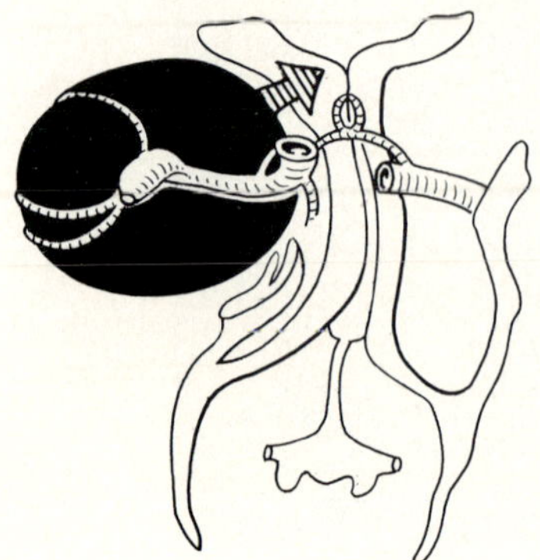

Fig. 36 Sylvian hematoma due to a ruptured middle cerebral artery aneurysm (from Hirano, A. Recent Advance in Research of the Nervous System (Tokyo), 5: 480, 1961)

Middle cerebral aneurysms usually occur at the first bifurcation of the middle cerebral artery in the Sylvian fissure. Unruptured aneurysms at this site are usually asymptomatic and may be missed unless specifically looked for by raising the temporal lobe during gross postmortem examination. When it ruptures, the resultant hematoma is primarily located in the Sylvian fissure but, as it expands, it penetrates into the brain substance and may rupture into the lateral ventricle.

for such aneurysms are the bifurcation at the anterior cerebral and anterior communicating arteries (Figs. 29,30), the internal carotid and posterior communicating arteries (Figs. 31—34) and at the bifurcation of the middle cerebral artery in the Sylvian fissure (Figs. 35,36). It is not uncommon for more than one aneurysm to be present (Fig. 34). The rupture of such aneurysms is the most common cause of subarachnoid hemorrhage.

REFERENCE

Hirano, A.: Ruptured intracranial aneurysms, A patho-anatomical analysis of intraventricular hemorrhage. Recent Advance in Research of the Nervous System (Tokyo), 5: 480-499, 1961.

CRANIAL NERVES (Fig. 37)

In most cranial nerves only the small proximal portion is part of the central nervous system. The *first and second nerves*, however, are true extensions of the central nervous system throughout their length. That is, the axons are surrounded by glial rather than Schwann cells and their myelin sheaths are of the central rather than peripheral type (see p. 237). Thus, *the optic nerve* is affected by central nervous system diseases such as multiple sclerosis in which demyelinated plaques are seen and gliomas rather than Schwannomas are formed.

Absence of the olfactory bulb is a well known finding in certain kinds of trisomy. However, in autopsies of infants one can sometimes inadvertently leave the nerve

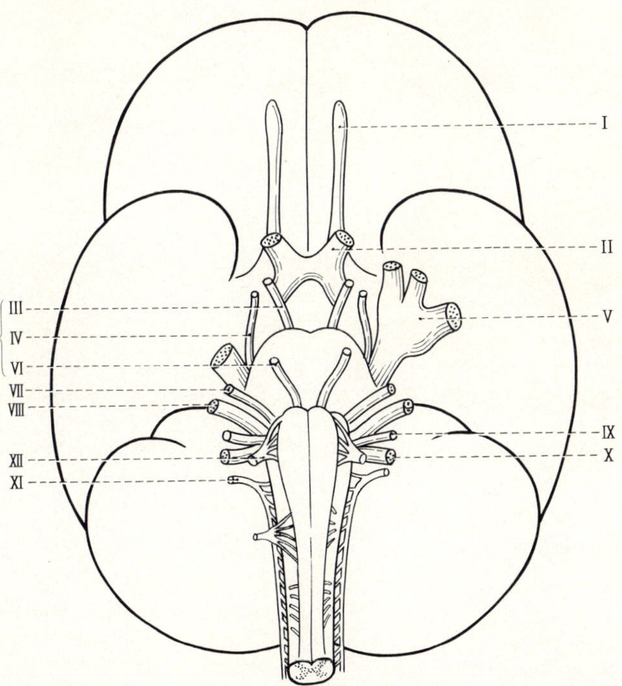

Fig. 37 Cranial nerves.

behind in the skull and thus mistakenly assume that *the olfactory nerve* was missing as a result of congenital anomaly.

Similarly, *the third nerve* is easily lost at the site of exit from the brain stem due to rough treatment during removal or subsequent handling of the brain. Because the third nerve passes in close proximity to the posterior communicating artery, it is particularly subject to compression as a result of aneurysm in this vessel. Similarly the third nerve is affected by any space-occupying lesion in this region as well as by uncal herniation due to increased intracranial pressure (see p. 33). Increased intracranial pressure can also result in downward displacement of the brain stem and blood vessels thereby causing compression of the third nerve between the posterior cerebral artery and the superior cerebellar artery.

The fourth and sixth nerves, especially the latter, are clinically very important but, in general, are not well known for gross prominent pathological alterations. The fourth nerve arises from the dorsal aspect of the brain stem and is quite small. *The sixth nerve* is easily detected and is known to have the longest intracranial course of any cranial nerve.

The fifth nerve is the largest in diameter. The proximal portion consists of a large amount of central nervous system tissue and is therefore subject to isolated plaques in multiple sclerosis. While not common, schwannomas have been seen in the gasserian ganglion. The fifth nerve may also be the object of various surgical procedures for the treatment of trigeminal neuralgia. Viral particles have been

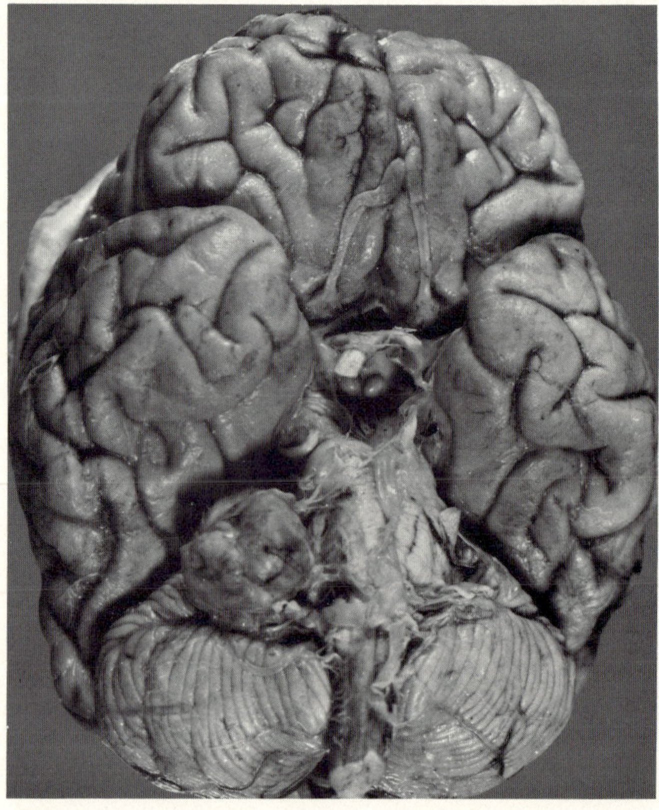

Fig. 38 Acoustic neuroma.

observed in the gasserian ganglion in cases of infection with herpes zoster.

Among the other cranial nerves the most common neuropathological changes are *schwannomas* (*acoustic neuromas*) of *the eighth nerve* (Fig. 38). Compared to most other cranial nerves the 8th has central-type myelin for relatively long distances after it exits from the neuraxis. Nevertheless, schwannomas are the most common neoplasm at the cerebellopontine angle. These benign tumors are derived from cells of peripheral nerve. The subarachnoid space at the cerebellopontine angle is relatively ample and other tumors may also be located in this area. These include tentorial meningiomas, metastatic tumors and cholesteatomas. In addition to compression of the brain stem, tumors at this site may obstruct the flow of cerebrospinal fluid and produce obstructive hydrocephalus. Schwannomas may be found in other cranial nerves in cases of von Recklinghausen disease.

In general, such conditions as meningitis, or metastatic tumor may involve any cranial nerve or nerves.

GROSS PATHOLOGY OF INCREASED INTRACRANIAL PRESSURE (Fig. 39)

The rigid skull provides an ideal protective nest for the delicate, fragile brain. However, in cases of increased intracranial pressure it becomes a liability, since it prevents the expansion of the brain, thus resulting in compression and damage to the tissue.

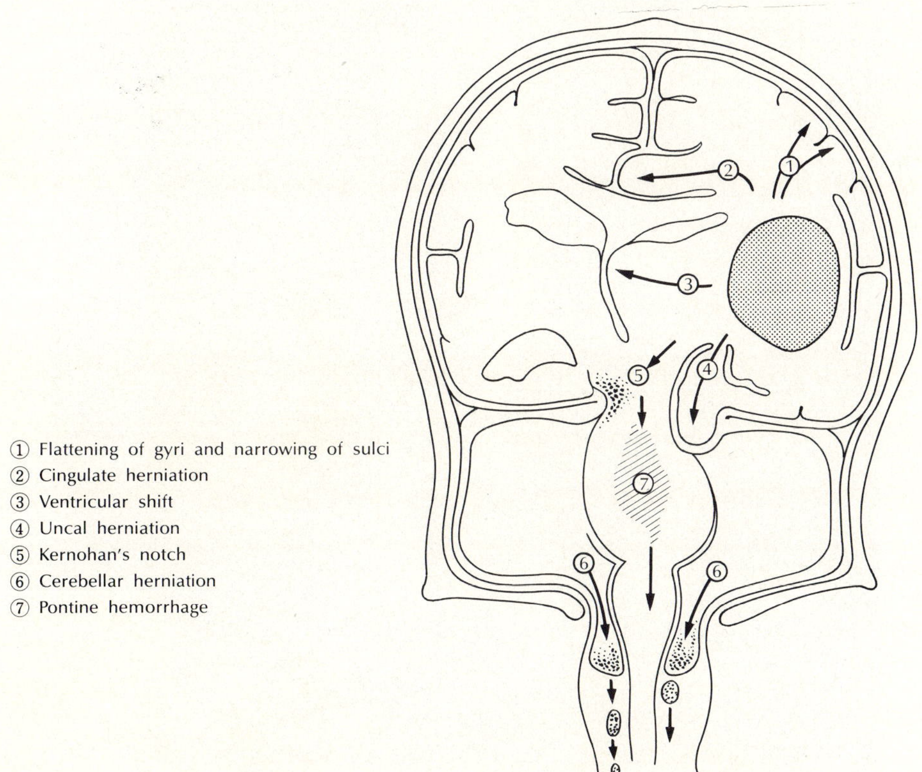

Fig. 39 Increased intracranial pressure.

Increased intracranial pressure is the most dangerous clinical problem in neurological medicine. It is found in virtually all space occupying lesions associated with head injury, tumors, inflammation and vascular pathology, etc. Brain edema, the abnormal increase of water content within the brain, is the most common mediator of increased intracranial pressure. The pathogenesis of cerebral edema will be described in detail later in this volume (p. 316). For the present we shall describe only the macroscopic changes one can expect to see as a result of increased intracranial pressure.

Both the size and weight of a swollen brain are increased. The gyri are widened and flattened while the sulci become narrowed. Depending on the location of the original lesion, various regions of the brain may be displaced. These are known as herniations.

Cingulate Herniation (Subfalx Herniation) (Figs. 40, 41)

The cingulate gyrus can be displaced under the falx cerebri and across the midline as a result of an expanding lesion in the upper portion of one hemisphere.

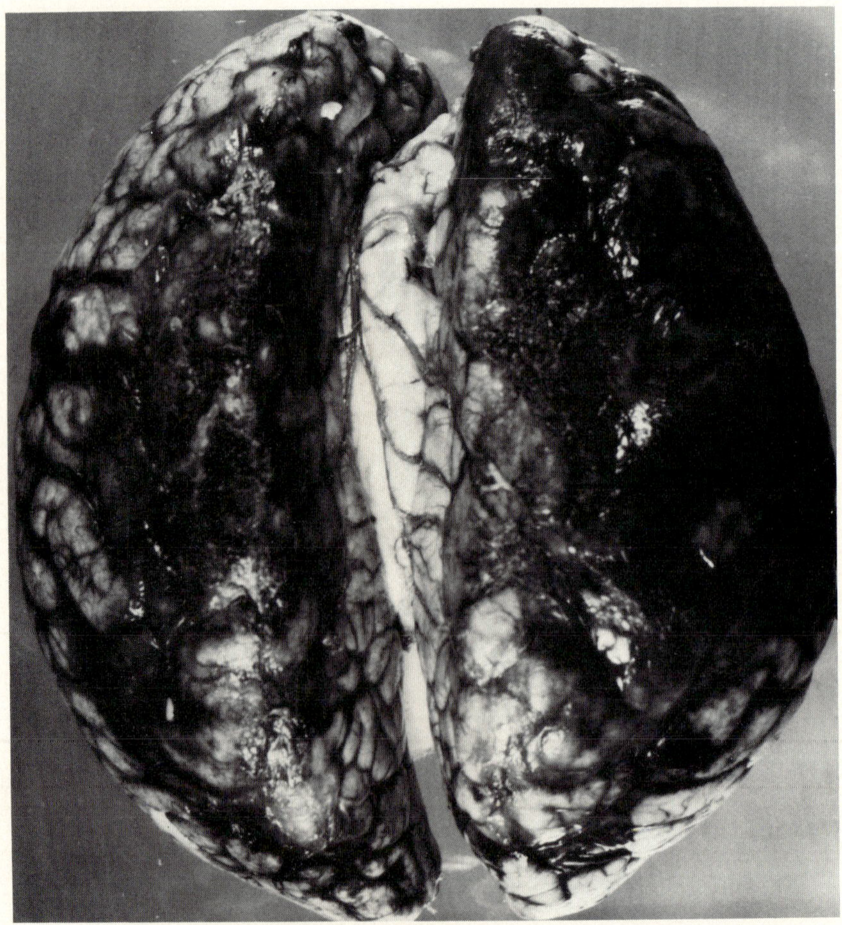

Fig. 40 Subarachnoid hemorrhage and cingulate herniation.

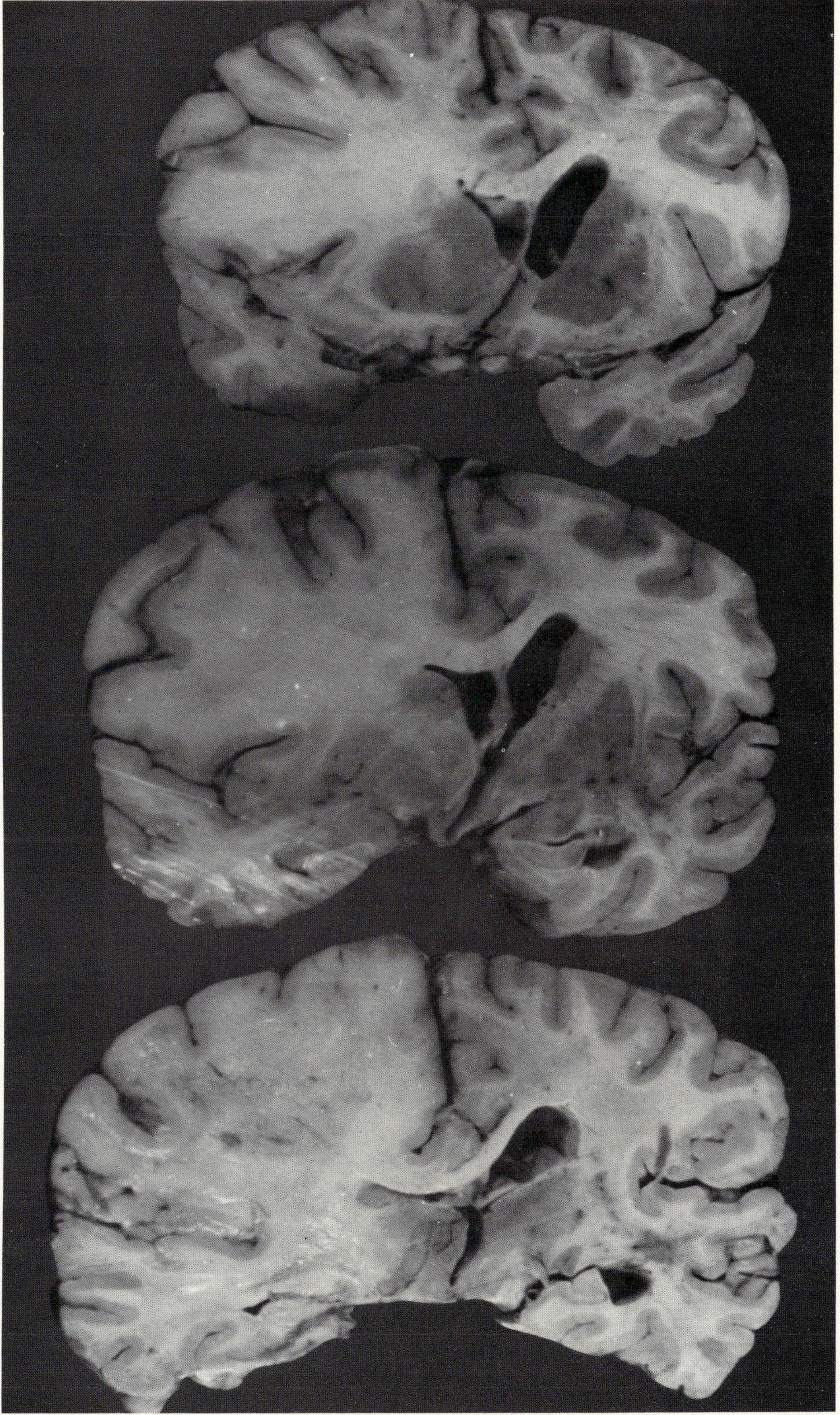

Fig. 41 Swelling is present predominantly in the white matter. Cingulate herniation is evident.

The movement of the tissue carries along the branches of the anterior cerebral artery resulting in characteristic "step signs" or "falx signs" in antero-posterior views in cerebral angiography. Due to the decreasing depth of the tough falx cerebri, the herniation is most severe in the anterior portion, but tapers off posteriorly, finally disappearing at the splenium of the corpus callosum where the falx cerebri comes close to the corpus callosum. The changing extent of the herniation is easily appreciated after removing the falx cerebri and widening the interhemispheric fissure as seen in Fig. 40. Coronal sections of the brain also clearly demonstrate this phenomenon (Fig. 41).

Tentorial Herniation (Uncal Herniation, Transtentorial Herniation, Hippocampal Herniation) (Fig. 42)

Expanding lesions in the cerebral hemisphere, especially in the temporal area, can cause tentorial herniation. In this case, a portion of the uncus is displaced downward towards the posterior fossa, past the tentorial edge (incisura tentorii).

This phenomenon can produce various, localized, important clinical symptoms and signs. First, it can compress the third nerve, resulting in its paralysis. Paralysis can arise by compression of the nerve between the uncus and the posterior communicating artery or between the displaced posterior cerebral artery and superior cerebellar artery. In addition, paralysis can be caused by the stretching of the third nerve itself due to the overall downward displacement of the brain stem.

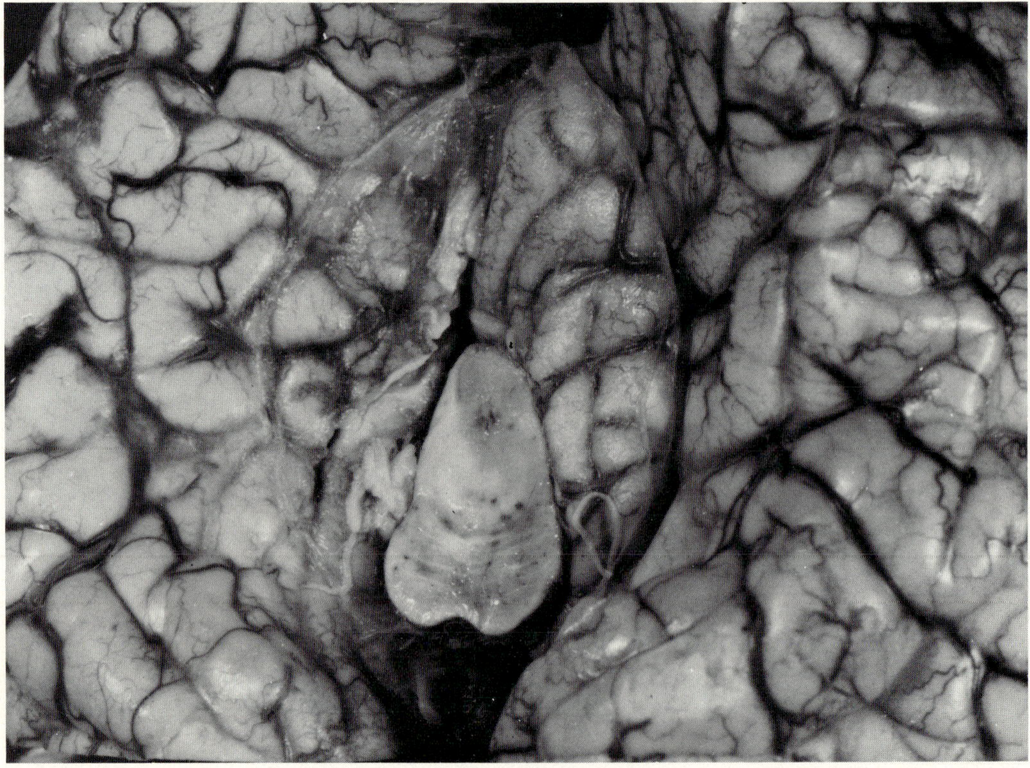

Fig. 42 Tentorial herniation.

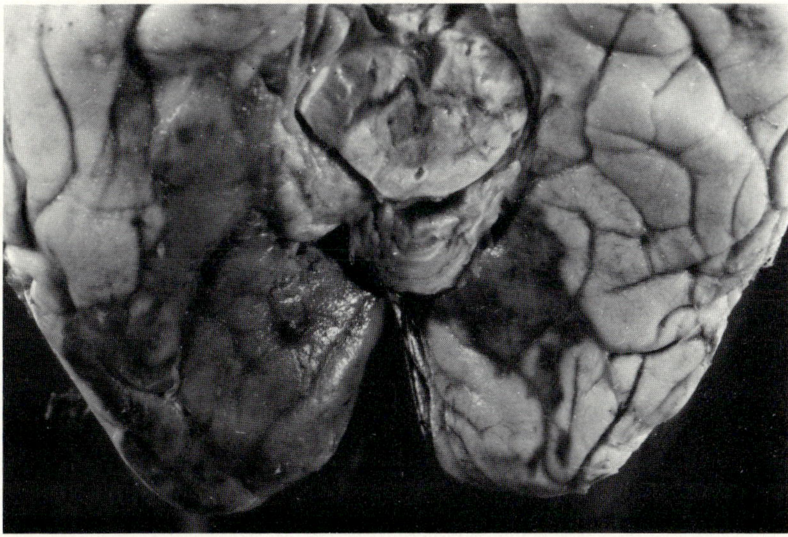

Fig. 43 Hemorrhagic infarcts in the bilateral occipital lobes and the midbrain secondary to increased intracranial pressure.

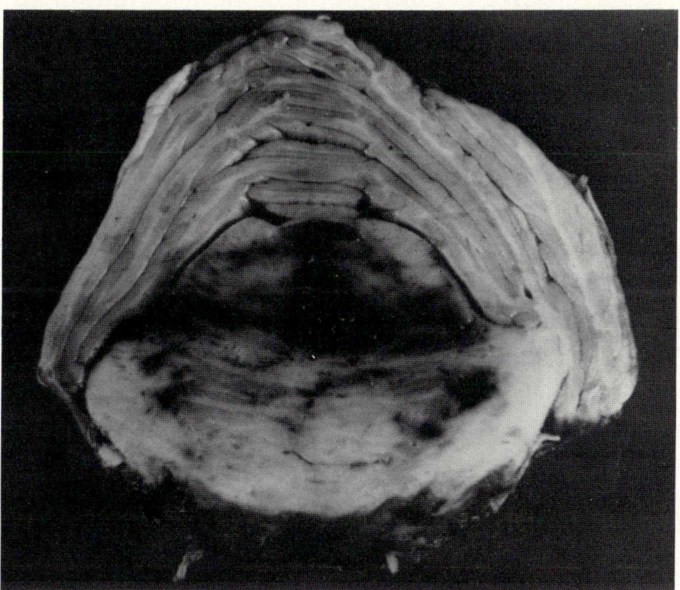

Fig. 44 Secondary pontine hemorrhage due to increased intracranial pressure.

Second, pyramidal signs on the same side as the lesion can develop as the result of a tentorial herniation. The lateral displacement of the tissue causes a wedge-shaped necrosis of the cerebral peduncle (*Kernohan's notch*) when it is pressed against the sharp, strong tentorial notch of the opposite side (Fig. 39). Thus the pyramidal tracts arising from the opposite hemisphere, traversing this area, are interrupted, producing signs on the same side as the lesion.

Third, because of compression of the posterior cerebral arteries, hemorrhage and infarcts can occur in the visual cortex (Fig. 43) and/or in the brain stem (Fig. 44). In the former, if the lesion is unilateral, homonymous hemianopsia is found,

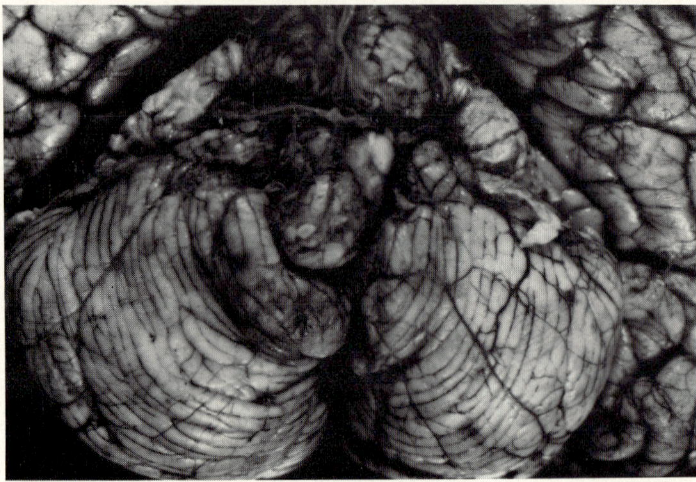

Fig. 45 Cerebellar tonsillar herniation.

and in the latter death usually ensues due to secondary brain stem hemorrhage. It is considered secondary since the hemorrhage is the result of the transtentorial herniation and not simply a primary hemorrhage originating within the brain stem.

Two opinions exist with regard to the pathogenesis of these lesions. The first is the traditional view that venous drainage is impeded by the pressure at the tentorial ridge resulting in infarct. The other is that the artery is temporarily occluded at the tentorial ridge. Recirculation within the damaged vessel then results in hemorrhagic infarct.

Tonsillar Herniation (Fig. 45)

In this lesion the cerebellar tonsils herniate downwards through the foramen magnum due to increased intracranial pressure. Downward displacement of the tonsils compresses the medulla thus interfering with the function of the vital centers, resulting in death. As in other herniations, the displaced tissue becomes necrotic due to the pressure and compression of the blood supply. When the patient's life is artificially prolonged by use of a mechanical respirator, the herniation can proceed to the point where cerebellar tissue can descend along the subarachnoid space of the spinal cord. In these "respirator brains" one can sometimes find necrotic Purkinje cells and cerebellar granule cells even at the level of the cauda equina.

Although "coning" of the cerebellum through the foramen magnum always accompanies tonsillar herniation, a certain degree of coning is normal. The degree of cerebellar coning varies greatly between individuals and is related to the size of the foramen magnum, etc. One must consider other aspects including the presence or absence of necrosis of the tonsils and other anatomical features of increased intracranial pressure before one can properly refer to the presence of a tonsillar herniation.

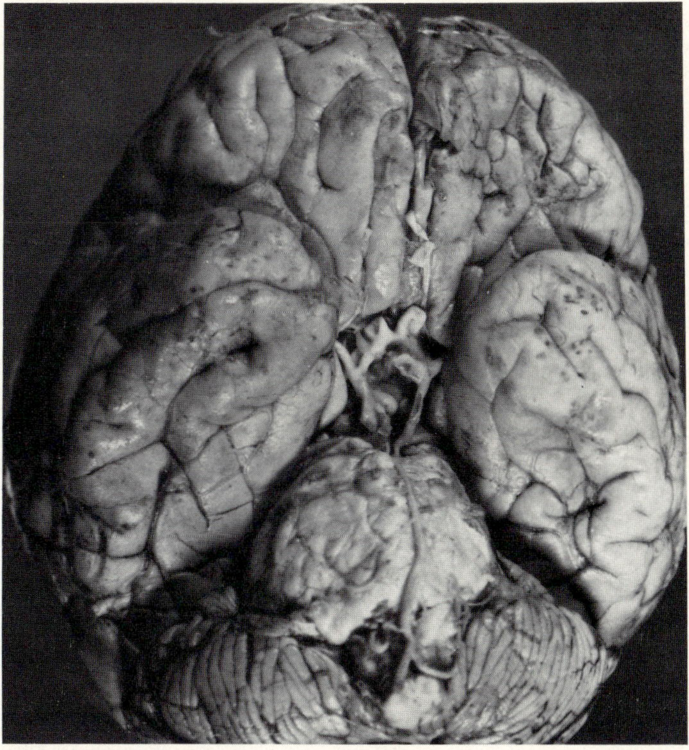

Fig. 46 Pits in temporal lobe associated with brain edema.

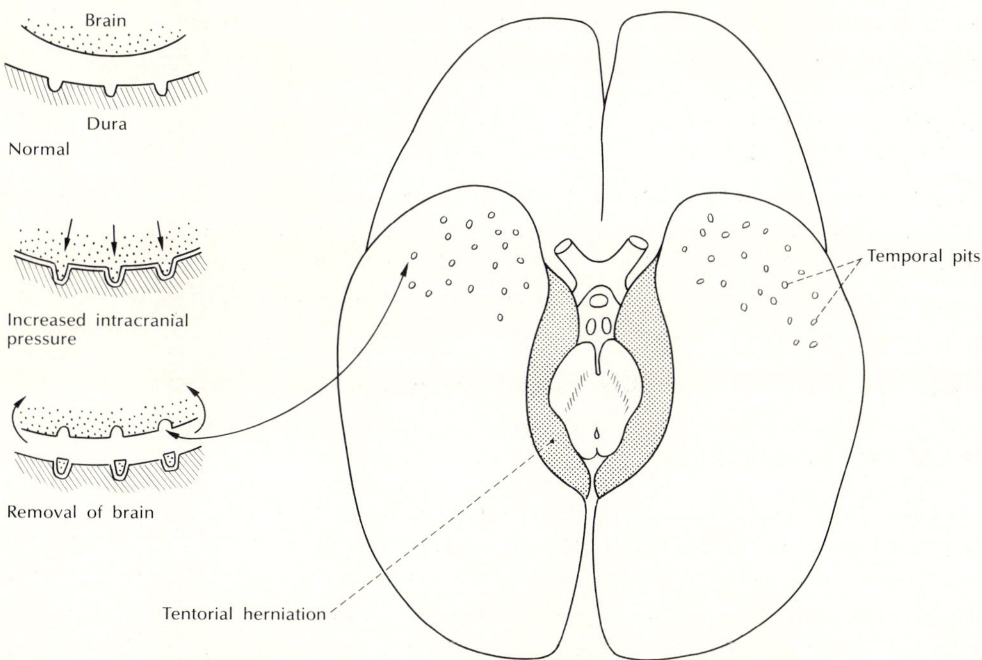

Fig. 47 Mechanism of formation of pits in the temporal lobes.

Other Herniations

Two other kinds of tissue displacement are sometimes seen in cases of increased intracranial pressure. In either case, however, despite morphological prominence, no clinical findings can be correlated with them.

In the first, the orbital gyri may press against the sphenoid ridge causing a prominent indentation in the tissue. In the second, many small pits can be found over the basal aspects of the anterior portion of the temporal lobes (Fig. 46). Microscopic section of the pits show torn out regions of missing tissue. A possible pathogenesis is illustrated in Fig. 47. Presumably, the increased intracranial pressure presses the surface of the temporal lobe into the rough dura mater. For some reason, when the brain is removed at autopsy small bits of tissue are left behind adhering to the dura mater. Generally, pits in the temporal lobe are most prominent at the site of the lesion but they are usually bilateral. Interestingly, no other part of the brain shows this phenomenon.

In contrast to the above two lesions which apparently have no clinical correlates, there exists a clinical term, "*central herniation*", with no clear cut anatomic correlation. Central herniation is a sequence of transient and changing clinical symptoms and signs implicating the diencephalon, cranial nerves, and brain stem, especially eye signs, and consciousness. Autopsies of these cases do reveal changes in these areas, but generally they are merely more advanced examples of alterations which are also seen in a wide variety of other areas as well.

Changes in the Ventricular System

Increased intracranial pressure can affect the ventricular system in various ways depending on the site of the space occupying lesion. For example, an expanding lesion in the right hemisphere will often cause compression of the right lateral ventricle, and, due to the displacement of tissue across the midline, compression and shift of the third ventricle (Fig. 39). This may result in dilation of the left lateral ventricle due to obstruction of the third ventricle as well as at the foramen of Monro. Tentorial herniation may compress the aqueduct resulting in dilation of the third and both lateral ventricles. A tonsillar herniation can result in the obstruction of the foramina of Luschka and Magendie with consequent dilation of the entire ventricular system above. In all cases, ventricular dilation will, in itself, cause increased intracranial pressure and thus, further aggravate the condition.

GROSS APPEARANCE OF THE UNSECTIONED BRAIN

General Considerations

Ideally, the normal, fixed brain is a well formed symmetrical structure in which the proportional sizes of the component parts are within reasonably close limits. Occasionally, however, improper fixation and handling result in some distortion, and the student must learn to distinguish between these artifactitious variations and those reflecting a real pathology. Moreover, a certain degree of individual variation can occur even within the normal brain. On the other hand, certain

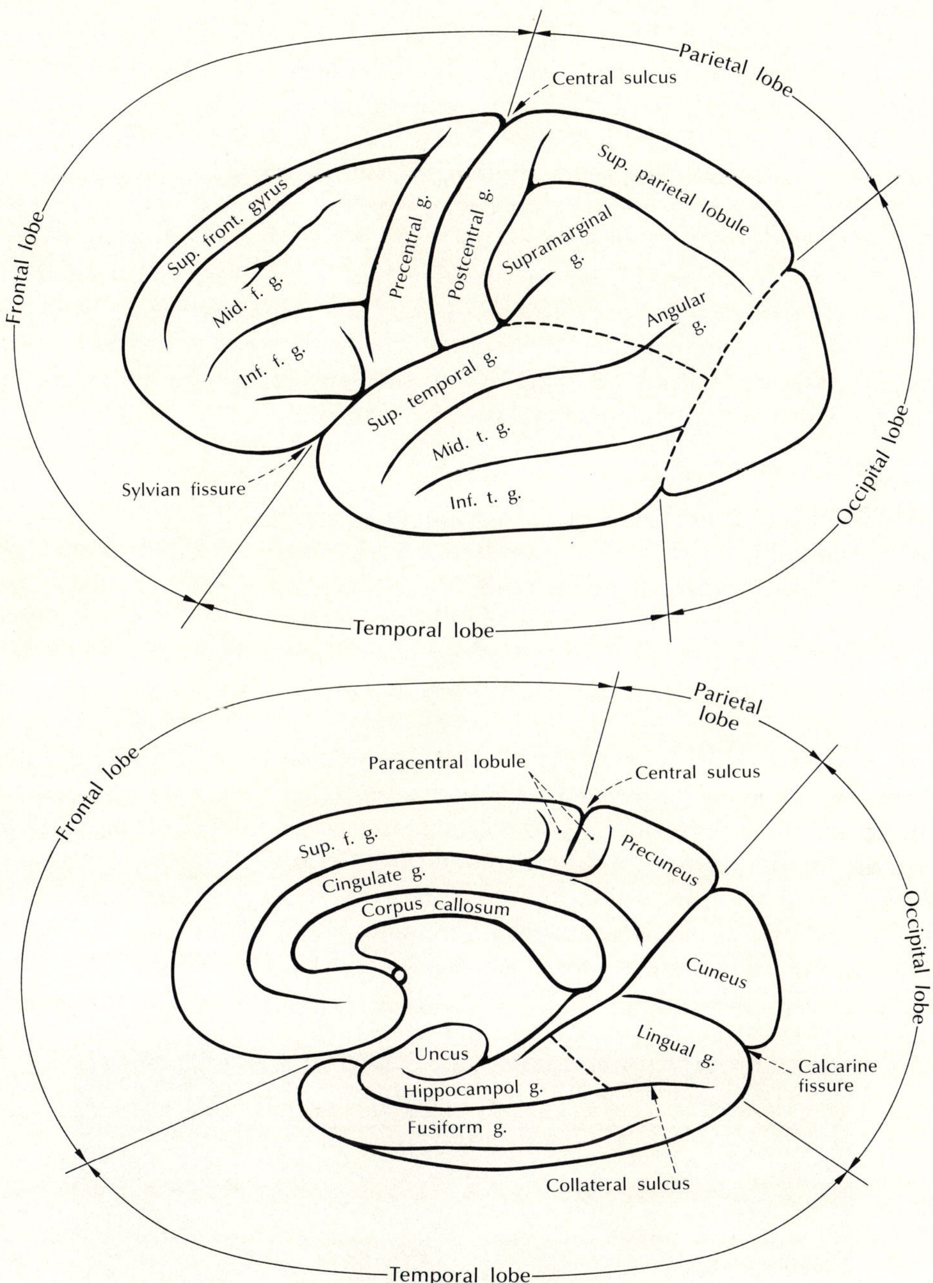

Fig. 48 Gyri and sulci.

pathological conditions, especially congenital deformities, can result in striking, gross deviations from the normal.

When examining the effect of pathological processes on the brain, one of its unique aspects become apparent. Unlike most other organs, the precise localization of the lesion is extremely important in correlating the anatomical changes with the clinical symptoms and signs. For example, as is well known, a lesion in the right hemisphere results in symptoms quite different from a similar lesion in a corresponding area of the opposite side. As a corollary, the underlying etiology of the lesion is often not as important with regard to the manifestation of the symptoms as is the topographical distribution. It is for these reasons that samples taken from the brain must be carefully identified as to their location as well as the side of the brain from which they are derived. The importance of these precautions cannot be overemphasized. A diagram of the surface of the brain with the identification of the gyri and sulci is shown in Fig. 48.

Diffuse Involvement

Generalized brain edema is a good example of a diffusely distributed lesion. The brains of individuals who died after being in a respirator often show diffuse swelling and discoloration (Walker, 1978).

Obstruction of the normal pathways of ventricular fluid may lead to "obstructive hydrocephalus" resulting in diffuse swelling of the brain. The cause and location of the underlying obstruction may vary and is more easily understood after section.

Another example, with essentially opposite effects, is the cerebral atrophy (Fig. 49) which accompanies senile and presenile dementia (Alzheimer's disease, Huntington's chorea, Parkinsonism-dementia complex, etc.) as well as other conditions affecting either the gray or white matter or both. Under these conditions the brain is small, the gyri are shrunken and the sulci widened.

Various developmental anomalies known as agenesis or dysgenesis result in deformities which are obvious during gross examination of the brain. Many such conditions occur. Well known among them is Arnold-Chiari malformation which is illustrated in Figs. 50—52.

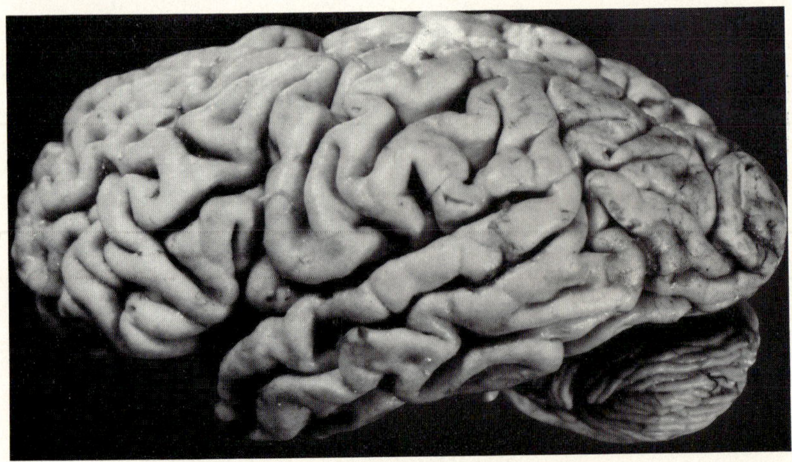

Fig. 49 Generalized cerebral atrophy.

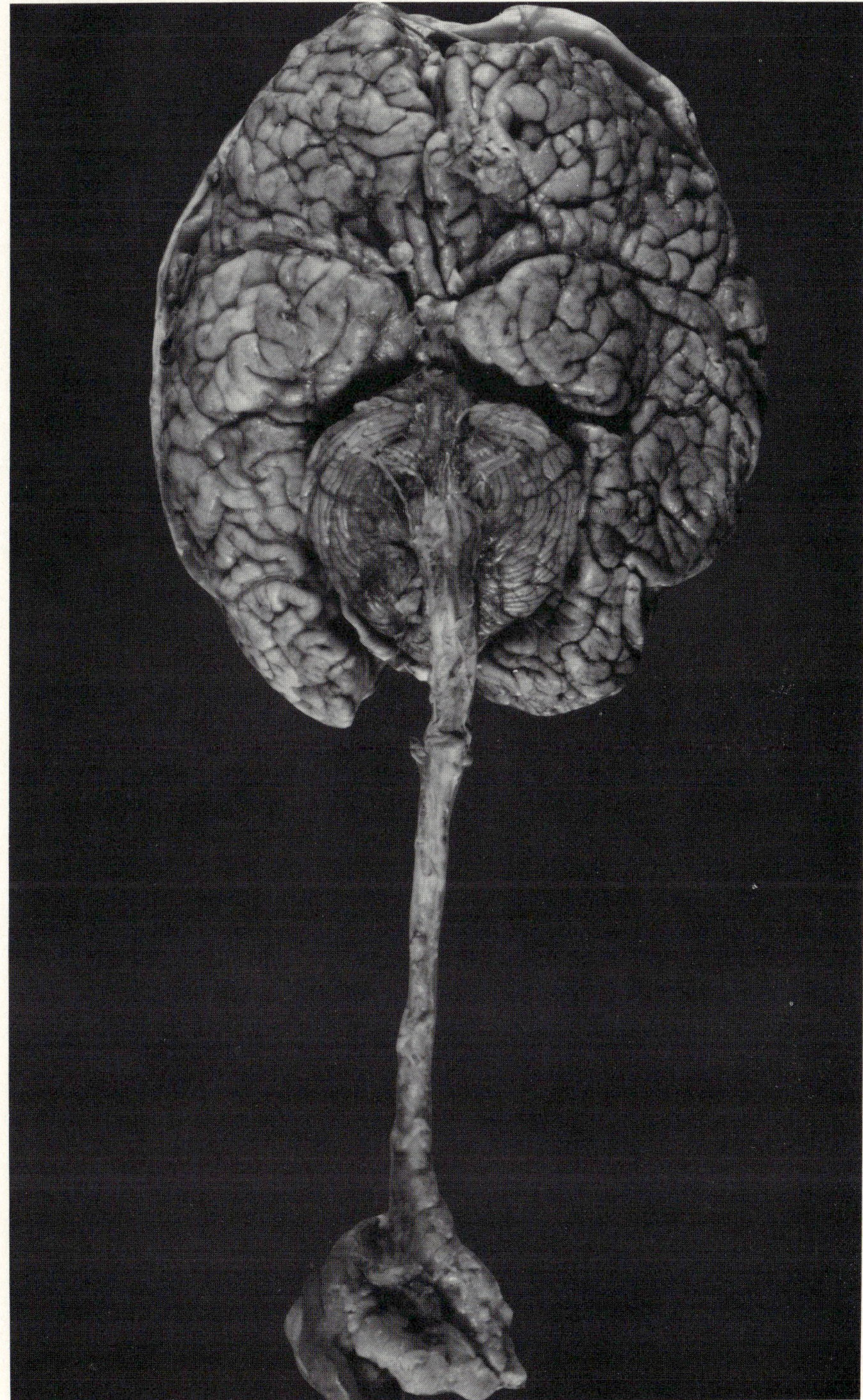

Fig. 50 Micropolygyria, Arnold-Chiari malformation and meningomyelocele.

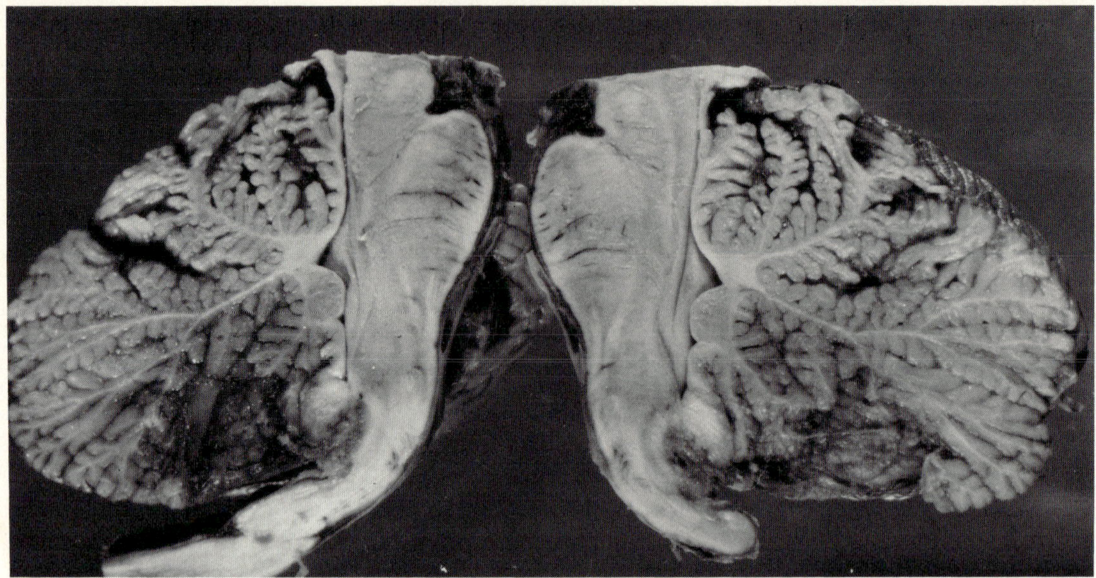

Fig. 51 Arnold-Chiari malformation.
A sagittal section through the cerebellum and brain stem of the same case as that illustrated in Fig. 50.

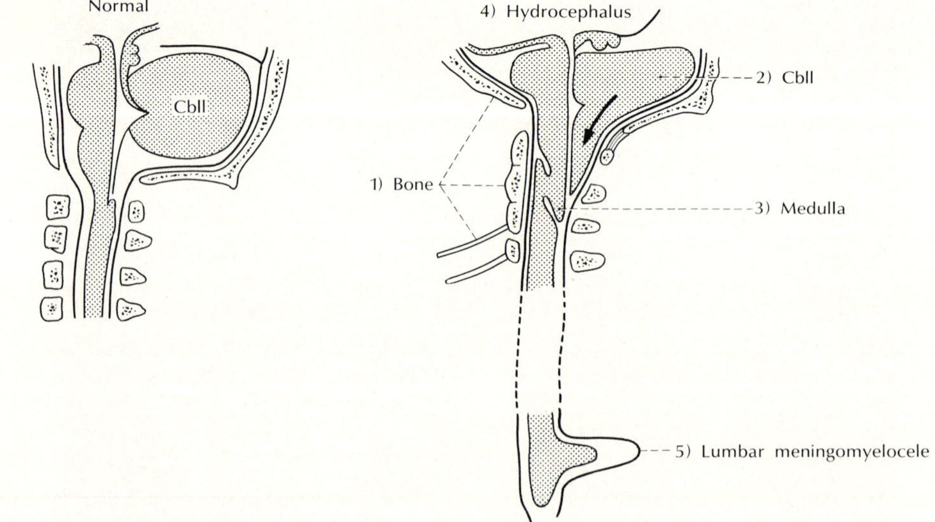

Fig. 52 Arnold-Chiari malformation.
Diagrammatic representation of the anatomical relationships commonly seen in Arnold-Chiari malformations. The base of the skull is flattened (platybasia) and cervical ribs may be present as well as fusion of some cervical vertebrae. The medulla displays an S-shaped kinking and the cerebellum shows a vertical elongation and tonsillar herniation. The fourth ventricle is compressed and the foramina of Luschka and Magendie are obstructed resulting in hydrocephalus.

REFERENCES

Walker, A.E.: Pathology of brain death. Ann. N.Y. Acad. Sci., 315: 272-280, 1978.

Iwata, M., Kawamoto, K., & Hirano, A.: Arnold-Chiari malformation. Neurol. Med. (Tokyo), 9: 86-88, 1978.

Focal Involvement

It is convenient to divide these changes into symmetrical and asymmetrical lesions. A good example of the former is the *boundary zone* or *watershed zone infarct* (Fig. 53). These are the result of transient ischemia or other insults usually due to some circulatory disturbance. In these cases, the areas furthest from a major arterial supply are most susceptible to infarct. Thus the infarct forms at the boundary between regions nourished by different major arteries. Variations in the circle of Willis, as already described, as well as the severity and duration of the insult, can modify the configuration and extent of a boundary zone infarct.

Other focal, symmetrical lesions are the result of *systemic degeneration* in which specific entire neuronal systems are selectively affected.

Pick's disease is a good example of a focal, symmetrical cerebral lesion. In this condition, also known as lobar atrophy, the frontal and temporal lobes are usually markedly atrophic while other areas are spared. Interestingly, often the motor strips and the posterior portion of the superior temporal gyri, as well as certain other specific gyri, are remarkably well preserved in contrast to the remainder of the lobes.

Symmetrical atrophy of the mammillary body, often accompanied by discoloration due to hemorrhagic lesions, is characteristic of *Wernicke's encephalopathy*. Unilateral atrophy of the mammillary body may indicate the presence of a long-standing destructive lesion in the ipsilateral fornix or the median aspect of the temporal lobe perhaps suggesting transsynaptic degeneration (Torch et al., 1977).

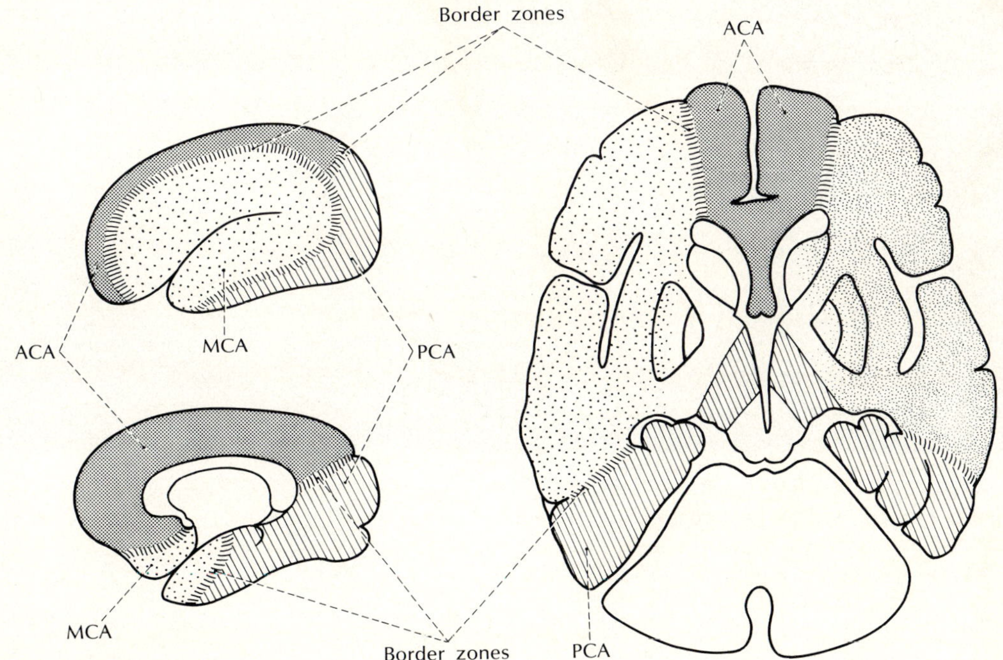

Fig. 53 Territories of anterior (ACA), middle (MCA), posterior (PCA) cerebral arteries and the border zones.

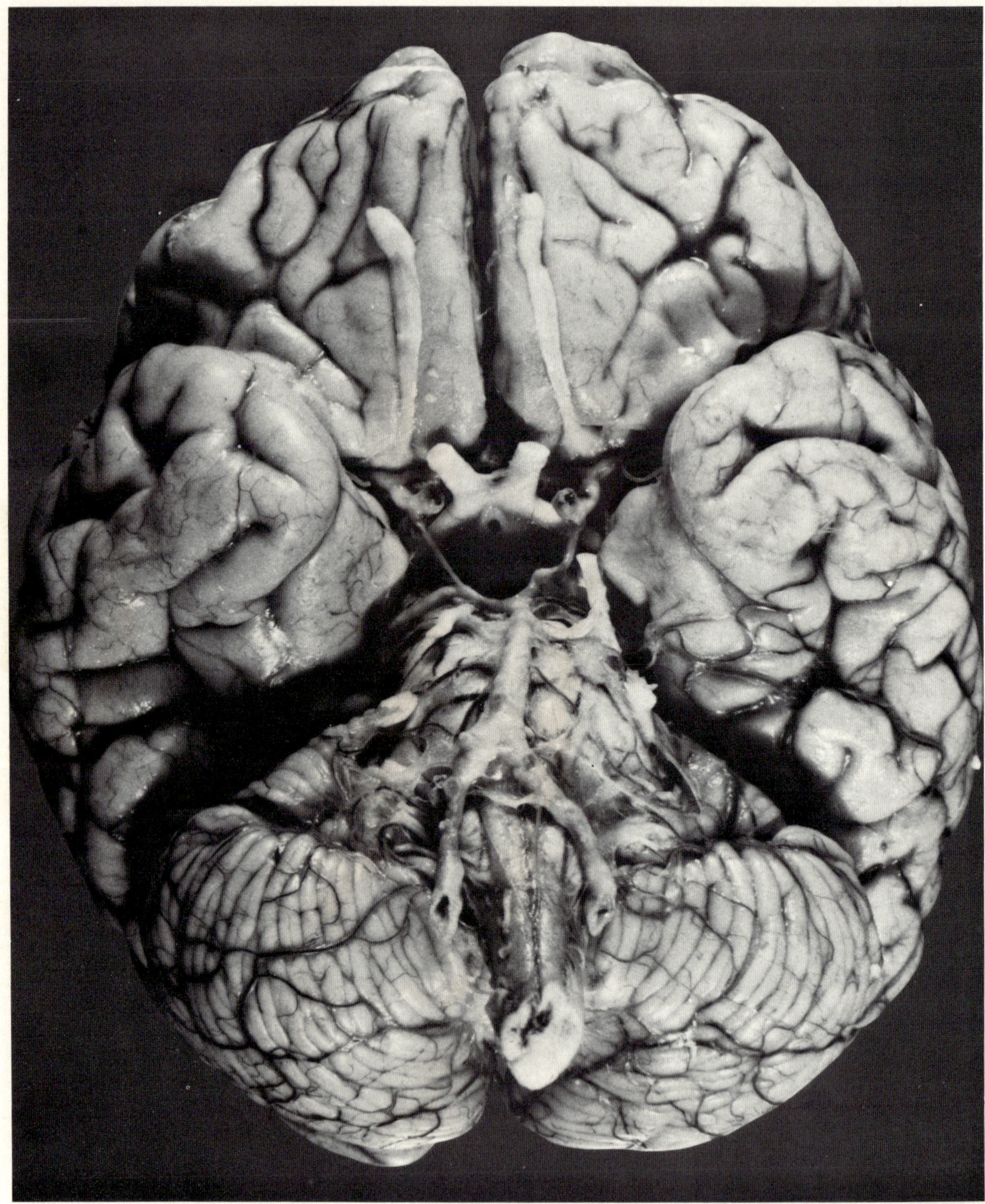

Fig. 54 Normal brain.

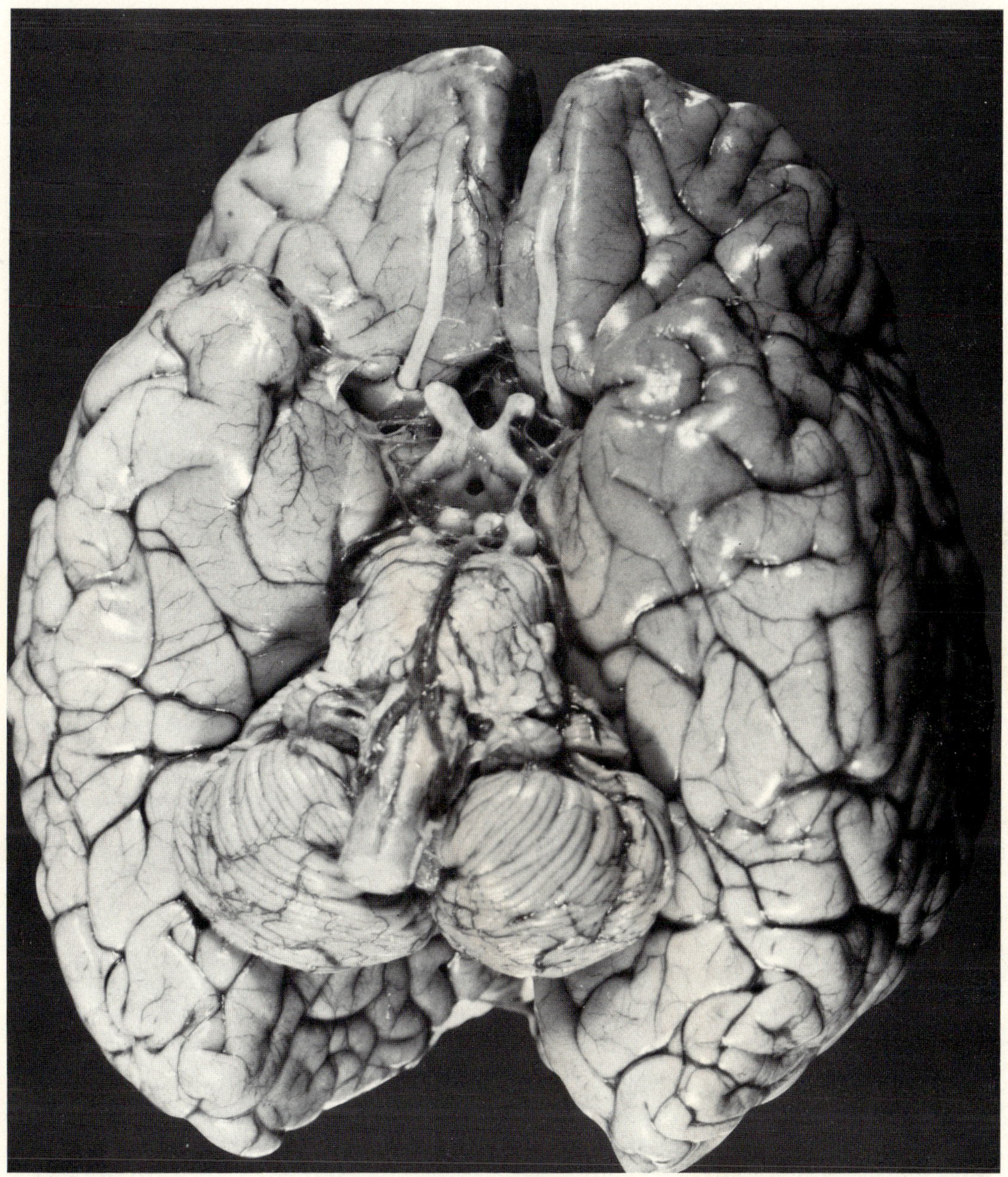

Fig. 55 Cerebellar atrophy (Compare with Fig. 54).

Other good examples of symmetrical focal lesions are various cerebellar degenerations. In the normal adult the cerebellum can approach the level of the occipital pole. In *cerebellar degeneration*, however, the cerebellum is disproportionately small (Fig. 54 and Fig. 55). In young infants, the cerebellum is still developing and is therefore very small even in the normal brain. When cerebellar degeneration is found one must examine the inferior olive and the pons as well as other nuclei and tracts connected to the cerebellum (Fig. 56).

More often, focal lesions, either single or multiple, are asymmetrical in distribution. In fact, most neuropathological alterations belong to this group. These are relatively easy to recognize because of the presence of built-in control areas.

Certain *infarcts* involving only single vessels (see Appendix I, Figs. 53, 57—63), intracerebral hematomas, *contusions* (Figs. 64—66), or *brain tumors* (see Appendix II, Figs. 67—70), are good examples of asymmetric focal lesions. Infection also may lead to obvious focal lesions. These include brain abscesses (see p. 274) and certain acute viral encephalites such as *herpes encephalitis* (Fig. 71).

Certain demyelinating diseases are often also focal in nature. Usually, because of the multiplicity of the old lesions the central nervous system appears atrophic. The demyelinated plaques themselves, however, cannot usually be detected on external examination and must await sectioning. Exceptions to this rule are some demyelinated plaques in the pons and optic chiasm where the white matter is not covered by gray matter (Fig. 72).

REFERENCES

Torch, W.C., Hirano, A., & Solomon, S.: Anterograde transneuronal degeneration in the limbic system. Clinical-anatomical correlation. Neurology, 27: 1157-1163, 1977.

Iwata, M., Kawamoto, K., & Hirano, A.: Chronic decortication state and wide-spread laminar necrosis of the cerebral cortex. Neurol. Med. (Tokyo), 8: 590-592, 1978.

Secondary Changes

Due to the extreme length of axons of many neurons, changes can appear in regions quite distant from the original lesion. Damage to the neuronal soma will ultimately result in the destruction of the entire axon. Conversely, damage to the axon will result in *Wallerian degeneration* and destruction of the distal portion. A good example is *pyramidal tract degeneration* (Fig. 73). In these cases damage to one hemisphere will result in degeneration of the pyramids in the medulla and ultimately in the spinal cord. The process, however, is slow so that gross atrophy of the pyramids of the medulla may not be conspicuous until several months after the original injury.

In addition to secondary changes which are confined to a single cell and its processes, transsynaptic degeneration may also be observed after damage to the afferent neurons or its processes. When significant lesions are present in the dentate nucleus of the cerebellum or the tegmentum of the pons involving the central tegmental tracts, the inferior olivary nucleus should be examined for changes. Under these circumstances the inferior olive may be hypertrophic due to pronounced vacuolation of the neuropil, and glial and neuronal changes due to

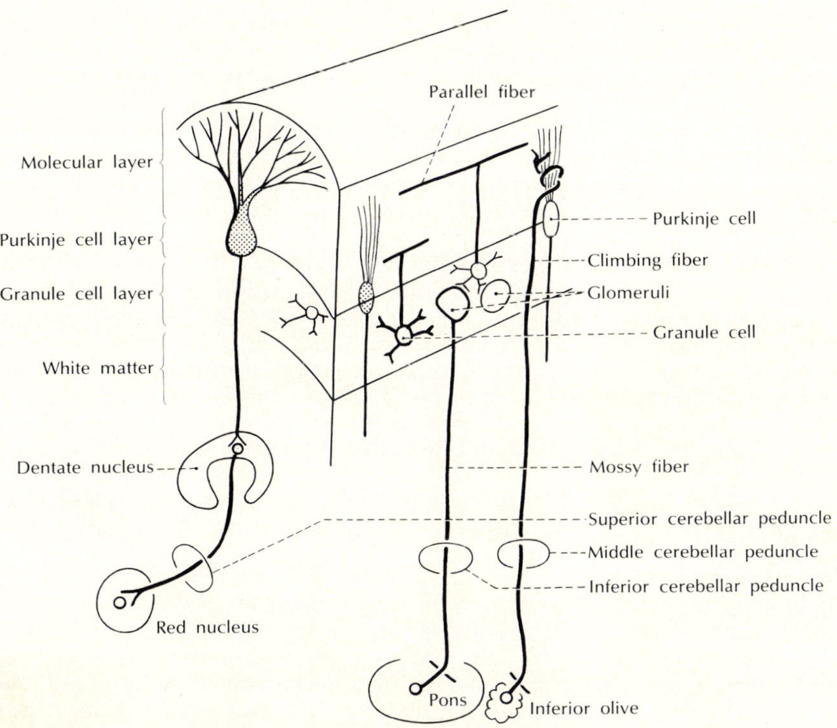

Fig. 56 Cerebellum.

transsynaptic effects. Similarly, lesions of the median aspect of the temporal lobe and the fornix may result in atrophy of the mammillary body.

It is worthwhile pointing out that the neuropathologist, because of his legitimate access to human pathological specimens and his concern with such processes as fiber tract degeneration, is in a unique position to be able to delineate the normal pathways in the human nervous system.

REFERENCE

Iwata, M., & Hirano, A.: Localization of olivo-cerebellar fibers in inferior cerebellar peduncle in man. J. Neurol. Sci., 38: 327-335, 1978.

Appendix I. Infarcts.

Infarcts represent the destruction of nervous tissue as the result of the compromise of the blood supply. Their gross as well as their histological appearance differs depending on whether or not there is an accompanying hemorrhage and on the interval between the onset of the lesion and examination.

In the so-called *"anemic infarct"* in which the blood vessel is merely occluded but no hemorrhage has occurred, no changes are detectable either grossly or microscopically until several hours after the clinical symptoms.

By two days the surface of the brain is pale and swollen. These changes are not especially obvious by visual inspection alone, especially for the inexperienced observer. Upon touching the infarct, however, it is immediately apparent that the brain is soft in this area as compared to the rest of the well-fixed, firm tissue. This phenomenon has given rise to the term "cerebral softening" often used to describe these changes. Microscopically, at this time one may find ischemic changes in the neurons, swollen astrocytes and other spongy changes of the tissue associated with infiltration of polymorphonuclear leucocytes.

By one week the swelling begins to subside but tissue necrosis is pronounced. At this time the infarct is easily visible by the discoloration and friable nature of the tissue. Histologically, numerous macrophages are present containing sudanophilic lipid granules. The astrocytes become markedly hypertrophic and filled with eosinophilic organelles.

Thereafter the lesion undergoes liquefaction and becomes concave as the tissue atrophies. By a month after onset cyst formation is underway. Microscopically the essentially healed lesion consists of a glial scar with small numbers of residual macrophages around the remaining blood vessels. In contrast to the cysts associated with other etiologies such as abscess, trauma, etc. the cysts formed after infarcts show relatively little connective tissue proliferation.

Hemorrhagic infarcts are easily identifiable by the presence of extravasated blood. They differ from hematomas in that the blood is interspersed among the tissue elements.

Location of the Infarct in Relation to the Site of the Occlusion

a) Carotid artery system (Anterior circulation) (Figs. 25 and 53).

(1) Infarcts in the territory of the internal carotid artery (Fig. 57).

Infarcts involving the entire territory of the internal carotid artery are signs of the complete and sudden occlusion of the artery and of poor collateral circulation provided by the anterior and posterior communicating arteries and sometimes the ophthalmic artery as well. The most common site of thrombosis of the internal carotid artery is the area of bifurcation from the common carotid artery.

(2) Infarcts in the territory of the middle cerebral artery (Figs. 58, 59 and 60).

These infarcts are the most common of all. When the entire field is involved it is an indication of occlusion of the middle cerebral artery somewhere between its origin from the internal carotid artery and the perforating branches. Such infarcts, however, may also be due to occlusion of the internal carotid artery itself. If only the caudate-putamen system is involved the presumption is that the perforating branches are occluded (Fig. 60). When the occlusion is situated in the distal branches of the middle cerebral artery the cortex and the underlying white matter are involved (Fig. 59). The size and severity of such infarcts depend upon the size of the occluded branches and the degree of anastomosis with other arteries. Cortical infarcts of this type may also be due to occlusion of the internal carotid artery as well.

(3) Infarcts of the territory of the anterior cerebral artery.

Because of the anastomosis of this vessel with the anterior communicating artery, occlusions in the anterior cerebral artery do not often result in infarcts when the obstruction is proximal to the site of the anastomosis.

b) Vertebrobasilar artery system (posterior circulation)

(1) Infarcts in the territory of the posterior cerebral artery (Fig. 43).

The territory of the posterior cerebral artery is largely hidden by the cerebellum. Small and old infarcts in this region may, therefore, be easily missed unless the cerebellum is lifted up and the occipital lobe inspected. This is a very common site of infarcts and they are often bilateral. Infarcts in this area may be due to occlusion in the basilar artery or to the simultaneous compression of both posterior cerebral arteries against the tentorial edge due to increased intracranial pressure. Unilateral infarcts in this territory may be due to occlusion of the ipsilateral posterior cerebral artery or of the posterior communicating artery when that vessel is the major source of blood supply to that region. The posterior cerebral artery and the posterior communicating artery both give rise to numerous small perforating branches which supply a large variety of areas within the posterior portion of the base of the brain including the thalamus, the lateral geniculate body, the hypothalamus and the midbrain among others. The areas most likely to result in obvious gross change and the most common are the visual cortex and part of Ammon's horn.

(2) Infarcts in the territory of the basilar artery (Fig. 61).

Occlusion of this artery results in infarction of the pons and adjacent brain stem. These lesions are responsible for the clinical symptoms related to basilar artery insufficiency.

(3) Infarcts in the territory of the posterior inferior cerebellar artery (PICA) (Figs. 62 and 63).

Occlusion of PICA results in Wallenberg's or lateral medullary syndrome. The infarct as indicated in Fig. 63 involves the lateral portion of the medulla oblongata and the posterior and inferior aspects of the cerebellum and results in characteristic clinical manifestations. It must be noted that actually the occlusion is much more likely to be found in the vertebral artery itself rather than in PICA.

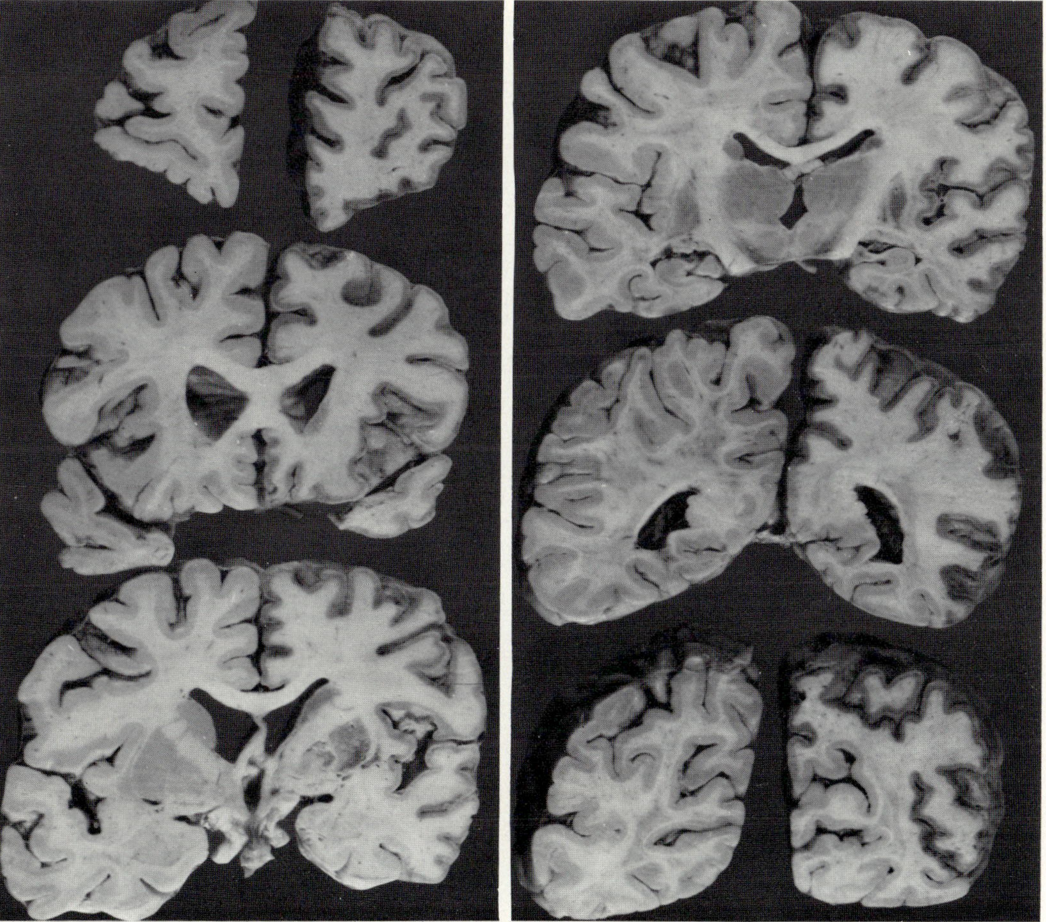

57-1 **57-2**

Fig. 57-1 Laminar necrosis in the cerebral hemisphere due to occlusion of the common carotid artery. Edematous white matter and necrosis of the basal ganglia are also evident.
Fig. 57-2 Laminar necrosis in the cerebral hemisphere due to occlusion of the ipsilateral common carotid artery.

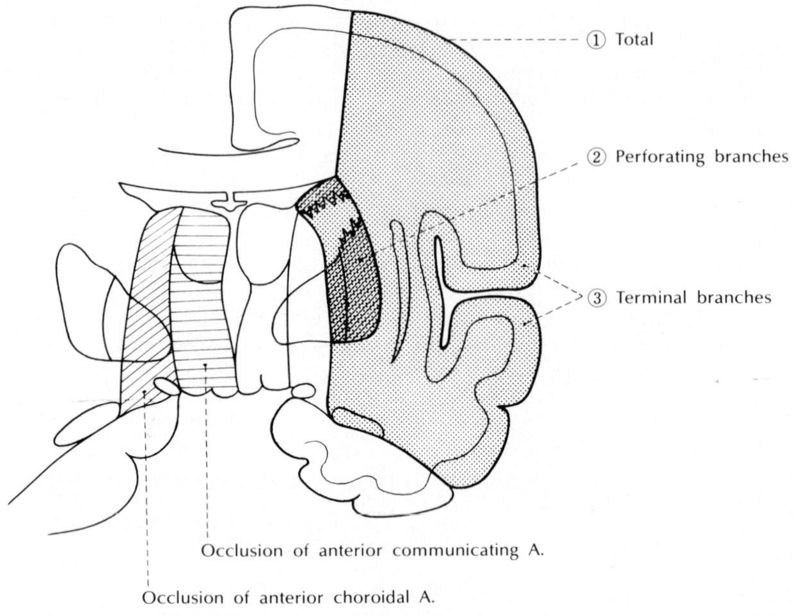

Fig. 58 Occlusion of the middle cerebral artery.

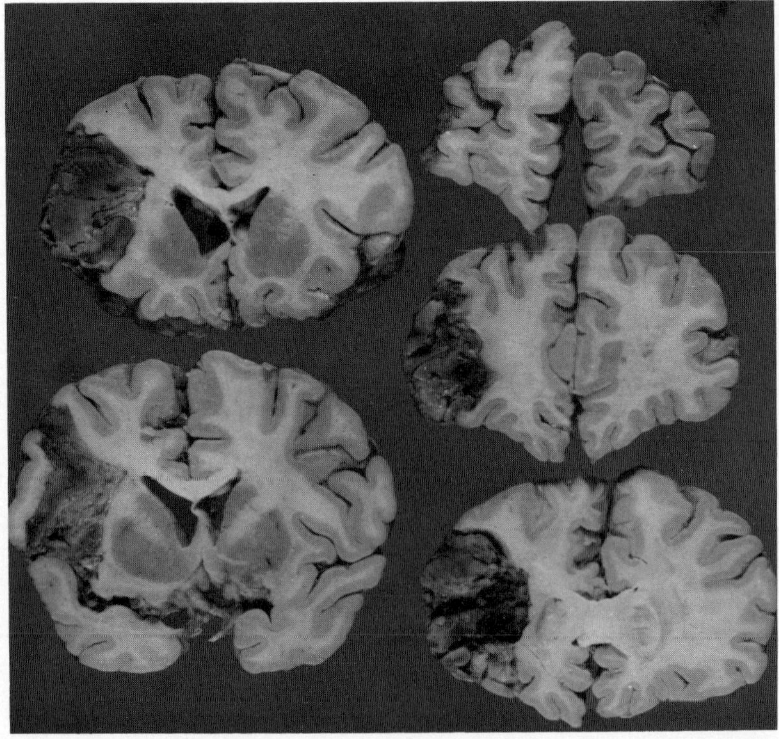

Fig. 59 Hemorrhagic infarct in the territory of the middle cerebral artery.

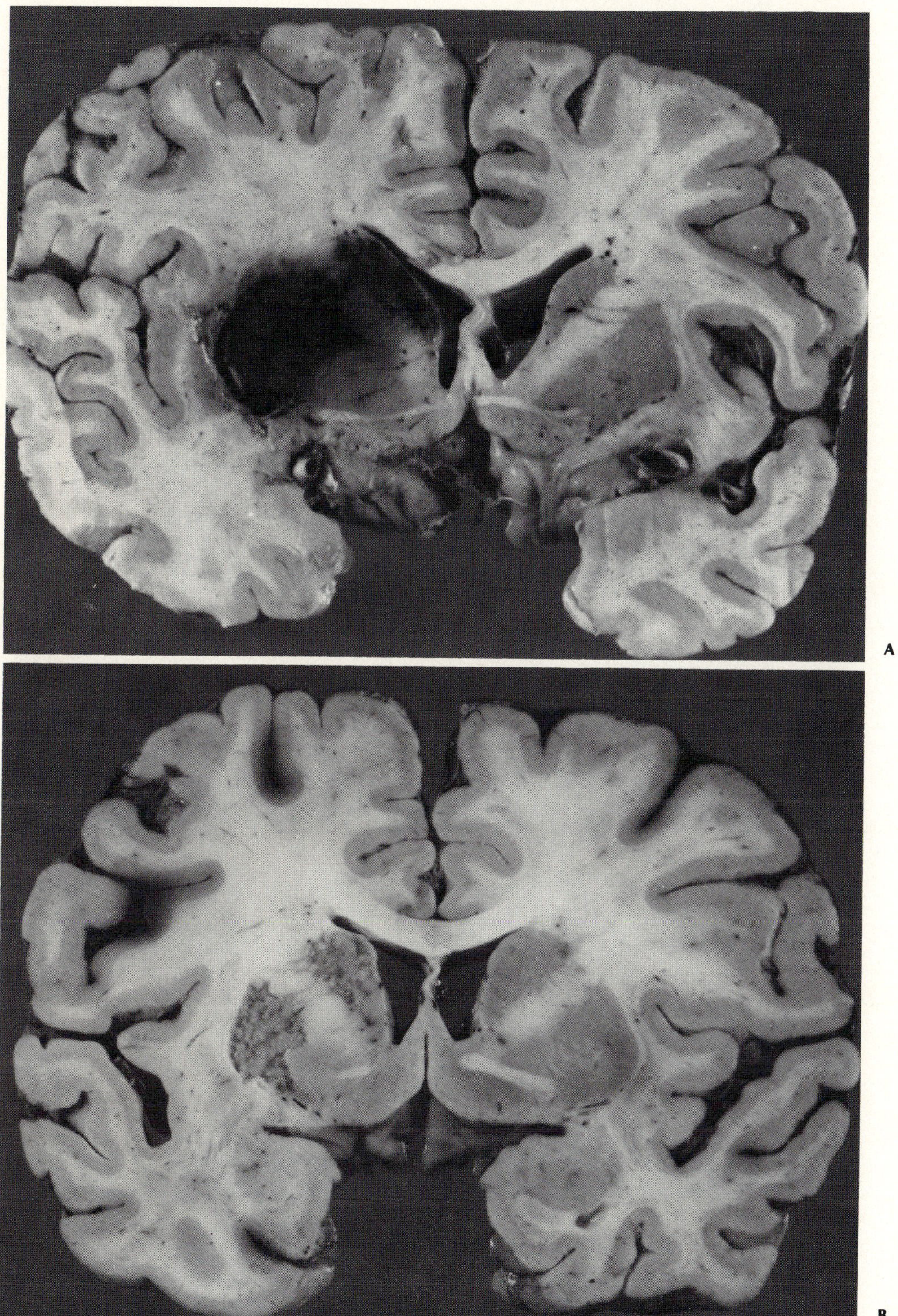

Fig. 60 Infarct in the caudate-putamen complex. A. Fresh hemorrhagic infarct. B. Old lesion.

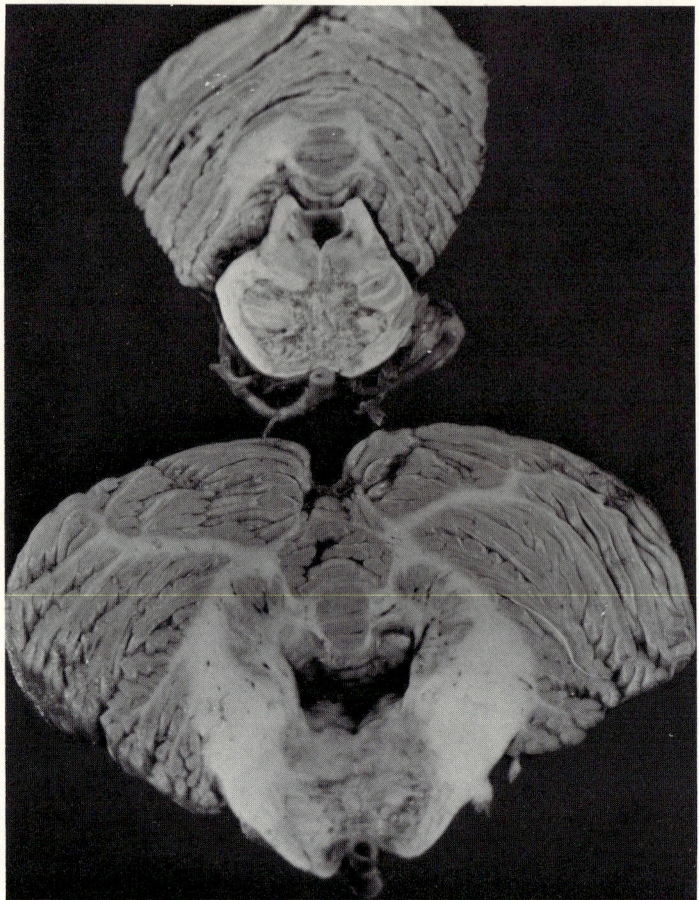

Fig. 61 Necrosis of the pons due to thrombosis of the basilar artery.

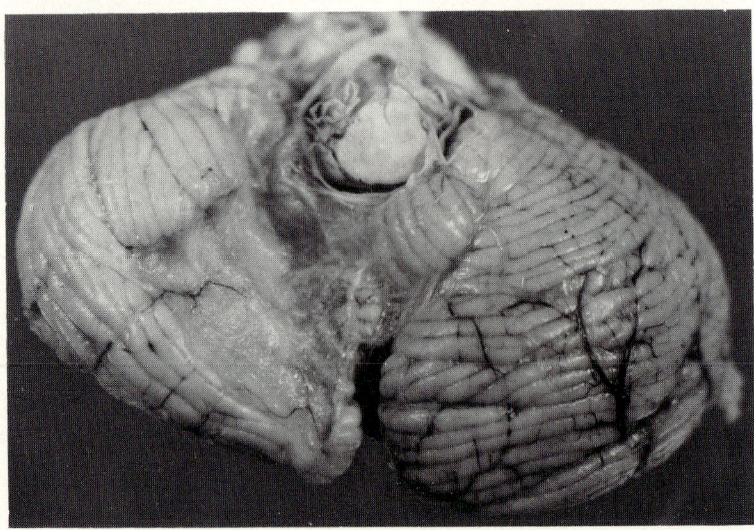

Fig. 62 Old infarct in the territory of the posterior inferior cerebellar artery.

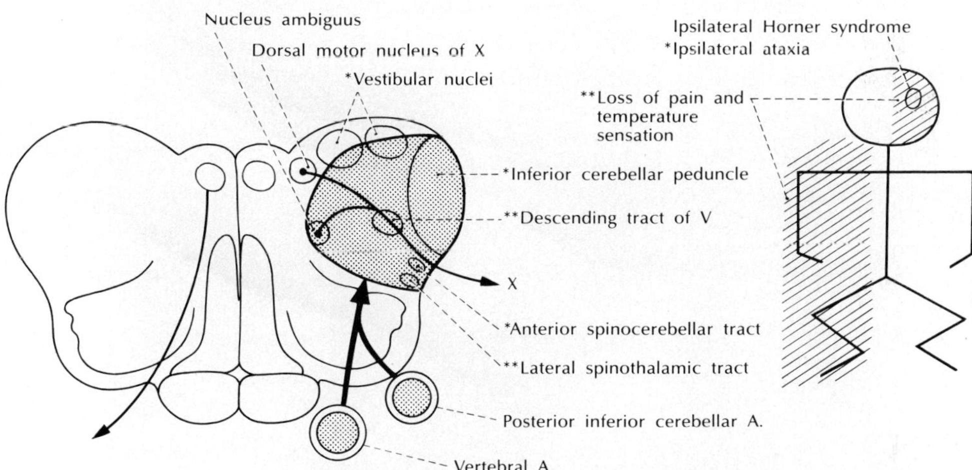

Fig. 63 Lateral medullary syndrome.

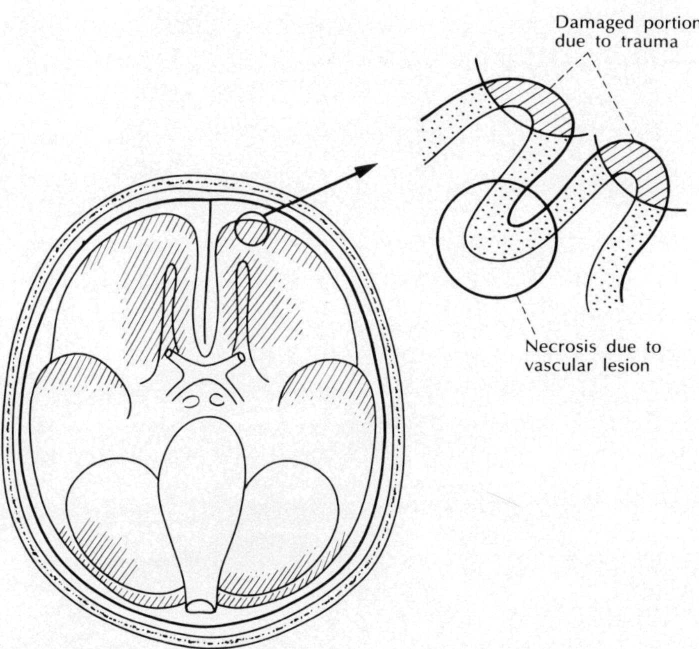

Fig. 64 Contusion.
In head injuries leading to contusion of the brain the tips of the gyri are more vulnerable than the depths of the sulci. Particularly likely to sustain such injuries are the frontal, temporal and occipital poles as well as the orbital gyri. When the lesion affects diagonally opposite poles it is known as a coup-countrecoup lesion.

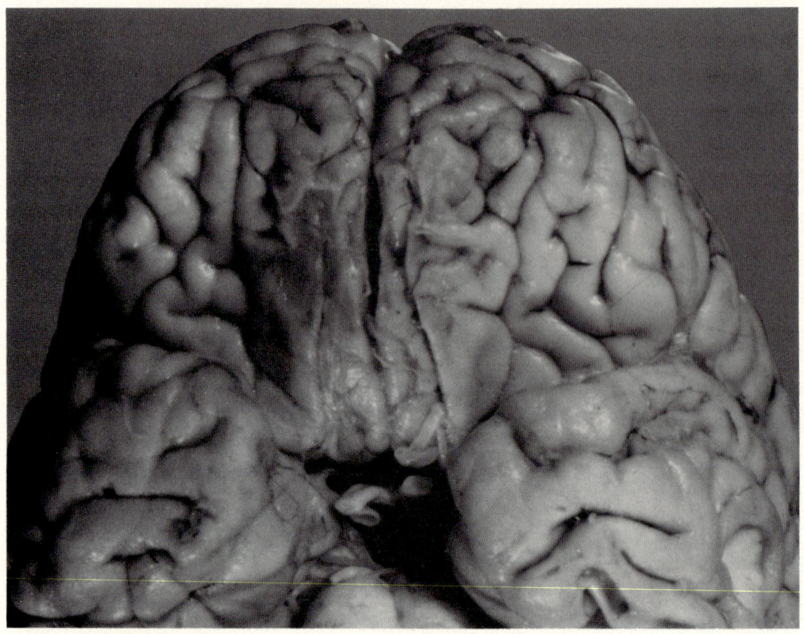

Fig. 65 Old traumatic lesion in the orbital and rectal gyri. The olfactory bulbs are destroyed.

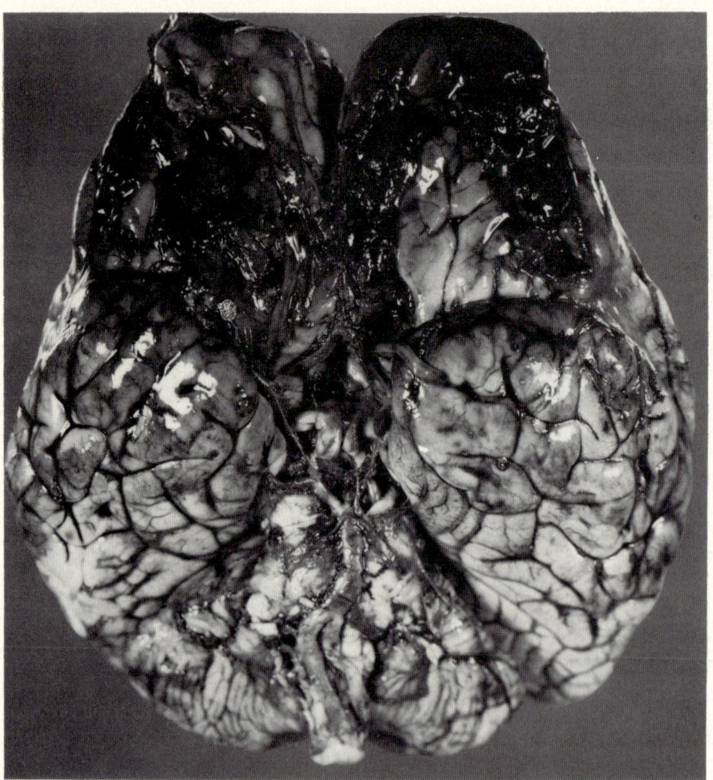

Fig. 66 A fresh contusion of the frontal and temporal lobes. A subarachnoid hemorrhage is apparent.

Appendix II. Brain Tumors.

Gliomas and metastatic tumors constitute the majority of the neoplasms involving the brain parenchyma.

Over half of the gliomas are *glioblastoma multiforme* which is the most malignant form of gliomas in adult life. It may occur in any area of the central nervous system, but most commonly it is found within the cerebral hemispheres (p. 222).

Due to the expanding mass and associated edema, necrosis, vascular congestion and occasional hemorrhages, the lesion is usually easily identified. On the other hand, the exact extent of the involvement is impossible to ascertain on external examination due to the infiltrative nature of the tumor and its location deep within the brain parenchyma.

Astrocytomas are the second most frequent gliomas. They may occur in any area in the central nervous system but in the adult they most commonly affect the cerebral hemispheres and are usually malignant. In children they usually affect the cerebellar hemispheres and tend to be cystic and more benign. Cerebellar astrocytoma and medulloblastoma are the most common intracranial tumors in children (p. 221).

Gliomas involving the optic nerve or pons (Figs. 67 and 68) are easily recognizable on external examination.

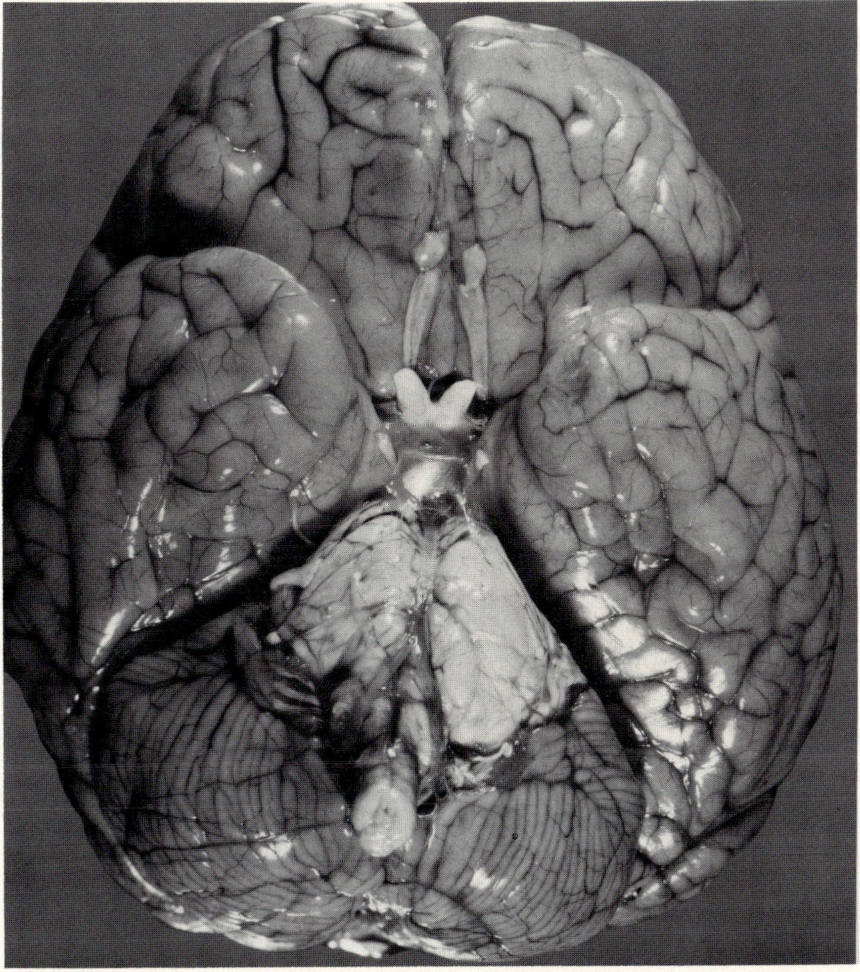

Fig. 67 Pontine glioma.

Metastatic tumors are usually multiple, but single lesions are by no means uncommon. The most common site of the primary tumor is the lung in men, and the breast in women. Other primaries include carcinomas of the kidney or gastrointestinal tract, melanomas and lymphomas. In general, metastatic neoplasms are not infiltrative and are well circumscribed from surrounding brain tissue (p. 337).

In the case of lymphomas, whether intracranial primary lymphomas or metastatic, the lesions may be circumscribed as are other metastatic tumors, but they may also infiltrate as do gliomas. Diffuse involvement of lymphomas may sometimes even resemble encephalitis or infarction.

Changes due to *delayed radiation* necrosis may be superimposed on the neoplastic lesion. It is, therefore, important to be aware of prior radiation therapy for proper evaluation of the pathology.

Two areas which are easily observed during external examination of the brain are the suprasellar region (Fig. 69) and the pineal region (Fig. 70). These sites have relatively ample subarachnoid space so that large masses such as tumors may develop insidiously.

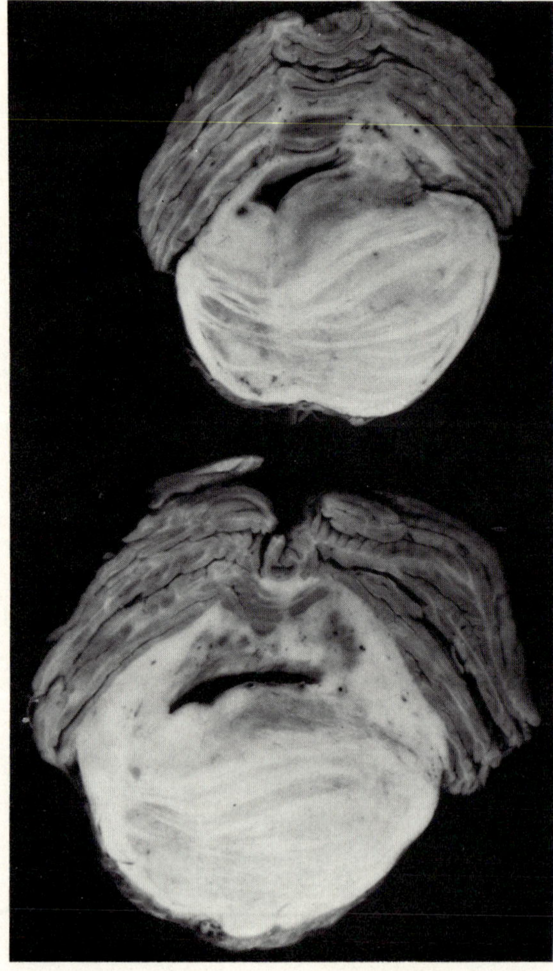

Fig. 68 Pontine glioma.

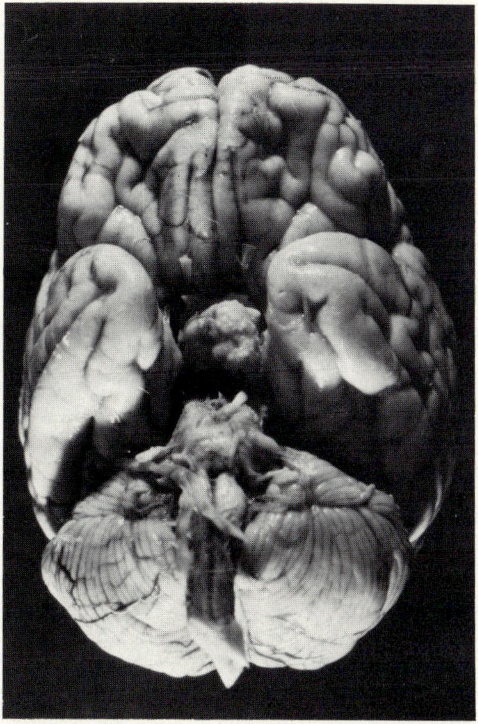

69

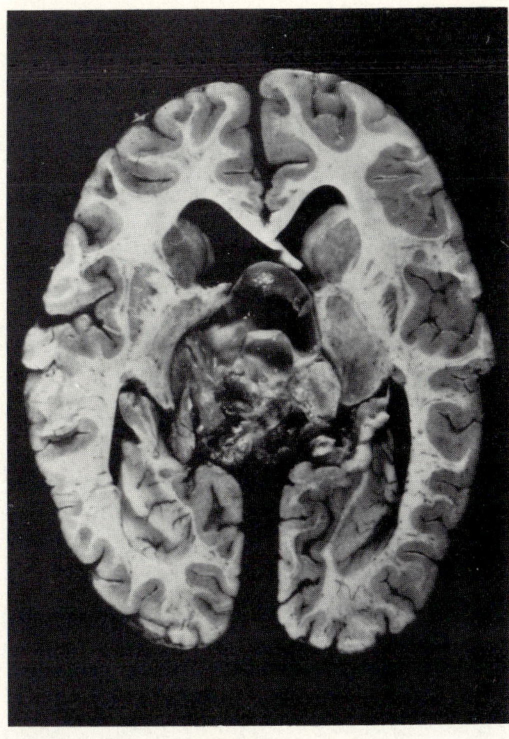

70

Fig. 69 Craniopharyngioma in a suprasellar position.

The suprasellar area has relatively ample subarachnoid space and tumors from adjacent areas may extend into the space to form relatively large masses before symptoms become apparent. The tumors may extend up into the hypothalamus, the third ventricle and involve the optic chiasm, the pituitary stalk and other structures. These tumors include:

pituitary adenomas (associated with endocrine disturbances)
craniopharyngiomas (associated with calcification and cysts)
germinomas (so-called ectopic pinealomas)
optic nerve gliomas (usually in childhood)
metastatic tumors
meningiomas
chordomas (from the clivus)
teratomas
epidermoid cysts (cholesteatomas)
granule cell myoblastomas

Fig. 70 Teratoma in the region of pineal gland.

The pineal gland occupies an area, where the ample subarachnoid space (see Fig. 76-2) may allow formation of large masses without obvious clinical manifestations. An aneurysm of the vein of Galen (Fig. 18) or large tumors in this location eventually produce compression of the quadrigeminal plate and the aqueduct causing obstructive hydrocephalus. These tumors include:

pinealomas
germinomas
yolk sac tumors
teratomas
gliomas
metastatic tumors

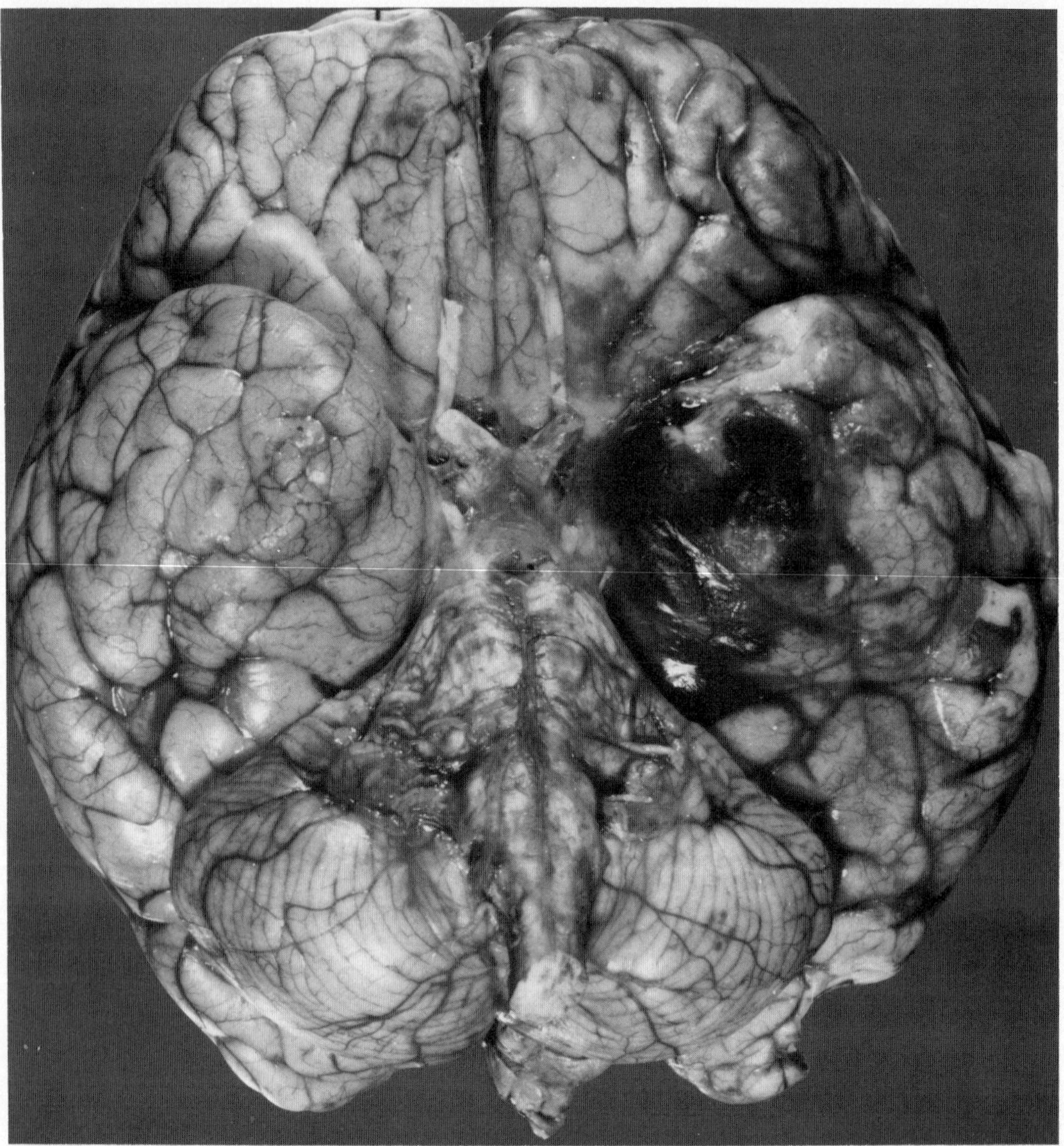

Fig. 71 Acute herpes (simplex) encephalitis.
A basal view of a brain with acute herpes encephalitis showing a characteristic lesion. The brain is edematous and congested and a hemorrhagic, necrotic area is visible on the median aspect of the anterior portion of the left temporal lobe.

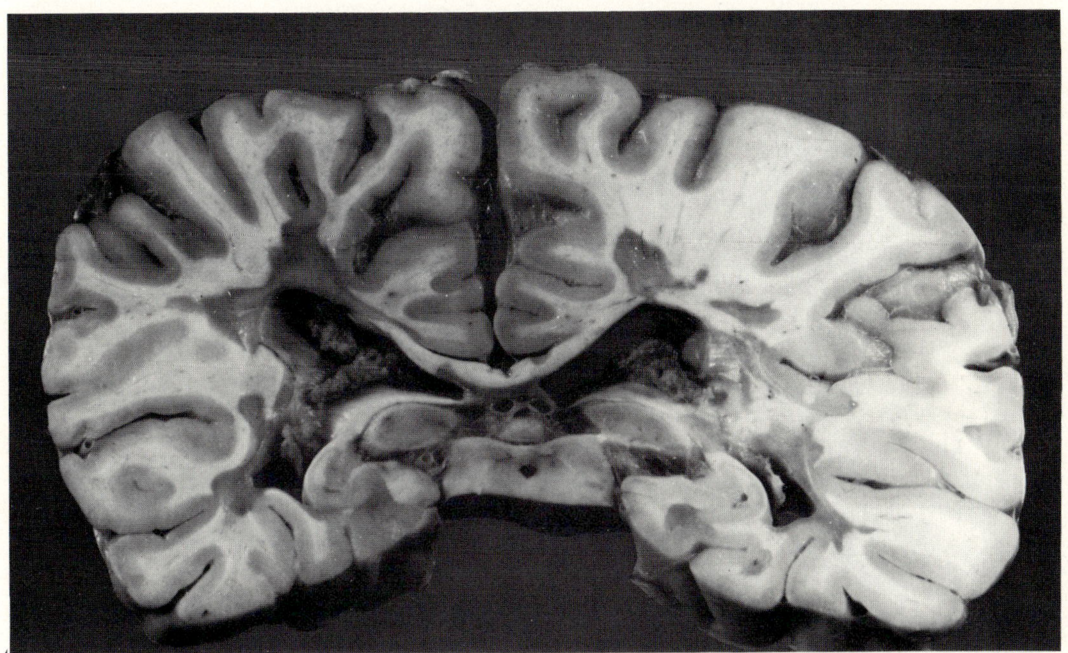

A

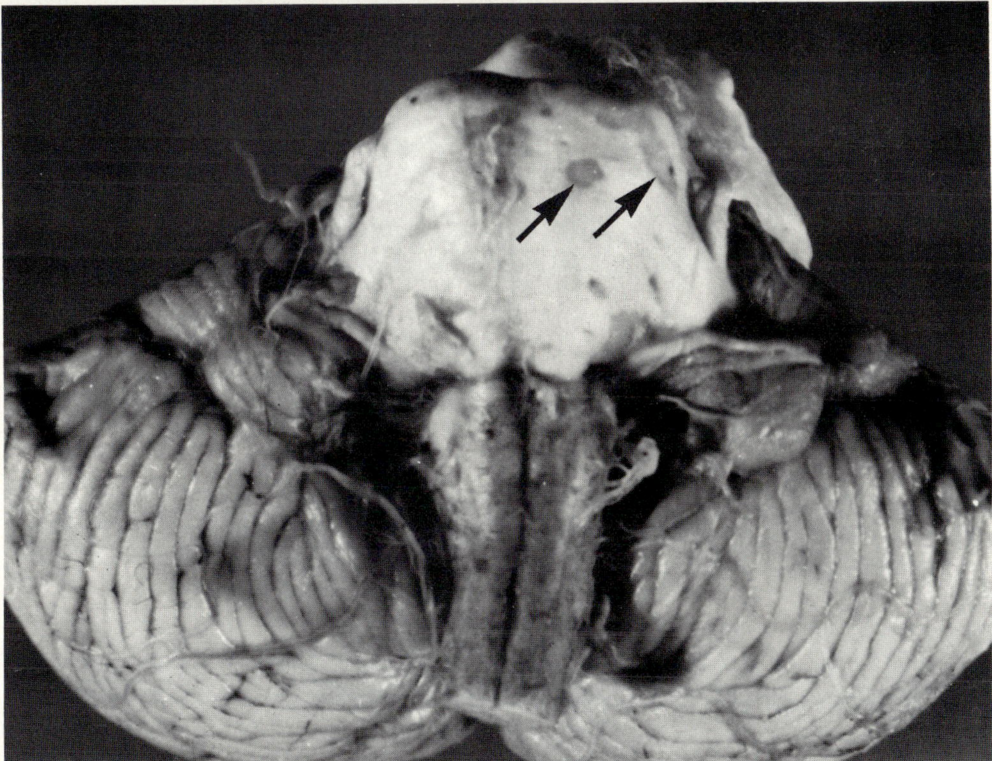

B

Fig. 72 The cerebrum and brain stem in multiple sclerosis (arrows indicate demyelinated plaques).

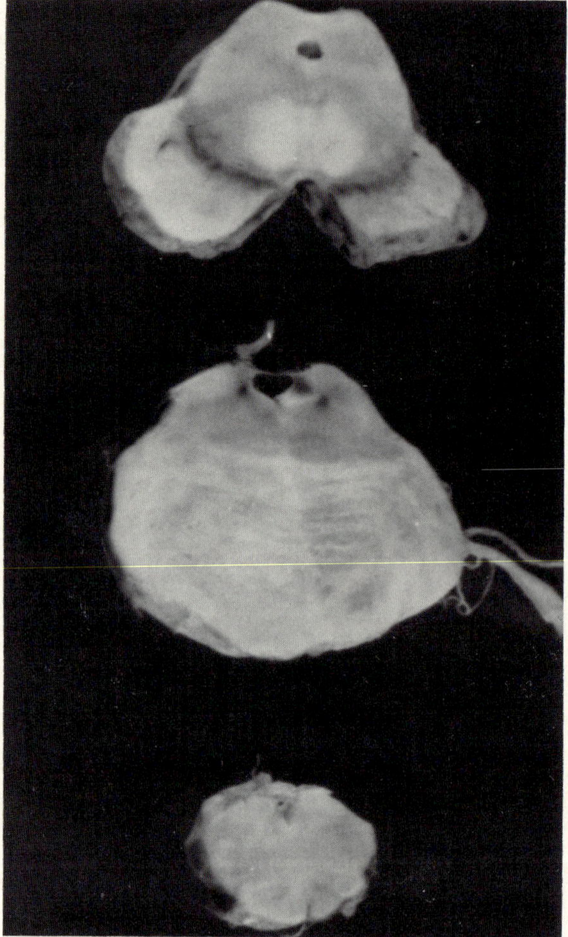

Fig. 73 Secondary, unilateral, descending degeneration of the pyramidal tract.

BRAIN CUTTING

Section Techniques

Coronal Sections

Coronal sections are the traditional sections studied in gross neuropathology. As a first step the brain stem and cerebellum are removed at the level of the midbrain and reserved for separate study. The brain is then placed on a cutting board with the base uppermost. It is steadied with one hand while the sections are made with a single, smooth cut of a well sharpened, long knife.

The cut must be continuous and must sever the section completely. For this reason a soft, cork or wood cutting surface is used. The cut is started from the basal aspect of the brain in order to be able to accurately place the knife with respect to the significant areas of the brain.

Section thickness may vary but, in general, we cut sections about one centimeter thick. When the brain is friable or is a "respirator brain" the section thickness is increased. The number of sections taken and the areas selected depend on the suspected findings. The following will describe the minimum number of sections we take, their levels, and the view offered by them (Figs. 74, 74-1, 74-2).

Sectioning is begun from the frontal lobes. Slice 1 of Fig. 74 is at the level of the temporal pole. This permits the maintenance of symmetry in the section and includes the tips of the anterior horns (Fig. 74-1). If the ventricles are visible in this section it is a sign of ventricular dilation.

The second level illustrated is through the anterior portion of the optic chiasm (2 of Fig. 74). This level reveals two additional commissure fibers, the corpus callosum and the anterior commissure (2 of Fig. 74-1).

The third slice is at the level of the mammillary body (3 of Fig. 74). This affords a good view of the mammillary body, globus pallidus and other basal ganglia (3 of Fig. 74-2).

The fourth cut illustrated in Fig. 74 is through the midbrain at the posterior ends of the substantia nigra. This section reveals a view of the lateral geniculate bodies and is ideal for removing specimens of Ammon's horn (4 of Fig. 74-2).

The fifth cut shown in Fig. 74 is in the occipital lobe and reveals the visual cortex including the posterior horns (5 of Fig. 74-2).

The cut surface of the separated brain stem, at the level of the midbrain, is examined before sectioning. This surface reveals the aqueduct and the substantia nigra among other structures (Fig. 75). The shape and size of the aqueduct is examined for evidence of stenosis or dilation. Stenosis of the aqueduct may be one of the causes of hydrocephalus. In the normal adult the substantia nigra is deeply pigmented. Depigmentation is a sign of the atrophy which usually accompanies parkinsonism. On the other hand, it should be remembered that the substantia nigra is not well pigmented in children and even in some adolescents. Furthermore, an asymmetric section may sometimes give the impression of unilateral depigmentation, erroneously suggesting hemiparkinsonism. The latter condition does, of course, occur and in those cases the clinical symptoms are always on the side opposite the lesion.

The separated brain stem is cut transversely along the long axis resulting in sections parallel to the mid brain. These are cut at about 7 millimeters thickness due to the greater number of small, significant structures.

Section Correlation with CT Scan Levels

In recent years the computerized tomography (CT) scanner has come to play an even more important role in diagnostic neuroradiology. It has therefore become necessary to devise a method by which the views offered by the scanner can be directly compared to sections of the brain. The following is a method currently being developed in our laboratory (Matsui and Hirano, 1978).

In conventional neuroradiology the x-rays are taken with reference to either the canthomeatal line (a line between the angle of the eye and the external auditory meatus) or to Reid's base line (a line from the inferior edge of the orbit through

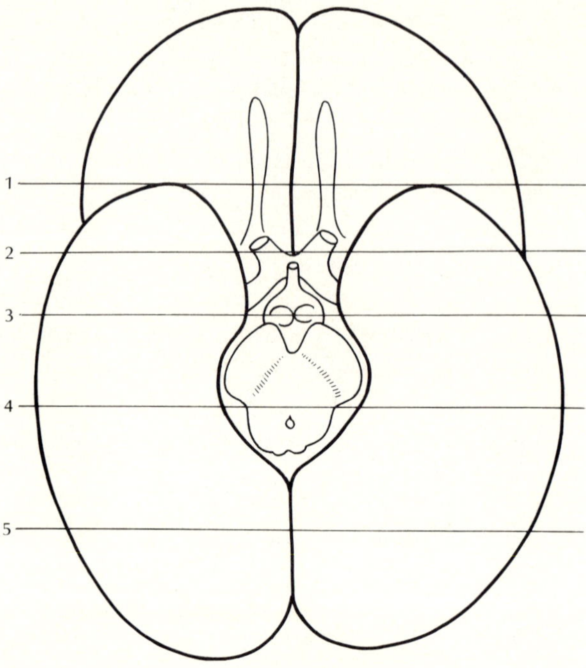

Fig. 74 Levels of coronal sections of the brain illustrated in Figs. 74-1 and 74-2.

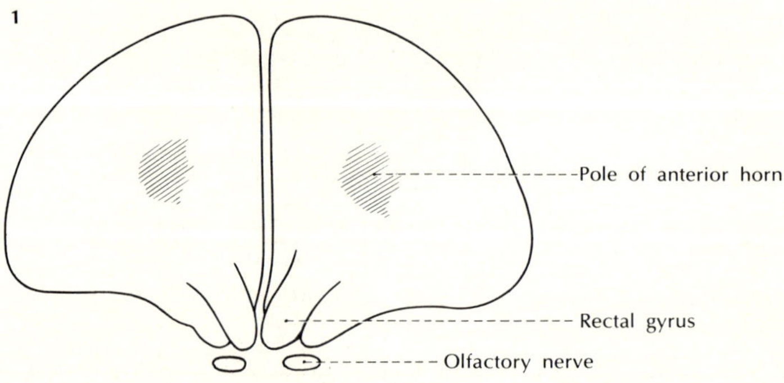

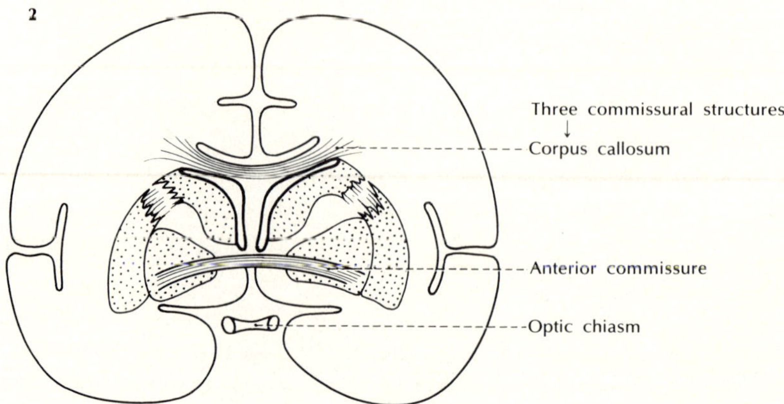

Fig. 74-1 Coronal sections of the brain (levels 1 and 2).

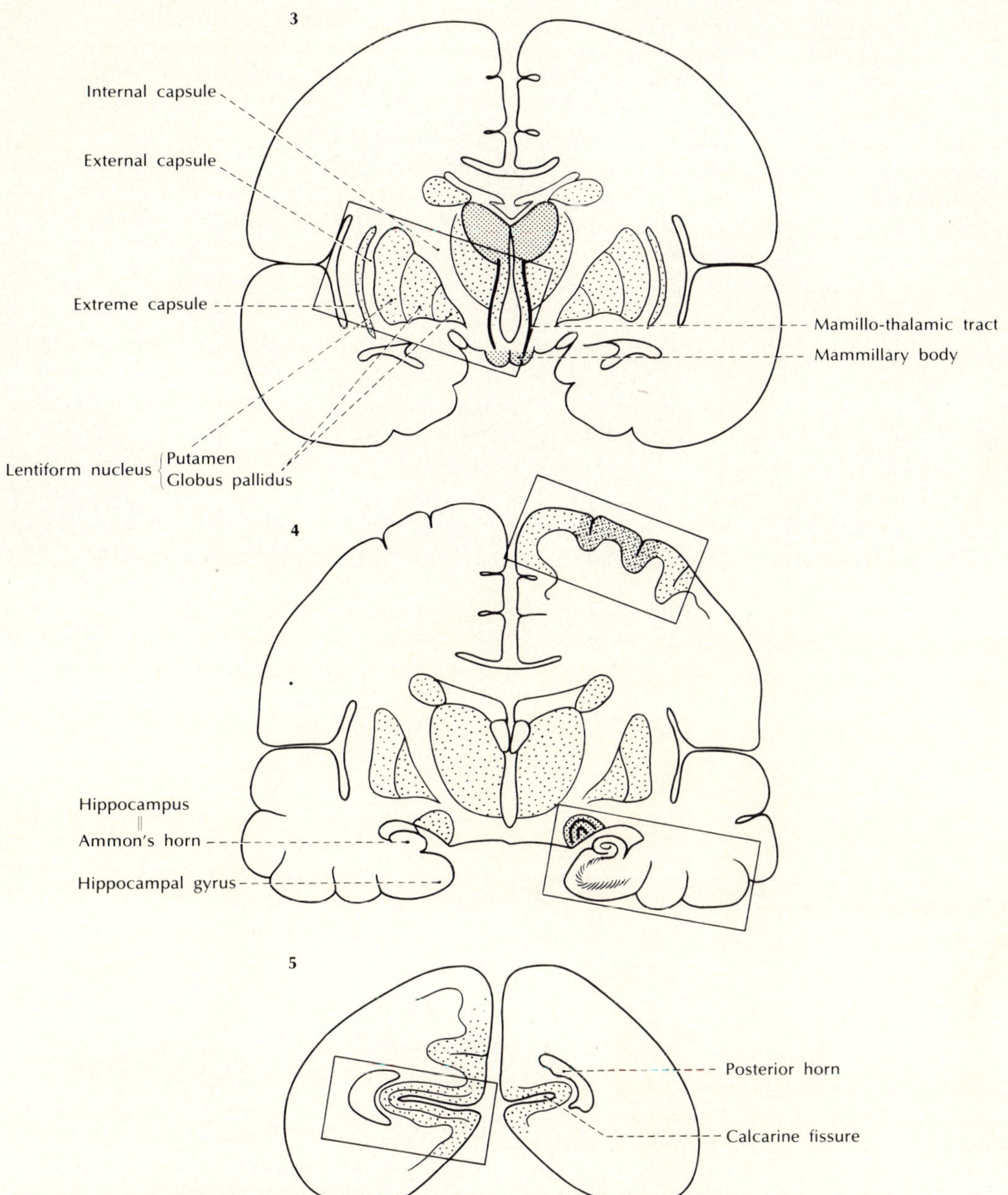

Fig. 74-2 Coronal sections of the brain (levels 3-5).

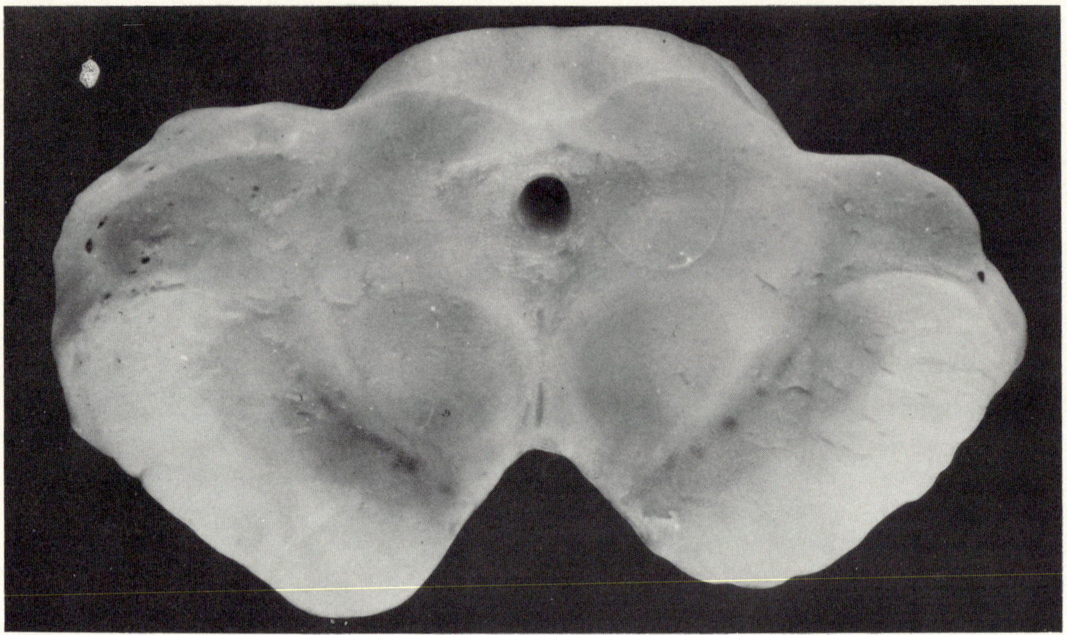

Fig. 75 Midbrain in Parkinsonism.

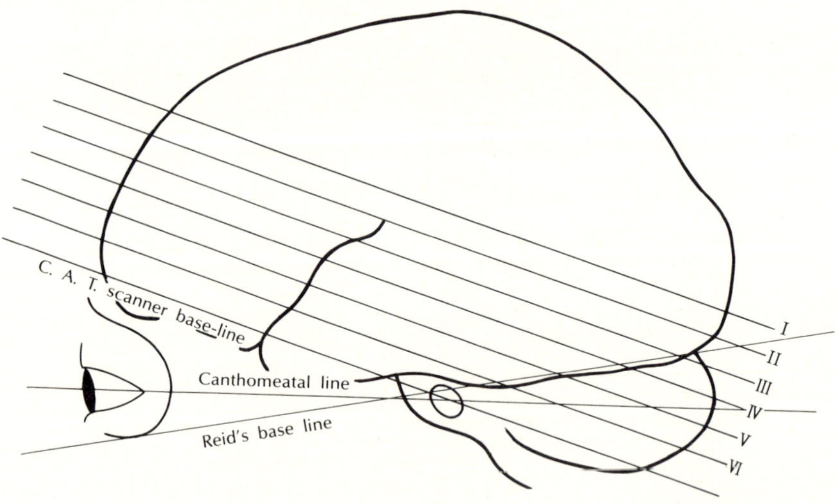

Fig. 76 Computerized tomography scanner levels through the brain, illustrated in Figs. 76-1 through 76-6.

the upper edge of the external auditory meatus). The angle used in CT scanning differs among neuroradiology laboratories. Presently, at Montefiore, an angle 15° from the canthomeatal line is used (Fig. 76). We, therefore, cut sections at about the same angle. This angle corresponds to a line between the preoccipital notch and a point along the pre-central gyrus seven millimeters above the Sylvian fissure.

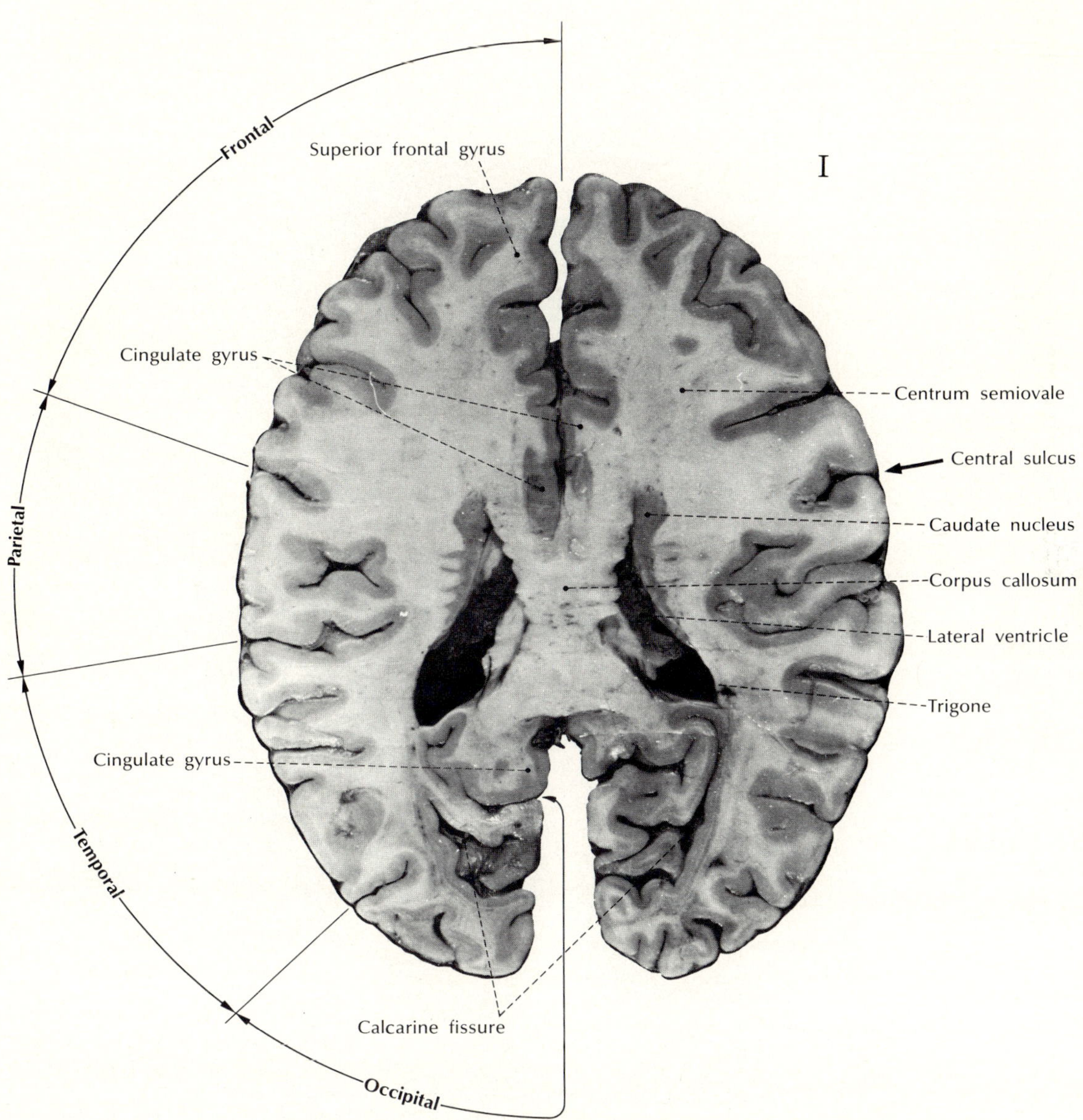

Fig. 76-1 Section of the brain corresponding to level I in Fig. 76.

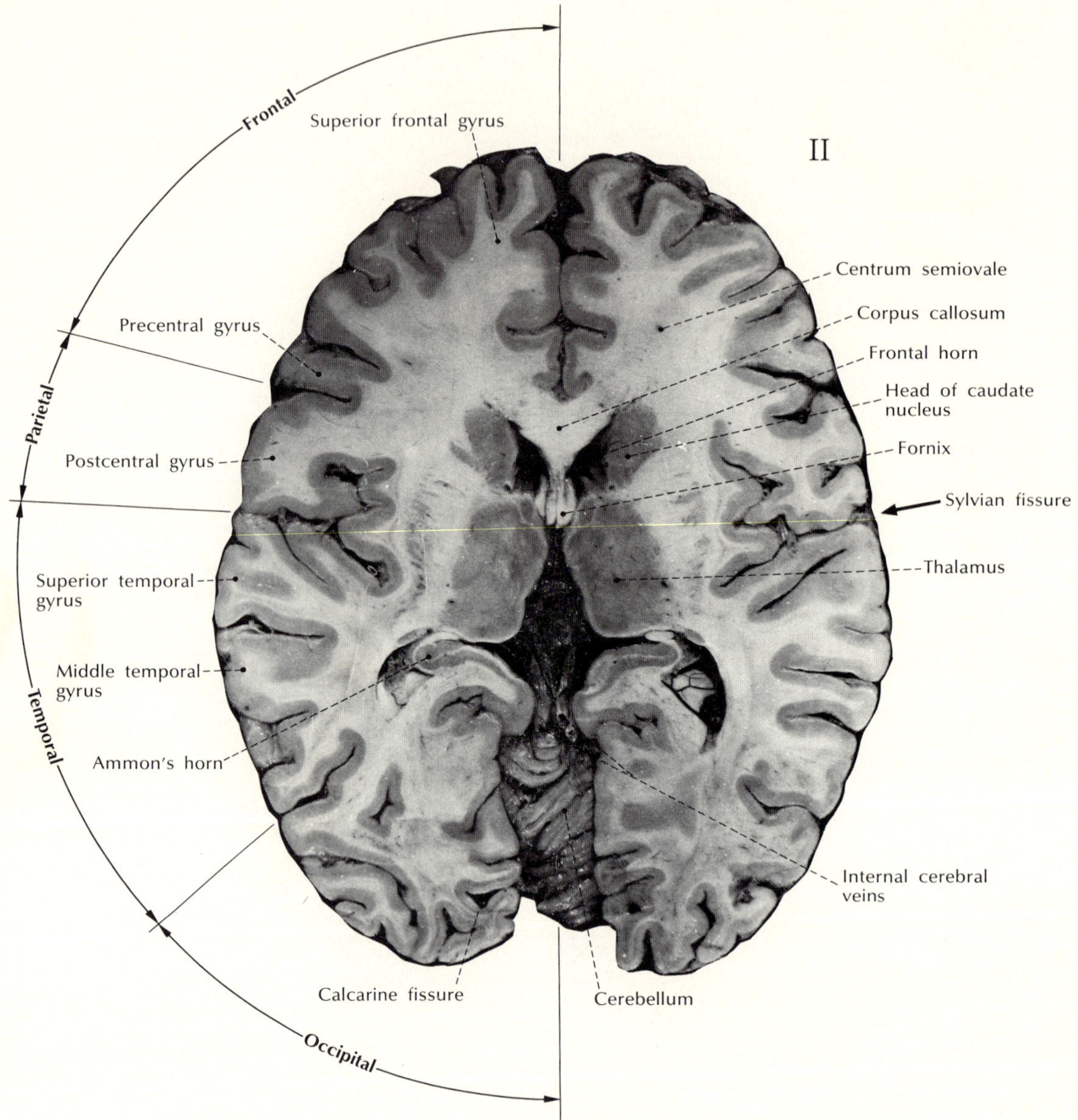

Fig. 76-2 Section of the brain corresponding to level II in Fig. 76.

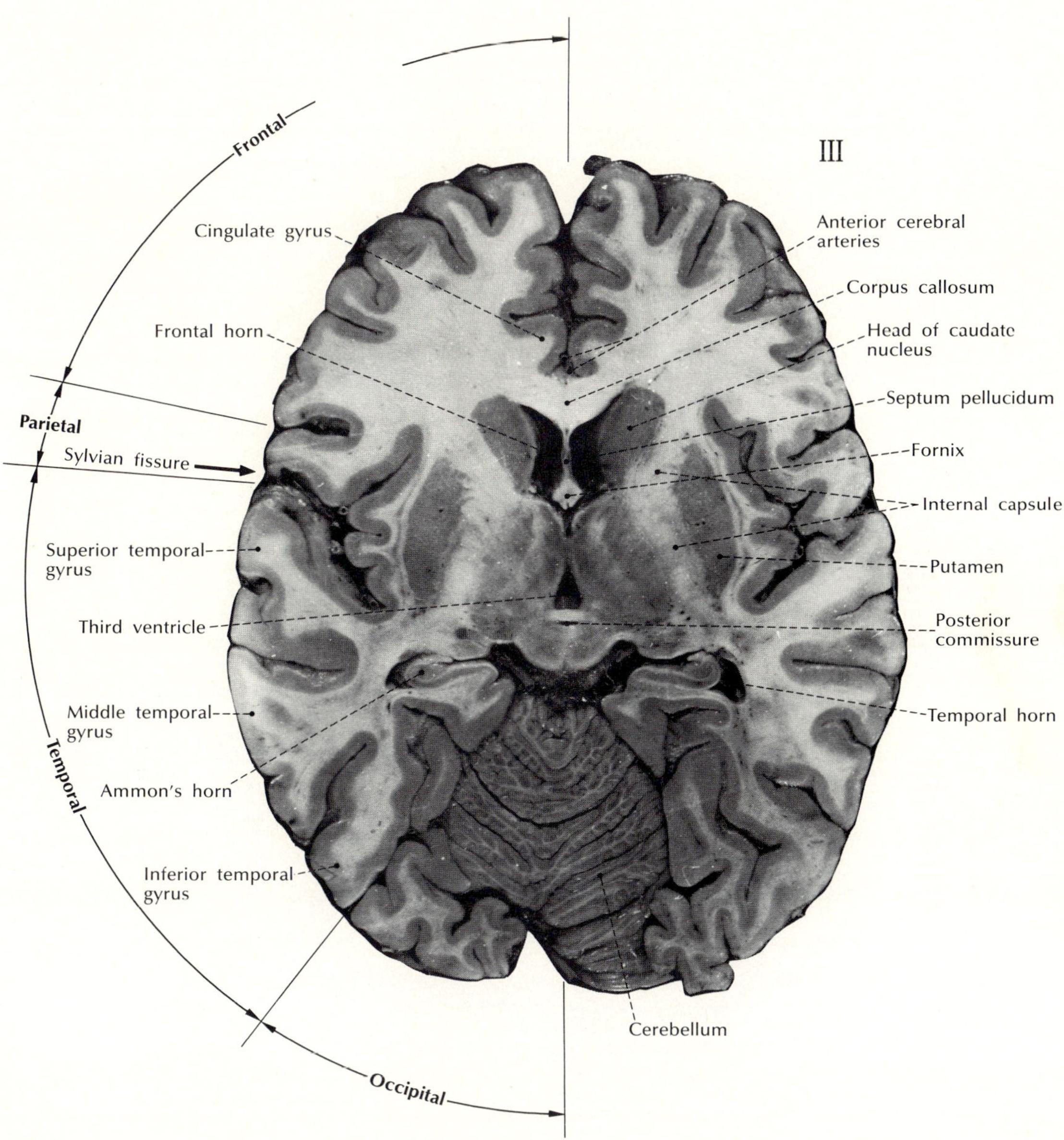

Fig. 76-3 Section of the brain corresponding to level III in Fig. 76.

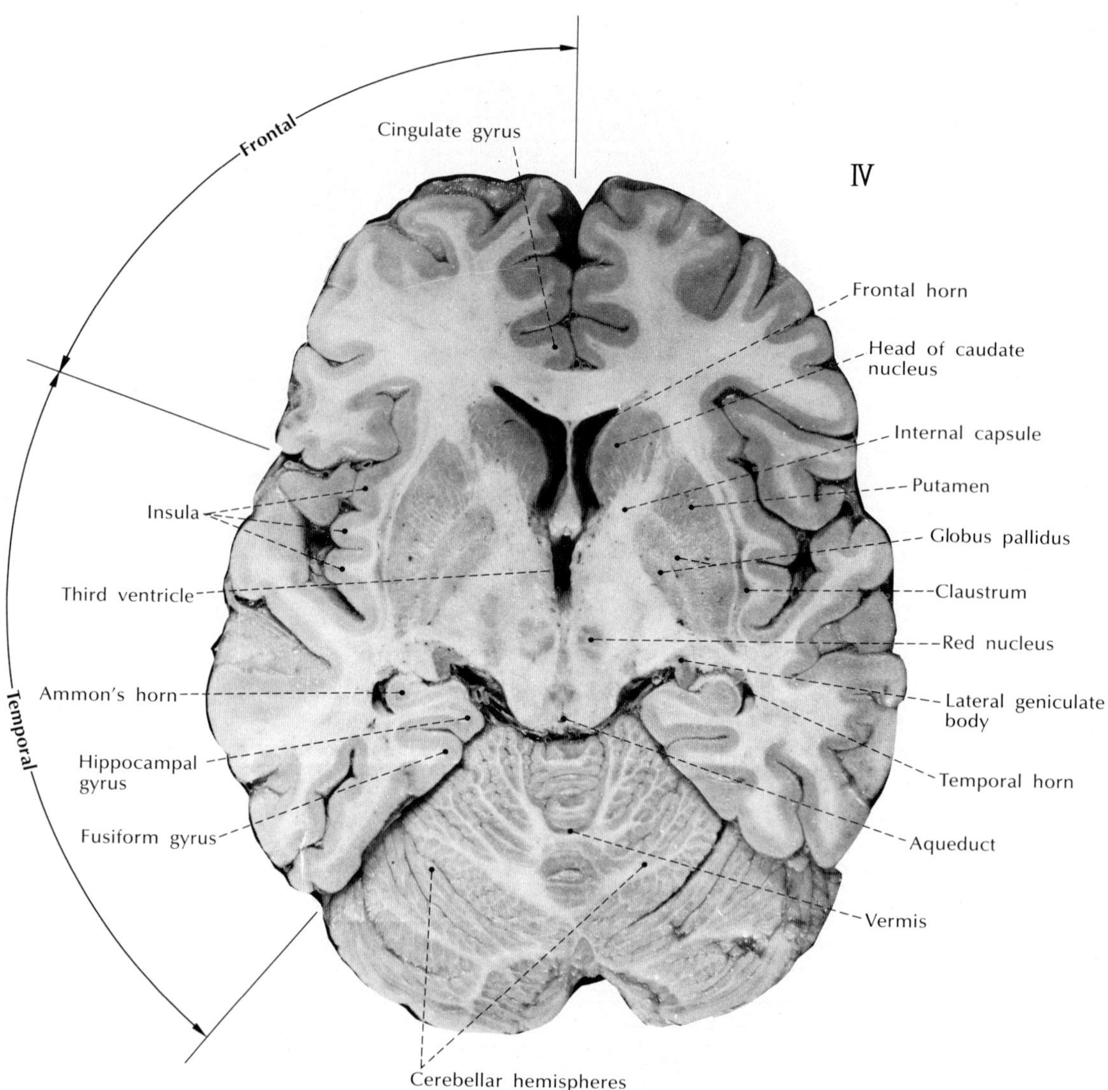

Fig. 76-4 Section of the brain corresponding to level IV in Fig. 76.

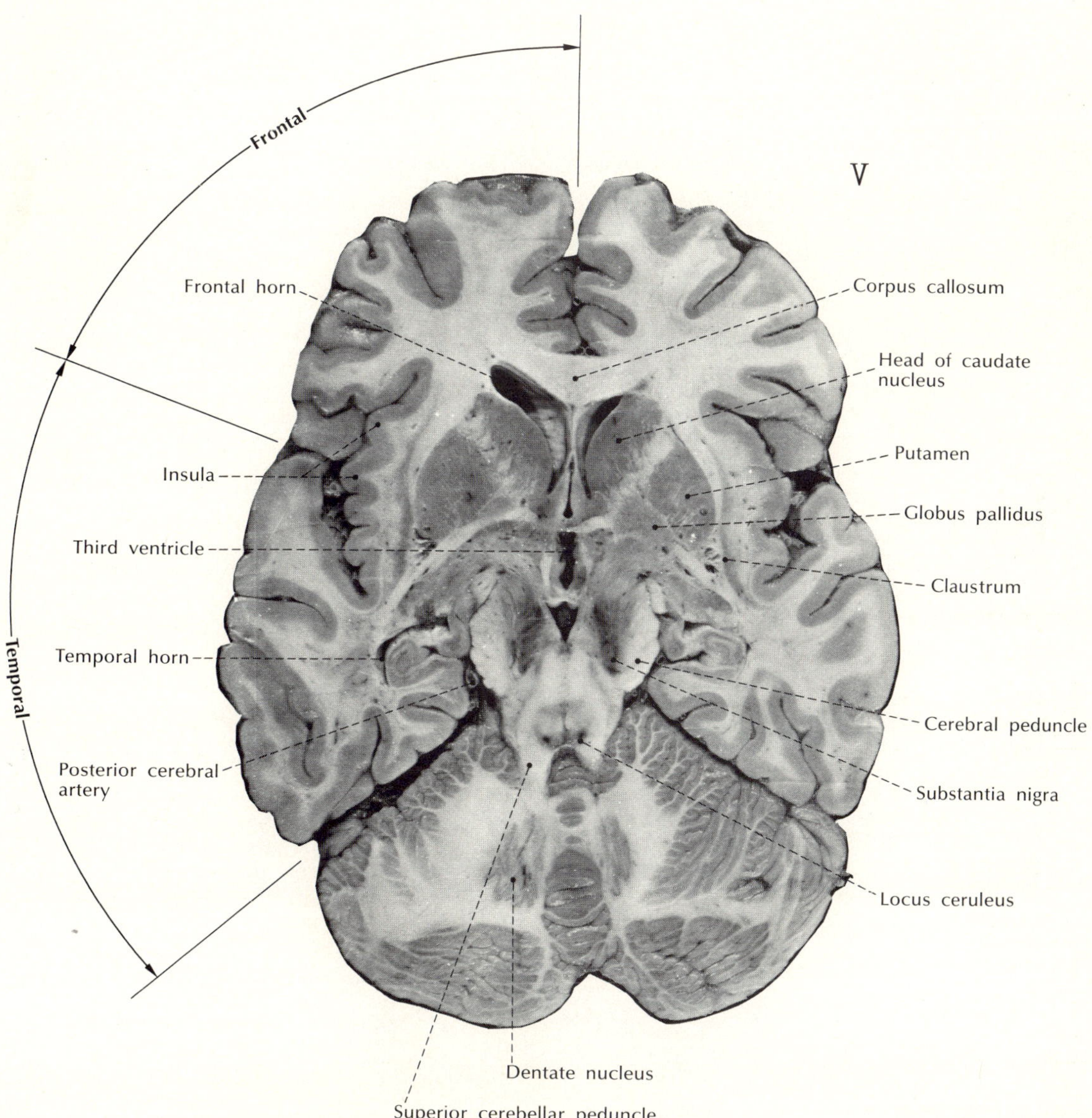

Fig. 76-5 Section of the brain corresponding to level V in Fig. 76.

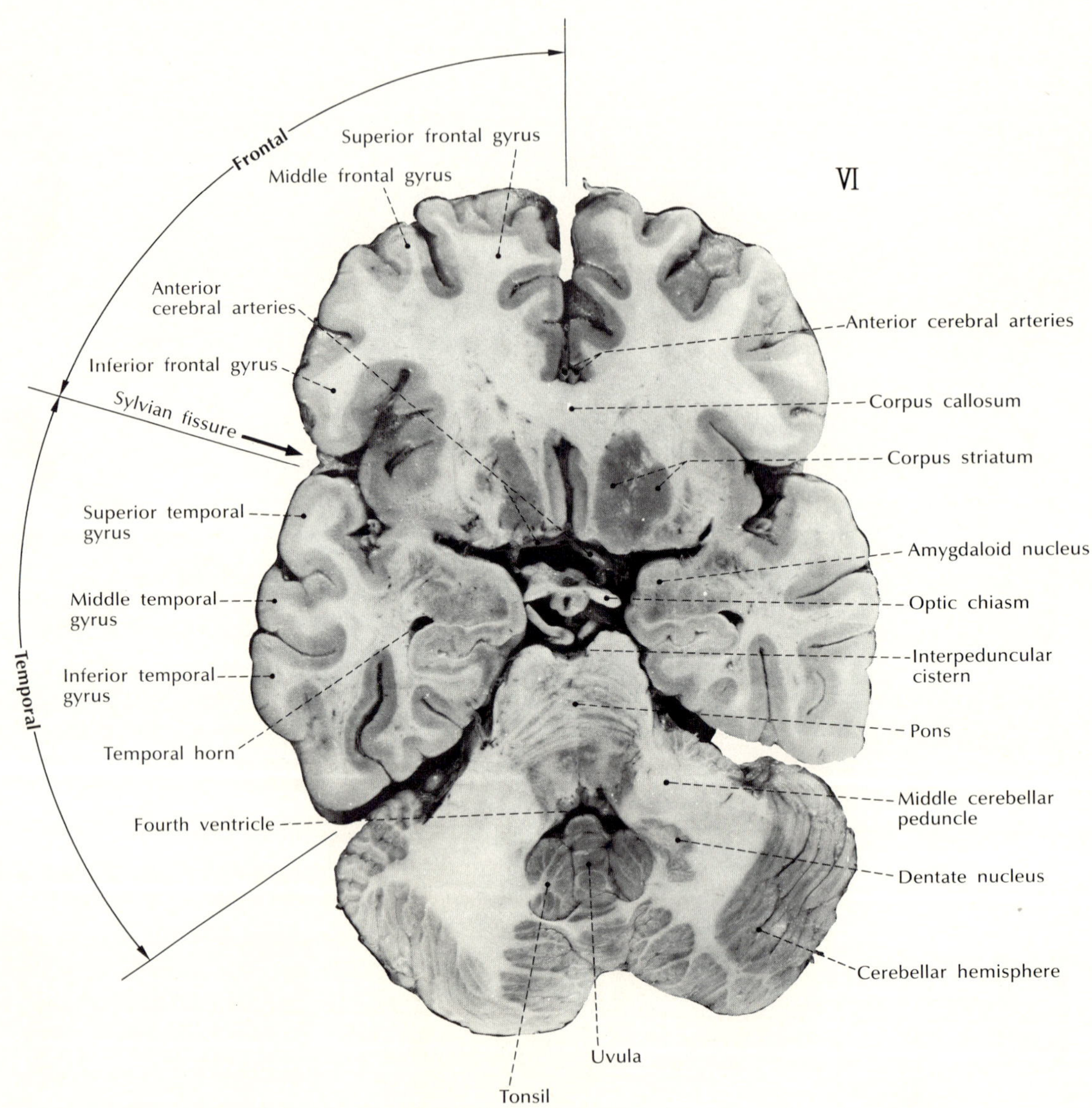

Fig. 76-6 Section of the brain corresponding to level VI in Fig. 76.

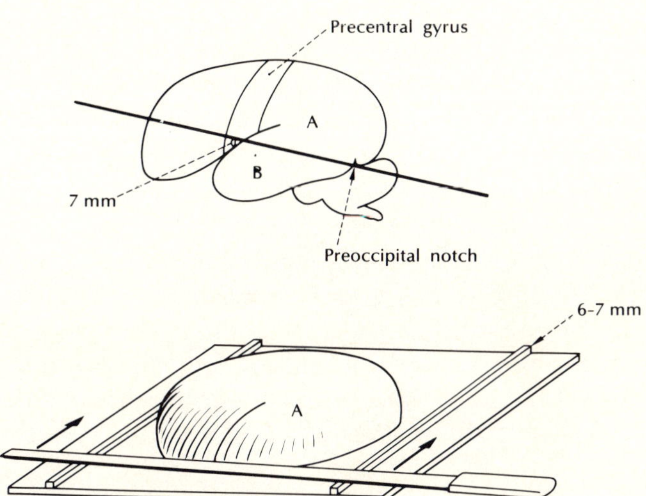

Fig. 77 A method to produce sections of the brain parallel to the CAT scanner base line (15° from the canthomeatal line).

This is the first cut we make which separates the brain into an upper, A, and lower, B portion (Fig. 77). Each portion is then placed on a device such as that pictured in Fig. 77, cut surface down, and sliced with the aid of two, 7 millimeter thick spacers, which roughly correspond to the thickness of the section of the CT scanner.

The six most important sections obtained in this manner are illustrated in Figs. 76-1 through 76-6.

Section I (Fig. 76-1) reveals the body of the corpus callosum and the upper edge of the caudate nucleus. In Section II (Fig. 76-2) we obtain the most useful view of the thalamus. Section III (Fig. 76-3) is useful for examining the internal capsule and its relationship to the basal ganglia, especially the putamen. This is also the level of the foramen of Monro and the superior colliculus. In Section IV (Fig. 76-4) we obtain further views of the basal ganglia, especially the globus pallidus. The occipital lobe is no longer seen at this level. Instead, the cerebellum becomes more prominent. The lateral geniculate body, red nucleus and aqueduct are also visible. Section V (Fig. 76-5) affords a view of the anterior commissure and the cerebellar peduncle. Both the substantia nigra and the locus ceruleus are identifiable at this level. In Section VI (Fig. 76-6) we see the optic chiasm, the circle of Willis, the amygdaloid nucleus as well as the cerebellum and pons.

REFERENCES

Matsui, T., Kawamoto, K., Iwata, M., Kurent, J.E., Imai, T., Ohsugi, T., & Hirano, A.: Anatomical and pathological study of the brain by CT scanner. 1. Anatomical study of normal brain. Computerized Tomography, Pergamon Press, 1: 1-44, 1977.

Matsui, T., & Hirano, , A.: An Atlas of the Human Brain for Computerized Tomography, pp. 1-570, Igaku-Shoin, Tokyo-New York, 1978.

Diffuse Alterations

Upon finding alterations at the cut surface of a section through the brain one must always be aware of the serious possibility of artifact. Artifactitous changes can be traced to two major sources. First, when the infolded surfaces of the cerebral hemispheres are cut the apparent relative thickness of the gray and white matter will vary depending upon the angle between the knife and the brain surface. Thus, before one can conclude that one portion or another is relatively thin one must be aware of the precise plane of the section. In addition, white matter bundles cut longitudinally always appear whiter than the same structures cut in cross section. Such effects are easily seen in coronal sections of the optic radiation which appear grayer than the surrounding white matter. Similar results are also seen when the pons is cut transversely and the pyramidal tracts appear darker. More subtle artifactitous changes can occur because of a dull knife causing smudging of the surface of the section which can mimic certain real pathologic changes.

The second source of artifact, and one which is commonly encountered, is the result of improper fixation. While preservation is improved by perfusion one can often find areas of poor preservation even under these best of circumstances. In general, the poorer preservation is found in those areas less exposed to the fixative, mainly the interior, especially the white matter in the cerebrum and the deeper layers of the cerebellar folia. The oligodendroglia of the white matter are apparently particularly sensitive to poor preservation and undergo rapid autolysis resulting in characteristic artifactitous halo-like configurations around the nucleus. In the cerebellum the granule cell layer can appear spongy and "washed out" (Fig. 78) (Ikuta et al. 1963). These autolytic changes are especially pronounced if there is excessive delay of the autopsy and are even more common in the summer months or in tropical areas, or if the patient died with high fever and/or infection.

Atrophy of the gray matter is probably the most well-known of the authentic diffuse changes seen in sections of the cerebral cortex. It is seen in presenile and senile dementia. Laminar necrosis, due to hypoxia is another common pathologic finding and is the result of differential sensitivities of the various layers of the cortex to lack of oxygen. Anoxic changes can also be seen in the border areas of major vessels or along the distribution of an occluded major artery.

Diffuse white matter changes are also well known. These include edema which causes an increase in the relative thickness of the white matter and demyelination which ultimately has the opposite effect. Diffuse demyelination is often a genetic defect as in Krabbe's disease or metachromatic leukodystrophy and others (Appendix III). Some interesting aspects of diffuse demyelination include the preservation of the so-called "U" fibers. These are the layers of myelinated fibers surrounding the bottom of the sulci that somehow avoid the demyelinating process going on around them. This effect can be seen in various conditions including demyelination resulting from long-standing edema as well as primary dysmyelination.

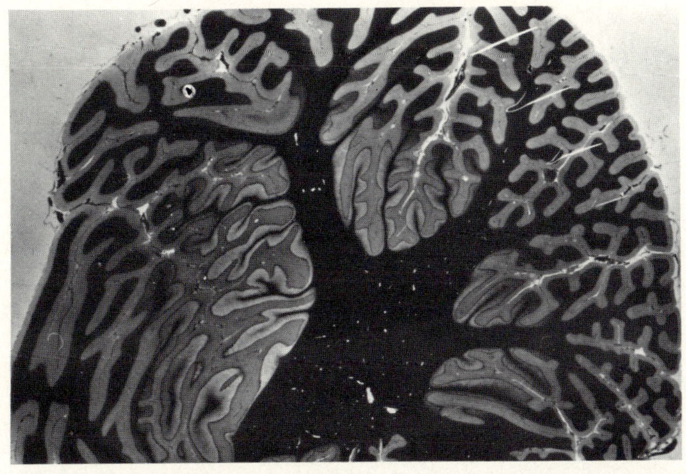

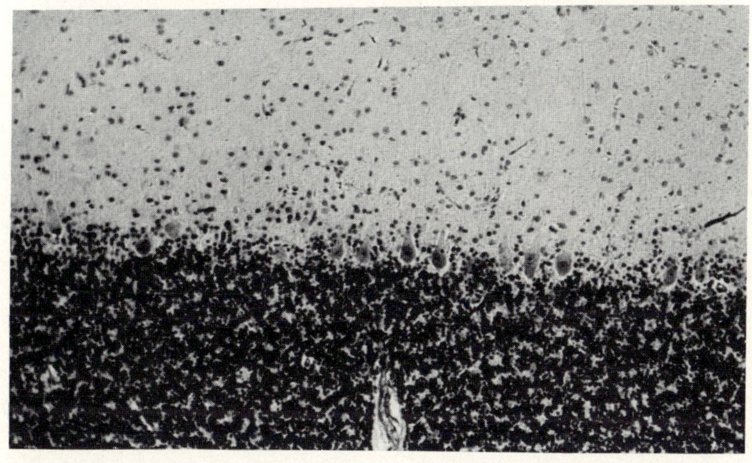

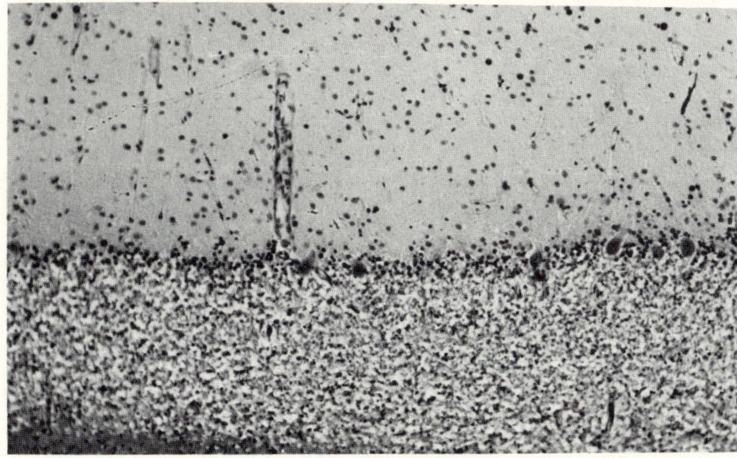

Fig. 78 A. Autolysis of granule cells in the cerebellum.
B. Intact superficial portion of the cortex.
C. Altered deeper portion of the cortex.

Hydrocephalus is easily visualized in sections. This alteration can usually be related to some change in the ventricular system and/or related structures (Figs. 79—81).

REFERENCE

Ikuta, F., Hirano, A., & Zimmerman, H.M.: An experimental study of postmortem alterations in the granular layer of the cerebellar cortex. J. Neuropathol. Exp. Neurol., 22: 581-593, 1963.

Appendix III. Dysmyelinating Disease (Leukodystrophy).

These rare conditions are the result of the failure of the proper developmental processes in the formation of myelin. In gross examination of sections they appear as a severe atrophy of the white matter and are usually observed in infants and children. Most often the lesion is genetic in origin.

The precise nature of the lesion depends on the specific developmental defect. Differentiation between the various conditions requires special studies utilizing both histological and biochemical techniques.

A. *Metachromatic leukodystrophy*. Due to defective arylsulfatase activity, excessive accumulations of sulfatides, which stain metachromatically, are found throughout the central and peripheral nervous systems.

Austin, J.H., Armstrong, D., & Shearer, L.: Metachromatic form of diffuse cerebral sclerosis. V. The nature and significance of low sulfatase activity: A controlled study of brain, liver and kidney in four patients with metachromatic leukodystrophy (MLD). Arch. Neurol., 13: 593-614, 1965.

Gregoire, A., Perier, O., & Dustin, P. Jr.: Metachromatic leukodystrophy, an electron microscopic study. J. Neuropathol. Exp. Neurol., 25: 617-636, 1966.

B. *Krabbe's globoid cell leukodystrophy*. Due to defective galactocerebroside β-galactosidase activity, excessive accumulations of galactocerebroside are found in globoid-appearing cells in the white matter.

Yunis, E., & Lee, R.E.: The ultrastructure of globoid (Krabbe) leukodystrophy. Lab. Invest., 21: 415-419, 1969.

Suzuki, K., & Suzuki, Y.: Globoid cell leukodystrophy (Krabbe's disease): Deficiency of galactocerebroside β-galactosidase. Proc. Nat. Acad. Sci. U.S.A., 66: 302-309, 1970.

Suzuki, K., & Grover, W.D.: Krabbe's leukodystrophy (globoid cell leukodystrophy). An ultrastructural study. Lab. Invest., 22: 385-396, 1970.

C. *Alexander's Disease*. The white matter is replaced by astrocytes which contain abnormal accumulations of strongly eosinophilic, thick bundles of altered glial fibrils (Rosenthal fibers). Unlike other leukodystrophies, this disease is usually sporadic rather than familial.

Herndon, R.M., Rubinstein, L.J., Freeman, J.M., & Mathieson, G.: Light and electron microscopic observation on Rosenthal fibers in Alexander's disease and in multiple sclerosis. J. Neuropathol. Exp. Neurol., 29: 524-551, 1970.

D. *Canavan's Disease*. Extensive vacuolar spaces are ubiquitous throughout the white matter resulting in a so-called "spongy" appearance.

Adachi, M., Wallace, B.J., Schneck, L., & Volk, B.W.: Fine structure of spongy degeneration of the central nervous system (van Bogaert and Bertrand type). J. Neuropathol. Exp. Neurol., 25: 598-616, 1966.

E. *Sudanophilic leukodystrophy*. Due to some unknown etiology, sudanophilic granules are found in cells in the white matter.

Watanabe, I., Patel, V., Gobel, H.H., Siakotos, A.N., Zeman, W., DeMyer, W., & Dyer, J.S.: Early lesion of Pelizaeus-Merzbacher disease: Electron microscopic and

biochemical study. J. Neuropathol. Exp. Neurol., 32: 313-333, 1973.
Schaumburg, H.H., Powers, J.M., Raine, C.S., Suzuki, K., & Richardson, E.P., Jr.: Adrenoleukodystrophy. A clinical and pathological study of 17 cases. Arch. Neurol., 32: 577-591, 1975.

F. *Lipidoses of the CNS.* Abnormal accumulations of various lipids are found within the neurons often accompanied by white matter alterations.

G. *Dysmyelination in experimental animals.* Severe paucity of central myelin is found in the murine mutants "jimpy" and "quaking."

Sidman, R.L., Dickie, M.M., & Appel, S.H.: Mutant mice (quaking and jimpy) with deficient myelination in central nervous system. Science, 144: 309-311, 1964.
Hirano, A., Sax, D.S., & Zimmerman, H.M.: The fine structure of the cerebella of jimpy mice and their "normal" litter mates. J. Neuropath. Exp. Neurol., 28: 388-400, 1969.
Berger, B.: Quelques aspects ultrastructuraux de la substance blanche chez la souris quaking. Brain Res., 25: 35-53, 1971.

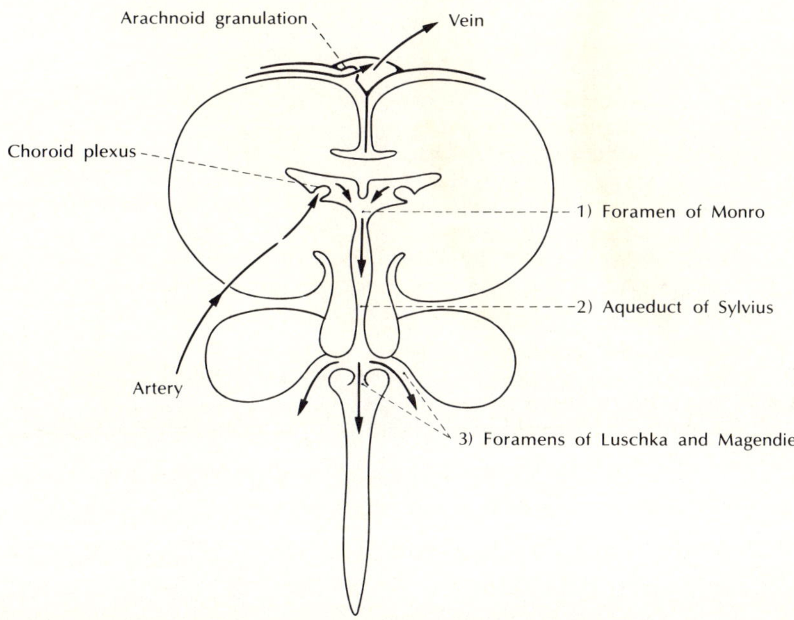

Fig. 79 Hydrocephalus.

Hydrocephalus may be of either the non-obstructive or the obstructive variety. The former, less common type, is the result of either an overproduction of cerebrospinal fluid as in choroid plexus papilloma or a defect in the absorption of cerebrospinal fluid such as may result from damage to the arachnoid granulations, meningitis, subarachnoid hemorrhage or subdural hematoma. Obstructive hydrocephalus is much more common. This condition is the result of interference with the normal pathways of flow of the cerebrospinal fluid. Obstruction of the foramen of Monro due to a tumor in this area such as a colloid cyst of the third ventricle or a glioma may result in obstructive hydrocephalus. The third ventricle may be compressed due to a large tumor in that vicinity such as a thalamic glioma or the upward extension of suprasellar masses. Stenosis of the aqueduct of Sylvius may also result in hydrocephalus as described in the legends to Figures 80 and 81. Obstruction of the foramens of Luschka and Magendie may result from chronic basal meningitis or tumor infiltration in the area of the fourth ventricle or the cerebellar pontine angle.

So-called "hydrocephalus ex vacuo" is, in reality, an abnormal enlargement of the ventricles due to generalized atrophy of the brain parenchyma.

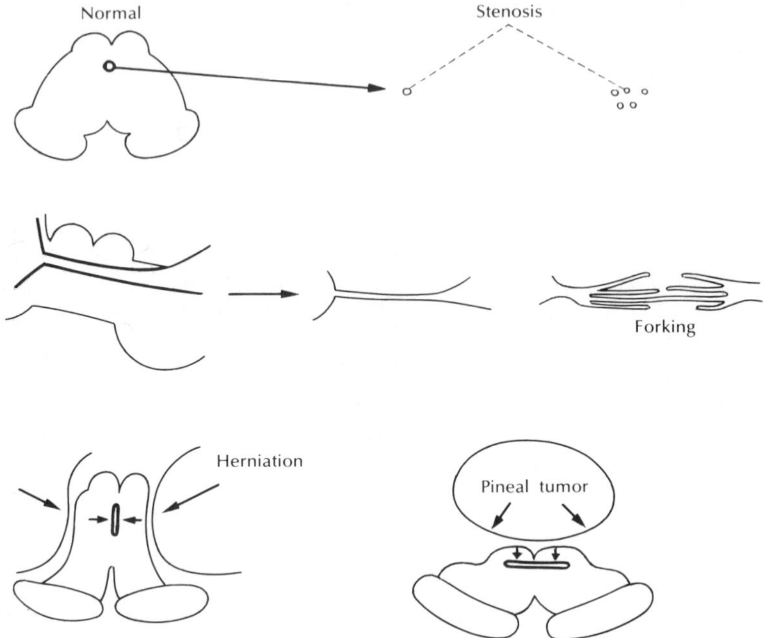

Fig. 80 Stenosis of aqueduct.

The aqueduct of Sylvius is the narrowest portion of the cerebrospinal fluid pathway. Obstruction of this structure results in hydrocephalus above the third ventricle. Stenosis may result in either a single very narrow canal or, because of "forking" several small canals may be visible on section. Compression of the midbrain may narrow and distort the shape of the canal. Pressure exerted from both sides due to transtentorial herniation causes a characteristic shape change as does pressure from above which might result from a mass lesion in the pineal region.

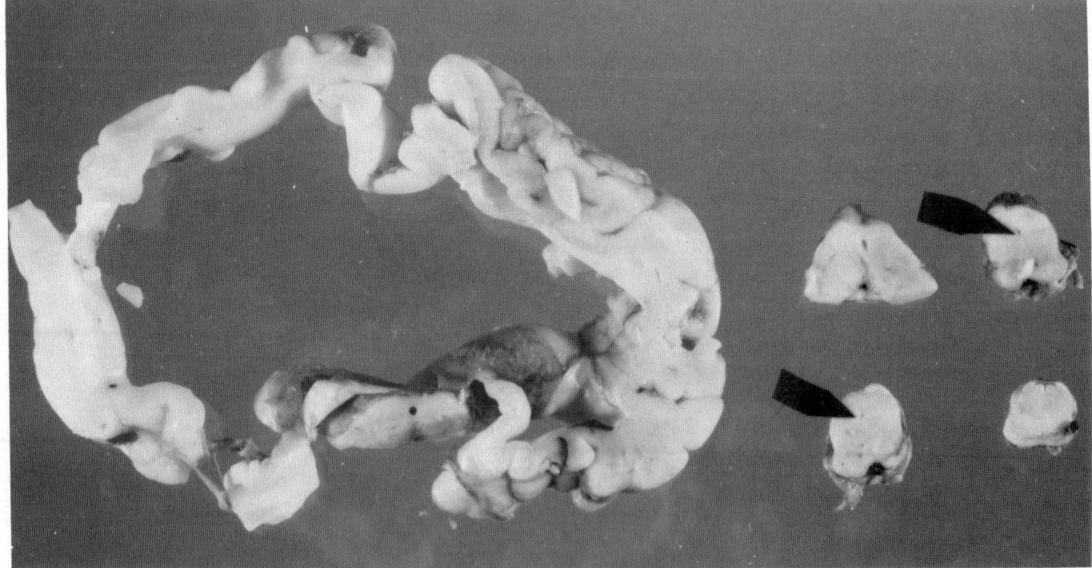

Fig. 81 Stenosis of aqueduct.

A dilated lateral ventricle and pinpoint narrowing of the aqueduct.

Focal Alterations

Focal alterations can be conveniently divided into two types. The first are the systemic changes which affect particular nuclei and tracts bilaterally. For example, in *Huntington's chorea* the putamen and caudate nucleus are severely atrophic leading to the characteristic macroscopic configurations including an enlarged ventricle (Fig. 82). Parkinsonism, parkinsonism-dementia complex on Guam, striatonigral degeneration, Hallervorden-Spatz disease, Wilson's disease, among many others, are good examples of systemic lesions involving the substantia nigra and/or the *basal ganglia* (Fig. 83). Two other conditions affecting the basal ganglia as well as certain other areas are Fahr's disease in which there is pronounced calcification in the globus pallidus and other areas and kernicterus which is seen in newborns and is characterized by a yellow discoloration of certain nuclei.

Sections of the brain of patients with *Wernicke's syndrome* and *Korsakoff's psychosis* reveal changes in various areas in addition to the mammillary bodies which were apparent from external examination. These areas are often hemorrhagic and, therefore, easily visualized (Fig. 84). In Pick's disease sections reveal that the lobar atrophy involves the underlying white matter as well as the gray matter which was apparent from external examination.

Generalized cerebellar atrophy may be seen in various degenerative conditions. Section allows one to determine the precise topography of the involvement. Predominant involvement of the anterior portion of the vermis, for example, is a characteristic feature in certain conditions such as chronic alcoholism. On the other hand, it is important to note that a similar macroscopic configuration is found in most elderly people, although usually to a lesser degree (Fig. 85).

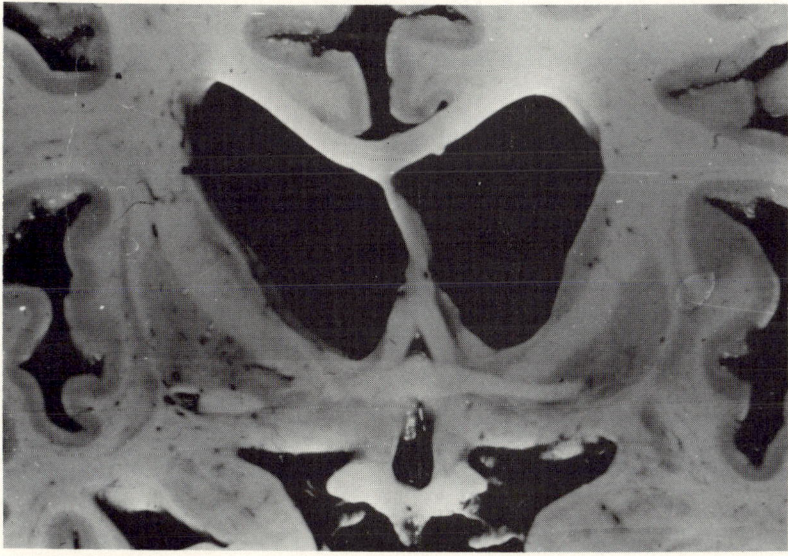

Fig. 82 Huntington's chorea.
Severe atrophy of the caudate nuclei and cerebral cortex associated with dilated ventricles.

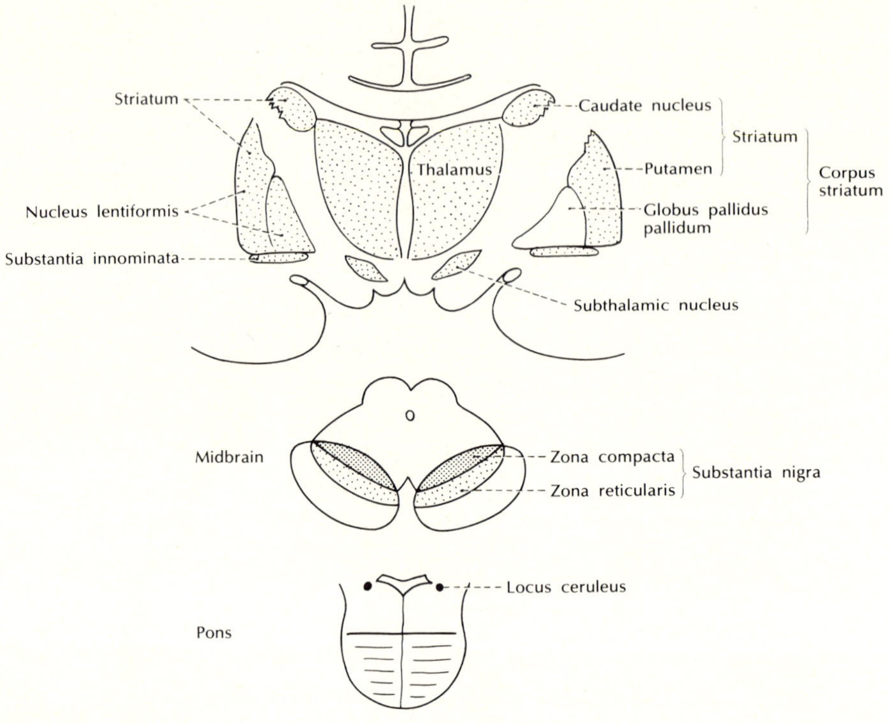

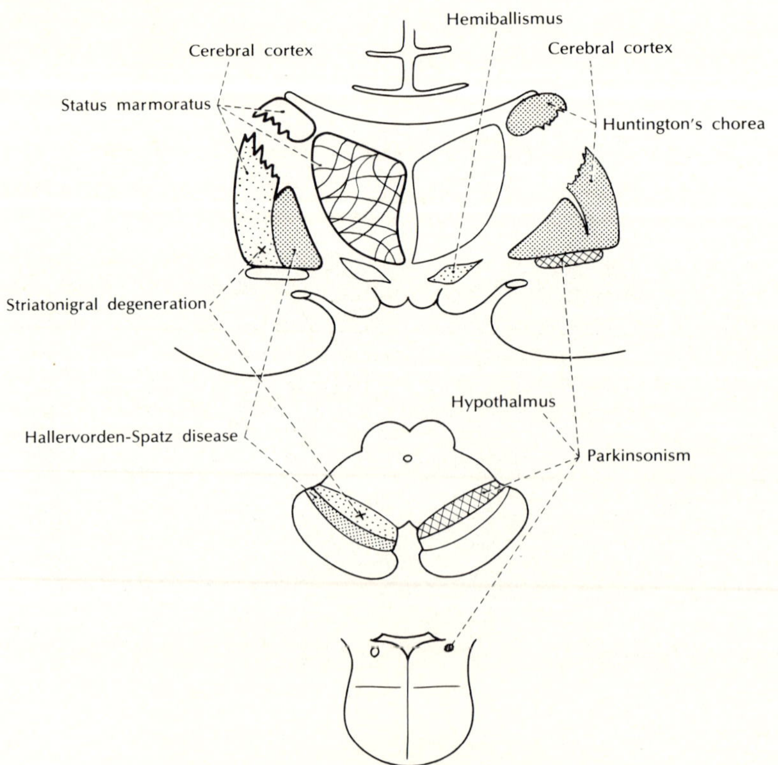

Fig. 83 Diseases affecting basal ganglia.

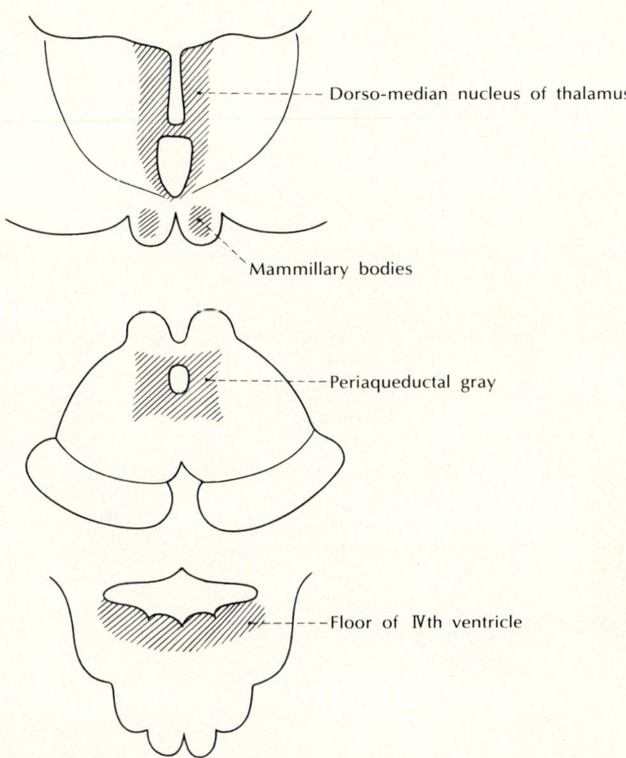

Fig. 84 Topographic distribution of lesions seen in Wernicke's syndrome and in Korsakoff's psychosis.

The second group of focal lesions are more haphazard in their distribution although a certain pattern of predilection can sometimes be detected. These include *infarcts* (Figs. 57-63), *hemorrhages* (Figs. 86, 87), *primary and metastatic neoplasms* (Figs. 88—99), abscesses, traumatic injuries, among many others. Often these lesions are well demarcated and circumscribed such as chronic abscesses or most metastatic tumors. In other cases, however, such as gliomas or certain lymphomas the borders are indistinct and seemingly normal tissue some distance from the apparent edge of the lesion can often be shown to contain infiltrating tumor cells.

Demyelinating diseases are also characterized by the occurrence of focal demyelinating plaques. These include *multiple sclerosis* (Figs. 100—102), *central pontine myelinolysis* (Fig. 103), *Marchiafava-Bignami disease* (Fig. 104), and post-infectious and post-exanthematous encephalomyelitis. Extensive white matter lesions are the main pathology in Binswanger's disease and carbon monoxide intoxication (Fig. 105).

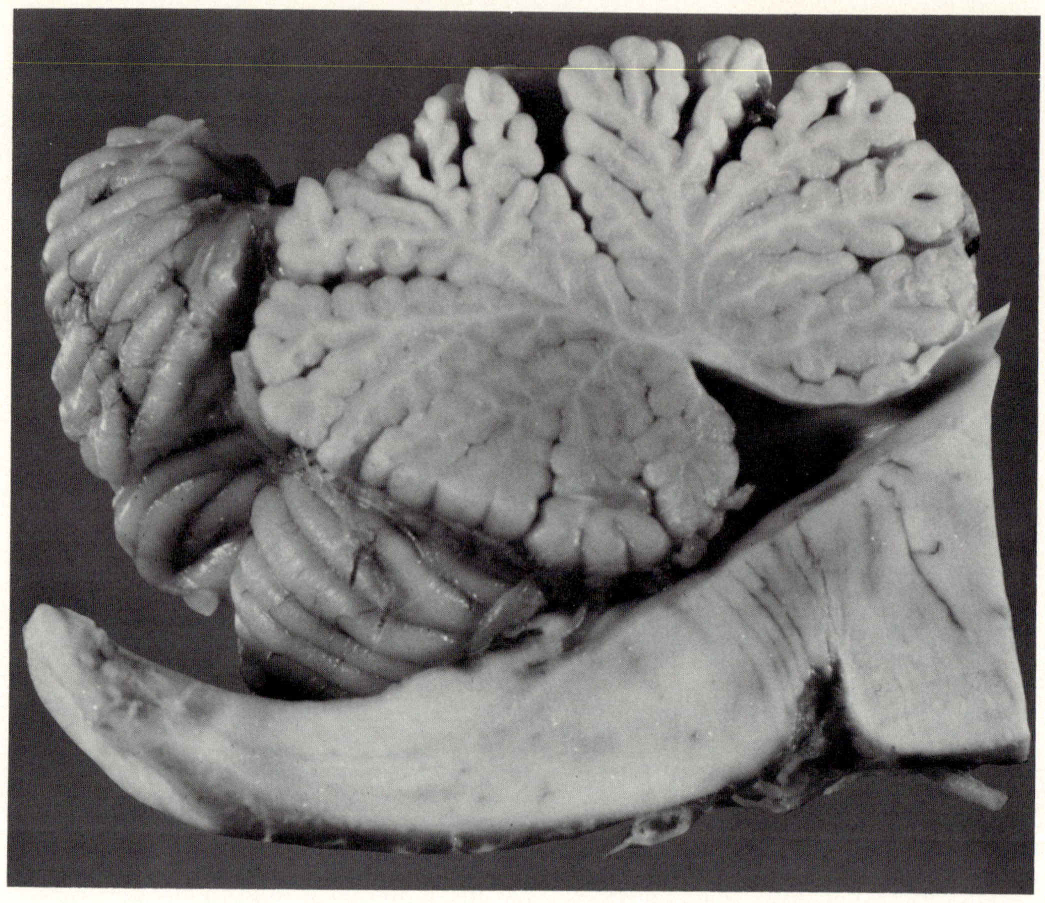

Fig. 85 Cerebellar vermis of a normal aged person.

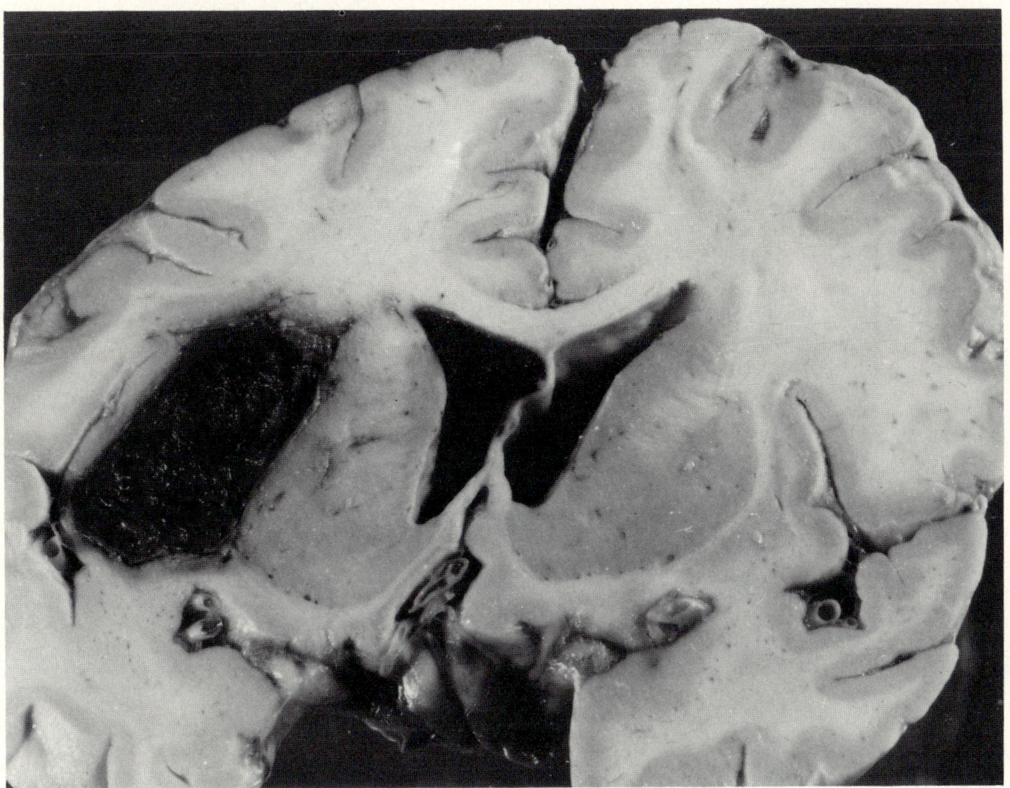

Fig. 86 Intracerebral hematoma between the insula and the basal ganglia.

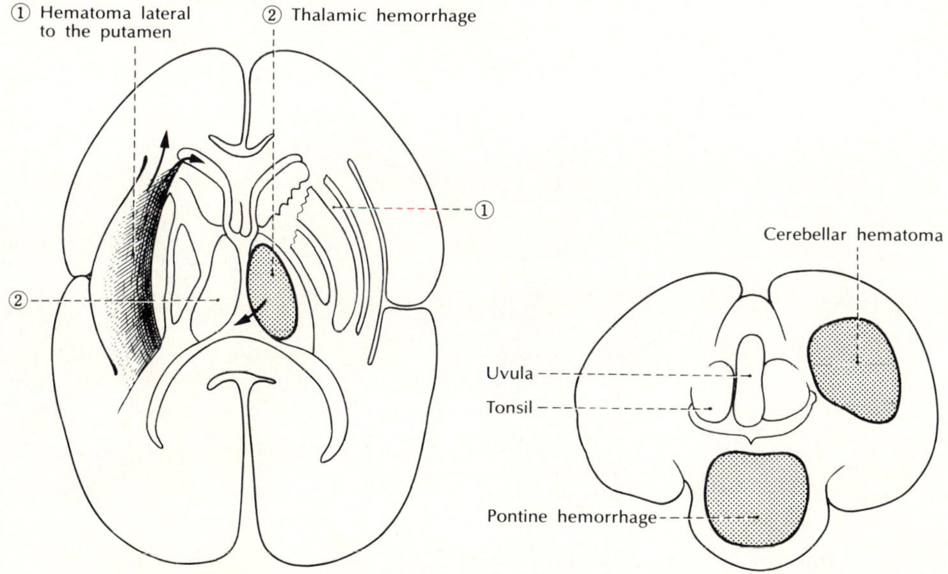

Fig. 87 Intracerebral hemorrhage.

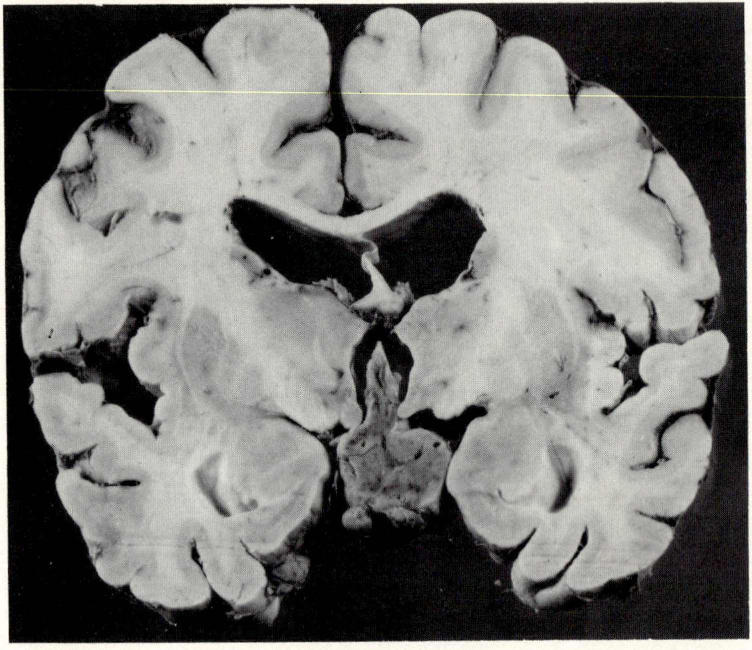

Fig. 88 Pituitary adenoma.
Most often pituitary adenomas are confined to the sella turcica. Frequently, however, the mass extends up into suprasellar regions and may protrude into the third ventricle as illustrated here.

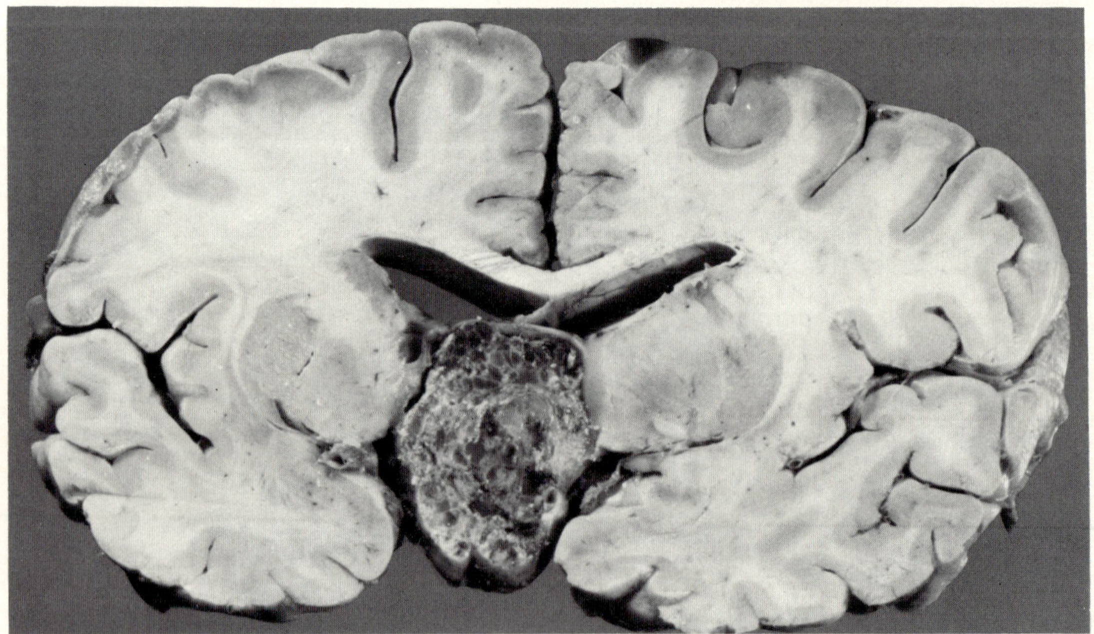

Fig. 89 Craniopharyngioma.
Craniopharyngiomas in the suprasellar region which may protrude upwards obstructing the third ventricle.

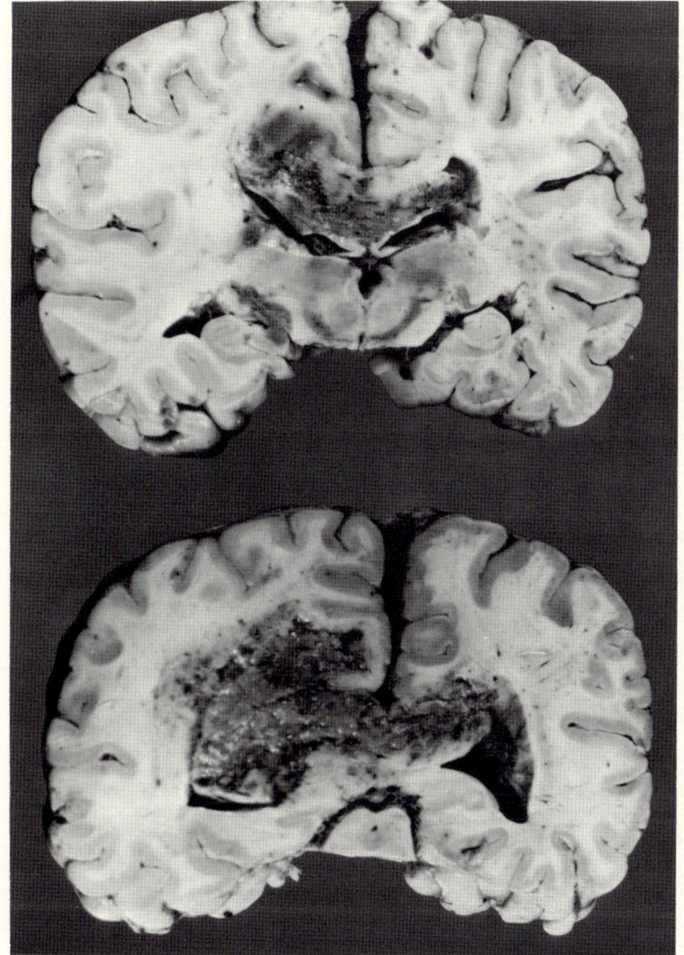

Fig. 90 Glioblastoma multiforme.

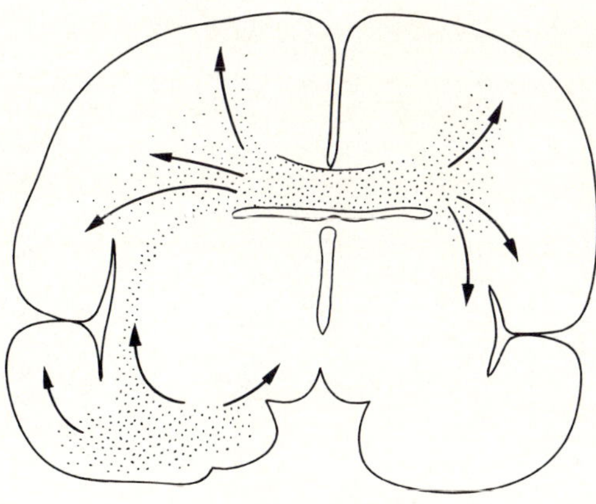

Fig. 91 Glioma.

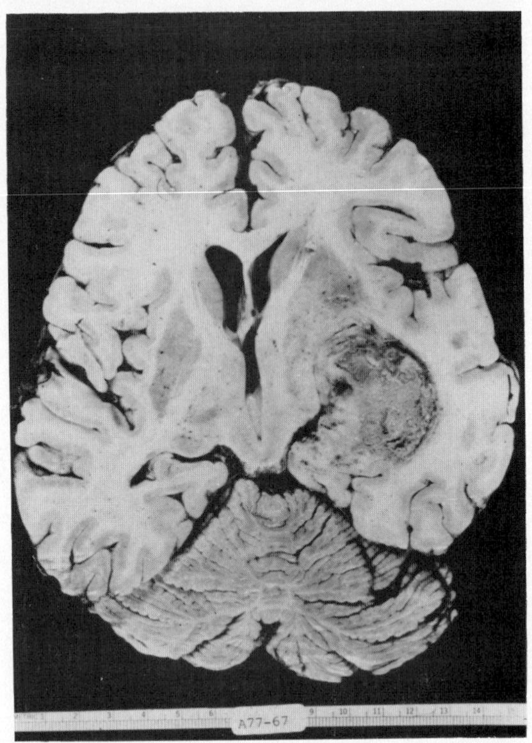

Fig. 92 A horizontal section corresponding to a CT scan of 15° from the canthomeatal line showing a glioblastoma multiforme involving the right temporal lobe.

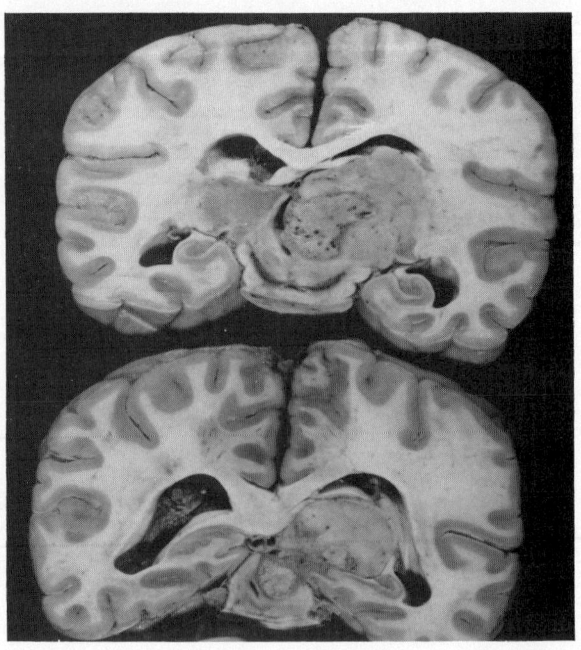

Fig. 93 Thalamic glioma (astrocytoma).

The tumor in this illustration compresses the midbrain and extends into the lateral ventricle and adjacent white matter.

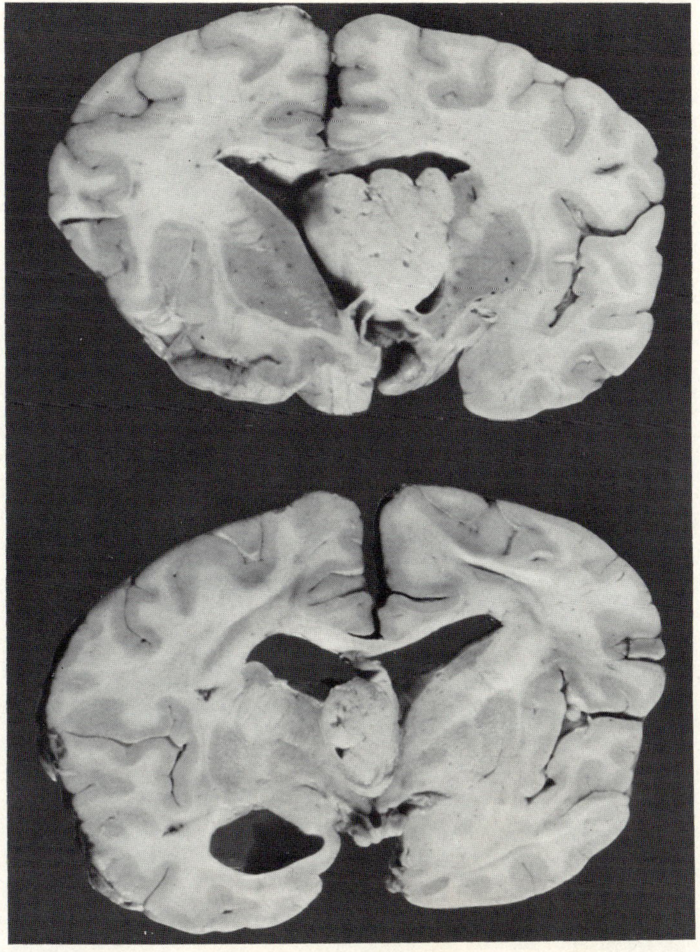

Fig. 94 Subependymal astrocytoma.

In this illustration the tumor is located in the anterior portion of the third ventricle near the foramen of Monro. Other tumors, as well, such as colloid cysts, may occur in this region. They may obstruct the ventricle and result in hydrocephalus.

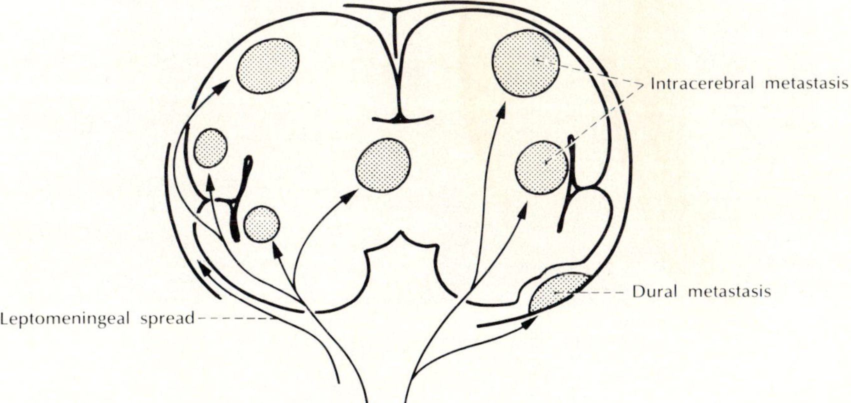

Fig. 95 Topographic distribution of metastatic neoplasms.

Metastatic tumors within the cranium may be found within the brain parenchyma, in the dura mater or diffusely spread in the leptomeninges, sometimes extending into the ventricular system.

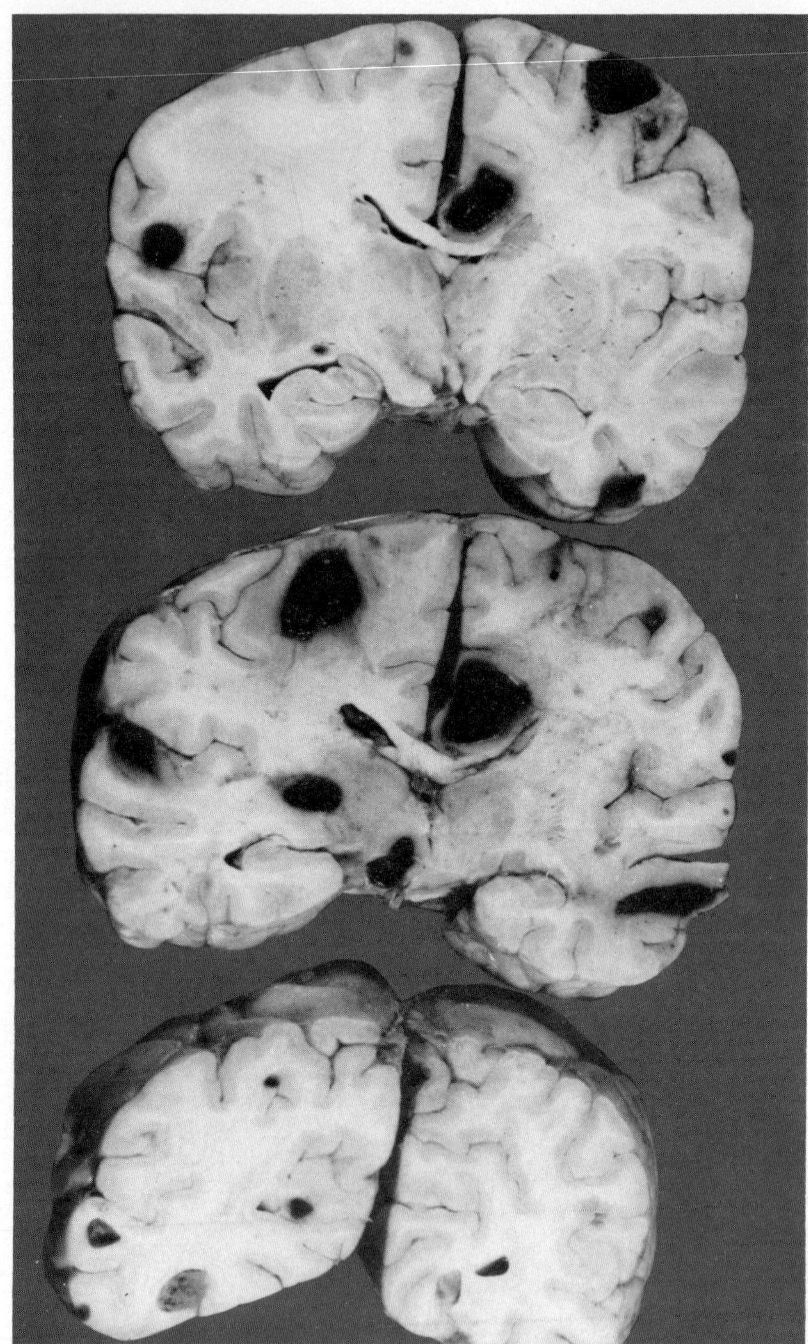

Fig. 96 Metastatic melanoma.

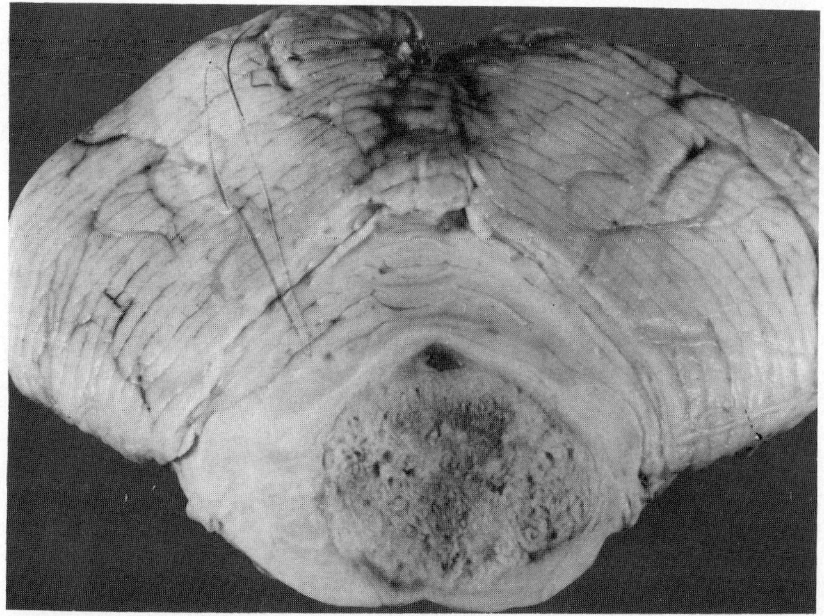

Fig. 97 Metastatic neoplasm in the pons.

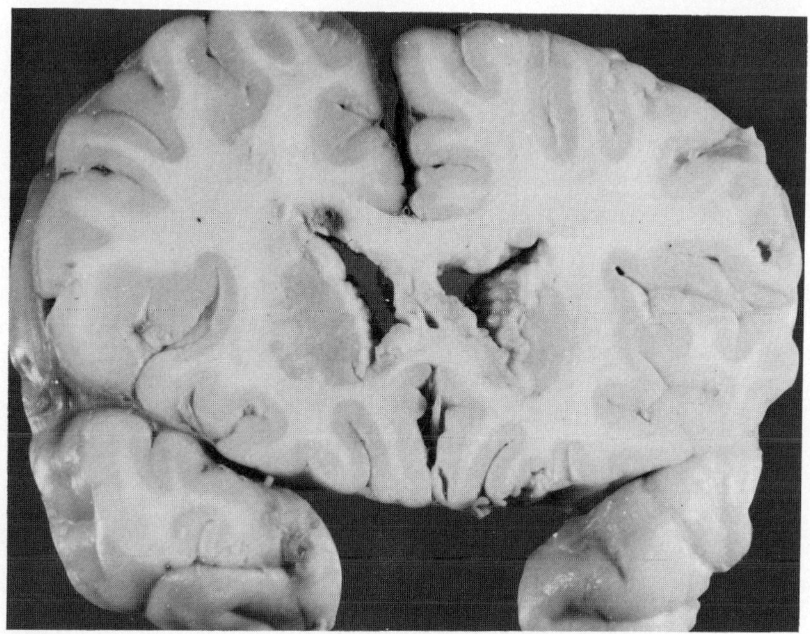

Fig. 98 Intraventricular spread of metastatic neoplasm.

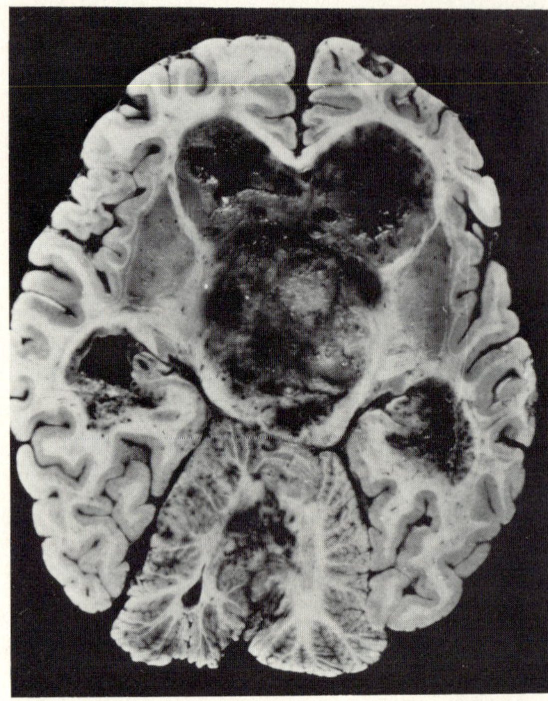

Fig. 99 A horizontal section corresponding to a CT scan at 15° from the canthomeatal line, illustrating an extreme example of the intraventricular spread of a medulloblastoma of the cerebellum.

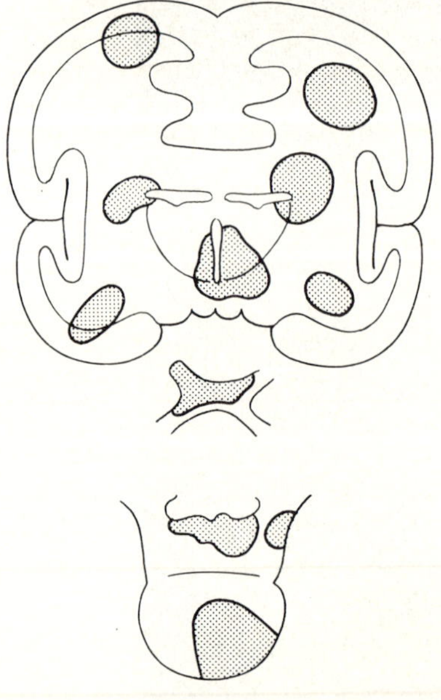

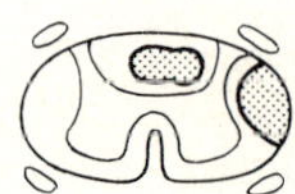

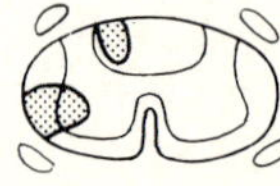

Fig. 100 Distribution of demyelinating plaques in multiple sclerosis.

The number, size and location of the demyelinating plaques in multiple sclerosis may vary greatly between individual cases. Areas of particular predilection, however, are periventricular regions, the optic chiasm and optic nerve and the other areas illustrated in this diagram.

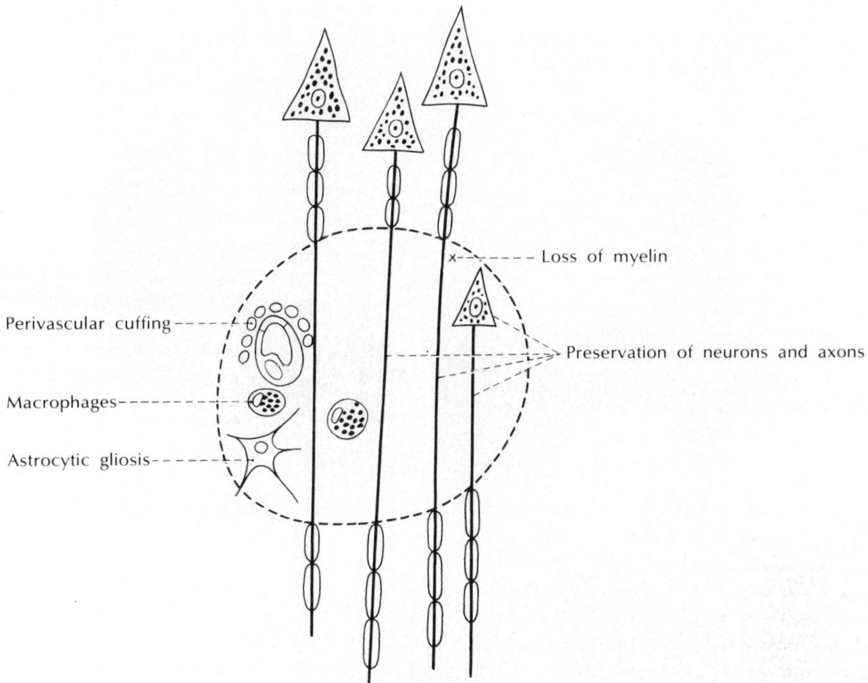

Fig. 101 Demyelinating plaque.
Schematic representation of histological changes in a demyelinating plaque in multiple sclerosis.

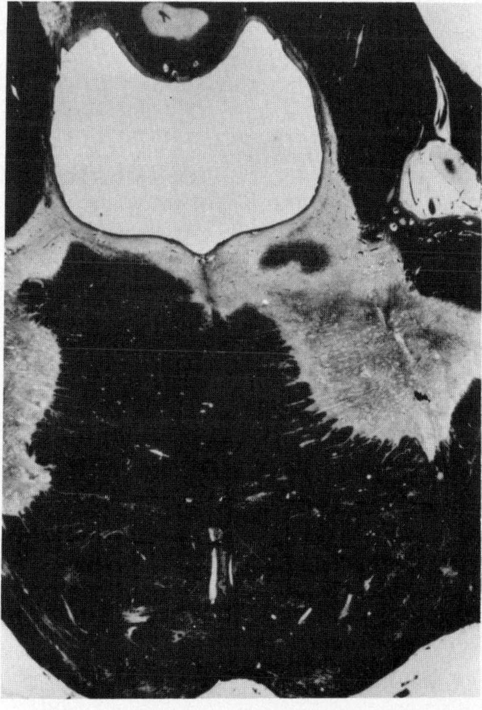

Fig. 102 Demyelinating plaques in the pons (myelin stain).

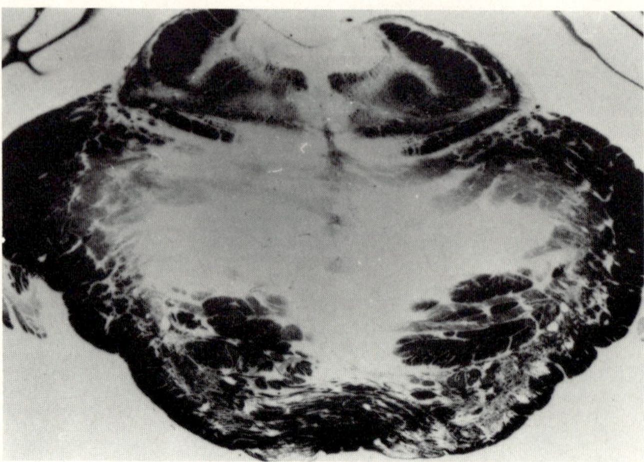

Fig. 103 Central pontine myelinolysis (myelin stain).

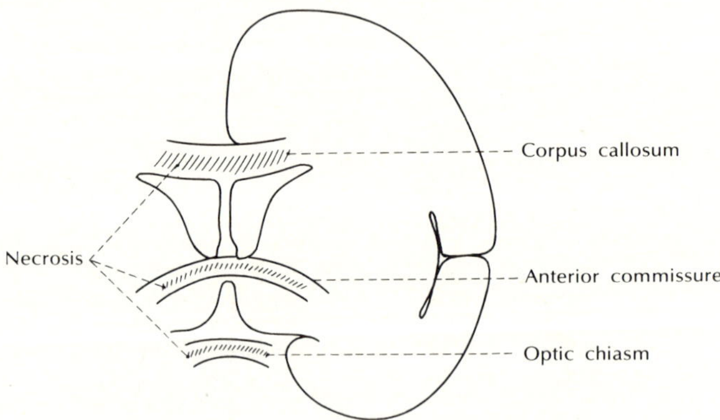

Fig. 104 Topographic distribution of lesions seen in Marchiafava-Bignami disease and in cyanide intoxication. In both of these conditions only the center of the commisural structures are affected while the periphery is spared. In Marchiafava-Bignami disease the changes consist of demyelination whereas necrosis and demyelination accompany cyanide intoxication.

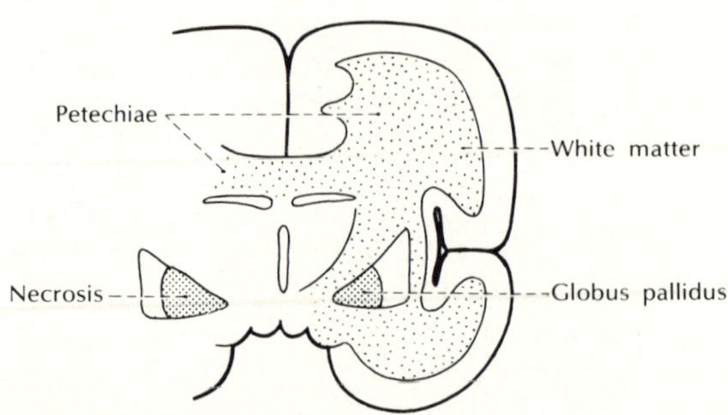

Fig. 105 Carbon monoxide intoxication.

Topographic distribution of changes associated with carbon monoxide intoxication.

Necrosis and atrophy are seen in either or both the globus pallidus and the white matter. Petechial hemorrhage is sometimes observed in the acute stages of intoxication. These alterations are similar to those seen in certain other anoxic conditions.

3. Examination of the Spinal Cord

THE SPINAL EPIDURAL SPACE

Unlike the epidural space under the skull, the spinal epidural space is a true space filled with blood vessels and connective tissue, especially fat. Lesions within the spinal epidural space can produce pain and x-ray changes resulting from small, localized lesions, followed by symptoms of cord or root compression. Today, *metastatic tumors* are the lesions most commonly encountered in the spinal epidural space (Fig. 106). Inflammation and abscess were the most common at one time, but the advent of antibiotics have diminished their frequency. Among the metastatic tumors, breast cancer, in women, and lung carcinoma, in men, are the two most frequently seen. They often differ in the initial symptoms associated with them. Symptoms due to metastatic breast cancer usually begin with back pain and multiple bony changes. These slowly progress finally leading to cord compression. In the case of metastatic lung carcinoma, however, signs of cord compression, occasionally acute, may be the first symptom noted. Regardless of the source of the tumor they generally remain epidural. Apparently the dura mater effectively prevents the infiltration of tumor cells directly into the cord.

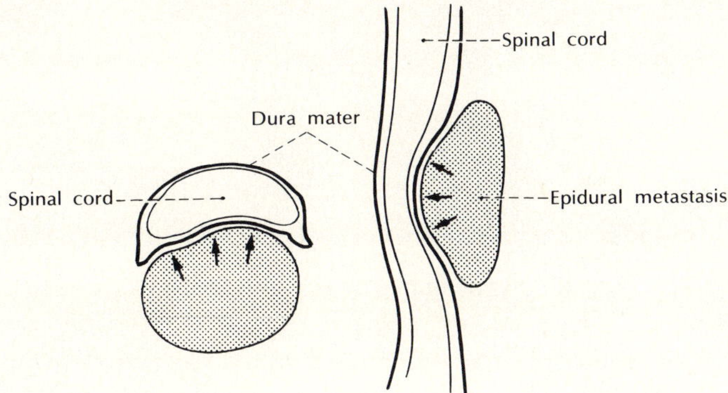

Fig. 106 Compression of spinal cord due to epidural metastasis.

In collecting specimens at autopsy from cords with metastatic lesions, it is important to remove not only the spinal cord alone but also the dura mater, epidural tissue, sometimes even bone, and the tumor itself. For this purpose it is best not to slit the dura mater but, instead, to cut the cord transversely at the appropriate level. This allows one to visualize the relationship between the growing tumor and surrounding tissue, especially the spinal cord root, and dura mater as well as the involvement of the nearby vasculature. Decalcification is needed whenever bone is involved.

REFERENCE

Barron, K.D., Hirano, A., Araki, S., & Terry, R.D.: Experience with metastatic neoplasms involving the spinal cord. Neurology, 9: 91-106, 1959.

THE SPINAL LEPTOMENINGES AND SUBARACHNOID SPACE

Fundamentally, the leptomeninges and subarachnoid space of the spinal cord are similar to those surrounding the brain. Brittle, calcified membranous plaques of various size are frequently seen in the normal adult spinal cord. In addition, large blood vessels in the subarachnoid space, especially the vein, are prominent. Both of these features are of no pathological significance although they frequently mislead the novice. They are not signs of arachnoiditis or vascular malformation both of which do indeed occur in this location but can be readily distinguished from these normal variations.

While spinal arachnoiditis is a term commonly used by clinicians, it is often difficult to discern associated pathological alterations. When they are found, the expected inflammatory changes or their residua are seen. When true arteriovenous malformations are present in the spinal subarachnoid space they are often quite profound and associated with significant cord changes such as malacia.

Thickening of the spinal leptomeninges is sometimes observed but it is not always a sign of pathology. Increased fibrosis is a normal aging phenomenon.

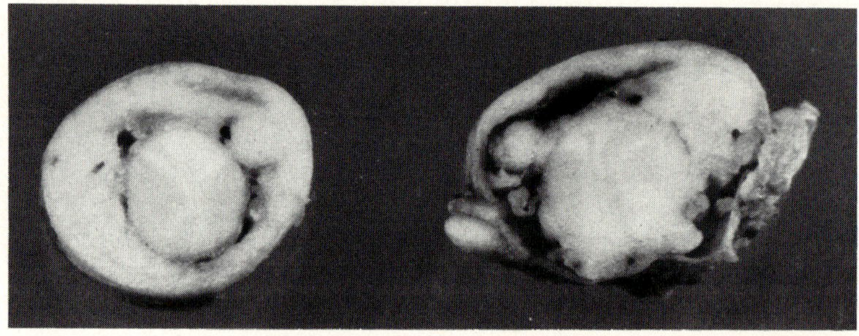

Fig. 107 Leptomeningeal carcinomatosis.

We have discussed the spinal subarachnoid space separately from that over the brain. It must be remembered, however, that the spinal and cerebral subarachnoid spaces are continuous so that pathological changes in the brain can easily enter the spinal subarachnoid space. For example, in a subarachnoid hemorrhage in the brain, blood will freely disseminate into the spinal subarachnoid space. Similarly, inflammation and tumors can spread along the neuroaxis (Fig. 107). In some cases necrotic brain tissue resulting from conditions such as a herniated cerebellar cortex can enter the spinal subarachnoid space. Because of the anatomy, these materials tend to accumulate in the area of the conus medullaris.

THE SPINAL CORD PROPER

Normal Anatomy

Proper orientation of the spinal cord is essential for the intelligent interpretation of morphological alterations. Once the cord is removed from its bony covering it is sometimes difficult for the uninitiated to distinguish between the *anterior (ventral)* and *posterior (dorsal) aspects*. The easiest way is to identify the anterior spinal artery lying in the subarachnoid space. The characteristic shape of the spinal cord as seen in transverse sections with its prominent anterior median fissure is also a simple way of determining the anterior-posterior orientation (Fig. 108). In addition, the dura mater of the dorsal surface of the cord is much thicker than that of the ventral surface.

The next step in orientation is to distinguish between the various *levels of the spinal cord*. In general, posterior roots are larger and more numerous than anterior roots at the cervical and lumbar levels. As one descends along the dorsal roots one notices a sudden change in caliber from quite thick to relatively narrow. The C8 root is the thickest. Th 1 is narrower but Th 2 and the lower ones are narrower yet.

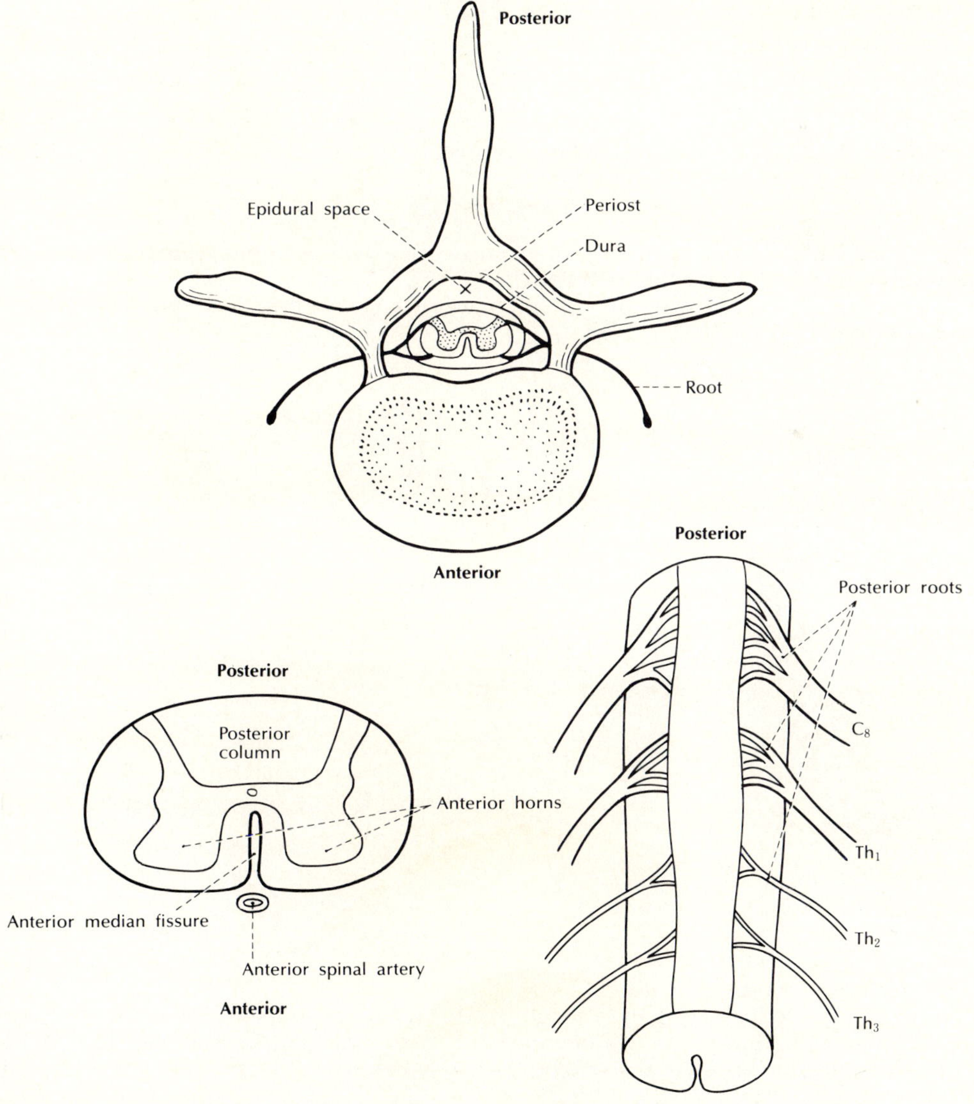

Fig. 108 Outline of the anatomy of the cervical cord.

A method for detecting S 1 has recently been suggested. The anterior roots change in caliber between S 1 and S 2. Normally, S 1 is distinctly larger than S 2, which is larger than S 3 and those below (Iwata and Hirano, 1977).

In the cervical cord the roots from each segment pass above the similarly numbered vertebra. However, there are only seven cervical vertebrae and eight cervical segments and roots of the spinal cord. Thus the C 8 root passes through the foramen between the C 7 and T 1 vertebrae. As a result all the remaining roots below this level pass below the similarly numbered vertebral body.

One must also be aware of the possible confusion that can arise in the use of the numbered designations to indicate *levels of the spinal cord.* Radiologists use the numbers to refer to the vertebral body seen in x-ray, but because the vertebrals are larger than the cord segments in the adult, the cord segment actually covered by a particular vertebral body is likely to be a very different segment from that designated by the number of the bone. Thus the L_1 cord segment, for example, is not covered by the L_1 vertebral body. Actually, the L_1 vertebral body covers the sacral cord. Spinal taps made between the L_3 and L_4 spinous processes enter the cauda equina. In the cervical region the correspondence is closer but the relationships change as the spinal roots elongate in the lower cord.

REFERENCES

Iwata, M., & Hirano, A.: A method for the macroscopic identification of human lumbo-sacral spinal cord level. Neurol. Med. (Tokyo), 7: 126-131, 1977.

Iwata, M., & Hirano, A.: Sparing of the Onufrowicz nucleus in sacral anterior horn lesions. Ann. Neurol., 4: 45-49, 1978.

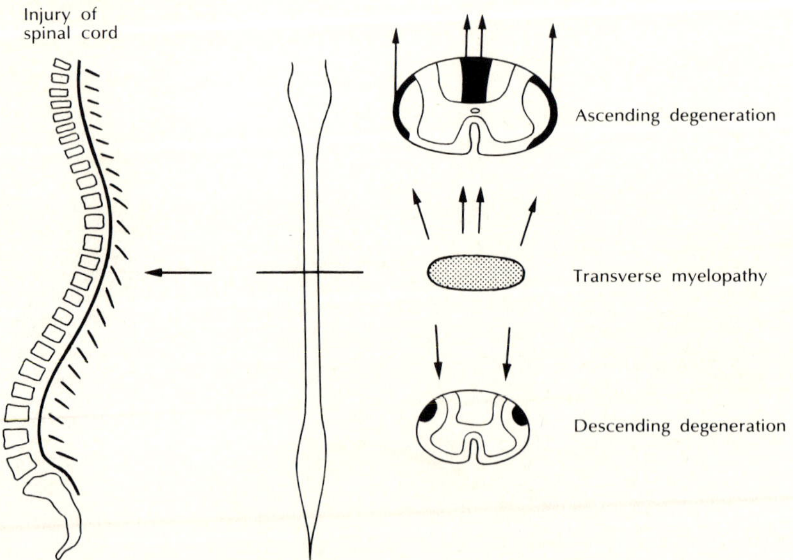

Fig. 109 Injury of the spinal cord.
Damage to the spinal cord may result in transverse myelopathy affecting the entire segment. This is followed by degeneration of ascending pathways above the affected segments and degeneration of descending pathways below.

Pathology of the Spinal Cord

Among the more common and easily recognizable pathological alterations of the spinal cord and roots are the neoplastic tumors, especially *meningiomas* and *schwannomas*. Meningiomas in the spinal canal are much more common in women than men. These are intradural and extramedullary in position and focal. In von

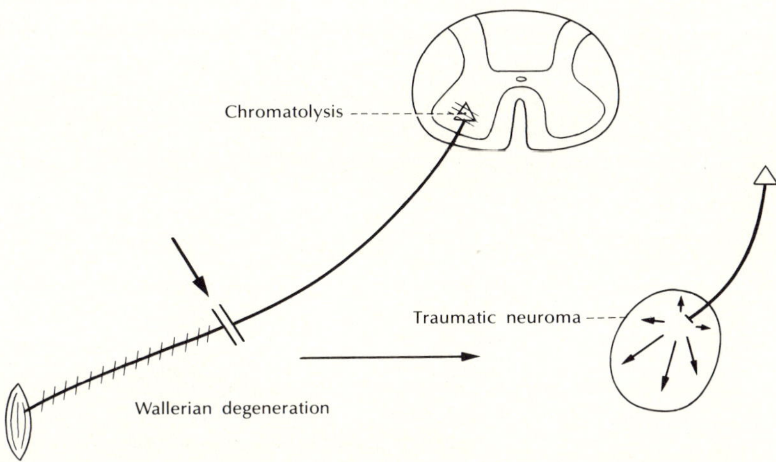

Fig. 110 Injury of peripheral nerve.
Damage to the peripheral nerves results in Wallerian degeneration peripherally and chromatolysis of the corresponding anterior horn cells. Sometimes the proximal stumps show evidence of traumatic neuroma.

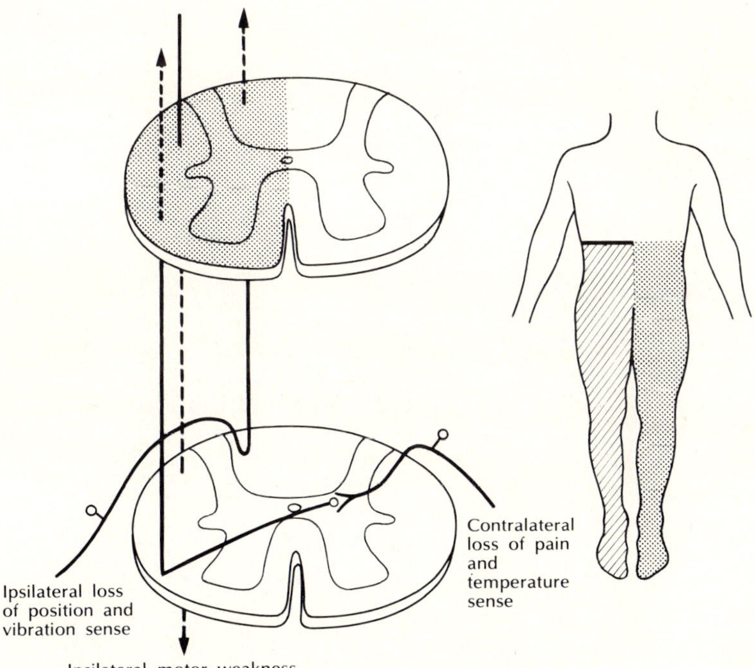

Fig. 111 Brown-Séquard syndrome.

Recklinghausen disease tumors may be found in many roots. Metastatic tumors, too, occasionally involve multiple roots.

Gliomas constitute most of the intramedullary tumors of the spinal cord. We must remind the beginner, however, not to confuse the "toothpaste" artifact described previously (p. 7) with actual neoplasms. In contrast to epidural or intracerebral metastases, intramedullary metastatic tumors are not common in the spinal cord although they do occur.

Other spinal cord changes which can be seen from the external surface include *injury* (Figs. 109—111) and *malformation* (Fig. 112).

The blood supply to the spinal cord is illustrated in schematic fashion in Figs. 113 and 114. Infarcts of the spinal cord tend to occur between T_4 and T_6, presumably because of the relatively poor collateral circulation.

Malformation of the blood vessels of the spinal cord may also be observed during gross external examination (Iwata et al., 1977).

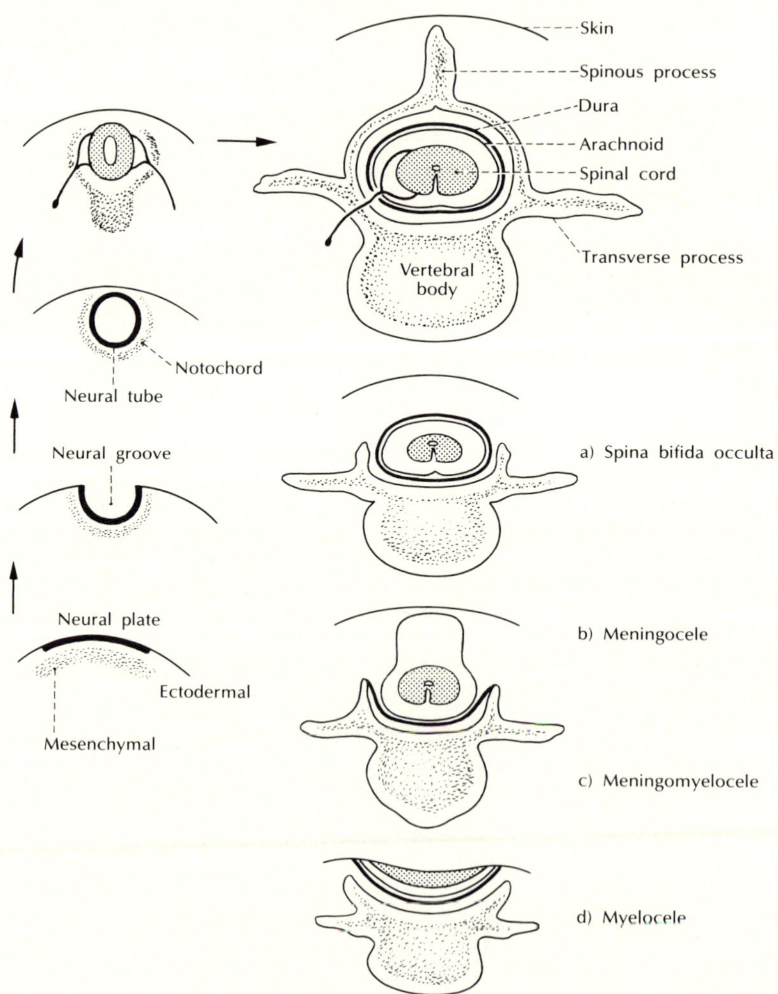

Fig. 112 Failure of fusion.

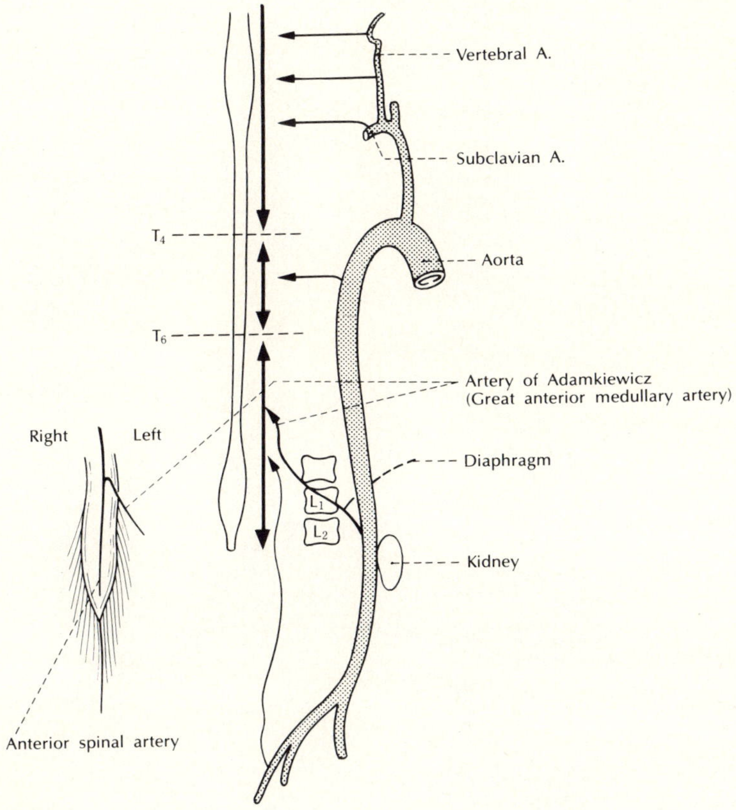

Fig. 113 Blood supply of the spinal cord.

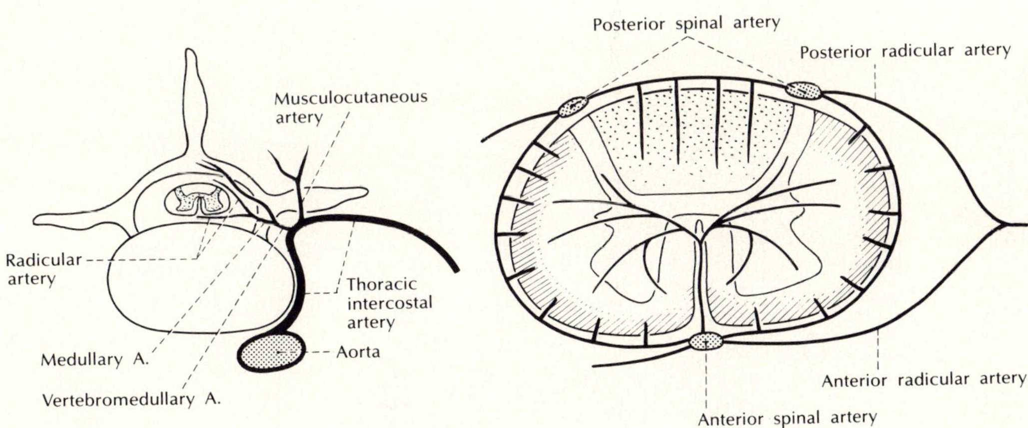

Fig. 114 Spinal arteries.

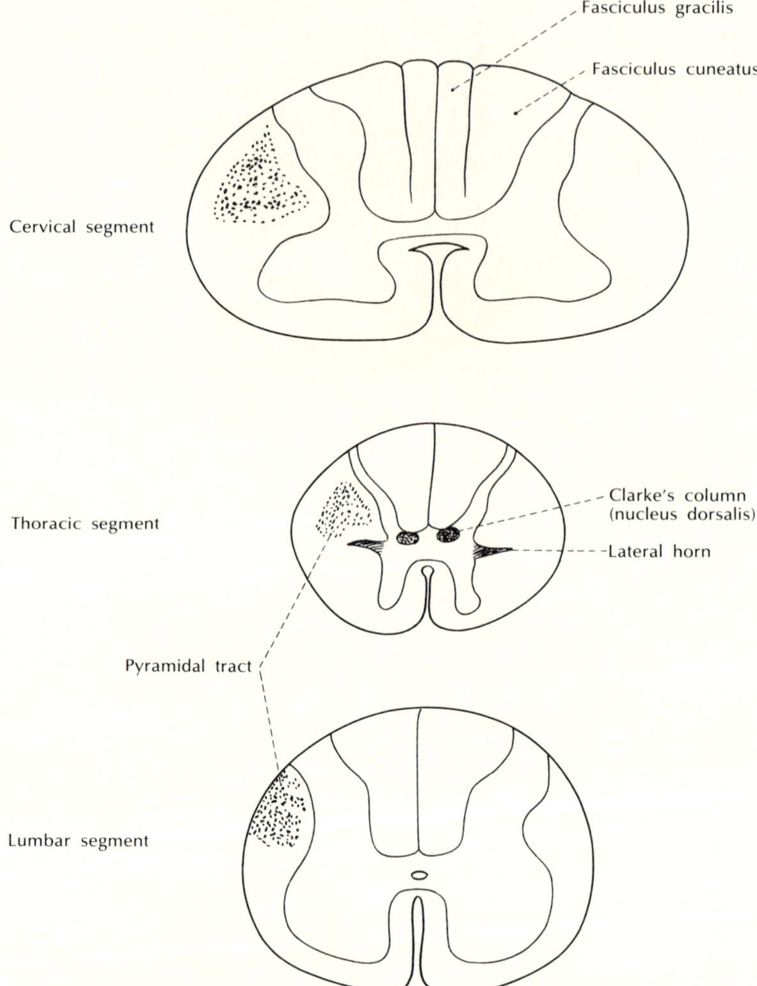

Fig. 115a Transverse sections of the spinal cord.

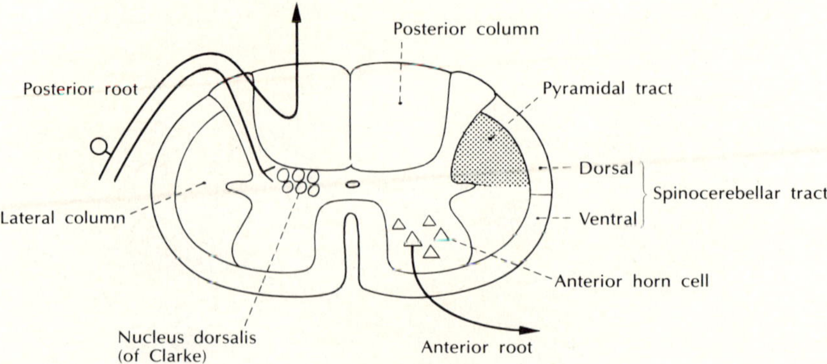

Fig. 115b Cross section of the spinal cord showing the major tracts.

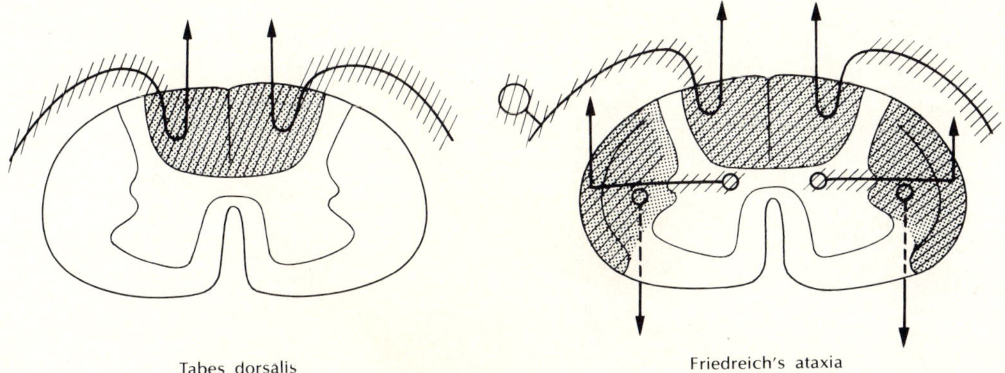

Fig. 116 Cross section of the spinal cord showing the major tracts, tabes dorsalis and Friedreich's ataxia.

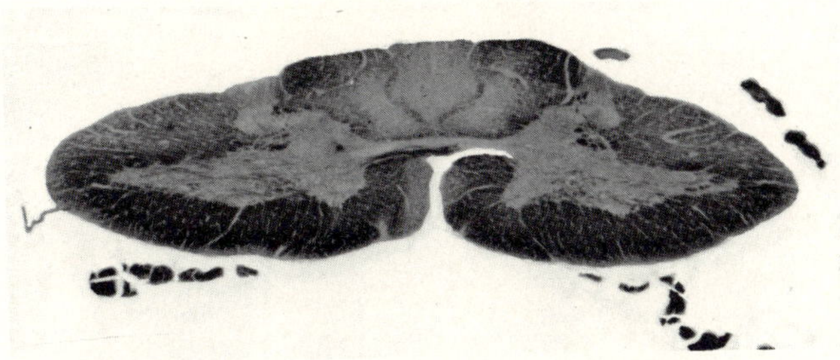

Fig. 117 Friedreich's ataxia (myelin stain).

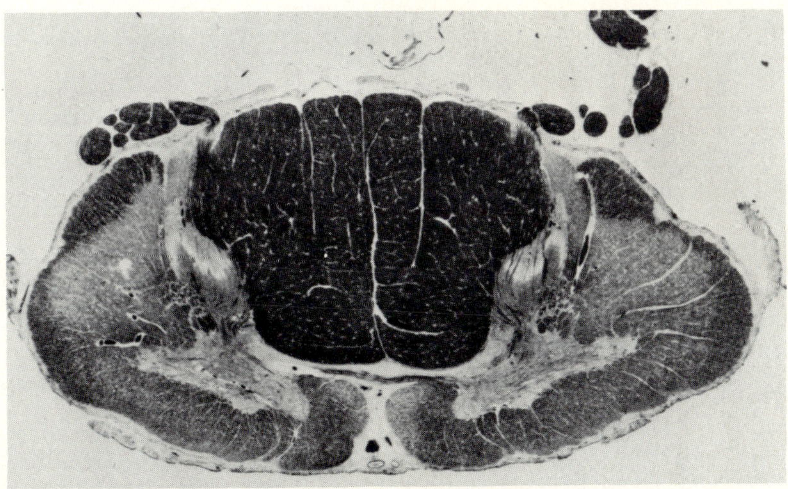

Fig. 118 Amyotrophic lateral sclerosis (ALS). Myelin stain of the cervical cord.

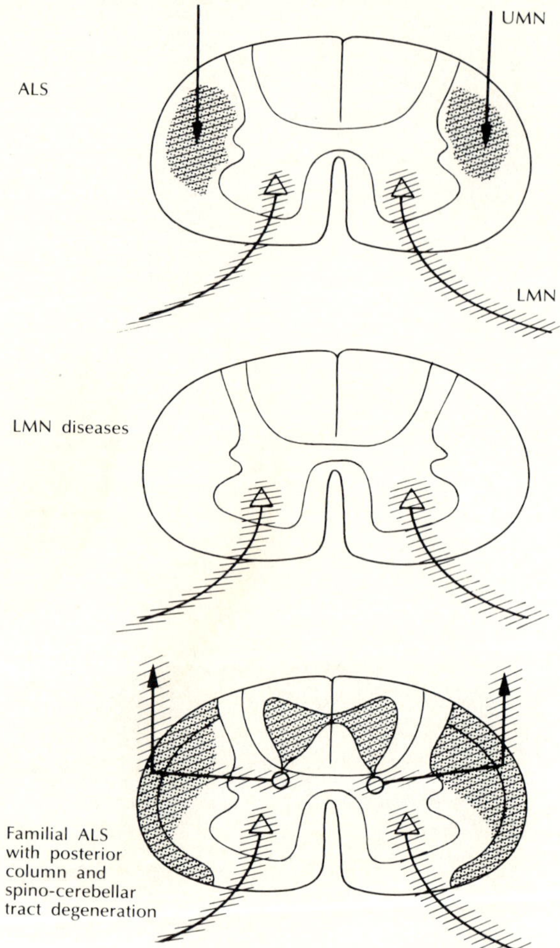

Fig. 119 Motor neuron disease.

REFERENCES

Hirano, A., Kurland, L.T., and Sayre, G.P.: Familial amyotrophic lateral sclerosis: A subgroup characterized by posterior and spinocerebellar tract involvement and hyaline inclusions in the anterior horn cells. Arch. Neurol., 16: 232-243, 1967.

Hirano, A., Malamud, N., Kurland, L.T., & Zimmerman, H.M.: A review of the pathological findings in amyotrophic lateral sclerosis. *In* Motor Neuron Disease: Research on Amyotrophic Lateral Sclerosis and Related Disorders, pp. 51-60. Norris, F.H. Jr., and Kurland, L.T. (eds.) Grune & Stratton, New York and London, 1968.

Metcalf, C.W., & Hirano, A.: Clinico-pathological studies of a family with amytrophic lateral sclerosis. Arch. Neurol., 24: 518-523, 1971.

Hirano, A.: Progress in the pathology of motor neuron diseases. *In Progress in Neuropathology,* Vol. II. pp. 181-225, Zimmerman, H.M. (ed.) Grune & Stratton, New York, 1973.

Ghatak, N.R., Hirano, A., & Zimmerman, H.M.: Rheumatoid arthritis with arteritis and neuropathy masking amyotrophic lateral sclerosis. Clin. Neurol. (Tokyo), 12: 186-204, 1972.

Hirano, A.: Some current concepts of ALS. Neuro. (Tokyo), 4: 43-52, 1976.

Andrews, J.M., Johnson, R.T., & Brazier, M.A.B. (eds.): Amyotrophic Lateral Sclerosis. Recent Research Trends. Academic Press, New York, 1976.

Hirano, A., and Iwata, M.: Pathology of motor neurons with special reference to amyotrophic lateral sclerosis and related diseases. *In* Symposium on Amyotrophic Lateral Sclerosis. pp. 107-133. Tsubaki, T. and Toyokura, Y. (eds.), Japanese Medical Research Foundation, Tokyo, 1979.

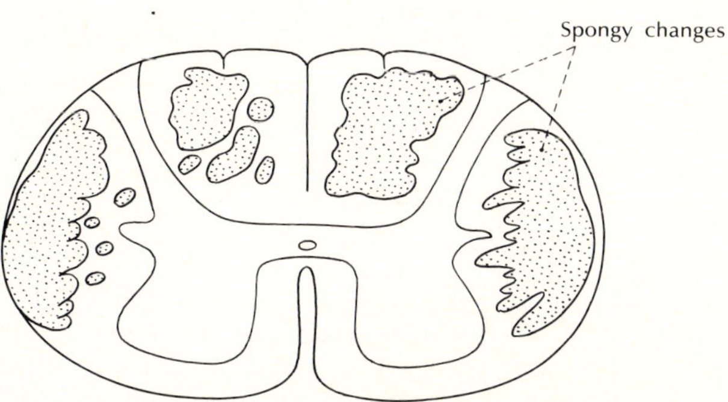

Fig. 120 Subacute combined degeneration.
Although this condition also usually involves the posterior and lateral columns it should not be confused with Friedreich's ataxia or certain forms of motor neuron disease. In addition to clear clinical and etiological differences, subacute combined degeneration results in spongy swelling rather than atrophy unless the patient has been subjected to a prolonged course of treatment. Furthermore, the involved areas do not correspond to specific fiber tracts as they do in Friedreich's ataxia and motor neuron diseases.

Sectioning the spinal cord (Fig. 115) reveals other features. Although it is common practice in some laboratories to routinely section the cord into regular, short segments, we feel that this procedure tends to obscure some of the pertinent anatomical relationships. We therefore usually remove material from the center of a lesion and from the border zone. Two or three additional sections are also taken from above and below the lesion, at some distance from it, in order to ascertain the presence or absence of tract degeneration. This principle is not to be maintained too rigidly. Occasionally, one can be surprised by the fortuitous discovery of occult lesions in the spinal cord not suspected from the clinical abstract and not visible externally. We have come across such changes as multiple sclerosis plaques (Ghatak et al., 1974) and fresh small infarcts in this way. Even in apparently normal spinal cords we usually collect at least one specimen each from the cervical, thoracic and lumbar cord (Fig. 115).

The spinal cord is the main site of involvement of certain systemic degenerative diseases. These include *Friedreich's ataxia* (Figs. 116 and 117) and various *motor neuron diseases* (Figs. 118 and 119). Other diseases whose primary site of involvement are in the spinal cord include *subacute combined degeneration* (Fig. 120) and syringomyelia.

When the history includes previous acute anterior poliomyelitis the appropriate areas of the spinal cord should be selected for microscopic study. In the past, these areas have been relatively neglected leading to a paucity of information regarding long-standing changes in poliomyelitis.

REFERENCES

Mackay, R.P., & Hirano, A.: Forms of benign multiple sclerosis with report of two "clinically silent" cases discovered at autopsy. Arch. Neurol., 17: 588-600, 1967.

Ghatak, N.R., Hirano, A., Lijtmaer, H., & Zimmerman, H.M.: Asymptomatic demyelinated plaque in the spinal cord. Arch. Neurol., 30: 484-486, 1974.

Iwata, M., Kawamoto, K., & Hirano, A.: Dilation and tortuosity of the anterior spinal artery and detritus of the cerebellar tissue displaced downward into spinal subarachnoid space. Neurol. Med. (Tokyo), 7: 84-86, 1977.

F. REMOVING TISSUE SAMPLES FOR MICROSCOPIC EXAMINATION (Fig. 121)

Because of the anatomical intricacy of the central nervous system and the uniqueness of each part due to its own particular position it is generally recommended to use as large a block as practical. Unlike the general organs such as liver or lung, the longer range anatomical relationships of the central nervous system are more important. For the same reason we try to include at least some surrounding, normal tissue when we take a pathological specimen. This procedure also allows us to properly evaluate the staining method and the status of the border zone between the "normal" and pathological regions.

Three types of preparations are used. These are celloidin, paraffin and frozen sections. Celloidin is not as commonly used in the United States as it had been at one time. Its major value is its ability to be sectioned over large areas thus permitting the retention of long range anatomical relationships. Additionally, one can easily cut 20-30 micron thick sections permitting excellent results with Nissl and myelin stain. On the other hand, celloidin embedding is slow and the larger blocks require individual processing rendering them expensive. In addition, thinner sections are difficult to obtain. When we do collect material for celloidin embedding, the specimen is usually about two and one half finger widths wide, three fingers long, and one centimeter thick. In order to preserve left-right orientation, a deep V-shaped notch is cut into the left side. The face of interest is indicated by a shallow notch cut into the opposite surface.

Paraffin is the most common embedding medium. For this purpose the width of the block is usually about a thumb's width, the length about three fingers and a third of a centimeter thick. As in the celloidin material, the block is notched on the left side and on the surface opposite to the one of interest. Sometimes when the tissue block is too small to conveniently notch as in specimens of the spinal cord, we place a fine nylon thread in the left side. When the tissue tends to ravel as in the cauda equina we retain the dura mater and loosely tie the specimen in a bundle.

For frozen sections, required for certain staining procedures, the specimens are much smaller and we cut relatively thin sections on the freezing microtome. Since there is no embedment used in this method, we must bear in mind that unattached parts included in a single section will separate when the section is floated on water during processing. This specimen must, therefore, be properly trimmed and oriented so that the knife cuts through material that is continuous in all planes.

All of the above techniques are, of course, used in conjunction with formalin-fixed material. In the case of certain surgical specimens, however, in which rapid diagnoses are required, the tissue is not fixed but is immediately frozen and sectioned in the cryostat. Relatively thin sections are cut and the section is collected directly onto the slide where it remains throughout processsing.

Once the specimen has been obtained from the brain and spinal cord, the question of the disposition of the remainder of the tissue arises. Practically

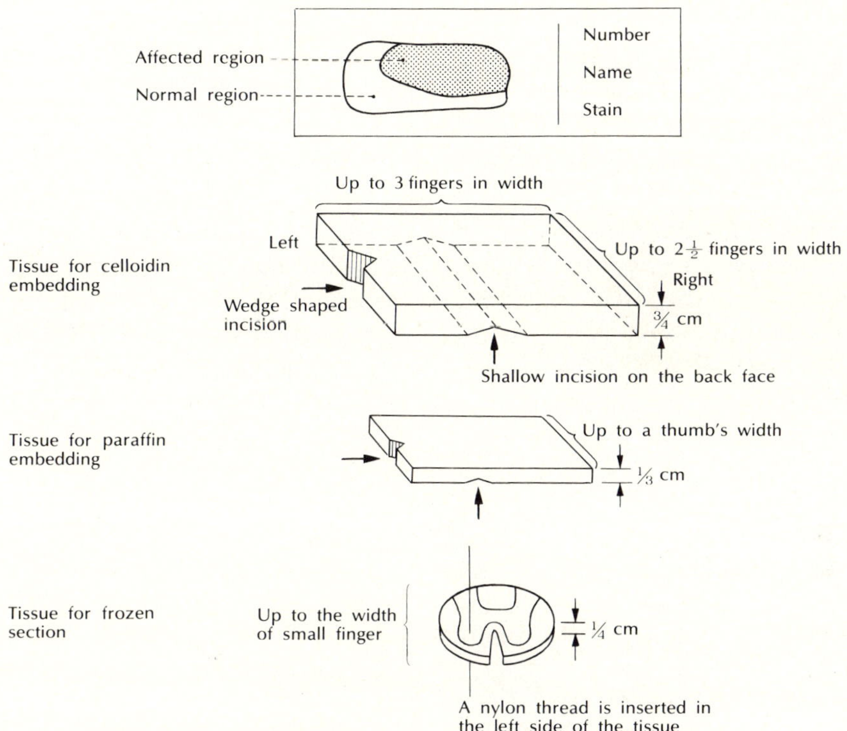

Fig. 121 Preparation of tissue blocks for embedding.

speaking, it is not feasible to retain all specimens in perpetuity. On the other hand, some material is valuable and should be kept. When, after gross examination, we judge a brain to be essentially normal or only of routine interest it is discarded in the proper manner. Other brains are temporarily stored in formalin until after microscopic examination of the embedded samples has been completed. If these are judged to be of sufficient interest the brain is kept indefinitely, otherwise it too is discarded in the prescribed manner.

G. STAINING

A wide variety of staining procedures are in use in various neuropathological laboratories. Many of these, however, are only rarely used or are confined to only certain laboratories. In the following, we shall describe only some of those stains which are most commonly used in the United States, especially at Montefiore Hospital.

The tissue components for which these stains are designed consist of neurons, glia, blood vessels and leptomeninges in the central nervous system (Fig. 122). In the peripheral nervous system Schwann cells replace the glia and there is a substantial amount of connective tissue. The stains to be described are all designed to stain some or all of these components and to enhance certain features with respect to others.

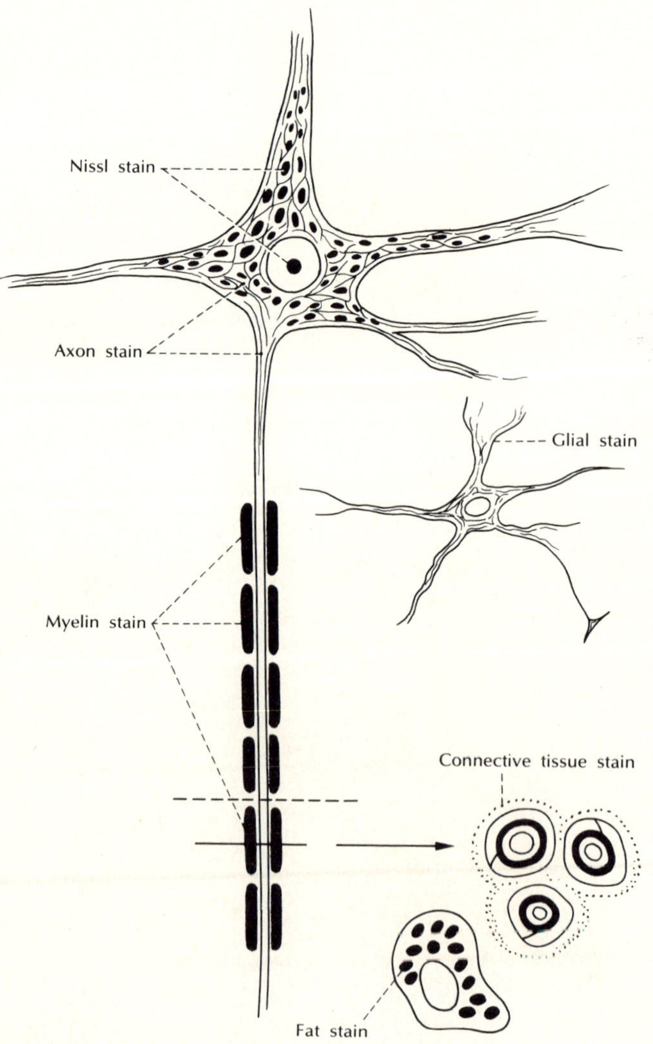

Fig. 122 Overall staining reactions in the nervous system.

REFERENCE

Luna, L.G. (ed.): Manual of Histologic Staining Methods of the Armed Forces Institute of Pathology. Third Ed. McGraw-Hill, New York, 1960.

1. Hematoxylin and Eosin Stain (H&E) (Fig. 123)

With some exceptions, this method stains all the tissue elements. The blue hematoxylin stains such structures as nucleoli and the Nissl substance. The eosin stains red blood cells, glial fibrils, muscle and collagen fibers red. Some materials such as lipofuscin are not stained by these dyes but retain their original color. Thus, based on the shape, color and anatomic relationship we can usually identify most of the cellular elements of the nervous system.

H&E staining, as in general pathology, is the basic method by which diagnoses are made. In most instances it suffices. With it we can diagnose various neoplasms, inflammations, vascular lesions, etc.

2. Special Stains

Often, however, one must turn to other techniques because hematoxylin and eosin stains some tissue components only poorly or not at all. These include myelin, senile plaques and the internal elastic laminae of the arteries. In addition, and perhaps more important, special stains are needed to differentiate between certain tissue components. For example, it is sometimes difficult to distinguish between connective tissue fibers and glial processes. Neurofibrillary tangles are difficult to distinguish from the background after hematoxylin and eosin staining, while other methods will stain these components more selectively.

NISSL STAIN (Fig. 123)

Nissl staining is most useful for evaluating the distribution and numbers of various cell populations. For this purpose it is recommended to use 15 micron rather than the more usual 7 micron paraffin sections. If celloidin is used 20 micron sections are cut.

The original method for Nissl preparations involved alcohol fixation, celloidin embedding and toluidine blue staining. Nowadays, however, other methods are used which give substantially the same results. These include formalin fixation, paraffin embedding or frozen sections and other aniline dyes such as cresyl violet or thionine.

These methods primarily stain the nucleoli and the Nissl substance blue, but other elements are also clearly stained. These include corpora amylacea and Lafora bodies among others which are rendered blue. The intracellular inclusions seen in metachromatic leukodystrophy stain red with toluidine blue stain, but one must remember to use a water soluble mountant instead of balsam to preserve the metachromasia.

Fig. 123-1
H&E and selected special stains.

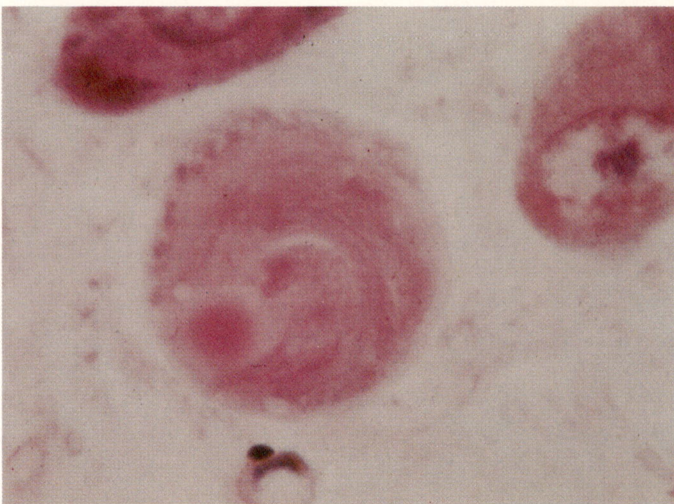

A. Neurofibrillary tangles and a Lewy body in a single neuron (H&E).

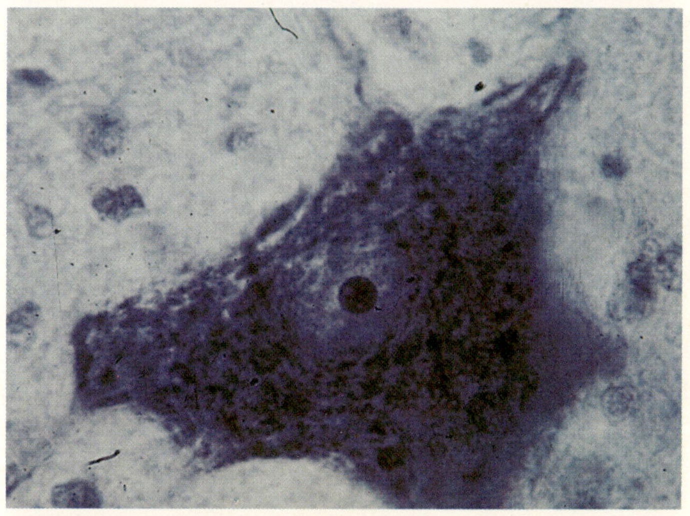

B. An anterior horn cell (Nissl stain).

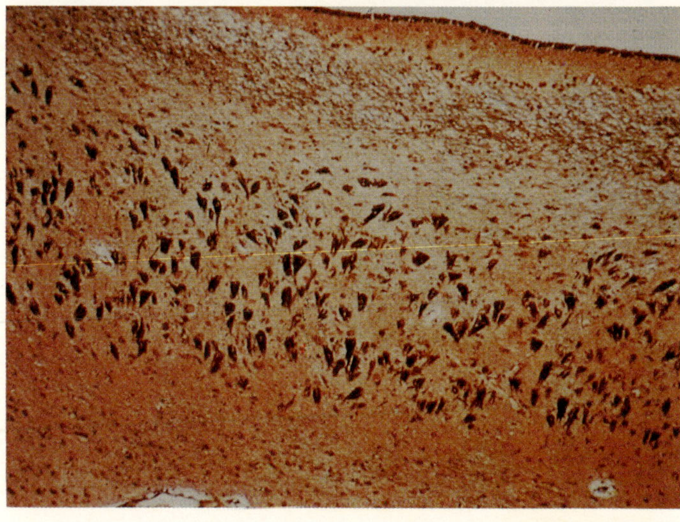

C. Neurofibrillary tangles in almost every neuron in Sommer's sector (modified Bielschowsky stain).

Fig. 123-2
Selected special stains.

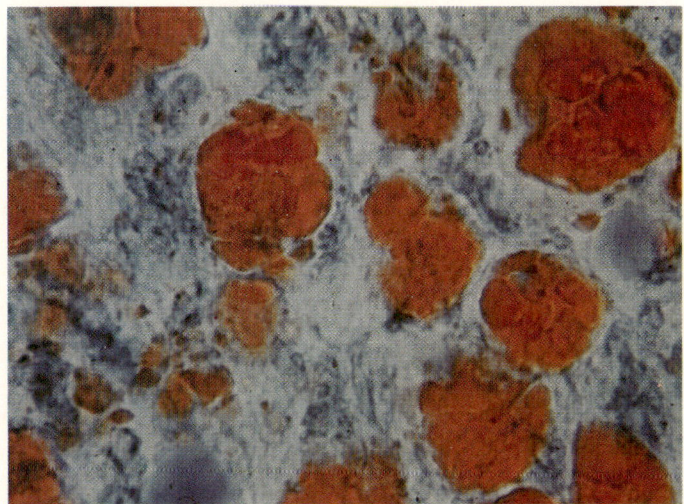

D. Macrophage containing sudanophilic lipid in a demyelinated pyramidal tract (sudan stain).

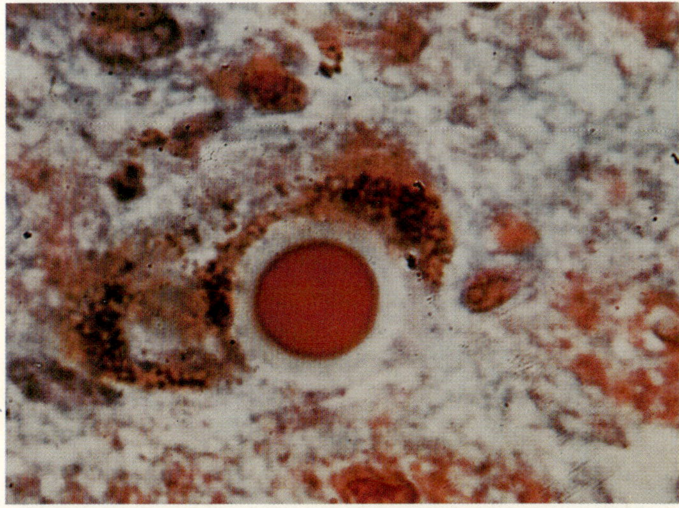

E. Lewy body in a neuron in a patient with Parkinson's disease (Masson stain).

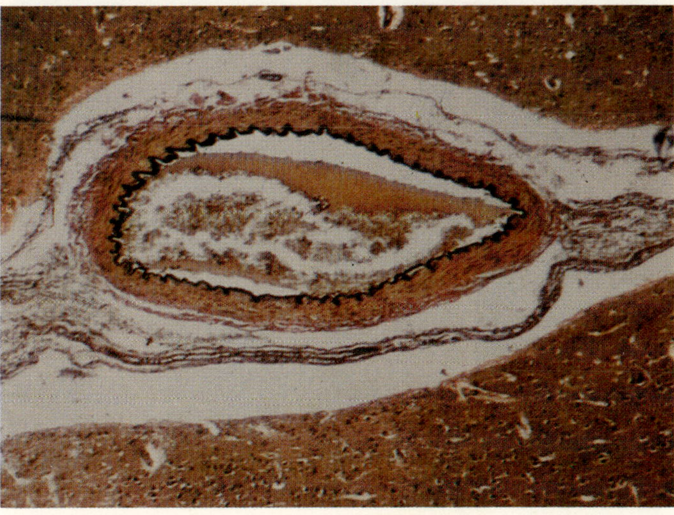

F. Anterior spinal artery showing the internal elastic lamina (van Gieson's elastic fiber stain).

BIELSCHOWSKY STAIN AND ITS VARIATIONS (AXON STAIN) (Fig. 123C)

The original Bielschowsky stain involved silver impregnation of frozen sections and it demonstrated neurofibrils in the cell body and in the processes, especially the axon. Today a number of variations are available which can use paraffin or celloidin sections in addition to frozen sections. These variations, notably the *von Brownmühl method* and *Bodian staining* are especially useful for the identification of altered neurofibrils. With these methods Alzheimer neurofibrillary tangles and abnormal accumulations of 100Å neurofilaments, as well as amyloid deposits, appear as prominent black fibrils against a light background. Because of these properties, such methods are especially useful for the demonstration of senile plaques.

Although used primarily as an axon stain these silver impregnation methods do not stain every axon. When they are small and immature containing only few neurofibrillary elements, some axons such as small parallel fibers are not stained by these methods.

REFERENCE

Hirano, A., & Zimmerman, H.M.: Silver impregnation of nerve cells and fibers in celloidin sections. Arch. Neurol., 6: 114-122, 1962.

STAINING FOR GLIAL FIBRILS

Glial fibrils are characteristic of astrocytes. Under normal conditions, however, it is difficult to demonstrate these fibrils in the light microscope. They become prominent only in reactive or neoplastic astrocytes, especially in chronic lesions.

Holzer staining is the most well known method for the demonstration of glial fibrils. Gliotic areas appear blue against a pale background by this method and can even become visible to the naked eye. One limitation of the Holzer stain is its ability to stain connective tissue even more strongly than glial fibrils. Therefore, in some parts of the nervous system such as peripheral nerve or leptomeninges, its usefulness is limited. Furthermore, a certain amount of experience is required to successfully apply the method.

Another widely used technique for the demonstration of glial fibrils is *Mallory's phosphotungstic acid hematoxylin (PTAH) stain.* Again, glial fibrils appear blue but myelin takes up the stain in the same way. PTAH is useful for distinguishing between gliomas and sarcomas since the connective tissue is rendered brown instead of blue. Reticulin staining (see below) is also used for this purpose since it stains the connective tissue fibers but not the glial fibrils.

One difficulty with PTAH staining is its tendency to fade after prolonged exposure to intense illumination. In addition, the tissue should be fixed in Zenker's solution. If formalin is used special variations must be applied for successful PTAH staining or the results may be variable. It should also be noted that the major constituent of the stain requires a six month period of storage for "ripening".

MYELIN STAINING (Fig. 102)

Luxol fast blue (LFB) is the most commonly used stain for myelin. Unlike most other myelin stains which render the myelin brownish-black, LFB results in blue-colored myelin sheaths. Usually, a red counterstain is used such as neutral red or PAS. Either will result in a purple color of the peripheral myelin, but the PAS does not stain central myelin so that it remains blue after *LFB-PAS* staining. LFB-PAS is, therefore, a useful method to distinguish between central and peripheral myelin (Feigin and Cravioto, 1961).

LFB can be used with paraffin, celloidin embedding or with frozen sections. In general, thicker sections are preferred for easy visualization of the myelin so that 15 micron sections are used rather than the usual seven microns.

Another advantage of LFB is its stability so that it can be used in combination with other stains such as Nissl staining. The combination of LFB and Nissl staining is usually referred to as *Klüver-Barrera staining*.

The classical methods in neuropathology for staining myelin such as Kultschitzky staining, require celloidin embedding. This method yields beautiful preparations, but it requires many days to perform and the blocks are not suitable for any other staining. The *Woelcke method* overcomes some of these difficulties. It requires only a few days to perform and the same block can be used for Nissl staining. It must be noted that central myelin always stains well with the Woelcke method but the reaction of peripheral myelin is more variable and sometimes it will not stain at all. Such results should not be construed as indicating demyelination. Woelcke staining can also be used for paraffin sections.

Other stains, too, can be used with paraffin. These include Heidenhain and Weil staining among a number of others. They all result in black-colored myelin.

REFERENCE

Feigin, I., & Cravioto, H.: A histochemical study of myelin. A difference in the solubility of the glycolipid components in the central and peripheral nervous systems. J. Neuropathol. Exp. Neurol., 20: 245-254, 1961.

SUDAN STAINING (Figs. 123, 124)

The central nervous system of the normal adult is devoid of sudanophilic lipid material. When present it is usually found within macrophages and is a sign of pathology. Sudan staining is a good method for the demonstration of myelin breakdown and is therefore often used in combination with a myelin stain.

Sudan staining requires frozen sections. Neutral fat stains red and a blue counterstain such as hematoxylin is usually used. For visualization of the myelin the use of frozen sections requires that nearby sections be treated with a method such as the Spielmeyer technique.

RETICULIN FIBERS AND CONNECTIVE TISSUE STAINING

Wilder's method is one of the most commonly used techniques for the demonstration of connective tissue fibers in the central nervous system. These fibers are rendered black by this method. Under normal circumstances Wilder-positive material is limited to the subarachnoid space and to the perivascular spaces. When found in the brain parenchyma it is a sign of pathology. Sarcomas in the parenchyma may be differentiated from gliomas by the presence of Wilder-positive material.

Masson trichrome staining is another useful connective tissue stain. It stains the connective tissue bluish green while muscles, red blood cells and myelin stain reddish-brown. The cores of Lewy bodies appear red (Fig. 123).

The internal elastic lamina of the larger blood vessels is stained a distinct black with the *elastic tissue van Gieson stain* (Fig. 123F). This is an effective method for differentiating between arteries and abnormally thickened A-V malformations. In parts of the sacs of most aneurysms the internal elastic lamina is either absent or fragmented. This phenomenon is clearly demonstrated by this technique.

OPTICAL STAINING FOR PLASTIC EMBEDDED MATERIAL (Fig. 125)

Conventional methods for the preparation of tissues for electron microscopic study include glutaraldehyde fixation followed by osmium tetroxide post-fixation, dehydration and embedding in a plastic such as Epon. This material can be used for optical study as well and results in some of the best preparations available. The method can also be used on formalin-fixed tissue even after prolonged storage but the preservation is less than excellent.

One drawback of this method is the small size of the sample since fixation adequate for electron microscopy requires small samples and it is extremely difficult to cut large sections of the hard plastic. In addition, special diamond or glass knives mounted on either an ultramicrotome or special adaptors for rotary microtomes are required.

The most convenient stain for the plastic tissue is toluidine blue. It must be noted that this is not a specific Nissl stain under these circumstances and that a great deal of the color is due to the osmification of the tissue. The image is therefore quite different from that perceived in paraffin or celloidin sections and some experience is required for proper interpretation.

The strong points of the method are the superb clarity with which tissue components can be visualized as well as the possibility of examining selected areas of interest in thin sections by electron microscopy. The latter must be stained with uranyl or lead salts, usually with both, for adequate contrast in the electron microscope.

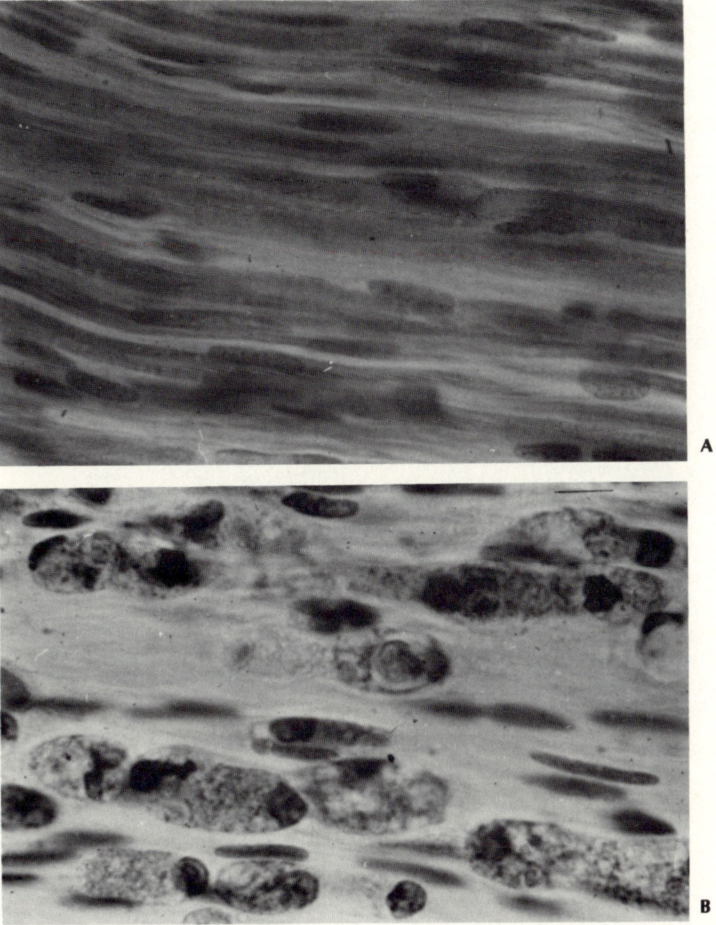

Fig. 124 Sudan stain of peripheral nerve.
A. Normal. B. Degeneration. Macrophages filled with sudanophilic lipid granules are visible.

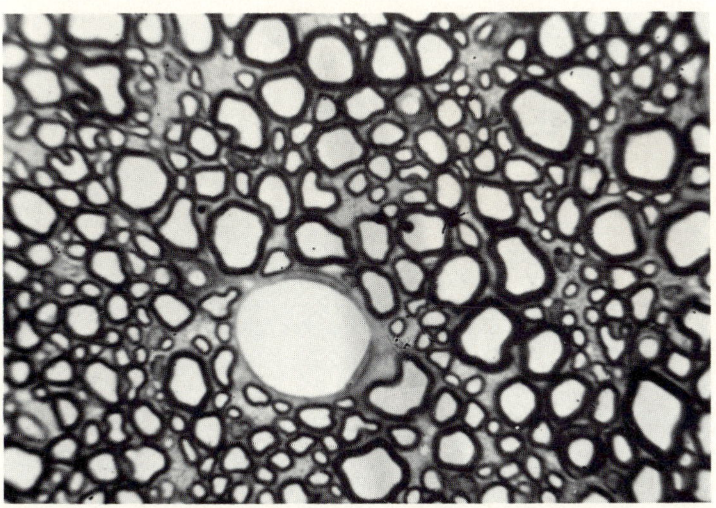

Fig. 125 Cross section of peripheral nerve (toluidine blue stain of an Epon embedded section).

IMMUNOHISTOCHEMISTRY

Recently, as in other fields, immunohistochemical methods have begun to be applied in neuropathology. This method depends on the use of a specific antibody for the localization of a tissue antigen. A marker such as fluorescein or peroxidase is attached either to the specific antibody or, in the indirect method, to another antibody directed against the specific antibody. The fluorescein or the peroxidase is then visualized by conventional means. The latter may also be detected in the electron microscope. These methods have been successfully utilized for the detection of glial fibrillary acidic protein, myelin basic protein, herpes virus and other antigens.

REFERENCES

Duffy, P.E., Graf, L., & Rapport, M.M.: Identification of glial fibrillary acidic protein by the immunoperoxidase method in human brain tumors. J. Neuropathol. Exp. Neurol. 36:645-652, 1977.

Deck, J.H.N., Eng, L.F., Bigbee, J., & Woodcock, S.M.: The role of glial fibrillary acidic protein in the diagnosis of central nervous system tumors. Acta Neuropathol. 42: 183-190, 1978.

Kumanishi, T., & Hirano, A.: An immunoperoxidase study on herpes simplex virus encephalitis. J. Neuropathol. Exp. Neurol., 37: 790-795, 1978.

Itoyama, Y., Sternberger, N.H., Webster, H.deF., Quarles, R.H., Cohen, S.R., & Richardson, E.P. Jr.: Immunocytochemical observations of the distribution of myelin-associated glycoprotein and myelin basic protein in multiple sclerosis lesions. Ann. Neurol. 7:167-177, 1980.

II
Neuropathology at the Cell Level

The central nervous system is composed of several cell types including neurons, glial cells and vascular cells, especially endothelium. It is our purpose in this section to describe the morphology of these cells at both the optical and electron microscopic levels and to illustrate some of their pathological alterations.

It is highly recommended for the student to become well acquainted with the normal histology of the nervous system which is necessary for the proper appreciation of pathological changes.

REFERENCE

Peters, A., Palay, S.L., & Webster, H. DeF.: The Fine Structure of the Nervous System. The Cells and Their Processes. Harper & Row, New York, 1970.

A. NEURONS (Fig. 126)

The neuron is the principal cell of the central nervous system. It is a stationary cell, incapable of division when mature and morphologically characterized by the presence of well-formed cell processes, an axon and dendrites. Functionally, the neuron is specialized for the propagation of impulses over its surface leading to the transmission of these impulses across synapses. This arrangement results in a

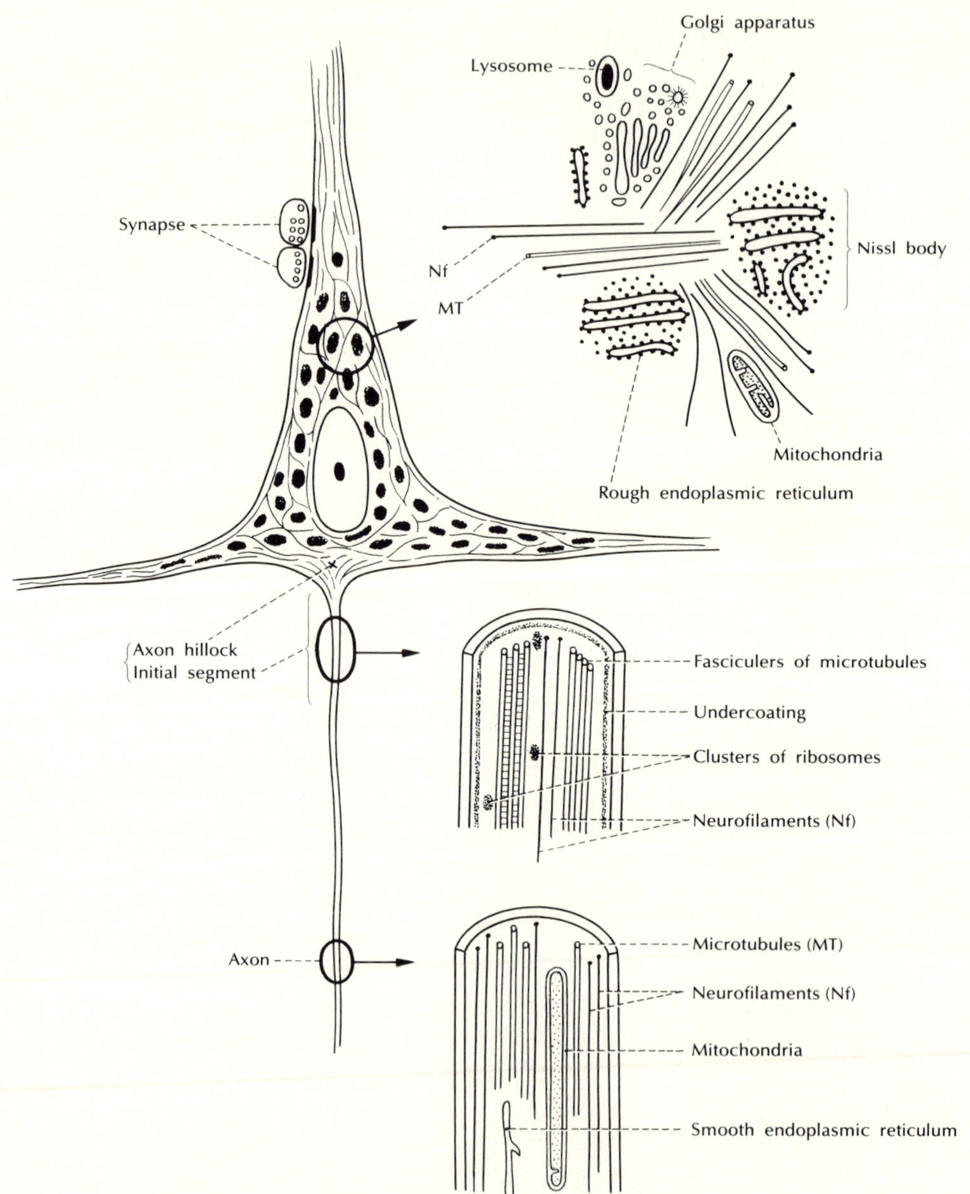

Fig. 126 A diagram of the fine structure of the neuron.

communicative network extending between individual neurons and between neurons and other target cells, especially muscles and glands.

Despite their fundamental similarities neurons display a wide range of morphological diversity in both form and size. Their shape can vary from the pyramidal to the spherical shape of the dorsal root ganglia. Some neurons, such as the Purkinje cells of the cerebellum have special shapes of their own. Their size varies from the large anterior horn cells of the cervical or lumbar cords and Betz cells, about 80 microns in width, to the tiny granule cells of the cerebellum which are only five or six microns in diameter.

The association of neurons with other cells of the nervous system can also vary. Certain neurons, such as Purkinje cells, are invariably associated with satellite cells which, in the central nervous system, are glia. In another, more important sense, the relationship of each neuron with other cells is different from that of any other neuron. Unlike other organs, the specific position of each neuron and its connection with other cells is unique.

1. Nucleus

The nuclei of neurons are not substantially different from those of other cells. Their size is generally proportional to the size of the neuron in which they reside. Usually the nucleus is in the center of the soma but, in certain neurons such as those in Clarke's column, the nuclei are most often at the periphery of the cell body.

In the large nuclei the usually single nucleolus is especially prominent in the relatively clear nucleoplasm. This results in a characteristic "fish eye" appearance which is a convenient feature differentiating neurons from the nearby astrocytes. The size and position of the nucleolus varies according to the functional state of the neuron. Nucleoli contain RNA, the amount of which varies with the activities of the cell unlike the DNA of the chromatin which remains constant in the neuron.

In the electron microscope the nucleoli can be shown to consist of a granulofilamentous network, the nucleolonema, and a fine granular ground substance, the pars amorpha. There is no limiting membrane separating the nucleolus from the nucleoplasm. The nucleus itself is surrounded by a characteristic double nuclear membrane which consists of two unit membranes. The internal membrane is generally smooth and closely applied to the nucleoplasm unlike the outer nuclear membrane which is studded with ribosomes and is part of the rough endoplasmic reticulum. The two membranes join in various places resulting in numerous nuclear pores, each of which is occluded by a fine diaphragm.

One of the most well-known pathological changes of the neuronal nucleus is the appearance of *eosinophilic intranuclear inclusion bodies*. These can sometimes serve as diagnostic criteria for certain kinds of viral encephalites. Often, in infections of herpes virus or in subacute sclerosing panencephalitis (SSPE) (p. 276), these inclusions are found to be accumulations of the specific viral particles themselves (Fig. 260). On the other hand, the eosinophilic inclusions in these conditions can sometimes be other abnormal products or even simple cytoplasmic invaginations into the nucleus. *The Marinesco body* (Fig. 127), which is apparently unrelated to viruses, is another eosinophilic inclusion often found in pigmented neurons of the substantia nigra in the normal aged brain. These are usually single, but sometimes a few are present in the same nucleus. They are often about the same size as the nucleolus, but are easy to differentiate because of their staining differences. They are also devoid of a limiting membrane and are composed of a fine granular matrix in which filaments are sometimes found in a lattice-like arrangement (Leestma and Andrews, 1969; Ikeda, 1974).

REFERENCES

Ikeda, K.: A study of the Marinesco body in monkey (Macaca fuscata). A comparative study to the Marinesco body in man. Folia Psychiatr. Neurol. Jpn., 76: 778-792, 1974.

Leestma, J.E., & Andrews, J.M.: The fine structure of the Marinesco body. Arch. Path., 88: 431-436, 1969.

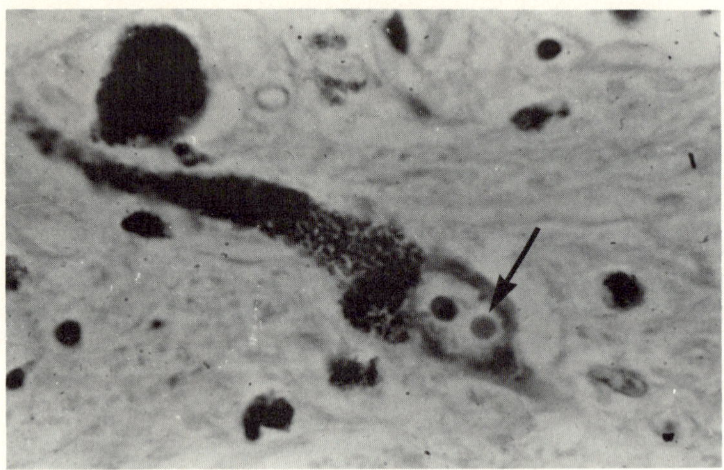

Fig. 127 A Marinesco body (arrow) in the nucleus of a pigmented neuron of the substantia nigra.

2. Nissl Substance (Fig. 128A, 129A)

Nissl substance is a characteristic feature of large neurons which stains blue with aniline dye (p. 107). It is found in the perikaryon and proximal portion of the dendrite but is absent in the axon hillock and the axon itself. Fine structural studies have revealed that Nissl bodies are, in fact, large, focal accumulations of rough endoplasmic reticulum. Bundles of microtubules and neurofilaments accompanied by other organelles, especially mitochondria may be found between the Nissl bodies. The rough endoplasmic reticulum consists of stacks of flattened, membrane-bounded cisternae, the surfaces of which are studded with ribosomes. The function of the Nissl body is apparently the same as that of the rough endoplasmic reticulum in other cells, namely, the production of protein for export.

In addition to the ribosomes attached to the membranes of the rough endo-

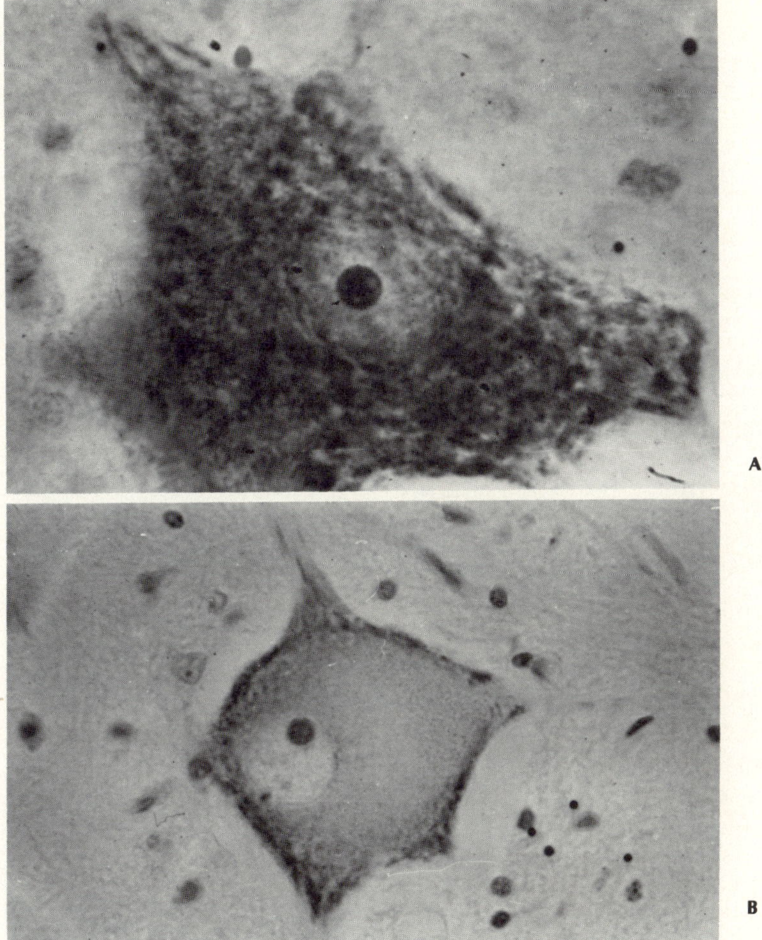

Fig. 128 Anterior horn cells (Nissl stain).
A. Normal (see Fig. 123-1, B) B. Chromatolysis.

plasmic reticulum, the neuronal cell body contains numerous *free ribosomes*, often arranged in rosette formations known as *polysomes*. The function of these ribosomes is presumably related to the synthesis of protein destined for use within the cell itself. This divergence of function between the free and the bound ribosome is reflected in the fine structure of developing neurons in which free ribosomes predominate and Nissl substance is relatively inconspicuous.

CHROMATOLYSIS (Figs. 128B, 129B)

A number of pathological processes affect the Nissl substance. Perhaps the most well known change of the Nissl substance is its loss known as *chromatolysis*, especially as seen in the large motor neurons such as the anterior horn cells or in the hypoglossal nucleus. This may be the result of trauma to the axon, also known as axonal reaction, or it may be associated with the acute stage of a number of

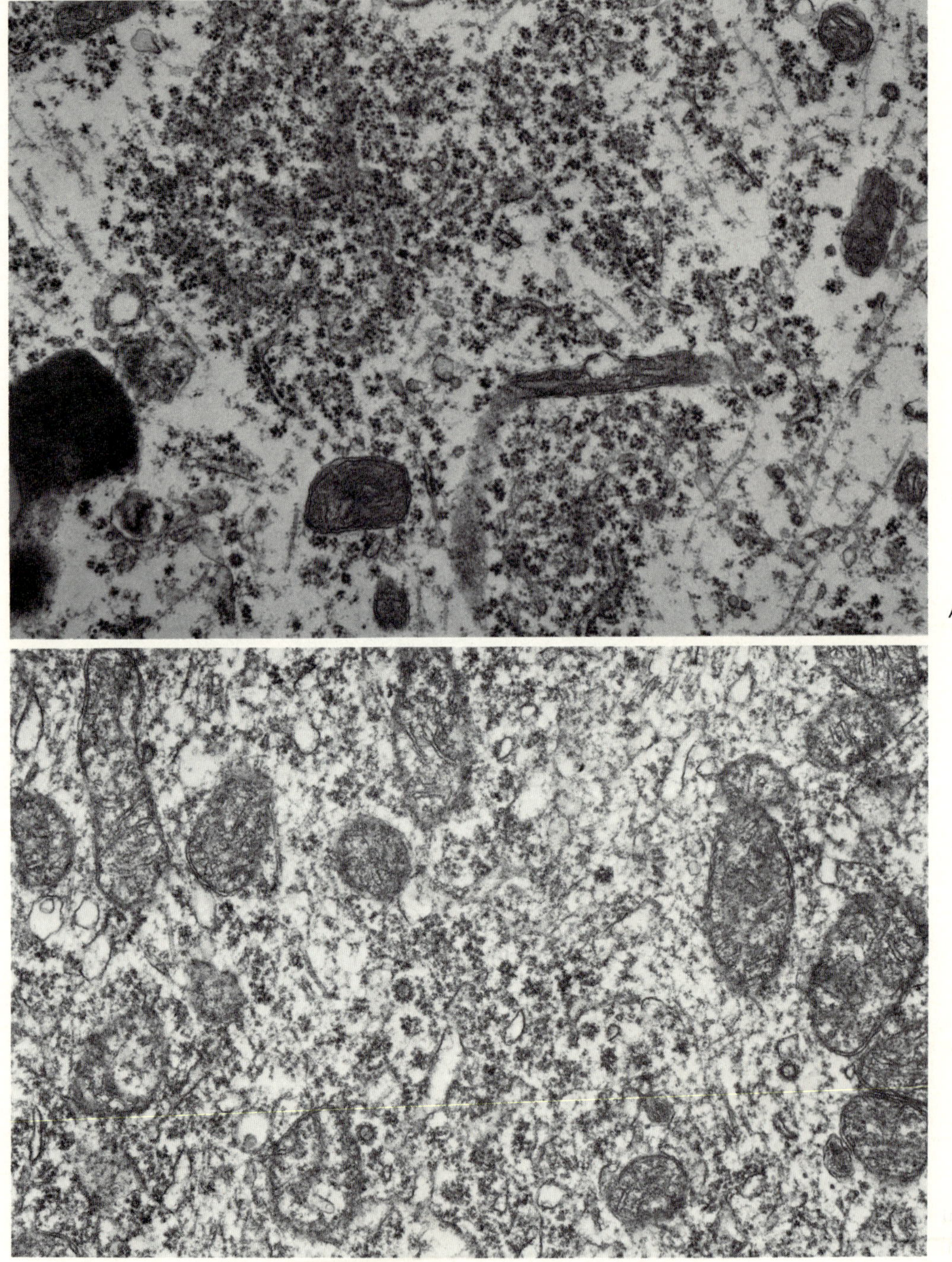

Fig. 129 Fine structure of anterior horn cells.
A. Nissl substance in the normal cell. × 30,000.
B. Chromatolysis in an affected cell. × 30,000.

diseases which have an effect on or near motor neurons such as poliomyelitis. Chromatolysis is characterized by swelling of the perikaryon, the eccentric position of the nucleus and the confinement of the small remnants of the Nissl substance to the margin of the cell. The bulk of the cytoplasm appears homogenous.

In the electron microscope the chromatolytic neuron is characterized by the relative absence of rough endoplasmic reticulum and, usually, the accumulation of filaments, tubules, smooth endoplasmic reticulum and mitochondria. Free ribosomes are abundant. Lysosomes are often present in increased numbers (Lieberman, 1971; Price and Griffin, 1976). On the other hand, some chromatolytic neurons do not show all of these changes. Betz cells, for example, show loss of Nissl substance after axonal section but some of the other changes described above such as filament accumulation may not be present (Barron and Dentinger, 1979).

The fate of chromatolytic neurons is not always certain. Apparently some can recover while others die.

Chromatolysis is sometimes accompanied by *satellitosis*, which is an increase in the number of satellite cells surrounding a neuronal perikaryon. Some workers regard this change as the first step in neuronophagia (see p. 196). On the other hand, the presence of these cells may represent a protective function of the glial cells. It should be pointed out that the presence of these cells virtually covering the neuronal surface implies that the numerous synaptic connections may be at least temporarily severed. The significance of this with regard to satellitosis and chromatolysis is not clear.

REFERENCES

Lieberman, A.R.: The axon reaction: a review of the principal features of perikaryal responses to axon injury. Internat. Rev. Neurobiol., 14: 49-124, 1971.

Price, D., & Griffin, J.W.: Structural substrate of protein synthesis and transport in spinal motor neurons. *In* Amyotrophic Lateral Sclerosis. Recent research trends. pp. 1-32, Andrews, J.M., Johnson, R.T., & Brazier, M.A.B. (eds.) Academic Press, N.Y., 1976.

Barron, K.D., & Dentinger, M.P.: Cytologic observations on axotomized feline Betz cells. 1. Qualitative electron microscopic findings. J. Neuropathol. Exp. Neurol., 38: 128-151, 1979.

In addition to its actual dissolution, Nissl substance may react in a variety of other ways.

LAMELLAR BODIES (Figs. 130, 131)

The lamellar body consists of short stacks of membranous cisterns. Ribosomes are present predominantly at the periphery of the body. It is seen predominantly in cerebellar Purkinje cells where it may be the result of poor preservation or other unknown causes. Lamellar bodies have been rarely seen in other neurons under certain conditions (Fig. 131), but only rarely.

REFERENCE

Herndon, R.M.: Lamellar bodies, an unusual arrangement of the granular endoplasmic reticulum. J. Cell Biol., 20: 338-342, 1964.

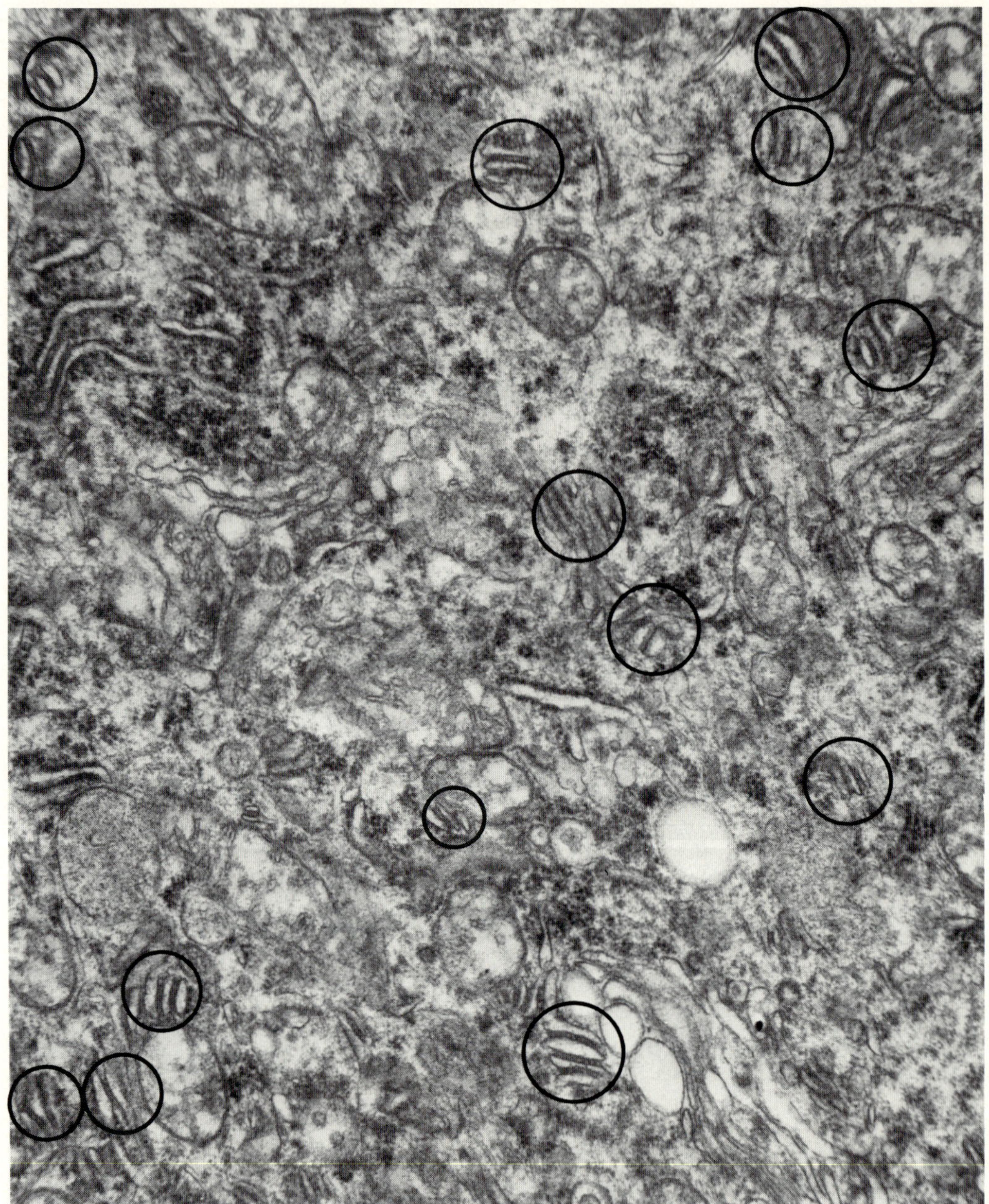

Fig. 130 Lamellar bodies (circles) in a Purkinje cell. × 36,000.

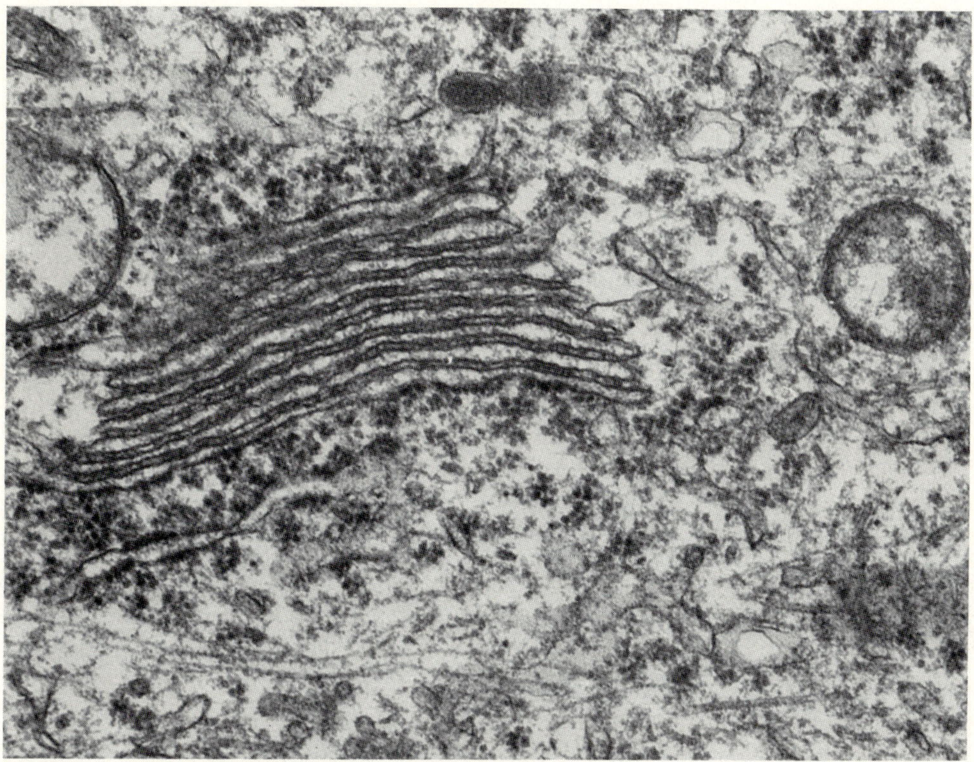

Fig. 131 A lamellar body in the dorsal root ganglion of a mutant hamster. × 50,000. (From Hirano, A.: J. Neuropathol. Exp. Neurol. 37: 75, 1978.)

ANNULATE LAMELLAE (Figs. 132, 133)

This stucture is similar in stucture to the lamellar body described above but, in addition, the membranes of adjacent lamellae apparently fuse forming numerous, regularly arranged pores similar to nuclear pores. Annulate lamellae are normal constituents of a variety of neuronal and non-neuronal cells such as oocytes. They are normally found in neurons of the lateral geniculate body and dorsal root ganglia in at least some species (Hirano, 1978). They are not uncommon in developing cells and can be found in pituitary adenoma and in germinoma among other neoplasms (Fig. 133). They have also been described in anterior horn cells undergoing retrograde degeneration in the cat and in humans with amyotrophic lateral sclerosis.

REFERENCE

Hirano, A.: Changes of the neuronal endoplasmic reticulum in the peripheral nervous system in mutant hamsters with hind leg paralysis and normal controls. J. Neuropathol. Exp. Neurol., 37: 75-84, 1978.

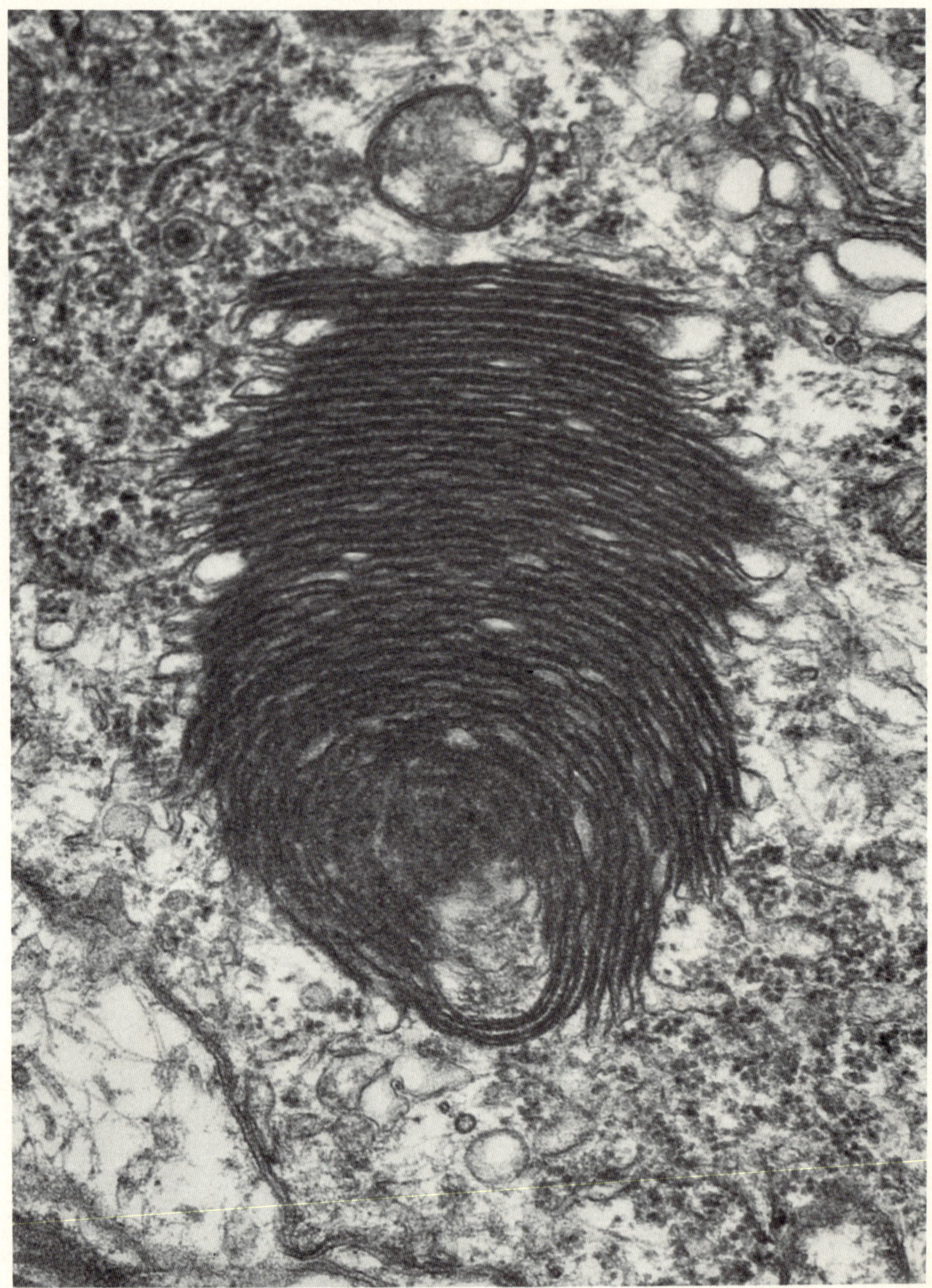

Fig. 132 An annulate lamellae-like structure in the dorsal root ganglion of a hamster. × 49,000.

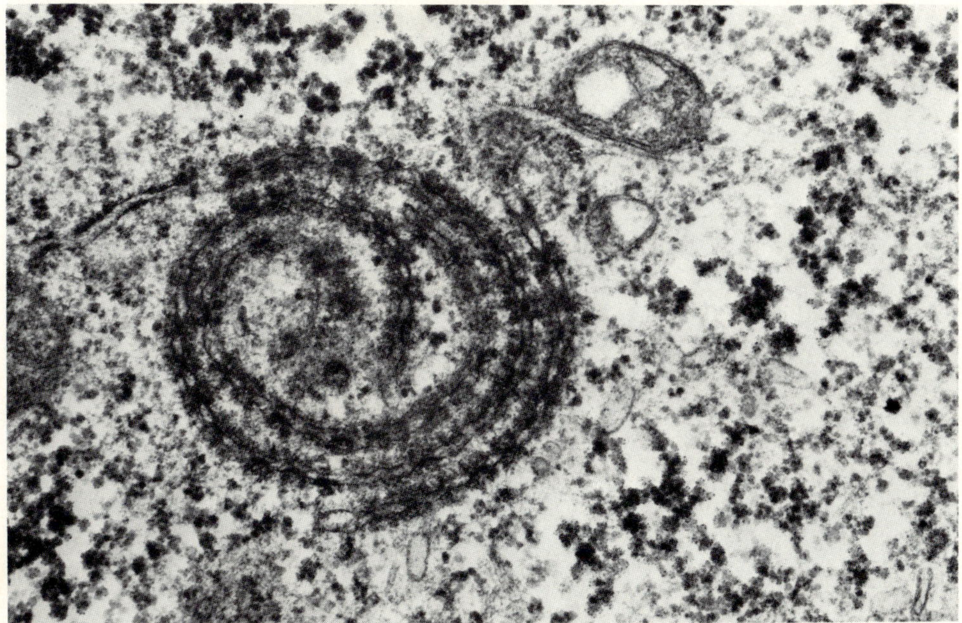

Fig. 133 A formation of annulate lamellae within a large polygonal cell in an intracranial germinoma. × 30,000.

MEMBRANE PARTICLE COMPLEXES (Fig. 134)

These bodies consist of stacks or concentric arrangements of membrane-bounded cisterns apparently derived from Nissl substance. They are found in the dorsal root ganglia of both normal (Pannese, 1969) and abnormal experimental animals. In these stuctures adjacent lamellae are separated by spaces containing single rows of dense granules, 200-300Å in diameter. Unlike ribosomes the granules are not attached to the membranes. They are generally considered to be glycogen so that the entire structure is sometimes referred to as a "glycogen-membrane complex".

The significance of all of these variations of the Nissl substance is not clear. While many such variations are present under normal conditions they are generally increased in number under pathological circumstances. In at least one condition, they may all be seen in a single structure (Fig. 135).

REFERENCE

Pannese, E.: Unusual membrane-particle complexes within nerve cells of the spinal ganglia. J. Ultrastruct. Res. 29: 334-342, 1969.

OTHERS

Other alterations of the Nissl substance include the presence of *virus* particles (Fig. 136), and the formation of large, lake-like distentions of the endoplasmic reticulum. The latter will be described below as an example of a cytoplasmic hyaline (colloid) inclusion (see p. 162).

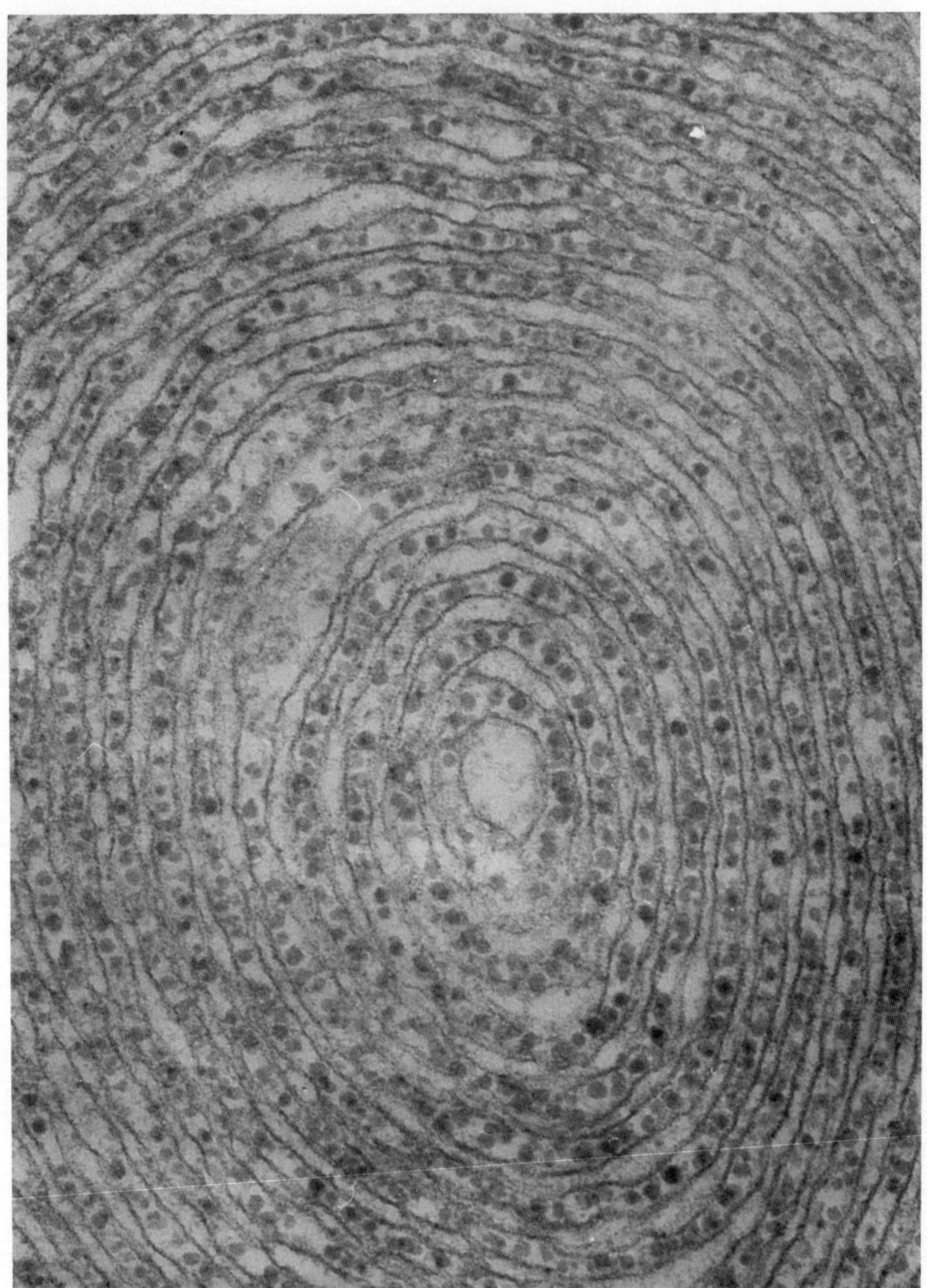

Fig. 134 A membrane-particle complex showing alternate rows of cisterns and granules. The latter are not attached to the cisternal membrane. × 100,000.
(From Hirano, A.: J. Neuropathol. Exp. Neurol. 37: 75, 1978.)

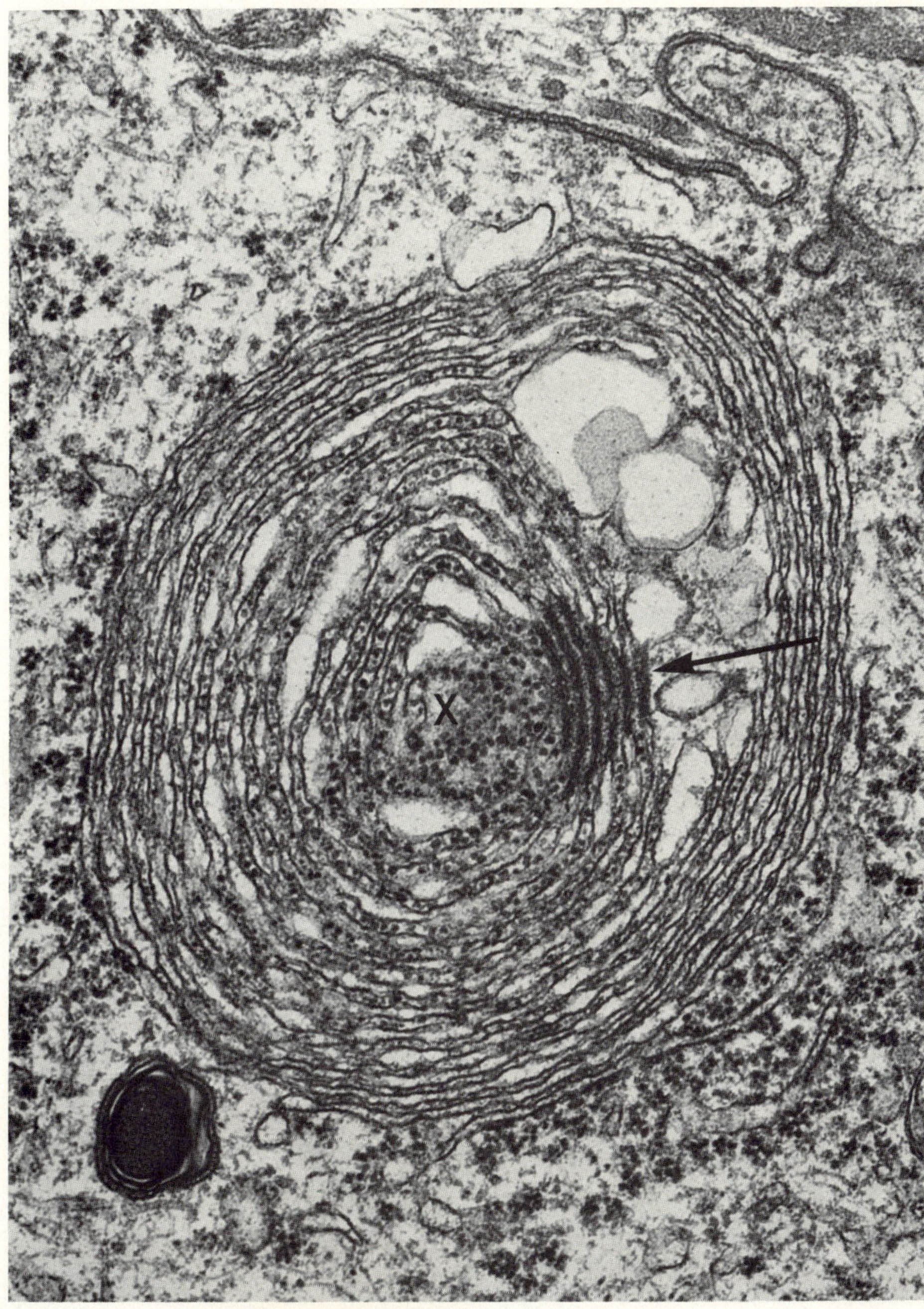

Fig. 135 Three types of alterations of the endoplasmic reticulum in a single structure. A lamellar body which includes a membrane-particle complex (X) and annulate lamellae (arrow). × 55,000.
(From Hirano, A.: J. Neuropathol. Exp. Neurol. 37: 75, 1978.)

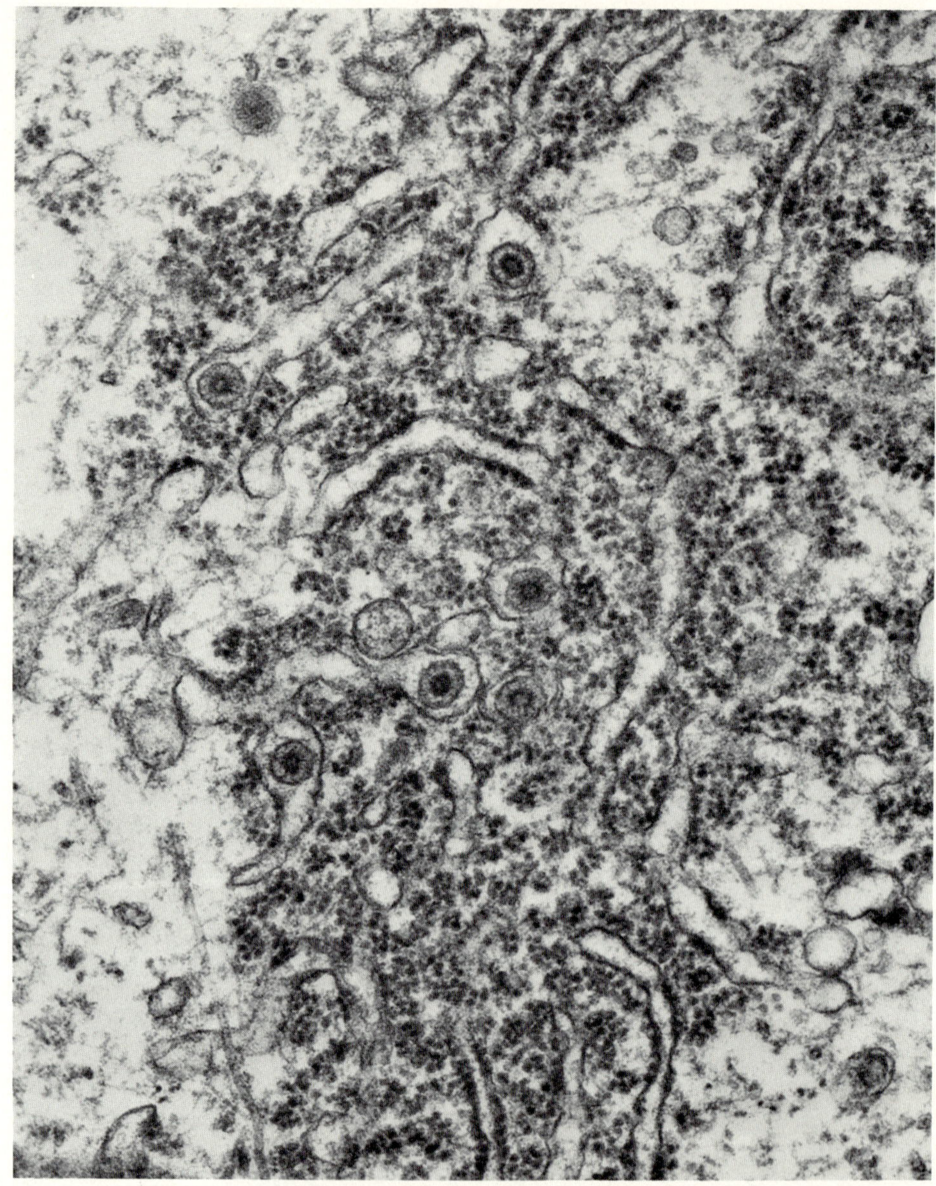

Fig. 136 Virus particles (R particles) within the cisterns of the rough endoplasmic reticulum in the dorsal root ganglion of a hamster. × 54,000.
(From Hirano, A.: J. Neuropathol. Exp. Neurol. 37: 75, 1978.)

In addition *glycogen granules* have been reported within distended cisterns of the endoplasmic reticulum in the neurons of the substantia nigra (Batty and Millhouse, 1976) and cochlear nucleus (Jew and Williams, 1977) of the Gunn rat. *Microtubule-like structures* have been described in PAS-positive, distended cisterns of the endoplasmic reticulum in cortical neurons of certain species of dogs (Suzuki et al, 1978).

REFERENCES

Batty, H.K., & Millhouse, O.E.: Ultrastructure of the Gunn rat substantia nigra. Acta Neuropathol., 34: 7-19, 1976.

Jew, J.Y., & Williams, T.H.: Ultrastructural aspects of bilirubin encephalopathy in cochlear nuclei of the Gunn rat. J. Anat., 124: 599-614, 1977.

Suzuki, Y., Atoji, Y., & Suu, S.: Microtubules observed within the cisterns of RER in neurons of the aged dog. Acta Neuropathol., 44: 155-158, 1978.

3. Lipofuscin and Other Pigments

LIPOFUSCIN (Fig. 137)

Lipofuscin granules are common features of a variety of neurons especially in aged brains. They remain their original yellow-brown color in H&E stain but are metachromatic and stain green in Nissl preparations. In silver impregnation techniques they remain unstained in contrast to melanin deposits. In neurons with large amounts of lipofuscin granules, silver impregnation can sometimes result in a honeycomb-like appearance in which the peripheries of the granules are outlined.

The topographical distribution of lipofuscin granules has always been considered quite distinct. They are prominent in the inferior olivary nucleus of the medulla, the dentate nucleus of the cerebellum, the dorsal root ganglia and the anterior horn cells of the spinal cord even in young individuals and they increase with age. In other neurons, however, such as the Purkinje cells of the cerebellum they were considered absent under normal conditions and were detected only during pathology. The electron microscope, however, has revealed the fact that they may be present, although in small numbers, even in normal Purkinje cells. Similarly, it was shown that, contrary to earlier belief, they are present in a number of experimental animals in addition to humans and other primates.

Lipofuscin granules consist of a membrane-bounded particle containing either dense, finely granular substance and/or a less dense, homogenous material often adjacent to one another in the same particle. Most workers consider these to be "residual bodies" or the remains of phagosomes which have been incompletely digested by lysosomes.

Accumulations of lipofuscin granules are prominent in certain parts of the central nervous system in senile dementia, Alzheimer's disease and in amyotrophic lateral sclerosis, etc. The effect of lipofuscin on neuronal function, however, remains unknown. In lipofuscinosis, a kind of lipidosis, there is an increase in the number of lipofuscin granules spread over a wider than normal distribution involving a number of neuronal systems. In other types of lipofuscinosis abnormal *curvilinear bodies* (Duffy et al, 1968; Gonatas et al, 1968) and *finger print-like* inclusions (Suzuki et al, 1968) have been seen.

The prominence of lipofuscin granules in aged neurons is presumably related to the fact that neurons do not turn over and so, like cardiac muscle, may accumulate residual bodies. Why certain neurons do so to a greater degree than others is a mystery. Tomlinson (1979) has published a concise review of current literature on lipofuscin and other changes associated with aging.

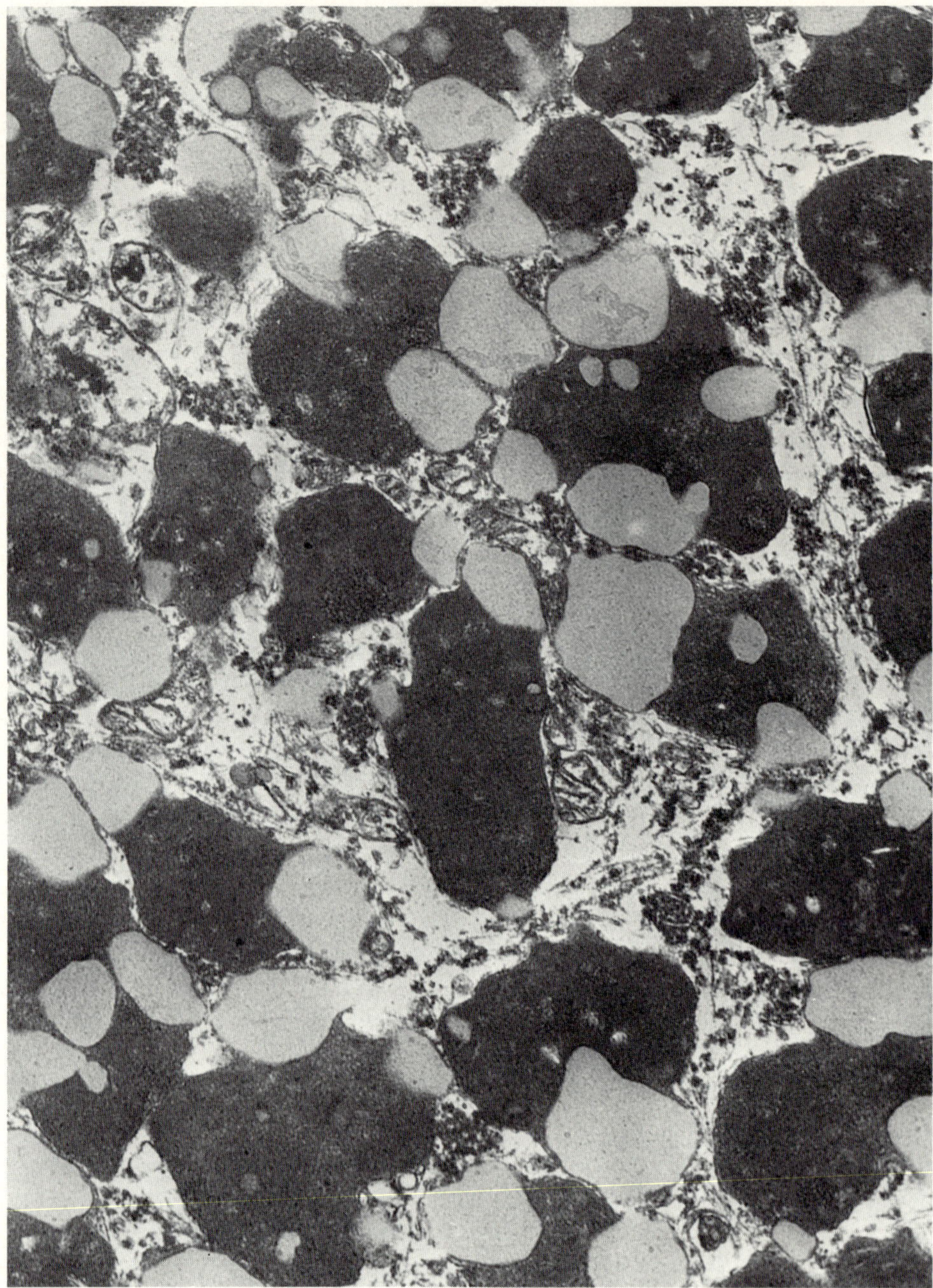

Fig. 137 Lipofuscin granules in the anterior horn cell of a patient with amyotrophic lateral sclerosis. × 36,000.

REFERENCES

Fine, D.I.M., Barron, K.D., & Hirano, A.: Central nervous system lipidosis in an adult with atrophy of the cerebellar granular layer: A case report. J. Neuropathol. Exp. Neurol., 19: 355-369, 1960.

Suzuki, K., Johnson, A.B., Marquet, E., & Suzuki, K.: A case of juvenile lipidosis: Electron microscopic, histochemical and biochemical studies. Acta Neuropathol., 11: 122-139, 1968.

Duffy, P.E., Kornfeld, M.D., & Suzuki, K.: Neurovisceral storage disease with curvilinear bodies. J. Neuropathol. Exp. Neurol., 27: 351-370, 1968.

Gonatas, N.K., Gambetti, P., & Baird, H.: A second type of late infantile amaurotic idiocy with multilamellar cytosomes. J. Neuropathol. Exp. Neurol., 27: 371-389, 1968.

Towfighi, J., Baird, H.W., Gambetti, P., & Gonatas, N.K: The significance of cytoplasmic inclusions in late infantile and juvenile amaurotic idiocy. An ultrastructural study. Acta Neuropathol., 23: 32-42, 1973.

Zeman, W.: Studies in the neuronal ceroid-lipofuscinoses. J. Neuropathol. Exp. Neurol. 33: 1-12, 1974.

Tomlinson, B.E.: The ageing brain. *In*, Recent Advances in Neuropathology. Vol. 1 Smith, W.T., & Cavanagh, J.B. (eds.) pp. 129-159, Churchill Livingstone, Edinburgh, 1979.

NEUROMELANIN (Fig. 138)

Neuromelanin is traditionally described in connection with lipofuscin because both are intraneuronal pigment deposits which tend to increase with age. There are, however, distinct differences between the two. Neuromelanin appears dark brown in H&E preparations but, unlike lipofuscin, is strongly argentophilic. Neuromelanin deposition is limited to only certain neuronal groups, whereas lipofuscin may be found in a wide variety of neurons. Neuromelanin is most conspicuous in the zona compacta of the substantia nigra and in the locus ceruleus where the pigmentation in the adult is obvious to the naked eye. It is also present in small amounts in the dorsal motor nucleus of the vagus nerve, spinal dorsal root ganglia, sympathetic ganglia, the tegmentum of the brain stem, and in scattered neurons in the roof of the fourth ventricle. Along with neuronal degeneration, pigmentation in the locus ceruleus and the substantia nigra becomes less obvious in the aged brain (Mann and Yates, 1974). In children, the substantia nigra appears pale, but neuromelanin can be demonstrated by histochemical methods. There are certain rare congenital conditions resulting in melanosis in specific nuclei such as the dentate nucleus of the cerebellum. However, these conditions are not known to be related to any progressive pathological process (Fan et al., 1978).

Neuromelanin appears very similar to lipofuscin in the electron microscope, but contains coarse, electron dense granules in addition to the finer granular material (Hirosawa, 1968).

The neuromelanin we have been discussing is distinct from true *melanin* which is seen in skin and in the eye. Electron microscopically true melanin differs from neuromelanin in its structure and in its extreme density. It is also found in the central nervous system, but it is limited to melanophores in the leptomeninges, especially areas covering the high cervical cord and the brain stem. It is more obvious in the darker races and is absent in albinos who, incidentally, retain pigmentation in the substantia nigra, etc. Primary melanomas of the central nervous system arise from leptomeningeal melanophores and not from the neuromelanin-containing neurons.

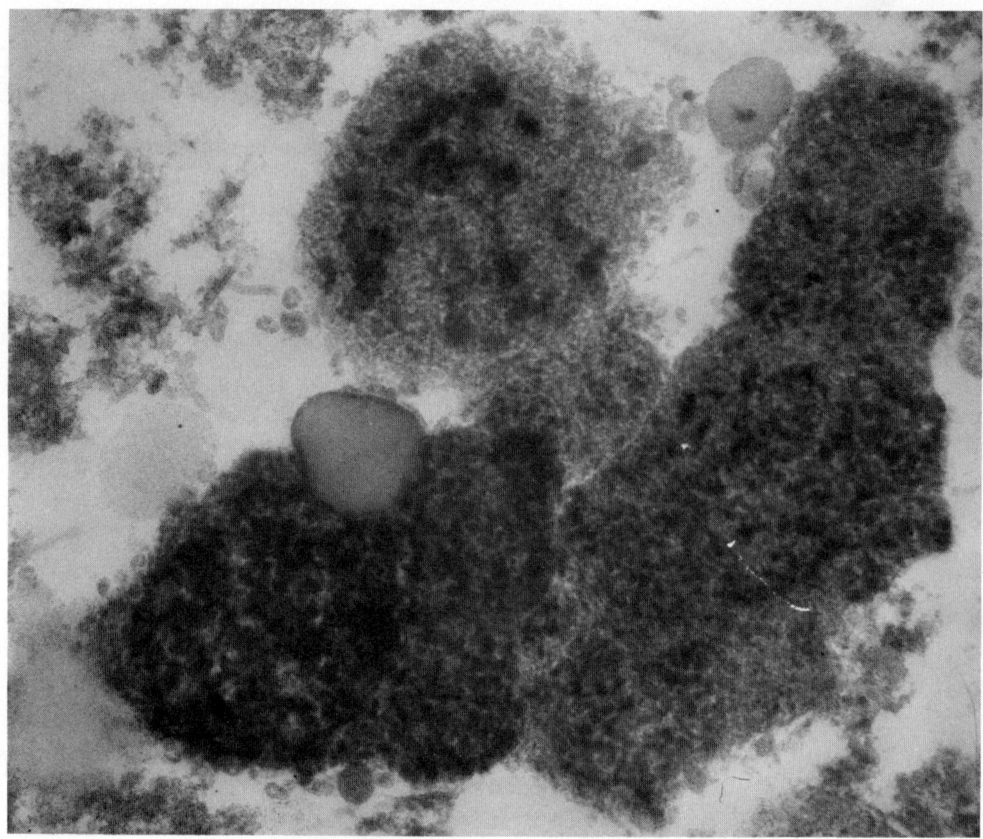

Fig. 138 Neuromelanin in the substantia nigra. × 74,000.
(From Hirano, A.: Progress in Neuropathology. Vol. 1, p. 1, Grune & Stratton, 1971.)

REFERENCES

Hirano, A., & Carton, C.A.: Primary malignant melanoma of the spinal cord. J. Neurosurg., 17: 935-944, 1960.

Hirosawa, K.: Electron microscopic studies on pigment granules in the substantia nigra and locus coeruleus of the Japanese monkey (Macca fuscata yakui). Z. Zellforsch., 88: 187-203, 1968.

Mann, D.M.A. & Yates, P.O.: Lipoprotein pigments—their relationship to aging in the human nervous system. II. The melanin content of pigmented nerve cells. Brain, 97: 489-498, 1974.

Fan, K.-J., Kovi, J., & Dulaney, S.D.: Melanosis of the dentate nucleus: Fine structure and histochemistry. Acta Neuropathol., 41: 249-251, 1978.

GRANULOVACUOLAR BODIES (Figs. 139, 140)

These structures, sometimes known as *Simchowicz bodies*, are seen in aged brains, in Alzheimer's disease, Pick's disease, and in Parkinsonism-dementia complex as seen on Guam among other conditions. They are essentially confined to the soma of the pyramidal neurons of Sommer's sector.

From a few to many of these 3-4 micron structures may be present within a

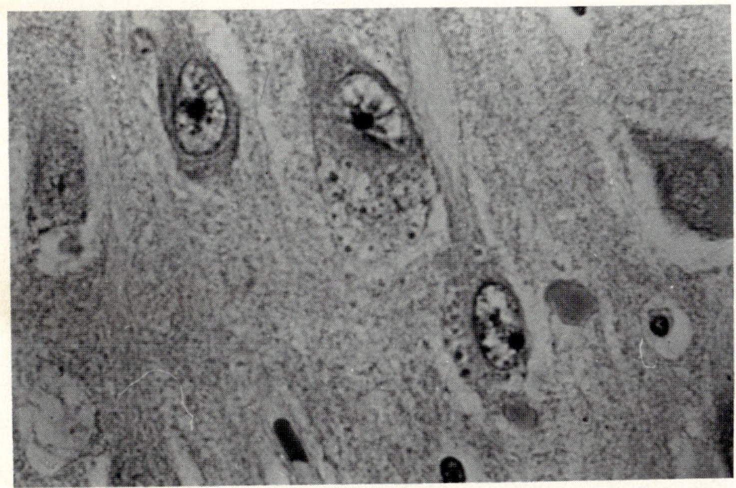

Fig. 139 Granulovacuolar bodies (H & E stain).

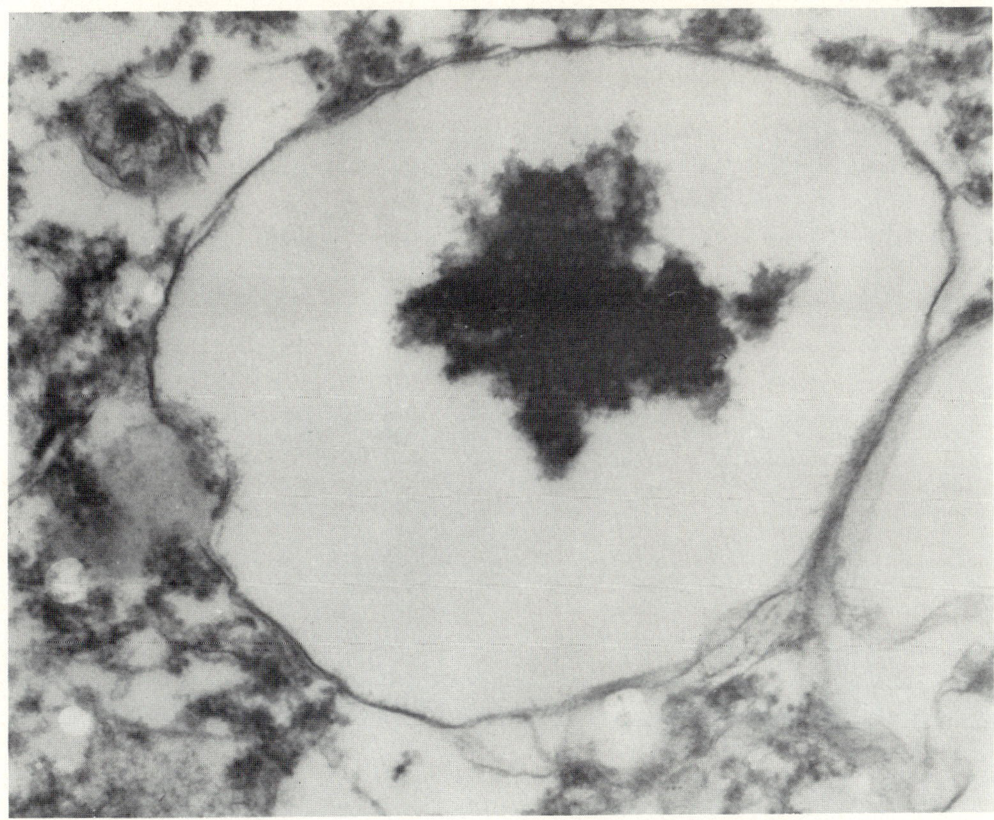

Fig. 140 Granulovacuolar body. × 45,000. (From Hirano, A. et al.: J. Neuropath. Exp. Neurol. 27: 167, 1968.)

single cell. They appear as round vacuoles with a dense core which stains blue in H&E and are argentophilic. Their fine structure consists of an outer limiting membrane enclosing a vacuolar space with a dense, granular central core.

The origin of granulovacuolar bodies is unknown. Some workers, on the basis of their morphology, believe that granulovacuolar bodies are lysosomal in nature. On the other hand, this does not explain why they are generally confined to only certain neurons in a limited area of the brain.

REFERENCE

Hirano, A., Dembitzer, H.M., Kurland, L.T., & Zimmerman, H.M.: The fine structure of some intraganglionic alterations. J. Neuropathol. Exp. Neurol., 27: 167-182, 1968.

ABNORMAL LIPID INCLUSIONS (Fig. 141)

Different lipidoses are the result of specific enzymatic deficiencies and different inclusions may be found within the neuron depending on the particular defect. The inclusions usually appear similar in H&E preparations or in Nissl staining, but they frequently show some subtle fine structural differences.

Membranous cytoplasmic bodies (*MCB's*) (Terry and Weiss, 1963) are found in Tay-Sachs disease (GM_2 gangliosidosis) among other conditions. (Fig. 142). They represent an abnormal accumulation of GM_2 gangliosides due to the lack of proper levels of hexoseaminidase A activity. *Zebra bodies* (Fig. 143) are characteristic features of Hurler's disease (Aleu et al., 1965). They consist of abnormal accumulations of mucopolysaccharides, chiefly chrondroitin sulfate B and heparan sulfate due to a decrease of α-L-iludonidase activity.

Certain intoxications may also result in the accumulation of lipids. In certain instances the inclusions may become so prominent and abundant as to mimic the true, inborn lipid storage diseases (Hirano and Llena, in press).

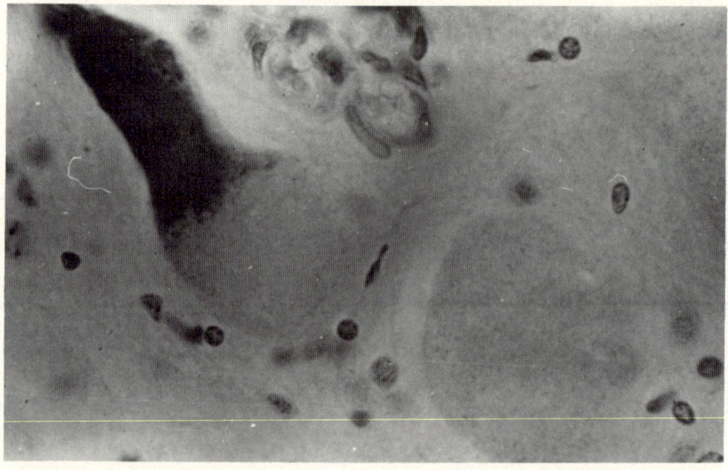

Fig. 141 Lipidosis. Anterior horn cells in lipidosis (Nissl stain).

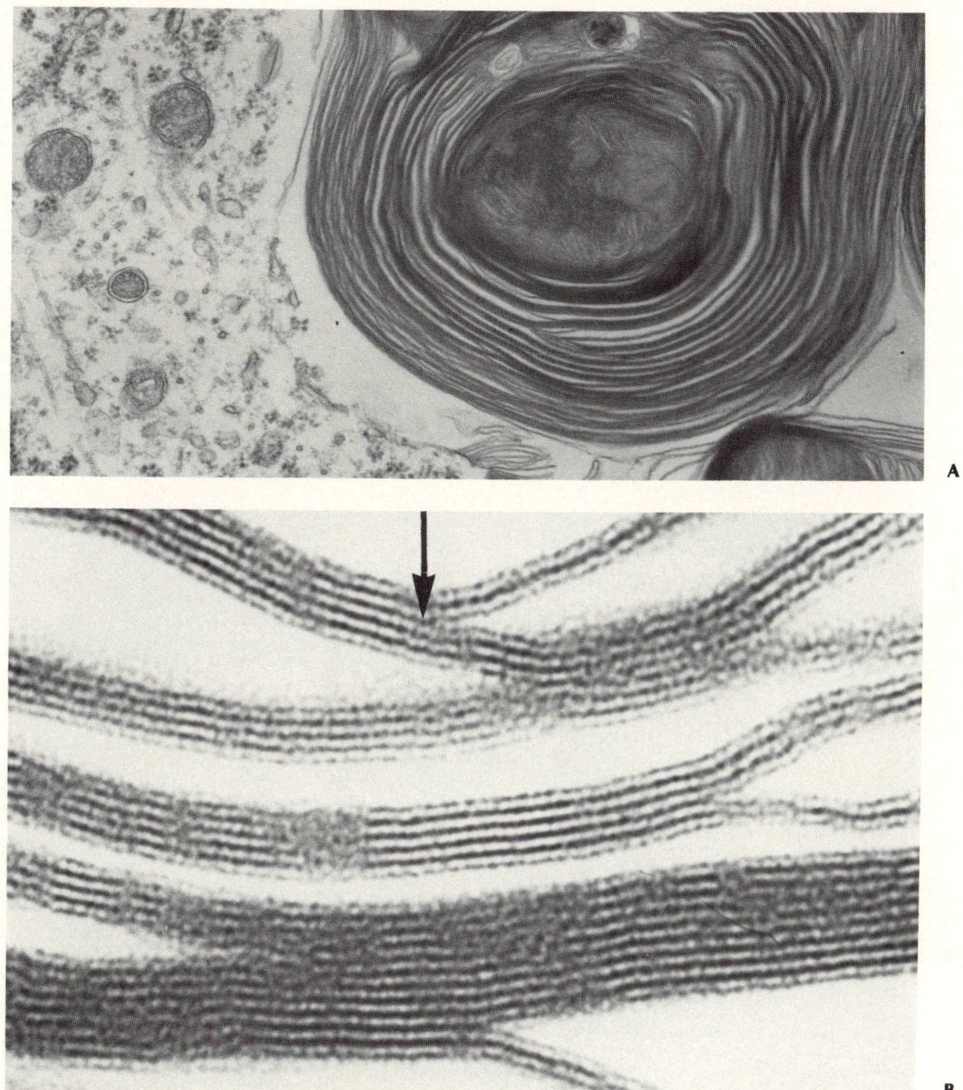

Fig. 142 Membranous cytoplasmic body (MCB). Arrow indicates fusion of two membranes. A. × 12,000. B. × 360,000.
(From Hirano, A. et al.: J. Neuropath. Exp. Neurol., 30: 470, 1971.)

REFERENCES

Korey, S.R., Terry, R.D., et al.: Studies in Tay-Sachs disease. J. Neuropathol. Exp. Neurol., 22: 2-104, 1963.

Terry, R.D., & Weiss, M.: Studies in Tay-Sachs disease. II. Ultrastructure of the cerebrum. J. Neuropathol. Exp. Neurol., 22: 18-55, 1963.

Aleu, F.P., Terry, R.D., & Zellweger, H.: Electron microscopy of two cerebral biopsies in gargoylism. J. Neuropathol. Exp. Neurol., 24: 304-317, 1965.

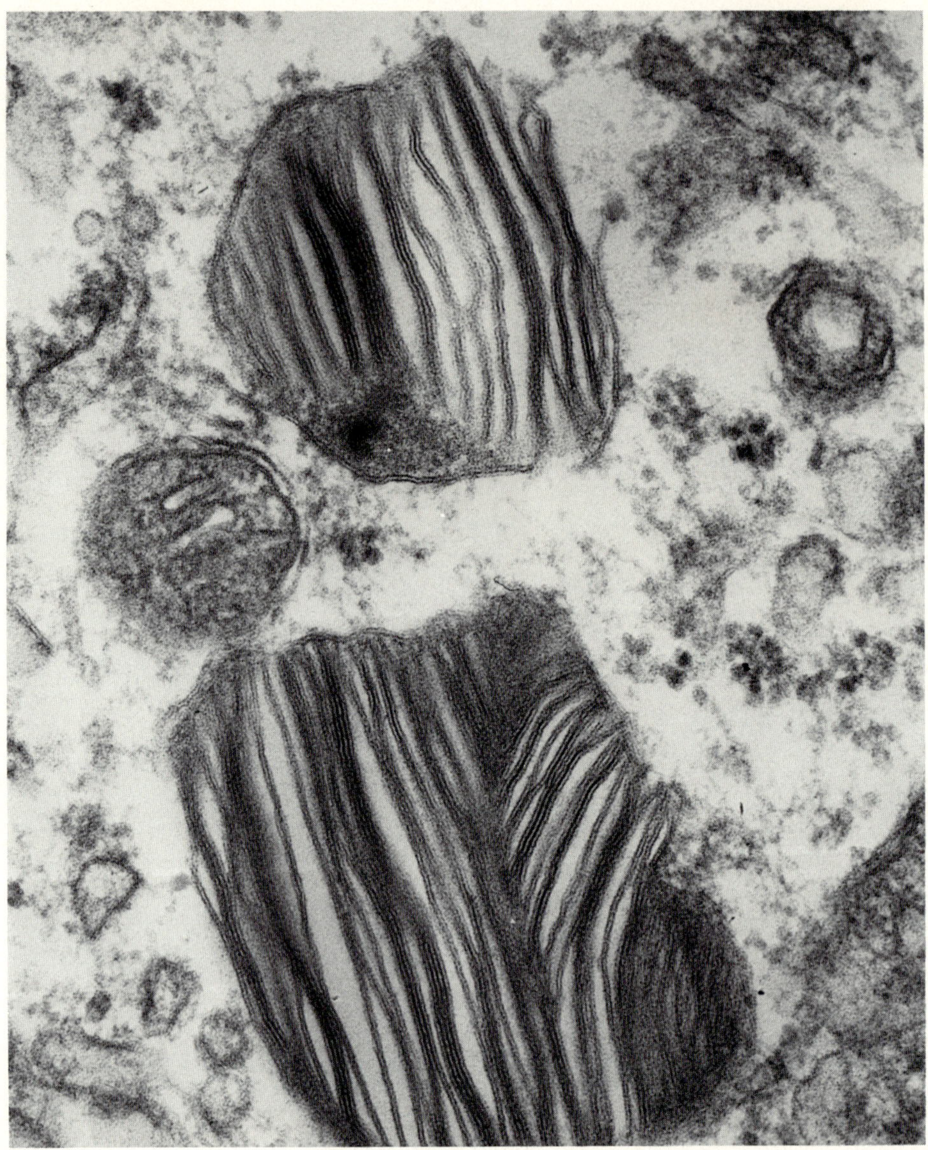

Fig. 143 Zebra bodies. × 112,000. (From Hirano, A.: Progress in Neuropathology. Vol. 1, p. 1, Grune & Stratton, 1971.)

Hirano, A., Zimmerman, H.M., Levine, S., & Padgett, G.A.: Cytoplasmic inclusions in Chediak-Higashi and wobbler mink. An electron microscopic study of the nervous system. J. Neuropathol. Exp. Neurol., 30: 470-487, 1971.

Volk, B.V., & Aronson, S.M.: Sphingolipids, Sphingolipidosis and Allied Disorders. Plenum Publishing Corp., New York, 1972.

Hirano, A., & Llena, J.F.: The central nervous system as a target site in toxic-metabolic states. *In* Experimental and Clinical Neurotoxicology. A Textbook of Environmental Neurobiology, pp. 24-34, Spencer, P.S., & Schaumberg, H.H. (eds.), The Williams and Wilkins Co., Baltimore, 1980.

4. Neurofibrils (Figs. 144, 145)

According to convention the term "nerve fiber" refers to an entire cell process such as an axon or dendrite. The term "*neurofibril*", however, is used to refer to three different fibrillar structures seen within normal neurons. These consist of microtubules, neurofilaments and the more recently described microfilaments. Microtubules and neurofilaments may be found in all parts of the neurons, i.e., the soma, the dendrites and the axons. Their proportional distribution and their arrangement may differ depending on the part of the neuron and the size of that part.

Microtubules in neurons were originally referred to as neurotubules. They are apparently, however, indistinguishable from microtubules seen in any other tissue, although they are unusually prominent in the characteristically long neuronal processes. Microtubules are circular in cross section where they appear as annuli about 240Å in diameter. Often, a central 50Å granule, the central density, may be seen in the lucent lumen of the tubule. The wall seems to be composed of helically arranged particles with thirteen particles per turn of the helix. Their length is indeterminate, but is thought to be quite long in the long neuronal processes. They maintain their width over their entire length and do not branch. Their function is not known with certainty but they are thought to be associated with intracellular transport and maintenace of cell shape.

Neurofilaments are only about 100Å in diameter although in cross section they also appear tubular in structure with a narrow central electron-lucent lumen. Their length is also unknown but they have short, fine side arms. Their function, too, is unknown but they may play the role of a cytoskeleton and be important in intracellular transport.

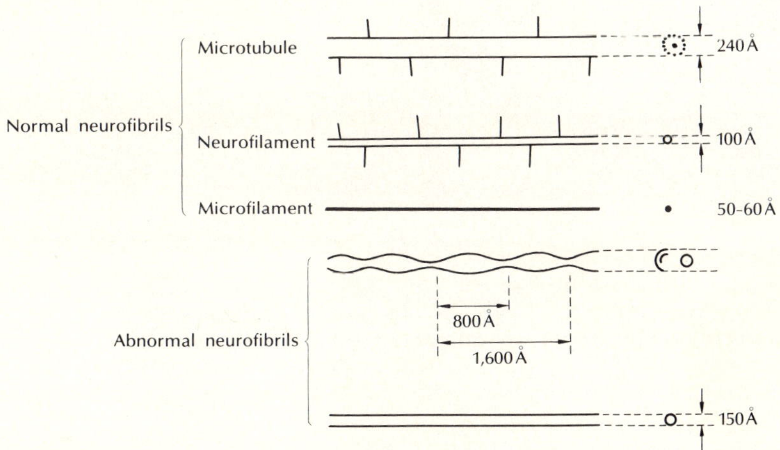

Fig. 144 Neurofibrils. (Modified from Hirano, A.: An Outline of Neuropathology, Igaku-Shoin, Tokyo, 1976, and Ishii, T.: Pathology of Dementia. Brain and Nerve (Tokyo), 31: 43, 1979.)

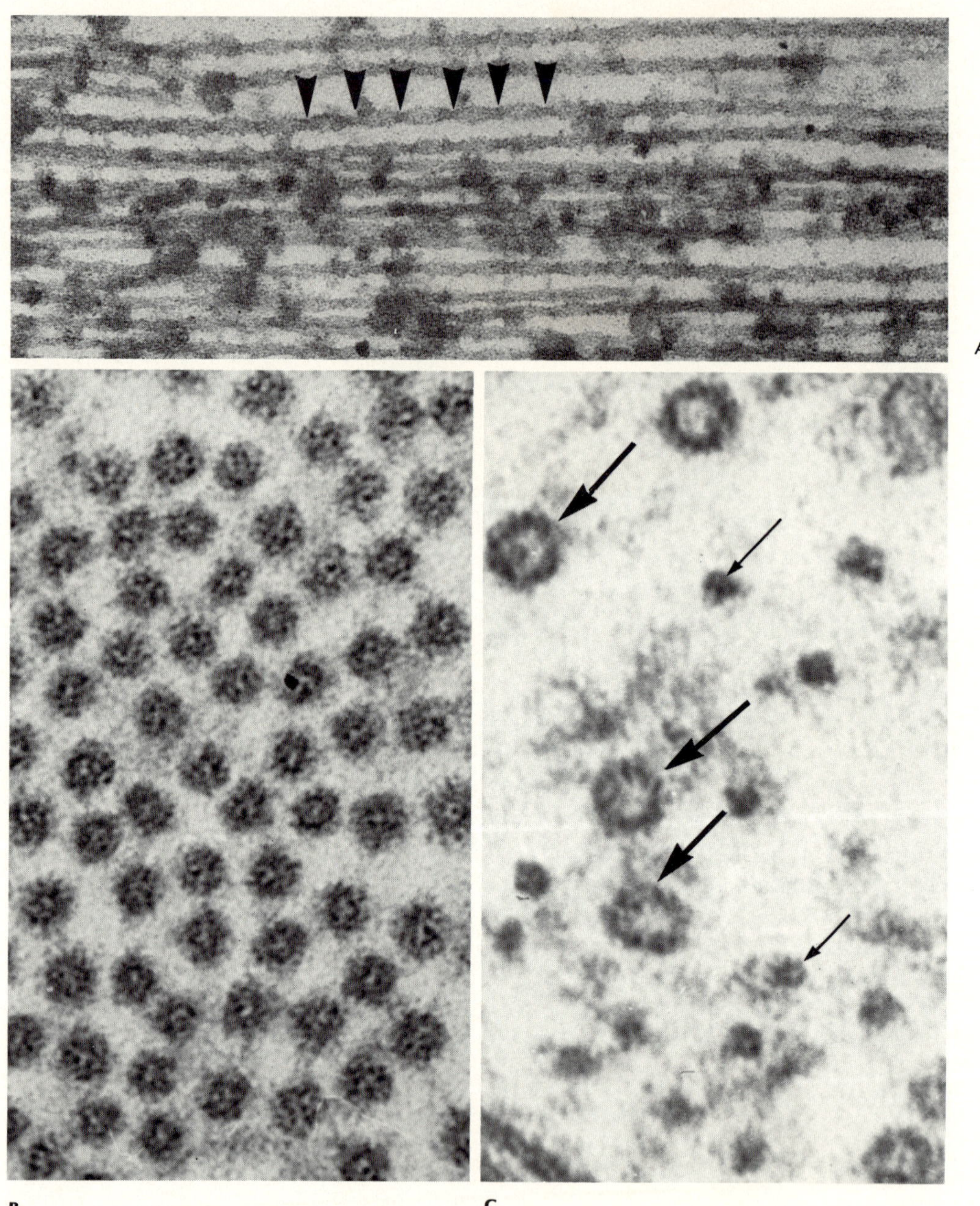

Fig. 145 Alzheimer's neurofibrillary changes. A. Longitudinal section. B. Cross section. C. Cross section of microtubules (large arrows) and neurofilaments of a normal neuron. Alzheimer's neurofibrillary tangles are characterized by regular constrictions at approximately 800Å intervals in longitudinal section. They are smaller than microtubules and larger than normal neurofilaments in cross section. (From Hirano, A.: Tokyo Igaku, 80: 438, 1973.)

Most recently, *microfilaments*, the smallest of the neurofibrillary elements, have been described. These are fine filaments, less than 60Å in diameter, and may be related to the actin filaments seen in other tissues. They are best seen in the growth cone of the developing neurite and in spines of mature neurons (Metuzals & Mushynski, 1974; Iqbal et al., 1978).

Microtubules and neurofilaments traverse the cell soma in all directions between Nissl substance and other organelles. In the neuronal process, however, the microtubules and neurofilaments are arranged parallel to each other and to the cell process itself. In general, the smaller the cell process, the greater the proportion of microtubules.

Current belief is that neurofibrillary protein is formed in the cell body and traverses the axon as part of the slow component of axonal flow (Hoffman and Lasek, 1975). Chemical analysis of neurofibrillary protein and the investigation of axonal flow are two areas of intense research at the present time.

REFERENCES

Wuerker, R.B.: Neurofilaments and glial filaments. Tissue & Cell, 2: 1-9, 1970.

Metuzals, J., & Mushynski, W.E.: Electron microscopic and experimental investigations of the neurofilamentous network in Deiters' neurons: Relationship with the cell surface and nuclear pores. J. Cell Biol., 61: 701-722, 1974.

Hoffman, P.N., & Lasek, R.J.: The slow component of axonal transport. J. Cell Biol., 66: 351-366, 1975.

Soifer, D. (ed.): The Biology of Cytoplasmic Microtubules. Ann. N.Y. Acad. Sci., Vol. 253, 1975.

Terry, R.D., & Gershon, S. (eds.): Aging, Vol. 3, Neurobiology of Aging, Raven Press, New York, 1976.

ALTERATIONS OF NEUROFILAMENTS (Figs. 146, 147)

Under certain pathological conditions the neurofibrils, especially 100Å neurofilaments, may increase in number. This abnormal accumulation may affect large parts of the soma or may be limited to a small segment of the cell process, especially in the axon.

A good example of this phenomenon is the effect of *aluminum intoxication* in which the cell soma and the proximal portion of the cell processes become engorged with neurofilaments (Terry and Peña, 1965). Similar changes in the proximal portion of the axon were seen after β-β′-iminodiproprionitrile *(IDPN) intoxication* (Chou and Hartman, 1964) and in hereditary canine spinal muscular atrophy (Cork et al., 1979). This experimentally-induced alteration mimics spheroids seen in anterior horn cells in certain motor neuron diseases (Carpenter, 1968).

Vinca alkaloids, which are mitotic spindle inhibitors, exert their effect on microtubules. In these intoxications the microtubules disappear and large filamentous crystalloids with a characteristic hexagonal honeycomb-like arrangement are formed (Fig. 148). Colchicine also causes the disappearance of microtubules, but does not induce crystalloid formation. These changes have been reported in both experimental animals and in patients subjected to these agents during cancer chemotherapy.

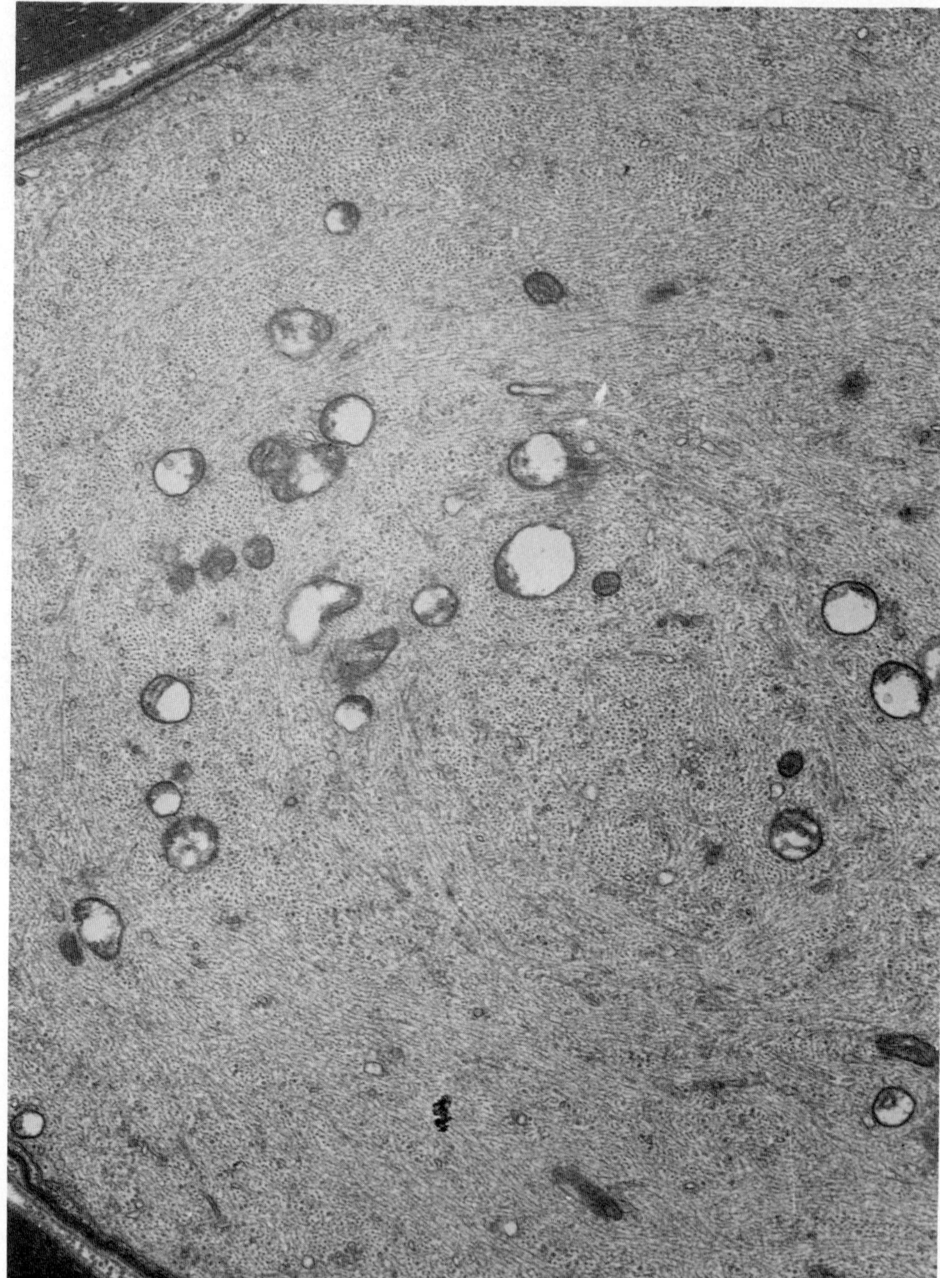

Fig. 146 Cross section of a distended myelinated axon in a mutant hamster with hindleg paralysis. Numerous neurofibrils and other organelles fill the axoplasm. × 15,000.

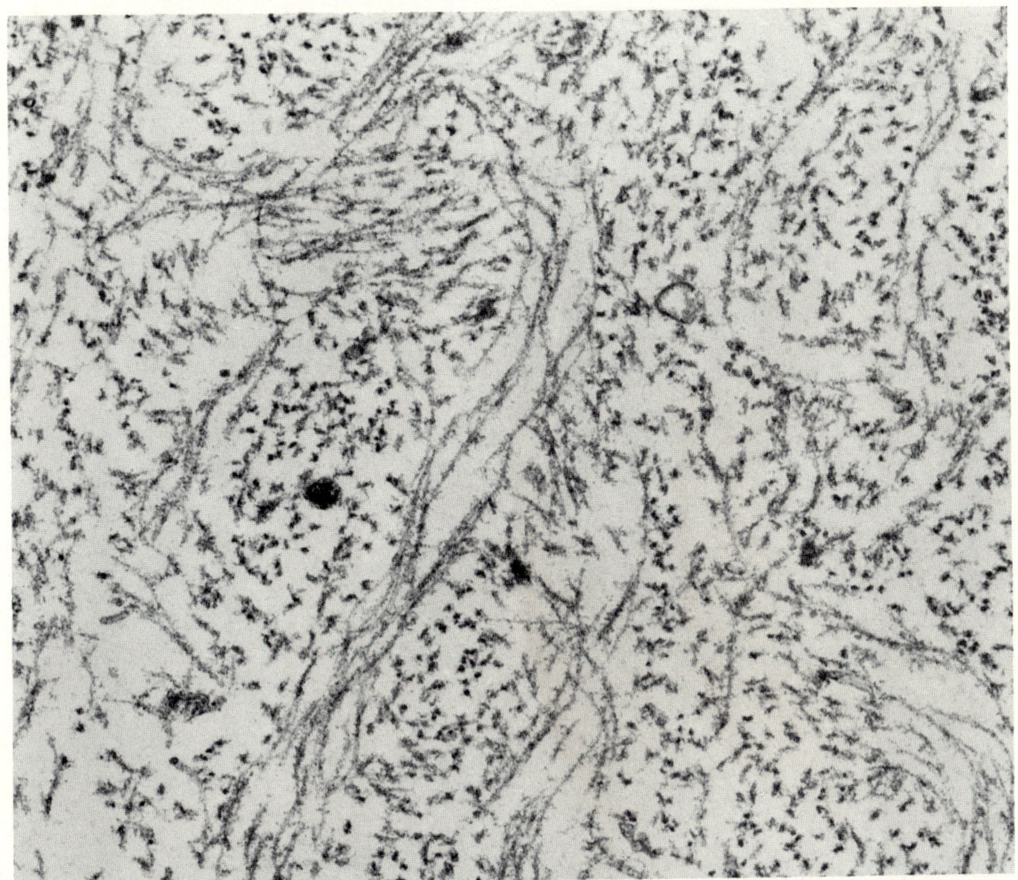

Fig. 147 A portion of a spheroid in the anterior horn cell of a patient with amyotrophic lateral sclerosis. 100Å neurofilaments are seen. × 36,000.

REFERENCES

Chou, S.M., & Hartman, H.A.: Axonal lesions and waltzing syndrome after IDPN administration in rats. With a concept—"Axostasis". Acta Neuropathol., 3: 428-450, 1964.

Terry, R.D., & Peña, C.: Experimental production of neurofibrillary degeneration. J. Neuropathol. Exp. Neurol., 24: 200-210, 1965.

Carpenter, S.: Proximal axonal enlargement in motor neuron disease. Neurology, 18: 84-851, 1968.

Hirano, A., & Zimmerman, H.M.: Some effects of vinblastine implantation in the cerebral white matter. Lab. Invest., 23: 358-367, 1970.

Hirano, A., & Iwata, M.: Pathology of motor neurons with special reference to amyotrophic lateral sclerosis and related diseases. *In* Amyotrophic Lateral Sclerosis. pp. 107-133, Tsubaki, T. & Toyokura, Y. (eds.), University of Tokyo Press, Tokyo, 1979.

Ghetti, B.: Induction of neurofibrillary degeneration following treatment with maytansine *in vivo*. Brain Res., 163: 9-19, 1979.

Cork, L.C., Griffin, J.W., Munnell, J.F., Lorenz, M.D., Adams, R.J., & Price, D.L.: Hereditary canine spinal muscular atrophy: J. Neuropathol. Exp. Neurol., 38: 209-221, 1979.

Inoue, K., & Hirano, A.: Early pathological changes of amyotrophic lateral sclerosis. A reappraisal of the spheroid, Bunina body and morphometry of the ventral spinal root. J. Neuropathol. Exp. Neurol., 39: 363 (abstract), 1980.

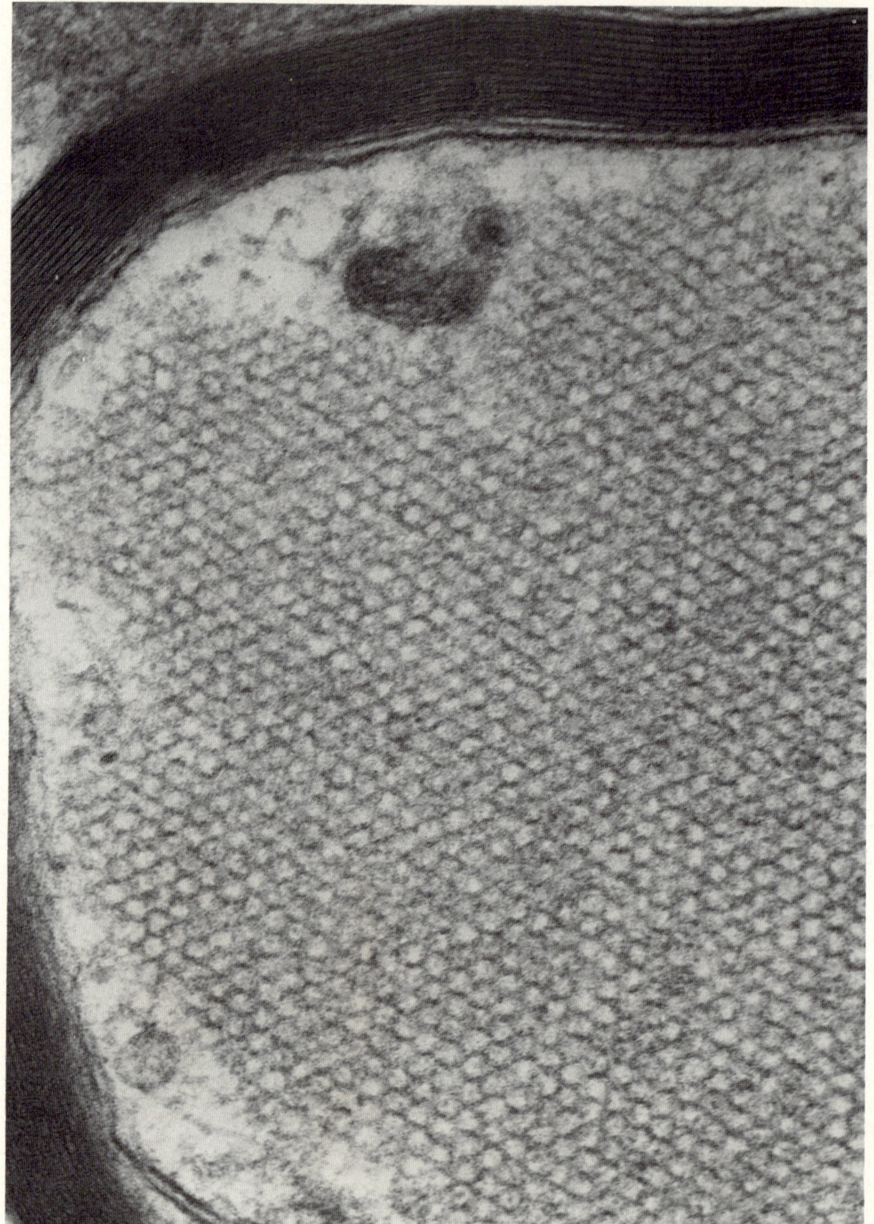

Fig. 148 Crystalloid within an axon after vinblastine treatment. A. Cross section. × 80,000. B. Longitudinal section. × 100,000. C. Longitudinal section (neurofilaments are also present). × 90,000. (From Hirano, A.: The Structure and Function of Nervous Tissue. Vol. 5, p. 73, Academic Press, 1972.)

B

C

ALZHEIMER'S NEUROFIBRILLARY TANGLES

Alzheimer's neurofibrillary tangles were among the first morphological changes of the neurons which could be correlated with clinical symptoms. More than half a century ago, Alzheimer, using Bielschowsky preparations, discovered argentophilic fibrillary changes in about one-fourth to one-third of the cerebral cortical neurons, as well as abundant senile plaques, in a 51 year old woman who had had a 4 ½ year history of progressive dementia. Alzheimer described three stages in fibrillary changes beginning with the appearance of unusual neurofibrillary tangles among the normal neuronal components and ending with the disappearance of the entire neuron leaving only the argentophilic tangles behind. These tangles, one of the best known alterations seen in neuropathology, came to be known as "Alzheimer's neurofibrillary tangles" and the disease, a type of presenile dementia, is now known as "Alzheimer's disease." Since their discovery Alzheimer's neurofibrillary tangles have been the subject of numerous, intensive research efforts.

Light Microscopic Demonstration of Alzheimer's Neurofibrillary Tangles (Figs. 149, 150)

The Bielschowsky method is still useful for demonstrating Alzheimer's neurofibrillary tangles. Today, however, the von Brownmühl modification, or equivalent methods, are preferred since they stain the tangles prominently while leaving the normal argentophilic fibrillary structure in the soma less conspicuous. It must be cautioned, however, that some of the silver methods tend to stain blood vessel

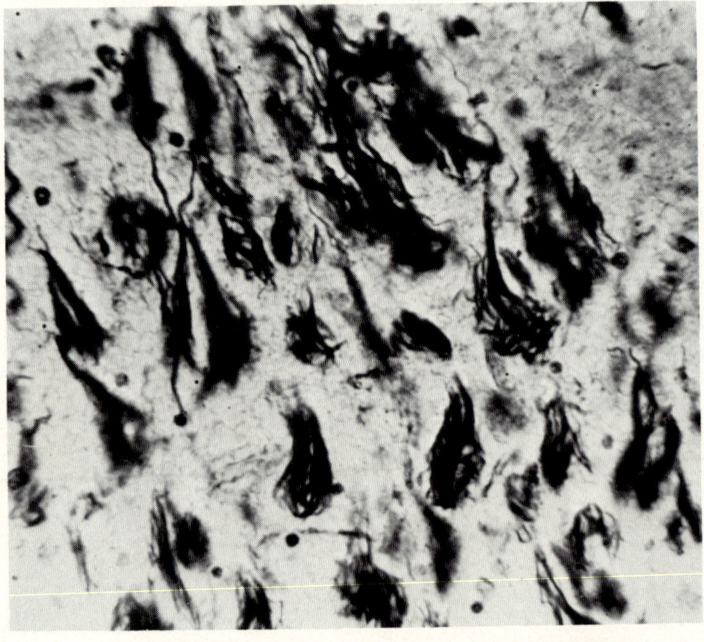

Fig. 149 Alzheimer's neurofibrillary changes in Sommer's sector (Silver stain). (From Hirano, A.: NINDB Monograph. No. 2, Slow, Latent, and Temperature Virus Infections. p. 23, 1965.)

walls prominently and the inexperienced observer may be confused when only small numbers of Alzheimer's neurofibrillary tangles are present.

After some experience, Alzheimer's neurofibrillary tangles become recognizable in ordinary H&E preparations. Most tangles stain blue, but the older ones may become weakly eosinophilic like the background. A source of possible confusion in H&E preparations is the eosinophilia of reactive glial fibrils which are also seen in Alzheimer's disease. These, however, may usually be easily distinguished from Alzheimer's neurofibrillary tangles by their different shape and orientation.

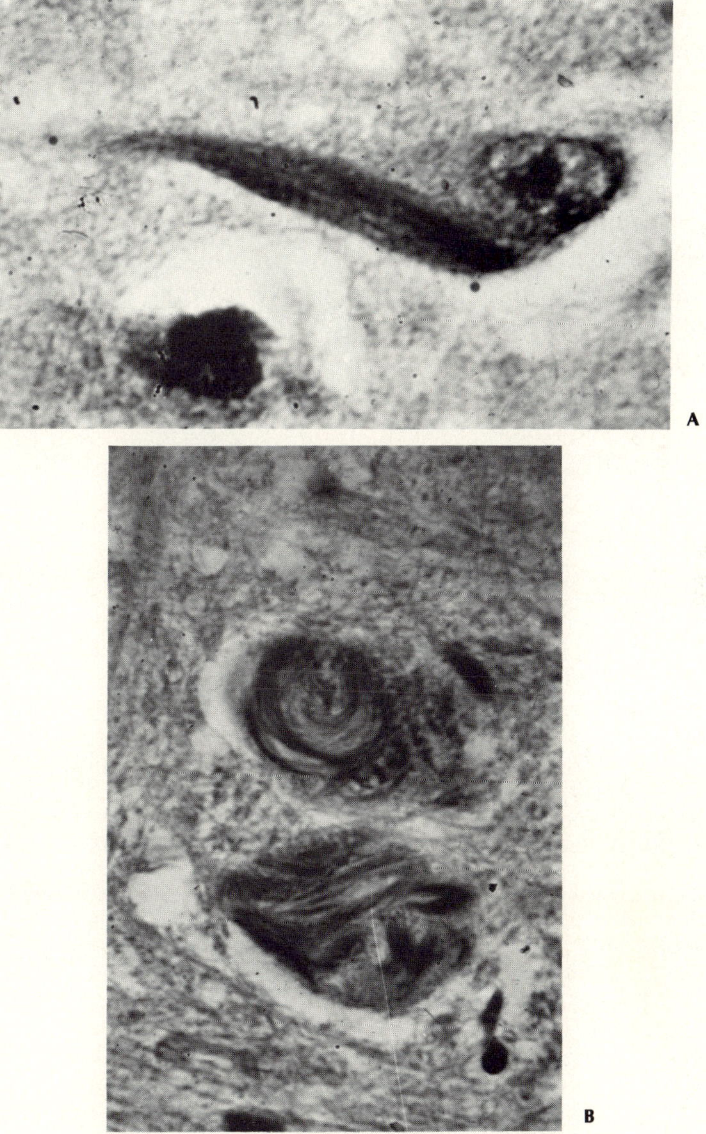

Fig. 150 Alzheimer's neurofibrillary changes (H&E stain). A. Pyramidal neuron in the cerebrum. B. Neurons in the brain stem.

Occurrence and Distribution of Alzheimer's Neurofibrillary Tangles (Fig. 151)

Alzheimer's neurofibrillary tangles are seen in a number of conditions and may be found in various parts of the central nervous system. The original description was in the cerebral cortex in Alzheimer's disease where large numbers of triangular or flame-shaped tangles were found. Later, globose-shaped tangles were seen in the basal ganglia and brain stem of patients with postencephalitic parkinsonism (Figs. 1 and 3 in Hirano, 1971). More recently Malamud described large numbers of Alzheimer's neurofibrillary tangles among all the ALS patients in the native Chamorro population on the island of Guam (Malamud et al., 1961). Somewhat later, even more tangles were seen among Chamorro patients with parkinsonism-dementia complex (P-D complex) (Hirano et al., 1961 a & b, 1966, 1974). In both of these groups of patients flame-shaped tangles were seen in pyramidal neurons of the cerebral cortex while the basal ganglia and the brain stem tended to have globose-shaped tangles.

Since those studies, aged brains of Caucasians have been shown to contain Alzheimer's neurofibrillary tangles. Furthermore, while usually fewer than in ALS or PD-complex patients, the tangles were present and distributed in a similar manner in Chamorros who died of other causes (Hirano et al., 1966; Brody et al., 1971; Anderson et al., 1979).

Other conditions in which Alzheimer's neurofibrillary tangles have been reported include subacute sclerosing panencephalitis, tuberous sclerosis (Hirano et al., 1968), Down's syndrome (Burger and Vogel, 1975), certain lipidoses (Horoupian and Yang, 1978) and in the brains of prize fighters (Corsellis et al., 1973).

REFERENCES

Malamud, N., Hirano, A., & Kurland, L.T.: Pathoanatomic changes in amyotrophic lateral sclerosis on Guam. Special reference to the occurrence of neurofibrillary changes. Arch. Neurol., 5:401-415, 1961.

Hirano, A., Kurland, L.T., Krooth, R.S., and Lessell, S.: Parkinsonism-dementia complex, an endemic disease on the island of Guam. I. Clinical Features. Brain, 84:642-661, 1961 a.

Hirano, A., Malamud, N., & Kurland, L.T.: Parkinsonism-dementia complex, an endemic disease on the island of Guam. II. Pathological Features, Brain, 84:662-679, 1961 b.

Hirano, A., Malamud, N., Elizan, T.S. & Kurland, L.T.: Amyotrophic lateral sclerosis and parkinsonism-dementia complex on Guam. Arch. Neurol., 15:35-51, 1966.

Hirano, A., Tuazon, R., & Zimmerman, H.M.: Neurofibrillary changes, granulovacuolar bodies and argentophilic globules observed in tuberous sclerosis. Acta Neuropathol., 11:257-261, 1968.

Hirano, A.: Electron microscopy in neuropathology. *In* Progress in Neuropathology Vol. 1, pp. 1-61, Zimmerman, H.M. (ed.), Grune & Stratton, New York, 1971.

Brody, J.A., Hirano, A., & Scott, R.M.: Recent neuropathologic observations in amyotrophic lateral sclerosis and parkinsonism-dementia on Guam. Neurology, 21:528-536, 1971.

Corsellis, J.A.N., Bruton, C.J., & Freeman-Browne, D.: The aftermath of boxing. Psychol. Med., 3:270-303, 1973.

Burger, P., & Vogel, F.S.: The development of the pathologic changes of Alzheimer's disease and senile dementia in patients with Down's syndrome. Am. J. Pathol., 73:457-468, 1973.

Horoupian, D.S., & Yang, S.S.: Paired helical filaments in neurovisceral lipidosis (Juvenile dystonic lipidosis). Ann. Neurol., 4:404-411, 1978.

Anderson, F.H., Richardson, E.P. Jr., Okazaki, H., & Brody, J.A.: Neurofibrillary degeneration on Guam. Frequency in Chamorros and non-Chamorros with no known neurological disease. Brain, 102:65-77, 1979.

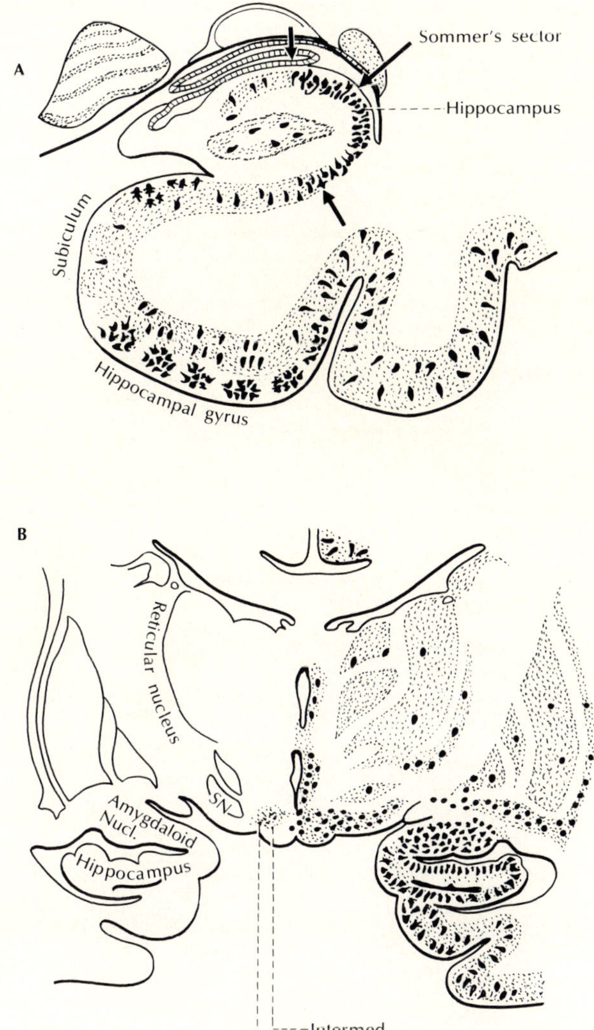

Fig. 151-1 Topography of Alzheimer's neurofibrillary changes. (From Hirano, A., & Zimmerman, H.M.: Arch. Neurol., 7: 227, 1962.)

In general, Alzheimer's neurofibrillary tangles show a rather striking predilection to affect particular areas in involved regions, although the intensity varies from disease to disease (Hirano & Zimmerman, 1962; Ishii, 1966). In those conditions affecting the cerebral cortex the glomerular formation of the hippocampal gyrus and the pyramidal neurons of Sommer's sector in Ammon's horn are especially vulnerable to fibrillary changes. Ball (1976) has reported that, in dementia, the severity of neurofibrillary change is greatest in the posterior portion of the hippocampus. When the basal ganglia are affected the hypothalamic nucleus, substantia innominata at the base of the lenticular nucleus, and the amygdaloid nucleus are special targets. In the brain stem the substantia nigra, locus ceruleus and neurons of the reticular formation are prone to these changes.

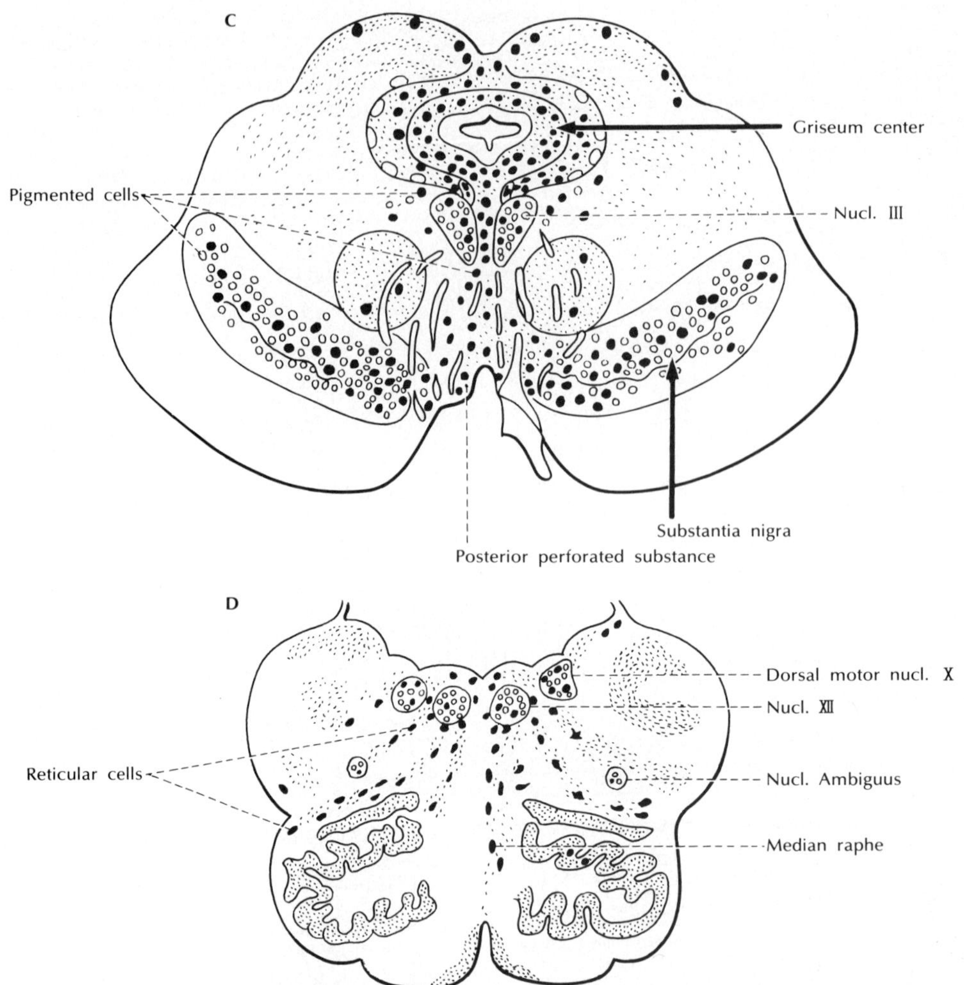

Fig. 151-2 Topography of Alzheimer's neurofibrillary changes in the brain stem.

On the other hand, certain neurons never seem to show Alzheimer's neurofibrillary tangles. These include Purkinje cells of the cerebellum, and neurons of the lateral geniculate body or the peripheral nervous system.

REFERENCES

Hirano, A., & Zimmerman, H.M.: Alzheimer's neurofibrillary changes. A topographic study. Arch. Neurol., 7:227-242, 1962.

Ishii, T.: Distribution of Alzheimer's neurofibrillary changes in the brain stem and hypothalamus of senile dementia. Acta Neuropathol., 6:181-187, 1966.

Hirano, A., Arumugasamy, N., and Zimmerman, H.M.: Amyotrophic lateral sclerosis. A comparison of Guam and classic cases. Arch. Neurol., 16:357-363, 1967.

Hirano, A.: Parkinsonism-dementia complex on Guam. Current status of the problem. *In* Proceedings of the Tenth International Congress of Neurology, pp. 348-357, Excerpta Medica, 1974.

Ball, M.J.: Neurofibrillary tangles and the pathogenesis of dementia. A quantitative study. Neuropathol. Appl. Neurobiol. 2:395-410, 1976.

Fine Structure of Alzheimer's Neurofibrillary Tangles (Figs. 144, 145)

Thin sections through the tangles present three views. The most characteristic is a longitudinal section in which fibrils are seen bearing regular constrictions at about 800Å intervals (Terry, 1963). Sometimes, however, regular constrictions as close as 500Å have been observed. The fibrils are approximately 250Å wide at their widest point midway between the constrictions. Some longitudinally sectioned fibrils appear straight and are approximately 150Å in diameter (Fig. 152) (Hirano et al, 1968; Oyanagi, 1974). Occasionally, circular profiles, 150Å in diameter are also seen. (Hirano et al, 1968). Another view results in characteristic arciform profiles (Terry, 1963).

Originally the fundamental fibrillar elements of Alzheimer's neurofibrillary tangles were considered to be twisted tubules (Terry, 1963). More recently Wiśniewski et al. (1976), have concluded that they represent two filaments twisted into a helix, termed "paired helical filaments" (PHF), as first postulated by Kidd (1963, 1964).

Up to the present, these structures have been reported only in certain neurons of the human central nervous system. Some recent reports have indicated that apparently similar structures may be seen in potassium chloride-incubated neurofilaments extracted from peripheral nerves (Schlaepfer, 1977). Another report describes the formation of paired helical filaments induced by the addition of an extract prepared from the brain of patients dying with Alzheimer's disease to cultured, human, fetal cerebral cortical neurons (De Boni and Crapper, 1978). The significance of these studies remains to be clarified.

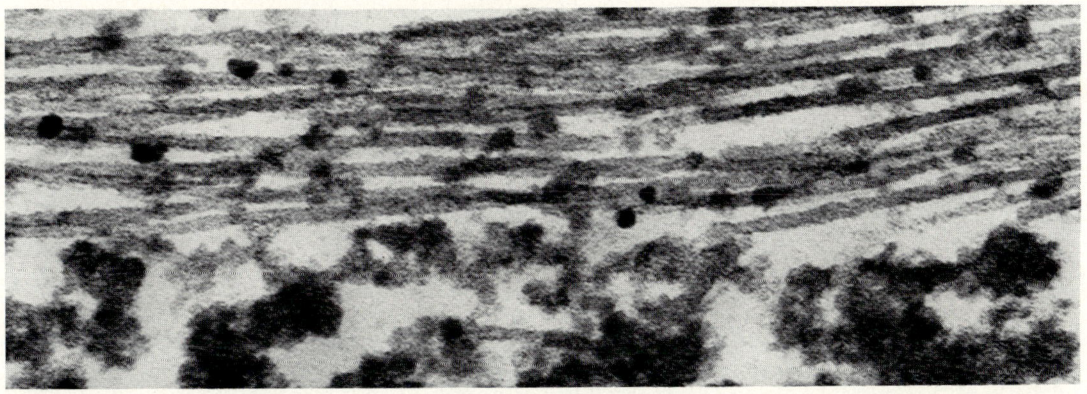

Fig. 152 Straight 150Å filaments in a cortical neuron of a patient with Alzheimer's neurofibrillary tangles. × 135,000.

REFERENCES

Terry, R.D.: The fine structure of neurofibrillary tangles in Alzheimer's disease. J. Neuropathol. Exp. Neurol., 2:629-642, 1963.

Kidd, M.: Paired helical filaments in electron microscopy in Alzheimer's disease. Nature, 197:192-193, 1963.

Kidd, M.: Alzheimer's disease. An electron microscopic study. Brain, 87:307-320, 1964.

Hirano, A., Dembitzer, H.M., Kurland, L.T., & Zimmerman, H.M.: The fine structure of some intraganglionic alterations. J. Neuropathol. Exp. Neurol., 27:176-182, 1968.

Hirano, A.: Neurofibrillary changes in conditions related to Alzheimer's disease. *In* Ciba Foundation Symposium. Alzheimer's Disease and Related Conditions. Wolstenholme, pp. 185-201, Wolstenholme, G.E.W., & O'Connor, M. (eds.) Churchill, London, 1970.

Wiśniewski, H., Terry, R.D., & Hirano, A.: A neurofibrillary pathology. J. Neuropathol. Exp. Neurol., 29: 163-176, 1970.

Oyanagi, S.: An electron microscopic observation on senile dementia, with special references to transformation of neurofilaments to twisted tubules and a structural connection of Pick bodies to Alzheimer's neurofibrillary changes. Adv. Neurol. Sci. (Tokyo), 18: 77-88, 1974.

Wiśniewski, H.M., Narang, H.K., & Terry, R.D.: Neurofibrillary tangles of paired helical filaments. J. Neurol. Sci. 27: 173-181, 1976.

Schlaepfer, W.W.: Studies of the substructure of mammalian neurofilaments. J. Neuropathol. Exp. Neurol., 36: 628 (abst.), 1977.

Shibayama, H., & Kitoh, J.: Electron microscopic structure of the Alzheimer's neurofibrillary changes in case of atypical senile dementia. Acta Neuropathol., 41: 229-234, 1978.

DeBoni, U., & Crapper, D.R.: Paired helical filaments of the Alzheimer type in cultured neurons. Nature 271: 566-568, 1978.

Terry, R.D.: Ultrastructural alterations in senile dementia. *In* Alzheimer's Disease: Senile Dementia and Related Disorders (Aging, Vol. 7), pp. 375-382, Katzman, R., Terry, R.D., & Bick, K.L. (eds.), Raven Press, New York, 1978.

Iqbal, K., Grundke-Iqbal, I., Wiśniewski, H.M., & Terry, R.D.: Neurofibers in Alzheimer's dementia and other conditions. *In* Alzheimer's Disease: Senile Dementia and Related Disorders (Aging, Vol. 7), pp. 409-420, Katzman, R., Terry, R.D., & Bick, K.L. (eds.), Raven Press, New York, 1978.

NEUROFIBRILLARY CHANGES IN STEELE-RICHARDSON-OLSZEWSKI SYNDROME

Argentophilic inclusions, reminiscent of Alzheimer's neurofibrillary tangles, have been described in certain brain stem nuclei in progressive supranuclear palsy (Steele-Richardson-Olszewski syndrome). The original description of the fine structure of these tangles indicated that they consisted of straight, 150Å wide, tubules with no constrictions. Subsequently, Tomonaga et al reported both straight and constricted tubules in another case of this disease.

REFERENCES

Steele, J.C., Richardson, J.C., & Olszewski, J.: Progressive supranuclear palsy: A heterogenous degeneration involving the brain stem, basal ganglia and cerebellum with vertical gaze and pseudobulbar palsy, nuchal dystonia and dementia. Arch. Neurol., 10: 333-359, 1964.

Hirano, A.: Discussion on Olszewski, J., Steele, J., & Richardson, J.C.: Pathological report on six cases of heterogenous system degeneration. J. Neuropathol. Exp. Neurol., 23: 188, 1964.

Tellez-Nagel, I., & Wisniewski, H.M.: Ultrastructure of neurofibrillary tangles in Steele-Richardson-Olszewski syndrome. Arch. Neurol., 29: 324-327, 1973.

Powell, H.C., London, G.W., & Lampert, P.W.: Neurofibrillary tangles in progressive supranuclear palsy. J. Neuropathol. Exp. Neurol., 33: 98-106, 1974.

Roy, S., Datta, C.K., Hirano, A., Ghatak, N.R., & Zimmerman, H.M.: Electron microscopic study of neurofibrillary tangles in Steele-Richardson-Olszewski syndrome. Acta Neuropathol., 29: 175-179, 1974.

Tomonaga, M.: Ultrastructure of neurofibrillary tangles in progressive supranuclear palsy. Acta Neuropathol., 37: 177-181, 1977.

OTHER NEUROFIBRILLARY CHANGES

In a case of quadriplegia of unknown etiology Kuroda et al (1979) have described abnormal, argentophilic, fibrillary accumulations throughout almost the entire motor neuron system as well as in certain other neurons. These inclusions are difficult to detect in routine light microscopic preparations. Their fine structure consists of wavy and parallel, or straight and randomly distributed, groups of tubules, 120Å in diameter.

REFERENCES

Kuroda, S., Otsuki, S., Tateishi, J., & Hirano, A.: Neurofibrillary degeneration in a case of quadriplegia and myoclonic movement. Acta Neuropathol., 45: 105-109, 1979.

EOSINOPHILIC ROD-LIKE STRUCTURES (HIRANO BODIES) (Figs. 153-155)

These structures were first described in patients with ALS or PD complex on the island of Guam. They are highly refractile eosinophilic structures which appear rod-like in longitudinal sections and circular or ovoid in cross sections. They are best seen in H & E preparations.

Eosinophilic rod-like structures are generally intraneuronal. They are most often found in cell processes in the neuropil but are occasionally seen in the perinuclear area. Most often they are confined to Sommer's sector and nearby areas (Hirano,

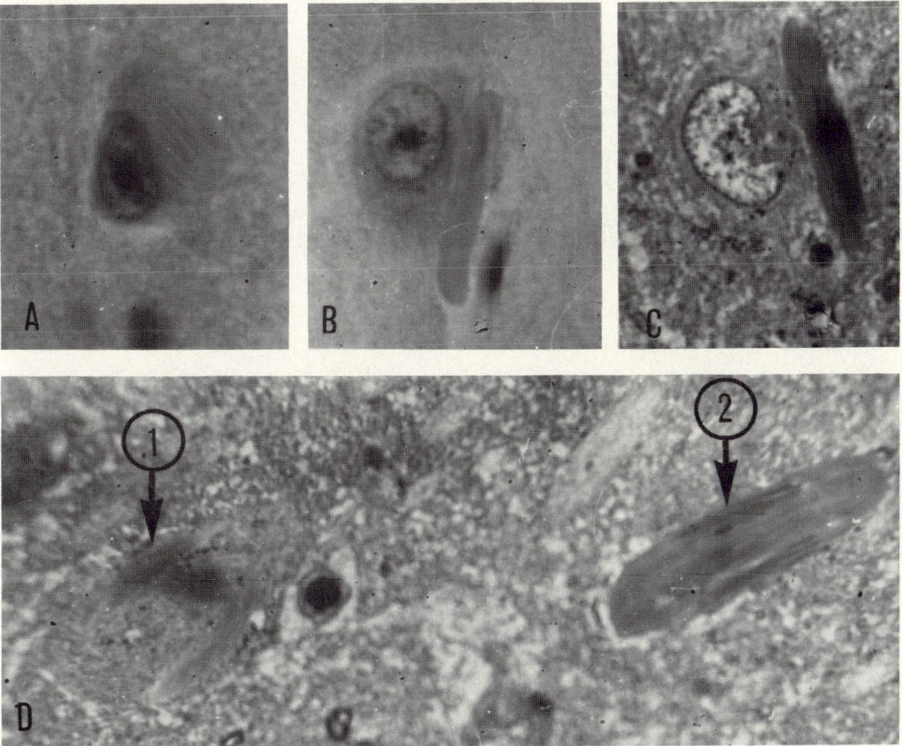

Fig. 153 Eosinophilic rod-like inclusions (Hirano bodies) in neurons of Sommer's sector. × 1,000. A. In the neuronal soma. B,C. In a neuronal process adjacent to a neuron. D. In a neuronal soma 1. In an apical dendrite 2. (From Hirano, A. et al.: J. Neuropath. Exp. Neurol., 27: 167, 1968.)

1965; Ogata et al, 1972; Gibbon and Tomlinson, 1977) but, as will be described below, have been observed in other parts of the nervous system.

Fine structural studies have confirmed their intraneuronal position by the occasional demonstration of synaptic terminals or Alzheimer's neurofibrillary tangles side-by-side with the eosinophilic rod-like structures within the same cell process. The rod-like structures consist of highly organized, crystalloid arrays of

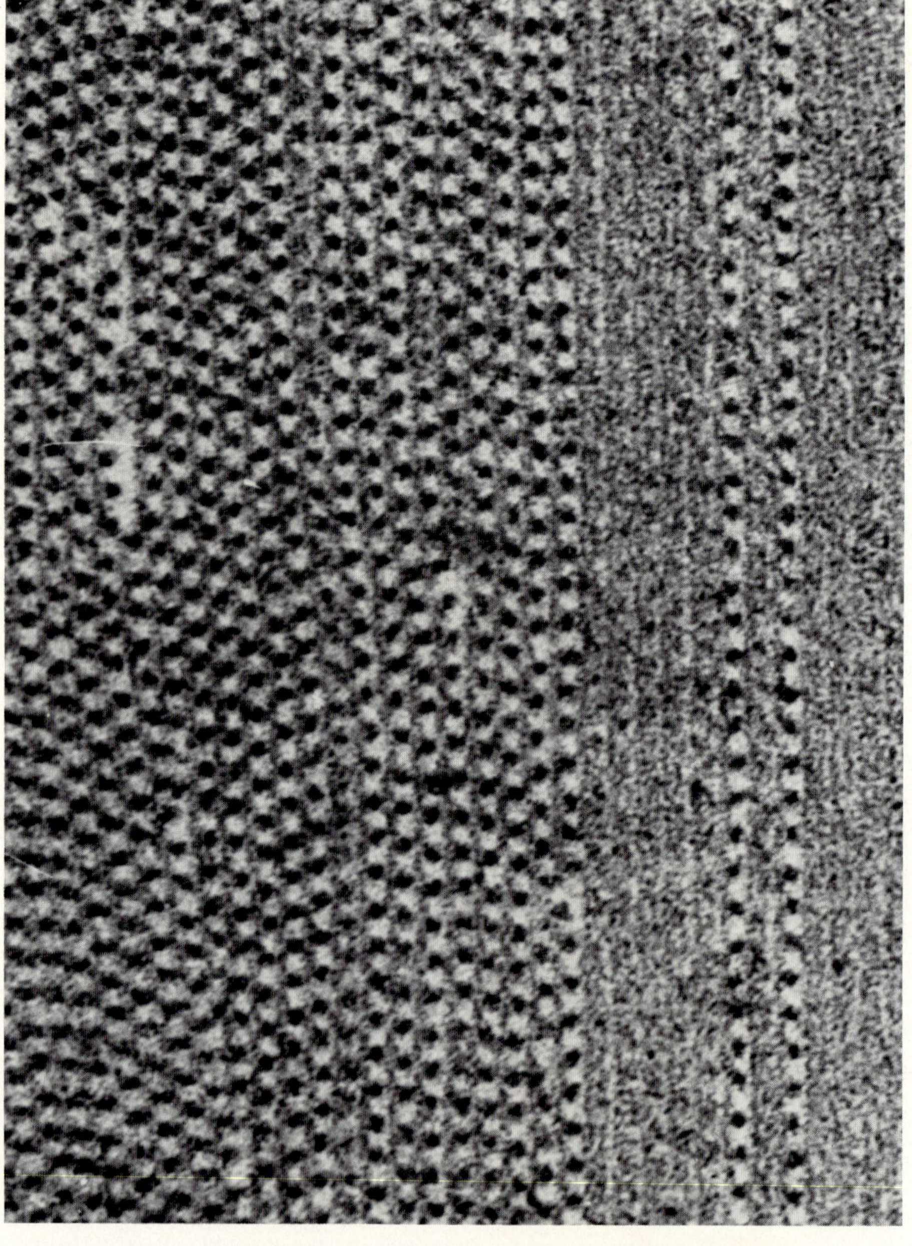

Fig. 154 Eosinophilic rod-like structure (Hirano body). × 270,000. (From Hirano, A., et al.: J. Neuropathol. Exp. Neurol., 27: 167, 1968.)

interlacing filaments displaying either a lattice-like or "herringbone" configuration (Hirano, 1965; Tomonaga, 1974). Homogeneous electron dense material may sometimes appear in patches permeating the fibrillar structures.

Since their first description, eosinophilic rod-like inclusions have been seen in a variety of conditions. They have been described in Sommer's sector in Pick's disease (Schochet et al, 1968), Alzheimer's disease, Creutzfeld-Jacob disease (Llena

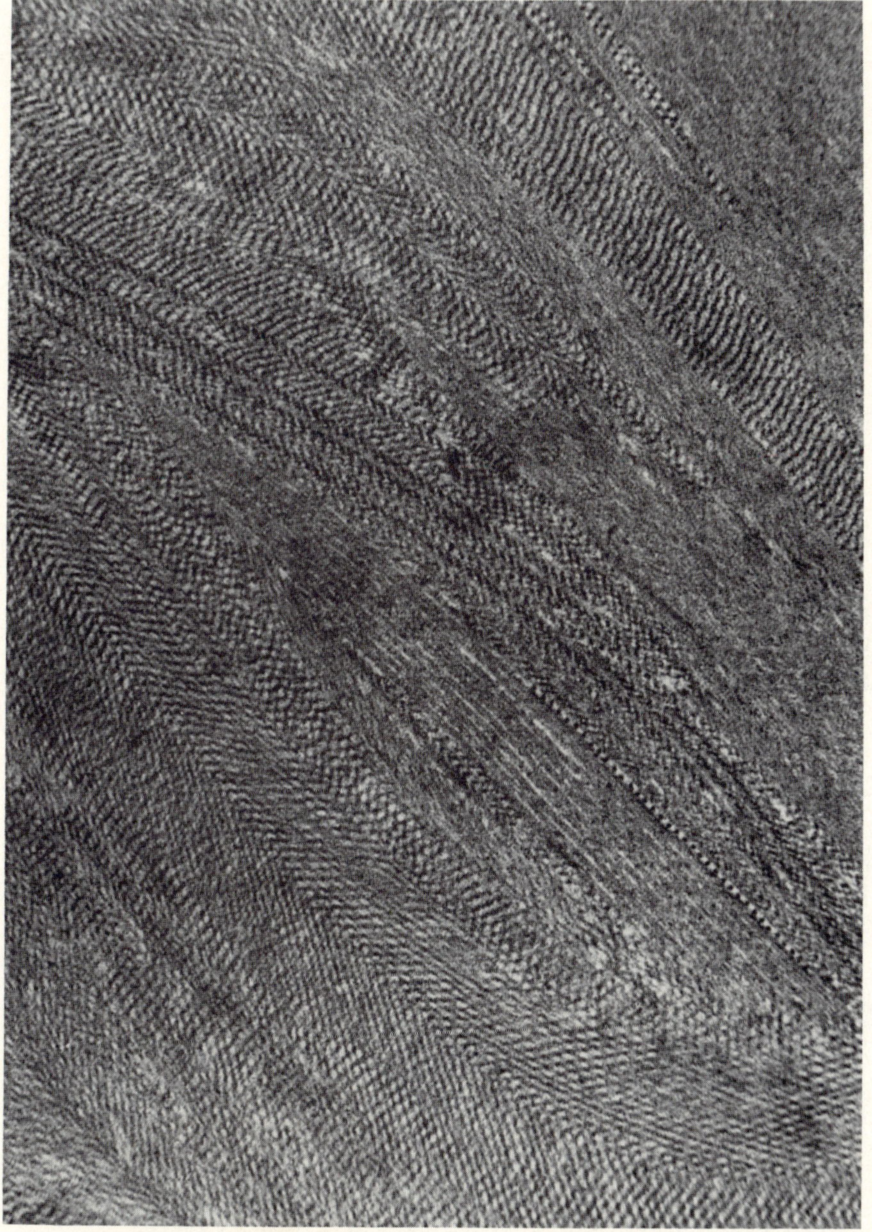

Fig. 155 Eosinophilic rod-like structure (Hirano body). × 96,000. (From Hirano, A.: NINDB Monograph No. 2, Slow, Latent, and Temperate Virus Infections. p. 23, 1965)

and Hirano, 1979), and in aged brain. In certain motor neuron diseases they may be found in anterior horn cells (Schochet et al, 1969). In other conditons rare examples were observed in other areas including the frontal cortex.

Some animals have also shown similar inclusions (Beal et al, 1977; Ohama et al, 1979). Aged primates show them in Sommer's sector. They have also been seen in scrapie-infected animals as well as in a number of other experimental disease conditions. More recently they have been observed in the inner loops of myelin-forming oligodendroglia (Cavanagh et al, 1971) or Schwann cells in certain experimental animals (Hirano and Dembitzer, 1972). In the mutant hamster showing hind-leg paralysis they seem to be related to demyelination of the peripheral nerve.

REFERENCES

Hirano, A.: Pathology of amyotrophic lateral sclerosis. *In* Slow, Latent, and Temperate Virus Infections, pp. 23-26, Gajdusek, D.C. & Gibbs, C.J. Jr. (eds.). NINDB Monograph, No. 2 National Institutes of Health, Washington, 1965.

Schochet, S.S. Jr., Lampert, P.W., & Lindenberg, R.: Fine structure of the Pick and Hirano bodies in a case of Pick's disease. Acta Neuropathol., 11: 330-337, 1968.

Schochet, S.S. Jr., Hardman, J.M., Ladewig, P.P., & Earle, K.M.: Intraneuronal conglomerates in sporadic motor neuron disease. Arch. Neurol., 20: 548-553, 1969.

Cavanagh, J.B., Blakemore, W.F., & Kyu, M.H.: Fibrillary accumulations in oligodendroglial processes of rats subjected to portocaval anastomosis. J. Neurol. Sci., 14: 143-152, 1971.

Schochet, S.S. Jr., & McCormick, W.F.: Ultrastructure of Hirano bodies. Acta Neuropathol., 21: 50-60, 1972.

Ogata, J., Budzilovich, G.N., & Cravioto, H.: A study of rod-like structures (Hirano bodies) in 240 normal and pathological brains. Acta Neuropathol., 21: 61-67, 1972.

Hirano, A.: Progress in the pathology of motor neuron disease. *In* Progress in Neuropathology, Vol. 2, pp. 181-225, Zimmerman, H.M. (ed.), Grune & Stratton, New York, 1973.

Tomonaga, M.: Ultrastructure of Hirano bodies. Acta Neuropathol. 28: 365-366, 1974.

Hirano, A., & Dembitzer, H.M.: Eosinophilic rod-like structures in myelinated fibers of hamster spinal roots. Neuropathol. Applied Neurobiol., 2: 225-232, 1976.

Ohama, E., Shibata, T., Yamamura, S., & Ikuta, F.: Hirano body-like crystallin structure in the Ammon's horn induced by chronic administration of 6-hydroxydopamine. Advances Neurol. Sci. (Tokyo), 20: 400-409, 1976.

Beal, J.A., Cooper, M.H., & LeQui, I.J.: Normal cytoplasmic inclusions in the dorsal horn and supraoptic nucleus of the squirrel monkey, *Saimiri sciureus.* Cell Tiss. Res., 176: 37-46, 1977.

Gibson, P.H., & Tomlinson, B.E.: Numbers of Hirano bodies in the hippocampus of normal and demented people with Alzheimer's disease. J. Neurol. Sci., 33: 199-206, 1977.

Llena, J.F., & Hirano, A.: Abundant eosinophilic rod-like structures in subacute spongiform encephalopathy. J. Neuropathol. Exp. Neurol. 38: 329 (abstract), 1979.

5. Mitochondria (Fig. 156)

The structure of neuronal mitochondria is fundamentally similar to those of other cells. They are surrounded by an outer, smooth membrane and an inner, folded membrane giving rise to the cristae which fill the interior of the organelle.

The overall size and shape of the neuronal mitochondria depend on their location within the cell. In the perikaryon, they are generally sausage-shaped, about 0.1 micron wide and 1.0 micron in length. In axons the mitochondria tend

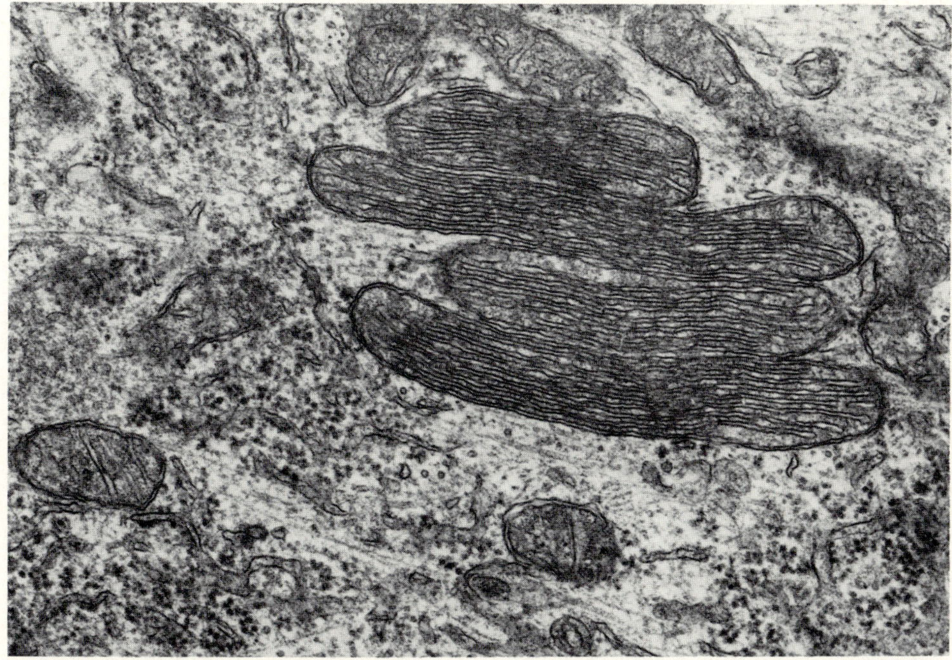

Fig. 156 Mitochondria in a neuron of the dorsal root ganglion in a hamster with hind leg paralysis. Note the variation in the orientation of the cristae between different mitochondria. × 40,000.

to assume a highly elongated shape, whereas they are more globoid in synaptic terminals. The mitochondria are motile structures and can sometimes be seen to branch. They are usually restricted from the Nissl substance, but otherwise may be found in virtually any other part of the cell except for spines from which they are excluded.

Under certain pathological conditions such as kinky hair disease the mitochondria increase dramatically in number in the perikarya of certain neurons (Ghatak et al, 1972; Yajima and Suzuki, 1979). In axonal pathology, such as Wallerian degeneration, the number of mitochondria, as well as that of other organelles, also increase in focal regions of the axon.

Mitochondria may swell to abnormal proportions under certain pathological conditions (Fig. 157). The matrix may become dense and contain large accumulations of electron dense deposits, presumably calcium, which are present normally in only small amounts. Pale and empty swelling or vacuolization of the mitochondria may be the result of ischemic insult which may be a reflection of an underlying pathology, but may well be the result of preparation artifact. In bilirubin encephalopathy of the Gunn rat these vacuolated mitochondria contain abnormal, membrane-bounded accumulations of glycogen granules (Schutta et al, 1970; Jew and Williams, 1977). In certain degenerative disorders many mitochondria appear which are shrunken and which have a dense matrix (Fig. 158).

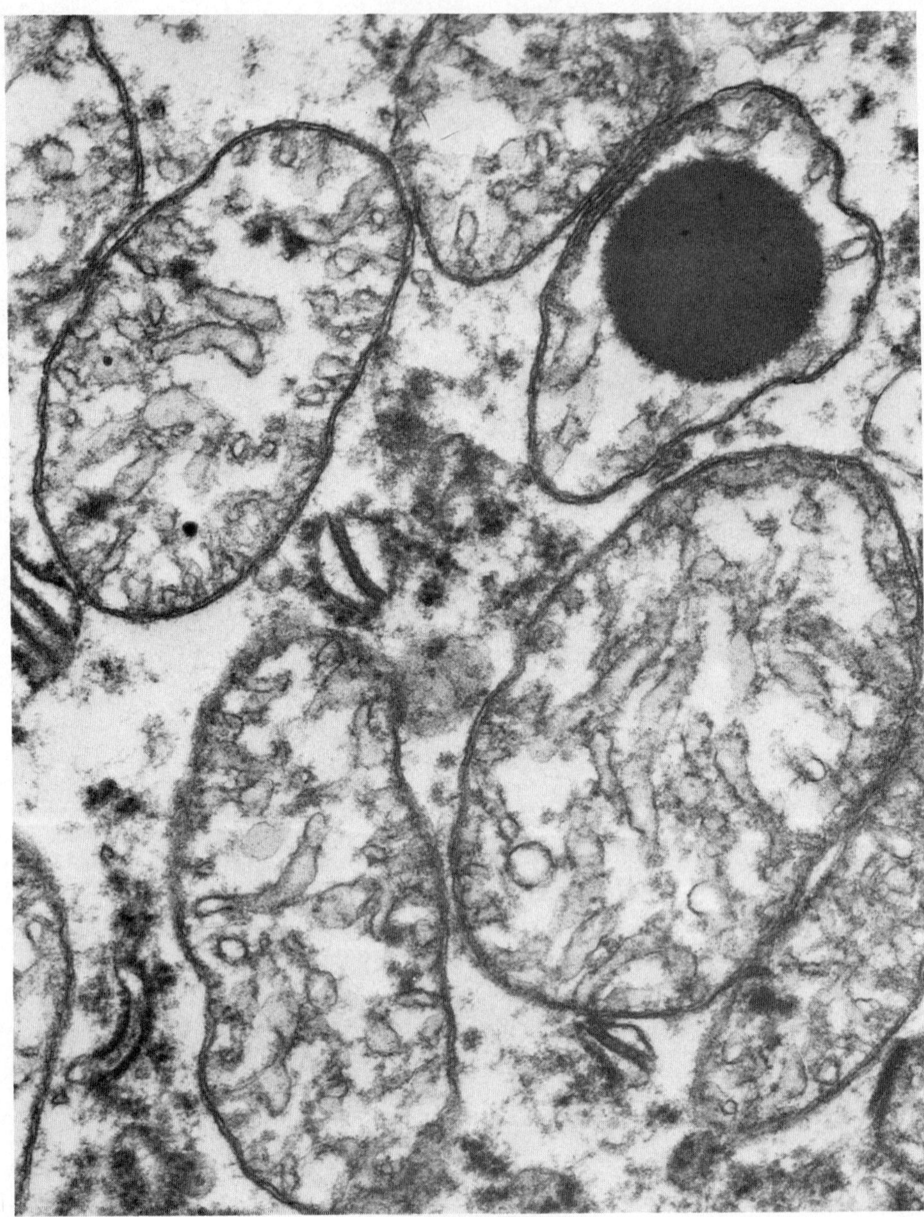

Fig. 157 Large mitochondria in the Purkinje cell of a patient with kinky hair disease. A dense intramitochondrial deposit is evident. × 45,000. (Hirano, A. et al.: Arch. Neurol. 34: 52, 1977.)

REFERENCES

Ghatak, N.R., Hirano, A., Poon, T.P., French, J.H.: Trichopoliodystrophy. II. Pathological changes in skeletal muscle and nervous system. Arch. Neurol., 26: 60-72, 1972.

Schutta, H.S., Johnson, L., Neville, H.E.: Mitochondria abnormalities in bilirubin encephalopathy. J. Neuropathol. Exp. Neurology., 29: 296, 1970.

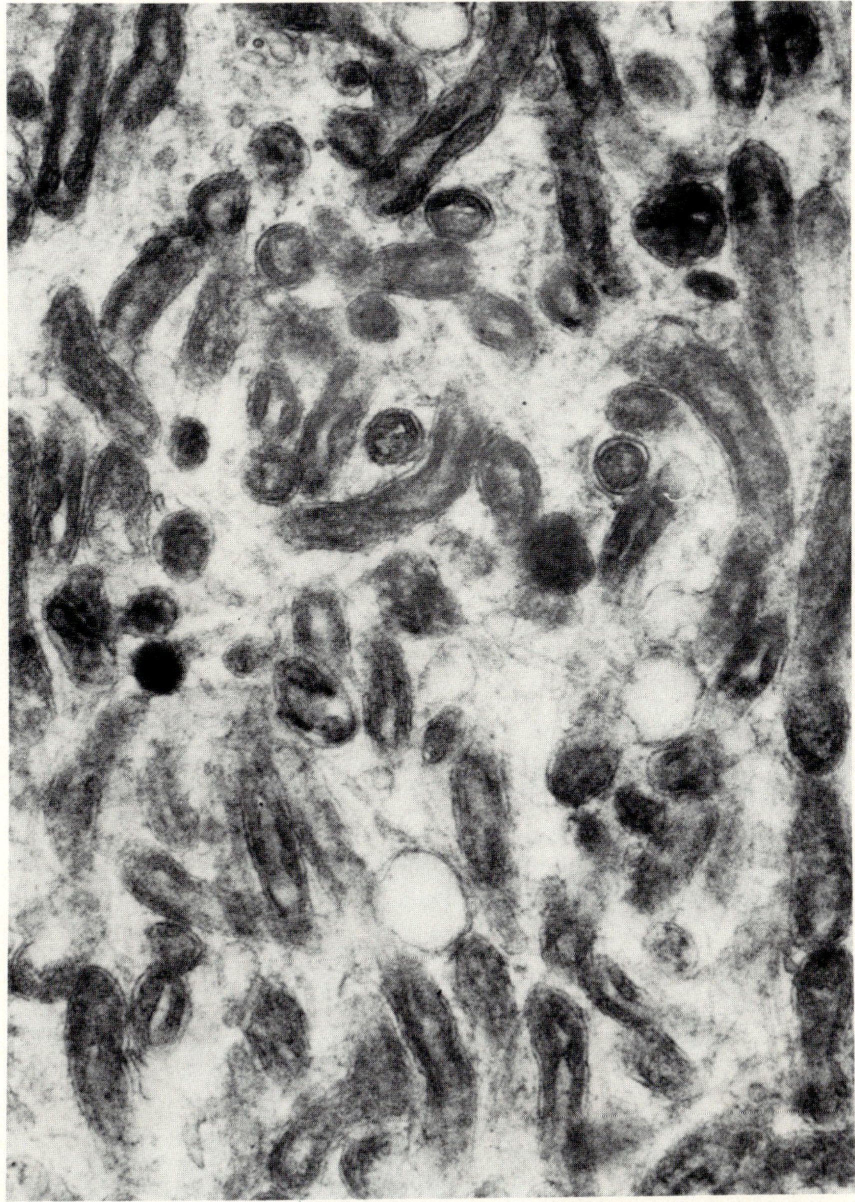

Fig. 158 Aggregate of shrunken mitochondria in a swollen axon in a chronic stage of cyanide intoxication in the rat. Compare with Fig. 157 at the same magnification. × 45,000. (Hirano, A. et al.: J. Neuropathol. Exp. Neurol. 30: 325, 1971.)

Jew, J.Y., & Williams, T.H.: Ultrastructural aspects of bilirubin encephalopathy in cochlear nuclei of the Gunn rat. J. Anat., 124: 599, 1977.

Yajima, K., & Suzuki, K.: Neuronal degeneration in the brain of the brindled mouse. An ultrastructural study of the cerebral cortical neurons. Acta Neuropathol., 45: 17-25, 1979.

6. Intracytoplasmic Inclusions

PICK BODIES (Fig. 159)

The entity known as Pick's disease was first described by Pick on clinical and macroscopic pathological bases alone. It is characterized by circumscribed, profound lobar cerebral atrophy. Later, Alzheimer, using the Bielschowsky silver technique, identified the characteristic argentophilic neuronal inclusions which he described as neurofibrillary changes despite the differences between these and those seen in Alzheimer's disease. It should be noted that Pick bodies are often not found in lobar atrophy.

Pick bodies are most often found in the pyramidal neurons of Sommer's sector and the small neurons of the fascia dentata. They appear singly and are about the size of the neuronal nucleus. They are usually found in the apical area of the cell and are always at a constant, narrow, but distinct distance from the nucleus. In addition to argentophilia, Pick bodies are mildly hematoxylinophilic and can, therefore, be easily identified in ordinary H&E preparations. Granulovacuolar bodies are frequently either within or, more often, surrounding the Pick body. Eosinophilic rod-like bodies are usually present in the nearby neuropil of Sommer's sector.

Wiśniewski et al (1972) and Brion et al (1973) have described the fine structure of the Pick body. Both these groups have pointed out the similarity between Pick bodies and chromatolysis. Pick bodies are nonmembrane-bounded regions containing large accumulations of fibrillary components such as neurofilaments and microtubules, as well as other organelles. Alzheimer neurofibrillary tangles, identical to those seen in Alzheimer's disease have been reported in a single case of Pick's disease by Schochet et al (1968).

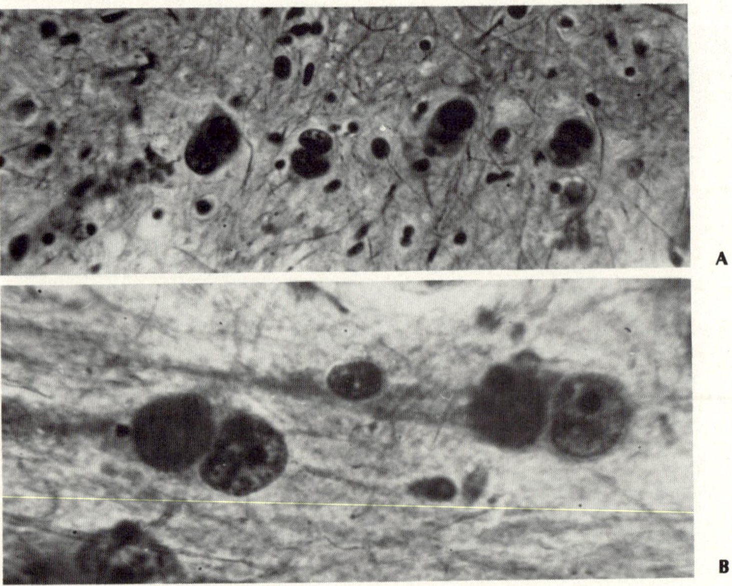

Fig. 159 Pick bodies (silver stain).

REFERENCES

Brion, S., Mikol, J., & Psimaras, A.: Recent findings in Pick's disease. *In* Progress in Neuropathology, Vol. 2, pp. 421-452, Zimmerman, H.M. (ed.), Grune & Stratton, New York, 1973.

Schochet, S.S. Jr., Lampert, P.W., & Lindenberg, R.: Fine structure of the Pick and Hirano bodies in a case of Pick's disease. Acta Neuropathol., 11: 330-337, 1968.

Wisniewski, H.M., Coblentz, J.M., & Terry, R.D.: Pick's disease. A clinical and ultrastructural study. Arch. Neurol., 26: 97-108, 1972.

LEWY BODIES (Fig. 160)

Lewy first described these cytoplasmic inclusions in the substantia innominata of a patient with idiopathic Parkinsonism. They are still considered a characteristic feature of that disease but have since been seen in the substantia nigra, locus ceruleus, and a variety of pigmented and nonpigmented neurons and in the spinal cord as well as in sympathetic ganglia (Ohama and Ikuta, 1976). In addition to idiopathic Parkinsonism, small numbers of Lewy bodies have been associated with

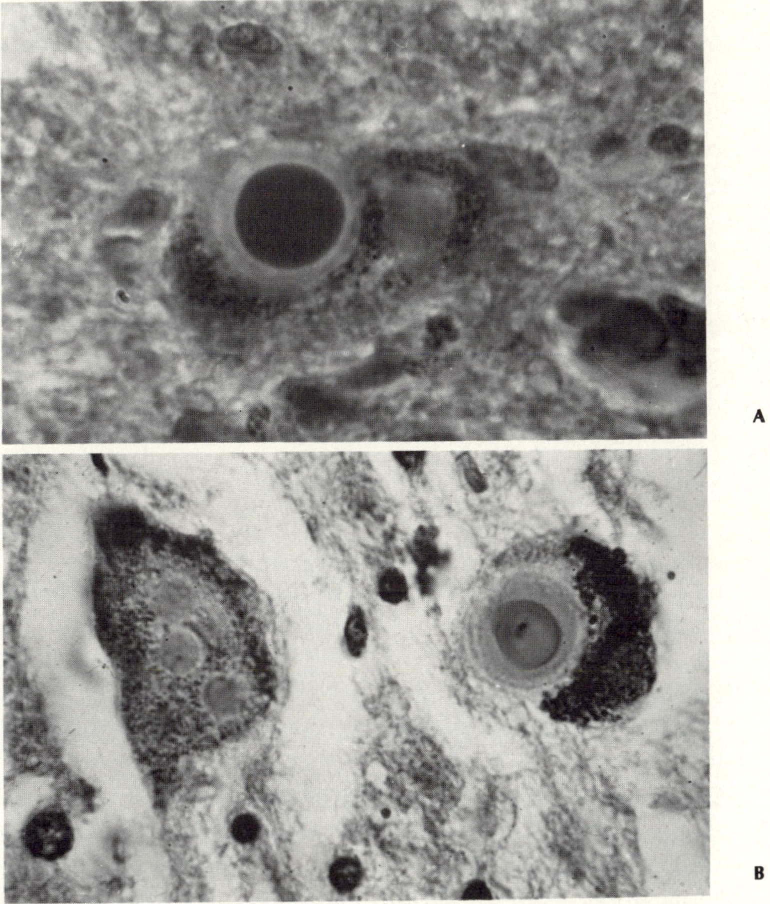

Fig. 160 Lewy bodies.
A. Masson stain (see Fig. 123.2E). B. H&E stain.

aging as well as with some cases of postencephalitic Parkinsonism where they are usually accompanied by neurofibrillary tangles. They have also been observed in a small fraction of patients with Parkinsonism-dementia complex on Guam where, again, neurofibrillary tangles, the main feature of the disease, are associated with them, sometimes even within the same cell (Figure 123-1A). Lewy body-like structures have also been seen in certain motor neuron diseases and in neuraxonal dystrophy.

Lewy bodies usually appear as single, round inclusions in the soma or processes of the neuron. Sometimes they are multiple and they may be elongated or sausage-like curving around the nucleus and extending into the cell process. The size is variable and they may be larger than the nucleus. They usually display a core and a less dense amorphous halo. They may sometimes display a concentric lamellar structure.

Lewy bodies do not stain in Nissl preparations where they appear amorphous or vacuolar. The cores are eosinophilic and stain a bright red in Masson's stain and blue in Holzer stain. They may be differentiated from Pick bodies by the latter's faint hematoxylinophilia and from Lafora bodies which stain blue in Nissl preparations among other differences.

Their fine structure was first elucidated by Duffy and Tennyson (1965) and since confirmed by a number of other workers. The core consists of a tangle of compactly arranged 70~80Å filaments sometimes with occasional interspersed minute vesicles. Despite the clear demarcation between the halo and core and between the halo and cytoplasm seen in the light microscope, no membrane separates these structures. Instead, at the boundary between the core and the halo the filaments are arranged in a radial pattern and become less densely packed.

REFERENCES

Duffy, P.O., & Tennyson, V.M.: Phase and electron microscopic observations of Lewy bodies and melanin granules in the substantia nigra and locus ceruleus in Parkinson's disease. J. Neuropathol. Exp. Neurol., 24: 398-414, 1965.

Okazaki, H., Lipkin, L.E., & Aronson, S.M.: Diffuse intracytoplasmic ganglionic inclusions (Lewy type) associated with progressive dementia and quadriparesis in flexion. J. Neuropathol. Exp. Neurol., 20: 237-244, 1961.

Roy, S., and Wolman, L.: Ultrastructural observations in parkinsonism. J. Pathol., 99: 39-44, 1969.

Schochet, S.S. Jr.: Neuronal inclusions. *In* The Structure and Function of Nervous Tissue, Vol. 4, pp. 129-177, Bourne, G.H. (ed.), Academic Press, New York, 1972.

Ohama, E., and Ikuta, F.: Parkinson's disease: Distribution of Lewy bodies and monoamine neuron system. Acta Neuropathol., 34: 311-319, 1976.

LAFORA BODIES (Fig. 161)

Lafora's disease is a rare (up to 1973 there were only 64 cases in the world literature), familial, progressive neurological disorder of children. It is characterized by myoclonic jerks and is sometimes referred to as myoclonic epilepsy. Pathological findings include the formation of Lafora bodies in neurons over widespread areas of the nervous system, especially in the substantia nigra and the

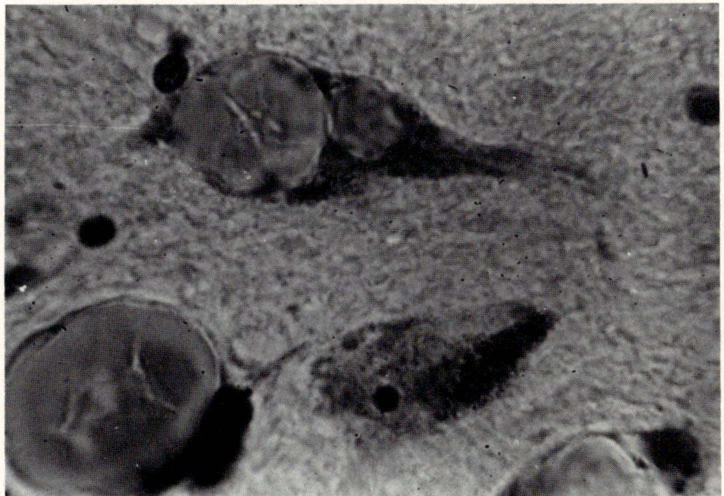

Fig. 161 Lafora bodies in neurons of the substantia nigra (Nissl stain).

dentate nucleus of the cerebellum. The mammillary bodies and subthalamic nuclei are reported to be free of these structures (Iwata, 1973).

Lafora bodies may appear either singly or multiply, and, while they are most often seen in the soma, they may also be found in the neuronal processes, including synaptic endings. In addition, large numbers are found in a certain strain of dogs which are used as a model for the disease (Holland et al., 1970). Apparently similar structures have been seen in diseases which are clinically distinct from Lafora's disease and in which the inclusions are confined to axons rather than soma (see p. 179).

Lafora bodies are easily recognized by their striking blue color in Nissl preparations in contrast to neurofibrillary tangles or Lewy bodies. They are PAS-positive.

The fine structure of the Lafora bodies consists of a nonmembrane-bounded accumulation of fine filaments interspersed with finely granular material. Both the light and electron microscopic findings suggest a virtually identical structure between the intraneuronal Lafora bodies seen in children and the corpora amylacea seen in astrocytes in adult and aged nervous systems.

Although a neurological disease, abnormal PAS-positive inclusions are also found in cardiac muscle and in hepatic cells in Lafora's disease. The fine structure of the myocardial inclusions have been shown to be very similar to that of the intraneuronal Lafora bodies.

REFERENCES

Nanba, M.: Lafora disease. Brain and Nerve (Tokyo), 20: 6-13, 1968.

Holland, J.M., William, C.D., Prieur, D.J., & Collings, G.H.: Lafora's disease in the dog. A comparative study. Am. J. Pathol., 58: 509-529, 1970.

Iwata, M.: Contribution a l'etude de la maladie de Lafora. Mémoire pour le titre dássistant étranger, Université de Paris VI, U.E.R. De Médecine Pitié-Salpetrière, Paris, 1973.

INTRACYTOPLASMIC HYALINE (COLLOID) INCLUSIONS

Intracytoplasmic hyaline inclusions are occasionally found in the hypoglossal nuclei or large anterior horn cells in elderly adults who may be apparently free of any neurological disorder. They are rare in children. They are easily identified by their sharp demarcation and distinct eosinophilia. Their size is variable and can sometimes fill and distend the soma. Nearby intracytoplasmic features of the cell appear unremarkable.

Fine structural studies reveal the hyaline inclusion to be widely distended elements of the rough endoplasmic reticulum. They are surrounded by ribosome-bearing membranes. These findings suggest that they represent unusual products of protein synthesis.

REFERENCES

Takei, Y., & Mirra, S.S.: Intracytoplasmic hyaline inclusion bodies in the nerve cells of the hypoglossal nucleus in human autopsy material. Acta Neuropathol., 17: 14-23, 1971.

Norman, M.G.: Hyaline ("Colloid") cytoplasmic inclusions in motoneurones in association with familial microencephaly, retardation and seizures. J. Neurol. Sci., 23: 63-70, 1974.

BUNINA BODIES

Bunina (1962) described a small, 1-2 micron eosinophilic granule in the anterior horn cell in patients with familial ALS. They appeared either singly or several at one time, sometimes arranged in a chain. These findings were later confirmed in a number of cases of ALS including sporadic and familial forms of the disease and in patients from Guam (Hirano, 1965).

Several attempts to analyze the fine structure have been made but, because of the rarity of the Bunina body, the results are uncertain. Most workers report that they consist of irregularly shaped, dense, granular material. The ill-defined border seems to be associated with nearby organelles including elements of the endoplasmic reticulum, vesicles, mitochondria, etc. The interior sometimes contains small islands of scattered fragments of filaments. In addition, on the basis of other fine structural studies it has been suggested that the Bunina body may be an autophagic vacuole (Hart et al., 1977) or an accumulation of annulate lamellae (Tomonaga et al., 1977).

The possibility of virus was originally suggested by Bunina (1962). This group also reported the induction of Bunina body formation in the anterior horn cells of monkeys who had tissue from ALS patients implanted into their brain (Zil'ber et al., 1963). Later, however, the appearance of Bunina bodies within the monkey anterior horn cells could not be confirmed and subsequent attempts to induce the ALS-like symptoms in experimental animals were not successful.

A variety of conditions not related to viral infection may lead to the formation of small eosinophilic inclusions in anterior horn cells (Figs. 162, 163). These include Chediak-Higashi disease in Aleutian minks, vinca alkaloid intoxication and neurolathyrism (Hirano et al., 1976). The fine structure of these inclusions are different from those of Bunina bodies.

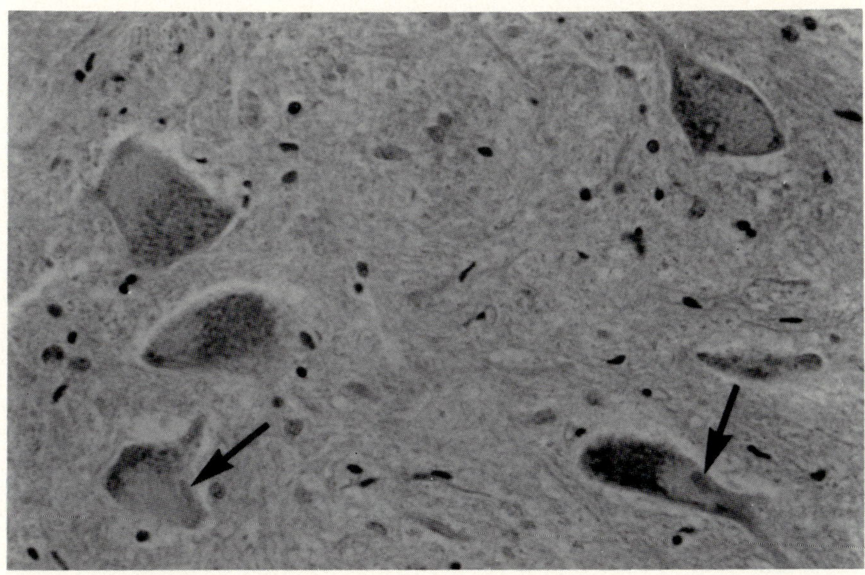

Fig. 162 A paraffin section of the spinal cord showing eosinophilic inclusions (arrows) in the cytoplasm of two anterior horn cells in a case of neurolathyrism. × 400. (From Hirano, A. et al: Acta Neuropathol. 35: 277, 1976.)

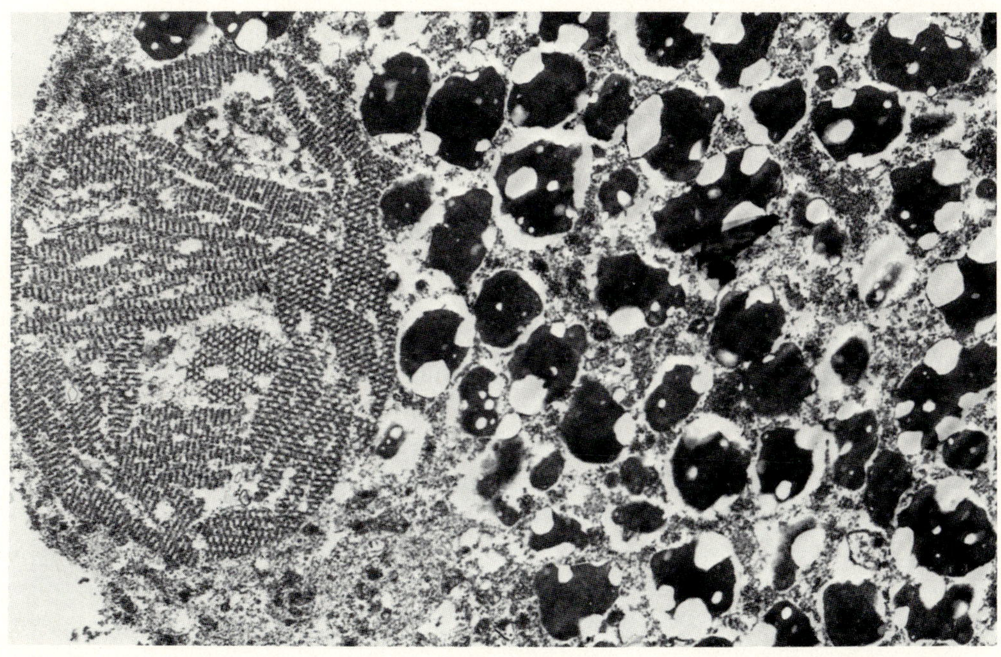

Fig. 163 A crystalloid inclusion (left) adjacent to a large accumulation of lipofuscin granules. × 10,000. (From Hirano, A. et al: Acta Neuropathol. 35: 277, 1976.)

REFERENCES

Bunina, T.L.: On intracellular inclusions in familial amyotrophic lateral sclerosis. Korsakov J. Neuropathol. & Psychiat., 62: 1293-1299, 1962.

Zil'ber, L.A., Bajdakova, Z.L., Gardas'jan, A.N., Konovalov, N.V., Bunina, T.L., & Barabadze, E.M.: Study of the etiology of amyotrophic lateral sclerosis. Bull. Wld. Hlth. Org., 29: 449-456, 1963.

Hirano, A.: Pathology of amyotrophic lateral sclerosis. *In* Slow, Latent and Temperate Virus Infection, pp. 23-37, Gajdusek, D.C., Gibbs, C.J. Jr., & Alpers, M. (eds.), NIH, Washington, D.C., 1965.

Hirano, A., Llena, J.F., Steifler, M., & Cohn, D.F.: Anterior horn cell changes in a case of neurolathyrism. Acta Neuropathol., 35: 277-283, 1976.

Hart, M.N., Cancilla, P.A., Frommes, S., & Hirano, A.: Anterior horn cell degeneration and Bunina-type inclusions associated with dementia. Acta Neuropathol., 38: 225-228, 1977.

Tomonaga, M., Saito, M., Yoshimura, M., Shimada, H., & Tohgi, H.: Intracytoplasmic inclusion (Bunina body) observed in amyotrophic lateral sclerosis. Neurol. Med. (Tokyo), 7: 160-163, 1977.

Asbury, A.K., & Johnson, P.C.: Pathology of Peripheral Nerve. Fig. 17-1D, W.B. Saunders Co., Philadelphia, 1978.

NEGRI BODIES

Negri bodies are spherical eosinophilic inclusions generally in the pyramidal cells of Ammon's horn or the Purkinje cells in patients with rabies. Their size is variable but usually approximately as large as the nucleoli. There may be one or several Negri bodies in a single neuron. Fine structural studies reveal that they consist of tubular shaped viral particles identical to those seen in experimental animals infected with rabies.

REFERENCE

Morecki, R., & Zimmerman, H.M.: Human rabies encephalitis. Fine structure study of cytoplasmic inclusions. Arch. Neurol., 20: 599-604, 1969.

SMALL EOSINOPHILIC GRANULES OF THE PIGMENTED NEURONS OF THE SUBSTANTIA NIGRA

Small eosinophilic granules are sometimes found in the melanin-containing neurons of the zona compacta of the substantia nigra. They are usually found in clusters and may be present at any age. They are of no known diagnostic significance and are seen in apparently normal nervous tissue.

Their fine structure consists of accumulations of parallel, 85Å diameter filaments connnected by finer filaments. Similar configurations may be seen in nearby distended cisternae of the rough endoplasmic reticulum and they are regarded as proteinacious products. Their fine structure renders them distinct from other cytoplasmic inclusions.

REFERENCE

Schochet, S.S. Jr., Wyatt, R.B., & McCormick, W.F.: Intracytoplasmic acidophilic granules in the substantia nigra. Arch. Neurol., 22: 550-555, 1970.

EOSINOPHILIC INCLUSIONS IN THALAMIC NEURONS

Eosinophilic intracytoplasmic inclusion bodies may be seen in thalamic neurons. Although they were observed originally in myotonic dystrophy (Culebras et al., 1973), they are nonspecific changes which may be seen in other conditions as well, including the normal thalamus. Although they are considered an aging change, their significance is unknown. Their fine structure has been examined and they are reported to be distended cisterns of the rough endoplasmic reticulum.

REFERENCE

Culebras, A., Feldman, G.R., & Merk, F.: Cytoplasmic inclusion bodies within neurons of the thalamus in myotonic dystrophy. J. Neurol. Sci., 19: 319-329, 1973.

7. Neuronal Cell Processes

DENDRITES

Dendrites arise from the cell body and, as their name suggests, proceed to branch in a tree-like fashion. In pyramidal cells the major trunks of the dendrites are classified as either apical or basal depending on the site of origin. Usually the arborization of the dendritic process is elaborate so that the cell surface covering the dendritic tree is much larger than that of the cell body. A great proportion of this surface is devoted to synaptic contacts which may be on either the smooth dendritic process itself or on small, specialized protrusions known as spines. That portion of the dendrite not involved in synaptic contact is, in many neurons, covered by "satellite cells", usually astrocytic processes. Unlike the axon, dendritic processes are not arranged in parallel bundles. Instead, each dendritic process seems to extend along its own pathway seeking its synaptic contact.

The interior of the proximal portions of the larger dendritic trunks are essentially the same as that of the perikaryal cytoplasm. They contain all the organelles including rough endoplasmic reticulum and the Golgi apparatus. As the branches get smaller, however, the organelles within them become limited to microtubules, filaments, mitochondria and occasional elements of the smooth endoplasmic reticulum. Except for the frequent presence of synaptic contacts, the smaller dendritic processes appear very similar to those of individual axons.

Relatively little attention has been paid to the pathology of the dendrite. This is, in large measure, due to the fact that routine optical preparations do not provide good visualization of the dendritic tree. Usually one sees only the cell soma and the proximal portion of the dendrite. Even in conventional silver impregnation preparations either only a portion of the dendritic processes are seen or only the filamentous elements are stained. Golgi methods allow visualization of much larger portions of the dendritic tree, but they suffer from certain serious drawbacks. Only a small number of cells become impregnated and the possibility always remains that some peripheral portion of the dendrites may not be visualized. Furthermore, the technique is difficult and can result in artifactitious metallic deposits.

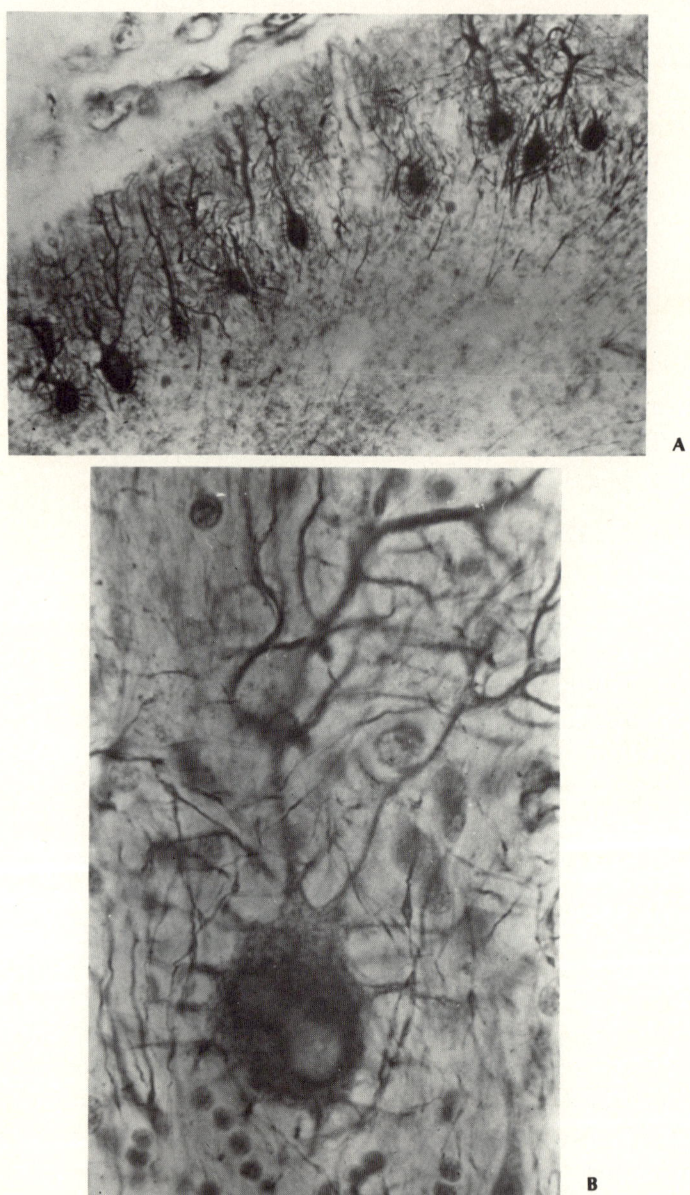

Fig. 164 Cerebellar cortex in kinky hair disease (silver stain). There are many somatic sprouts on the Purkinje cells.

Nevertheless, some pathological changes of the dendritic trees are known. The so-called "*stellate body*" or "*cactus*" is an expansion of segments of the peripheral portions of the dendritic processes of the Purkinje cells. Individual expansions can sometimes assume the size of the cell body itself and they display numerous radiating processes. They are seen in various lipidoses (Fine et al., 1960) and in a variety of other conditions such as granule cell type cerebellar degeneration, kinky hair disease (Menkes et al., 1962; Aguilar et al., 1966; Ghatak et al., 1972; Iwata et al., 1979), organic mercury poisoning (Hunter and Russell, 1954), etc.

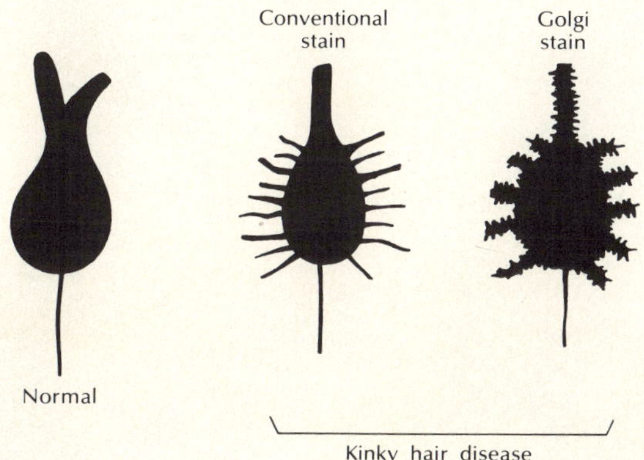

Fig. 165 Diagram of the Purkinje cells of the cerebella of normal (left), and kinky hair disease (center and right) patients. (From Hirano, A.: *In*: Neurobiology of Neurons and Glia. Kyoritsu Pub. Co., Tokyo, p. 65, 1977.)

Depending on the condition, when stellate bodies are present on dendrites the soma may also show similar changes. Indeed, in kinky hair disease the *somatic sprouts* are one of the main features of the disease (Figs. 164-168). In certain lipidoses, structures, termed *meganeurites*, have been found at the basal pole of the perikarya which are reminiscent of cactus-like enlargements of the dendrites.

Another well-known pathologic change seen in senile dementia and in normal aging is the reduction of dendritic arborization in cortical neurons (Scheibel, 1978; Mervis, 1978). In dementia paralytica due to syphilis the orientation of the dendritic trees of the cerebrum is severely distorted. Purkinje cell dendrites are also profoundly diminished and distorted in kinky hair disease and in other genetic disorders in humans and in mice (Hirano, 1978).

REFERENCES

Hunter, D., & Russel, D.E.: Focal cerebral and cerebellar atrophy in a human subject due to organic mercury compounds. J. Neurol. Neurosurg. Psychiat., 17: 235-241, 1954.

Fine, D.I.M., Barron, K.D., & Hirano, A.: Central nervous system lipidosis in an adult with atrophy of the cerebellar granular layer: A case report. J. Neuropathol. Exp. Neurol., 19: 355-369, 1960.

Menkes, J.H., Alter, M., Steigleder, G.K., Weakley, D.R., & Sung, J.H.: A sex-linked recessive disorder with retardation of growth, peculiar hair, and focal cerebral and cerebellar degeneration. Pediatrics, 29: 764-769, 1962.

Aguilar, M.J., Chadwick, D.L., Okuyama, K., & Kamoshita, S.: Kinky hair disease. 1. Clinical and pathological features. J. Neuropathol. Exp. Neurol., 25: 507-522, 1966.

Ghatak, N.R., Hirano, A., Poon, T.P., & French, J.H.: Trichopoliodystrophy. II. Pathological changes in skeletal muscle and nervous system. Arch. Neurol., 26: 60-72, 1972.

Kreutzberg, G.W. (ed.): International Symposium on Physiology and Pathology of Dendrites. Raven Press, New York, 1975.

Mervis, R.: Structural alterations in neurons of aged canine neocortex: A Golgi study. Exp. Neurol. 62: 417-432, 1978.

Hirano, A.: Aberrant synapses in the cerebellum. Advances Neurol. Sci. (Tokyo), 22: 1279-1295, 1978.

Scheibel, A.: Structural aspects of the aging brain: Spine systems and the dendritic arbor. *In* Alzheimer's Disease: Senile Dementia and Related Disorders (Aging, Vol. 7), pp. 353-373. Katzman, R., Terry, R.D., & Bick, K.L. (eds.), Raven Press, New York, 1978.

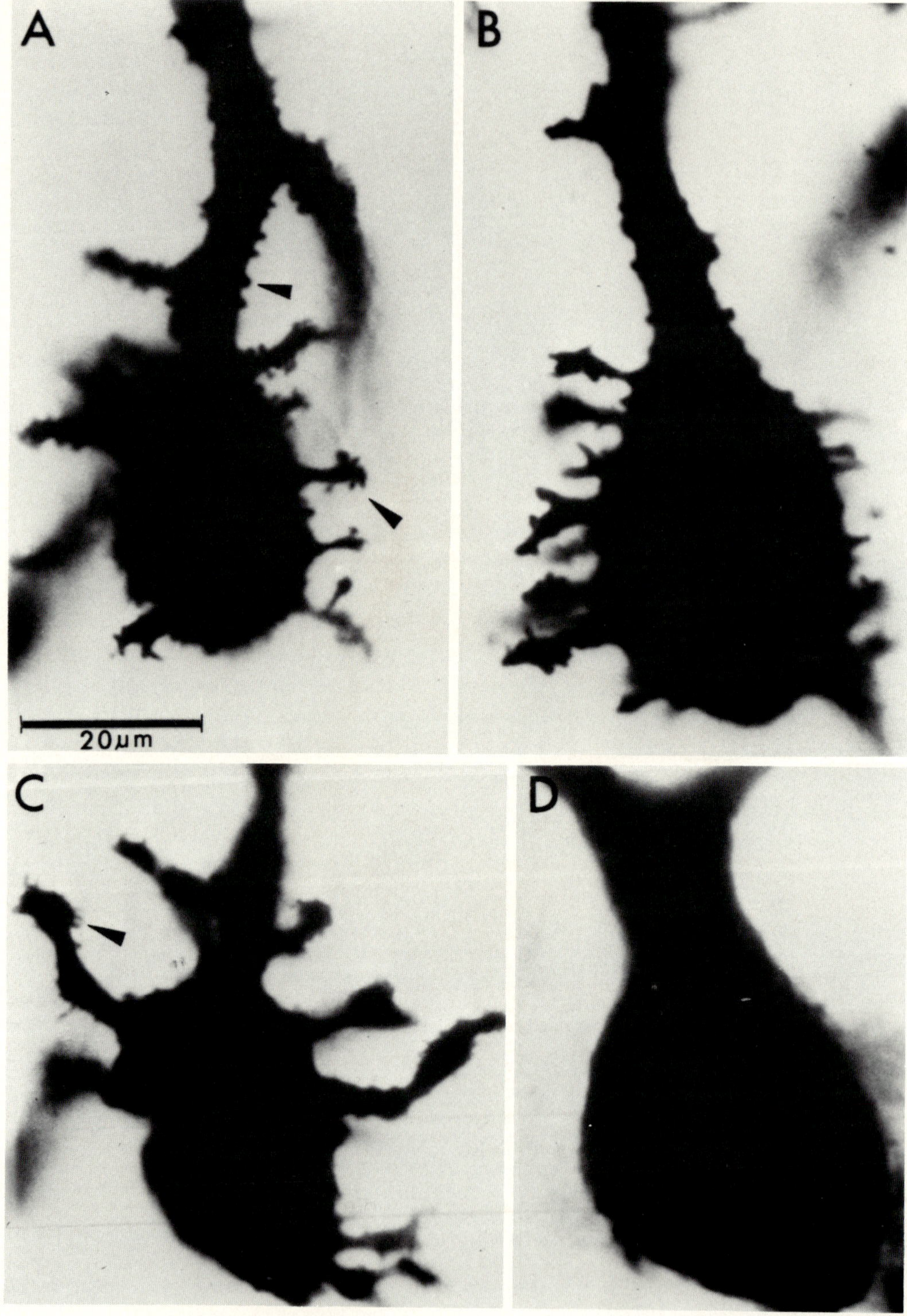

Fig. 166 A, B and C. Purkinje cells from a 21 month old child with Menkes' kinky hair disease. D. A normal Purkinje cell from a 2-year old child with a negative neurological history. (From Purpura et al., Brain Res. 117;125, 1976.)

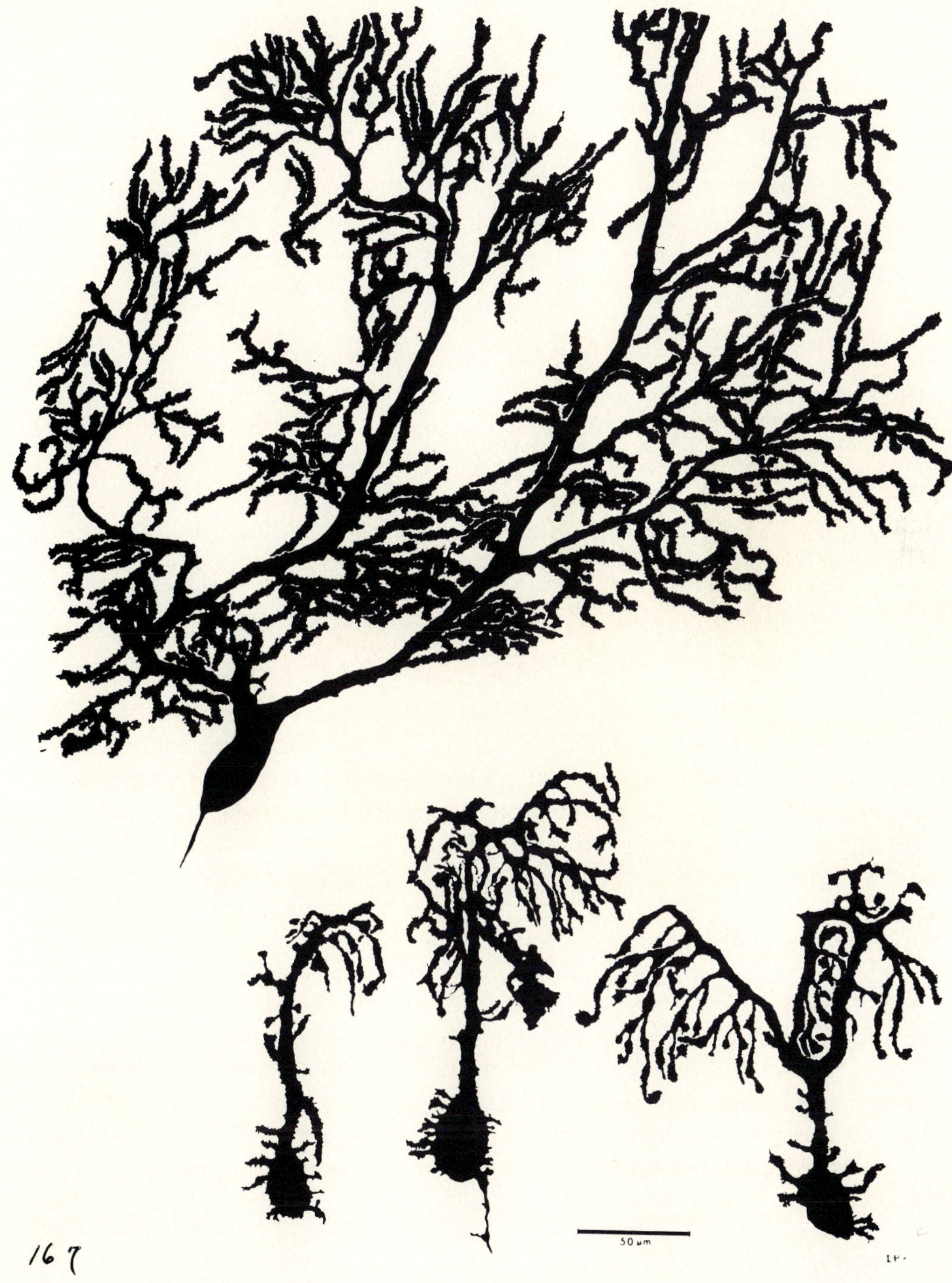

Fig. 167 Camera lucida drawings of Purkinje cells. The lower three are the same cells as A, B and C of Fig. 166. The dendritic arborization is small and distorted. The upper drawing is of a normal Purkinje cell from a 1 year old child. (From Purpura et al.: Brain Res. 117: 125, 1976.)

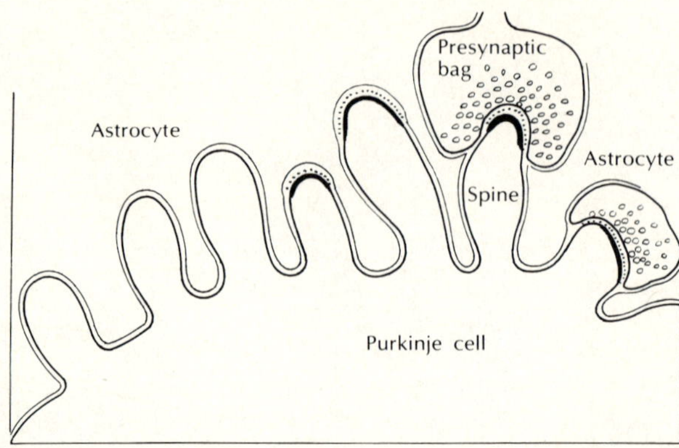

Fig. 168 A diagram of the electron microscopic view of the surface of a Purkinje cell soma or dendrite of a patient with kinky hair disease. (From Hirano, A.: *In*: Neurobiology of Neurons and Glia. Kyoritsu Pub. Co., Tokyo, p. 65, 1977.)

Iwata, M., Hirano, A., & French, J.H.: Degeneration of the cerebellar system in X-chromosome-linked copper malabsorption. Ann. Neurol., 5: 542-549, 1979.
Iwata, M., Hirano, A., & French, J.H.: Thalamic degeneration in X-chromosome-linked copper malabsorption. Ann. Neurol., 5: 359-366, 1979.

AXONS (Fig. 126)

In most neurons axons are long, unbranching processes. Their caliber may be quite small but it remains rather constant over most of its length until it approaches the target organ where it may branch into fine terminals. Some variations occur. In Purkinje cells, for example, the axon branches and gives rise to a recurrent fiber.

Axons stain faintly blue in H & E preparations. They are much more easily seen after silver impregnation for axons in which they appear dense and black.

The electron microscope has contributed substantially to our understanding of the axon. The *axoplasm* is surrounded by a plasma membrane, the *axolemma*, which is apparently identical to the rest of the neuronal plasma membrane except for three regions: the axon hillock and initial segment, the nodal and paranodal region and the synapses. At the axon hillock and initial segment and at the nodes of Ranvier the region subjacent to the axolemma contains a finely filamentous electron dense layer, the *undercoating*, separated from the inner leaflet of the plasma membrane by a narrow electron-lucent area. The structure of the axonal surface in the paranodal regions and the synapses will be discussed later.

The interior of the axon is relatively simple under normal conditions. Microtubules and neurofilaments, oriented parallel to the long axis of the axon are constant features. These may be related to axonal flow, a subject of intense, current investigation (Ochs and Worth, 1978). Occasional elongated mitochondria oriented in the same direction are also encountered. Elements of the smooth endoplasmic reticulum are common.

The *axon hillock* and *initial segment* display certain additional features.

Although Nissl substance is not seen in these areas, clusters of ribosomes are present. In addition, the microtubules are connected to one another by fine filaments and form fascicles.

REFERENCES

Palay, S.L., Sotelo, C., Peters, A., & Orband, P.M.: The axon hillock and the initial segment. J. Cell Biol., 38: 193-201, 1968.

Peters, A., Proskauer, C.C., & Kaiserman-Abramof, I.R.: The small pyramidal neuron of the rat cerebral cortex. J. Cell Biol., 39: 604-619, 1968.

Hirano, A.: The pathology of the central myelinated axon. *In* Structure and Function of the Nervous Tissue. Vol. 5, pp. 73-162, Bourne, G.H. (ed.), Academic Press, New York, 1972.

Hirano, A., & Dembitzer, H.M.: Fine structure of normal myelin. *In* International Encyclopedia of Neurology, Psychiatry, Psychoanalysis and Psychology. pp. 413-416, Wolman, B.B. (ed.) Van Nostrand, Reinhold, New York, 1977.

Hirano, A., & Dembitzer, H.M.: Morphology of normal central myelinated axons. *In* Physiology and Pathology of Axons, pp. 65-82, Waxman, S.G. (ed.) Raven Press, New York, 1978.

Ochs, S., & Worth, R.M.: Axoplasmic transport in normal and pathological systems. *In* Physiology and Pathobiology of Axons. pp. 251-264, Waxman, S.G. (ed.), Raven Press, New York, 1978.

Loss of Organelles (Fig. 169)

After a variety of insults it is not uncommon to encounter fibers in which segments of the axon have swollen and lost all of their organelles except for the distended axolemma. This is a nonspecific change and may accompany anoxia, hypoglycemia, acute cyanide intoxication and others. In Wallerian degeneration, the empty axon may collapse giving rise to bizarre configurations of the fiber (Fig. 170).

Changes of the Fibrillary Organelles

In certain conditions such as IDPN (β-β′-iminodiproprionitrile) intoxication or in giant axonal neuropathy, among other conditions, the axon becomes focally distended by abnormal accumulations consisting predominantly of 100Å filaments. This leads to marked argentophilia in silver preparations. The so-called *torpedoes* sometimes seen in Purkinje cells are, in fact, accumulations of the filaments in the Purkinje cell axons within the granule cell layer (Fig. 171).

Microtubules, too, may accumulate in abnormal amounts under certain pathological conditions (Fig. 172) including neuroaxonal dystrophy. *Vinca* alkaloid intoxication leads to the destruction of the microtubules and the associated appearance of a crystalloid formation composed of a hexagonal array of closely packed elements (Fig. 148). A tubulo-vesicular material often accumulates in association with these changes (Fig. 173).

Changes of the Smooth Endoplasmic Reticulum (Figs. 174,175)

In certain pathological conditions, most notably triorthocresyl phosphate intoxication and in neuroaxonal dystrophy, the smooth endoplasmic reticulum may proliferate in abnormal amounts forming bizarre, whorl-like or lamellar structures. Another variation, which has been shown to be continuous with the smooth

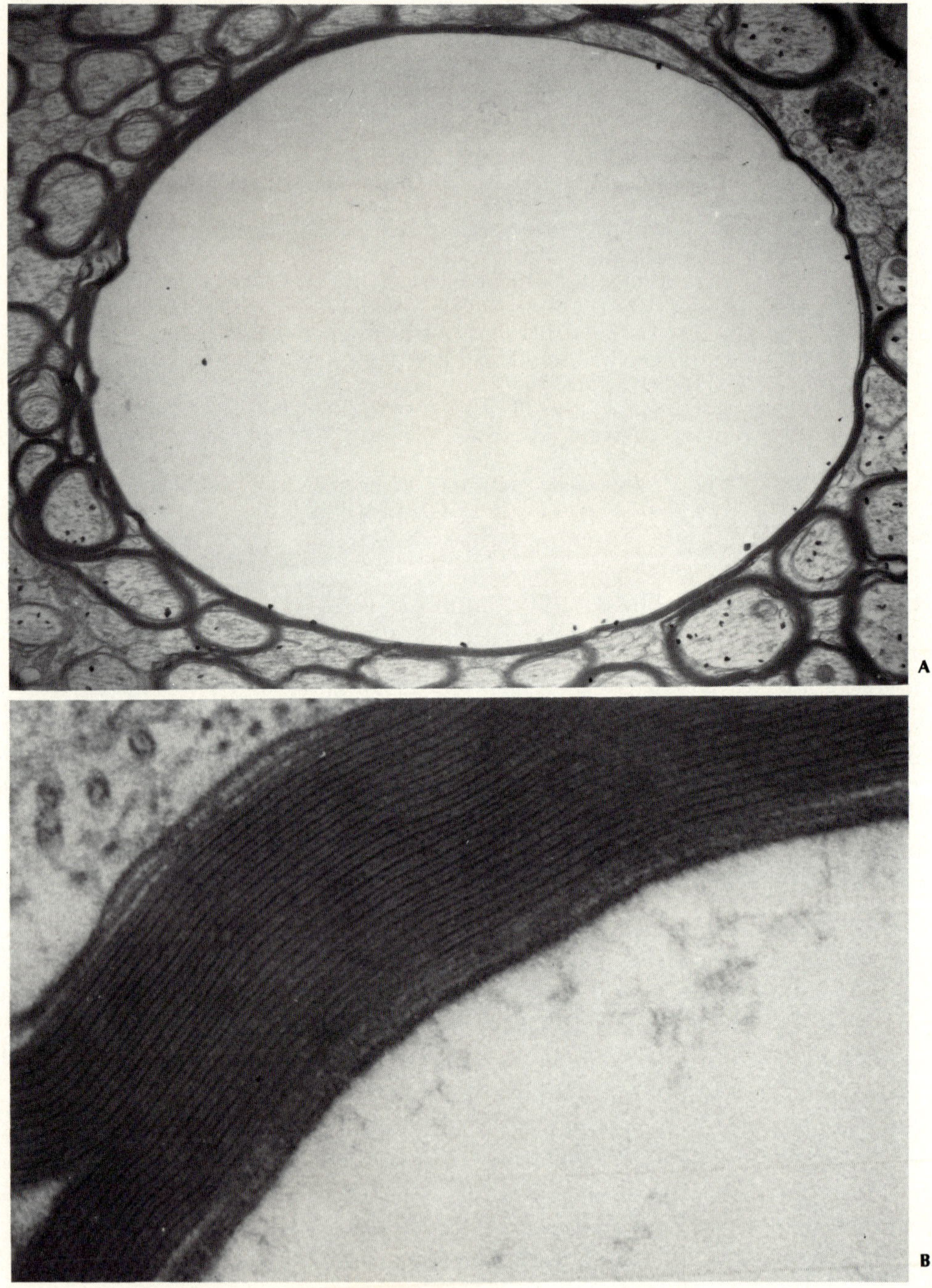

Fig. 169 A. Vacuolar distension of a myelinated axon in the cerebral white matter. × 20,000. B. Higher magnification of a similar area. The myelin sheath of the affected nerve fiber is identical to that of the adjacent normal fiber. × 180,000. (From Hirano, A. et al.: J. Neuropathol. Exp. Neurol., 26: 200, 1967.)

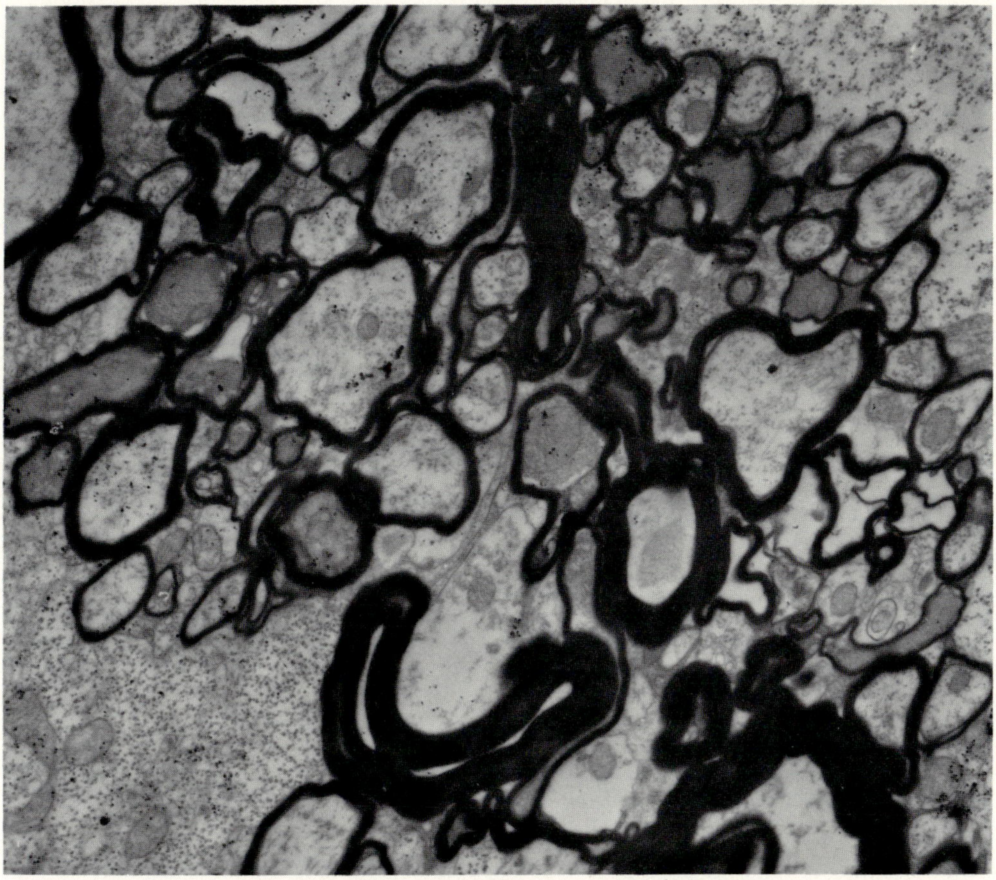

Fig. 170 Wallerian degeneration of the cerebral white matter. × 15,000 (From Hirano, A.: The Structure and Function of Nervous Tissue. Vol. 5, p. 73, Academic Press, 1972.)

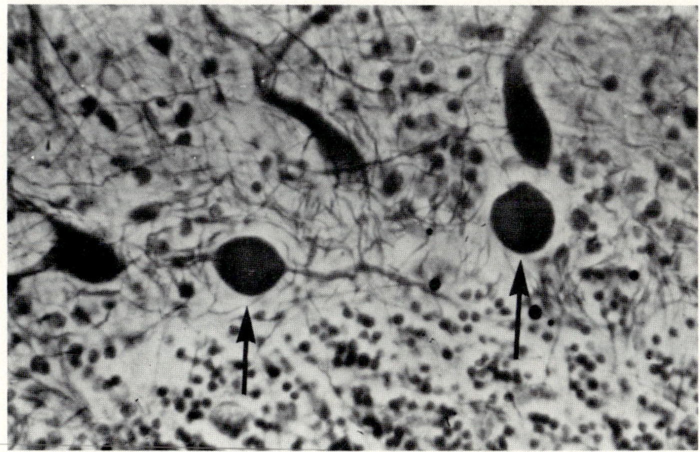

Fig. 171 Torpedoes (arrows) in the granule cell layer of the cerebellum (silver stain).

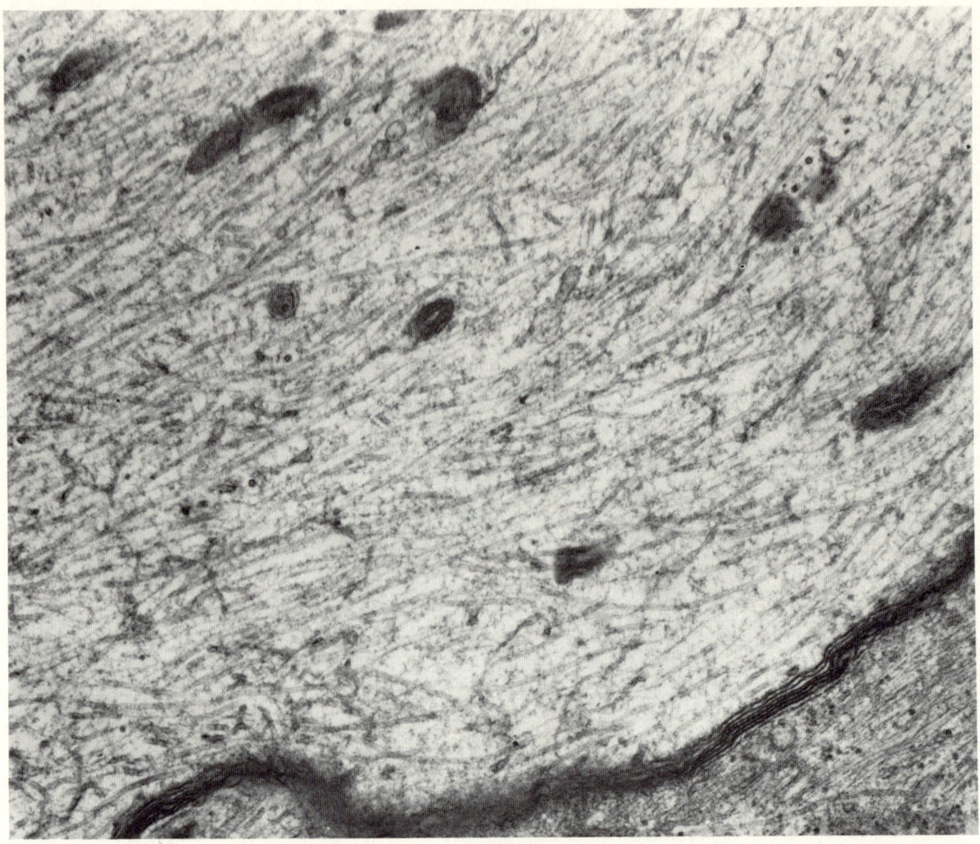

Fig. 172 Increase of microtubules in the myelinated axon. Neurofilaments are also evident. × 33,000. (From Hirano, A.: The Structure and Function of Nervous Tissue. Vol. 5, p. 73, Academic Press, 1972.)

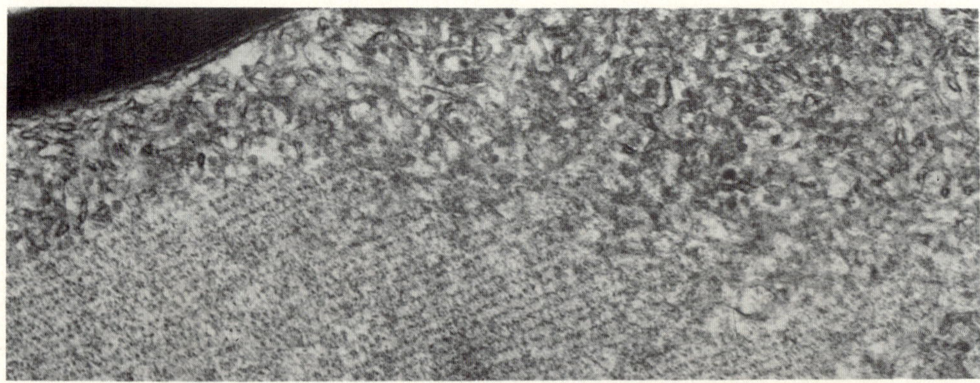

Fig. 173 Crystalloid and tubulo-vesicular structures in a myelinated axon of the cerebral white matter after vinblastine treatment. × 50,000. (From Hirano, A.: The Structure and Function of Nervous Tissue. Vol. 5, p. 73, Academic Press, 1972.)

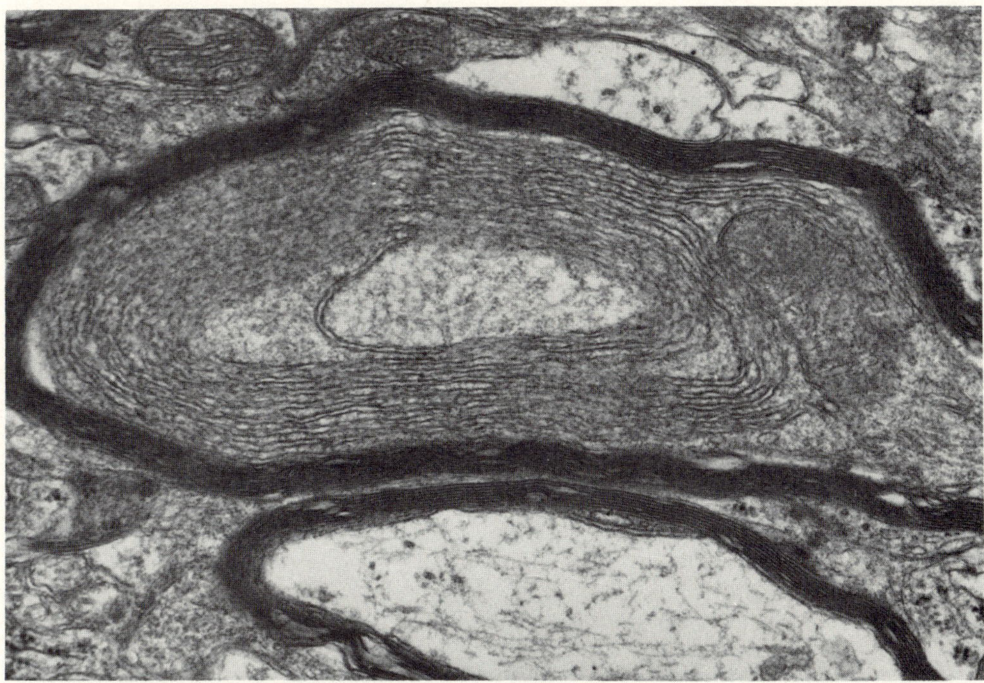

Fig. 174 A myelinated axon in the cerebellar granule cell layer of the jimpy mouse. A whorl-like arrangement of the endoplasmic reticulum is visible. × 31,000. (From Hirano, A. et al.: J. Neuropathol. Exp. Neurol., 28: 388, 1969.)

endoplasmic reticulum is the honeycomb-like tubular structure seen, for the most part, in myelinated axons in the cerebellar granule cell layer. These structures have been observed in apparently normal cerebella but are more common in a variety of pathological conditions where they are found in unmyelinated fibers as well. Some workers consider the honeycomb-like tubular bodies to be confined to the recurrent axon of the Purkinje cell. On the other hand the same structure has been seen in axons in the vestibular nucleus of thiamin-deficient rats. They have even been seen in myelinated and unmyelinated axons in the cerebrum of rats with intracranial lead or carcinogenic hydrocarbon implantation.

REFERENCES

Hirano, A., Rubin, R., Sutton, C.H., & Zimmerman, H.M.: Honeycomb-like tubular structure in axoplasm. Acta Neuropathol., 10: 17-25, 1968.

Hirano, A., Sax, D.S., & Zimmerman, H.M.: The fine structure of cerebella of jimpy mice and their "normal" litter mates. J. Neuropathol. Exp. Neurol., 28: 388-400, 1969.

Sotelo, C., & Palay, S.L.: Altered axons and axon terminals in the lateral vestibular nucleus of the rat: Possible example of axonal remodeling. Lab. Invest., 25: 653-671, 1971.

Hirano, A., & Kochen, J.A.: Experimental lead encephalopathy. Morphologic studies, Chapter II. *In* Progress in Neuropathology, Vol. III. pp. 319-342, Zimmerman, H.M. (ed.), Grune & Stratton, New York, 1976.

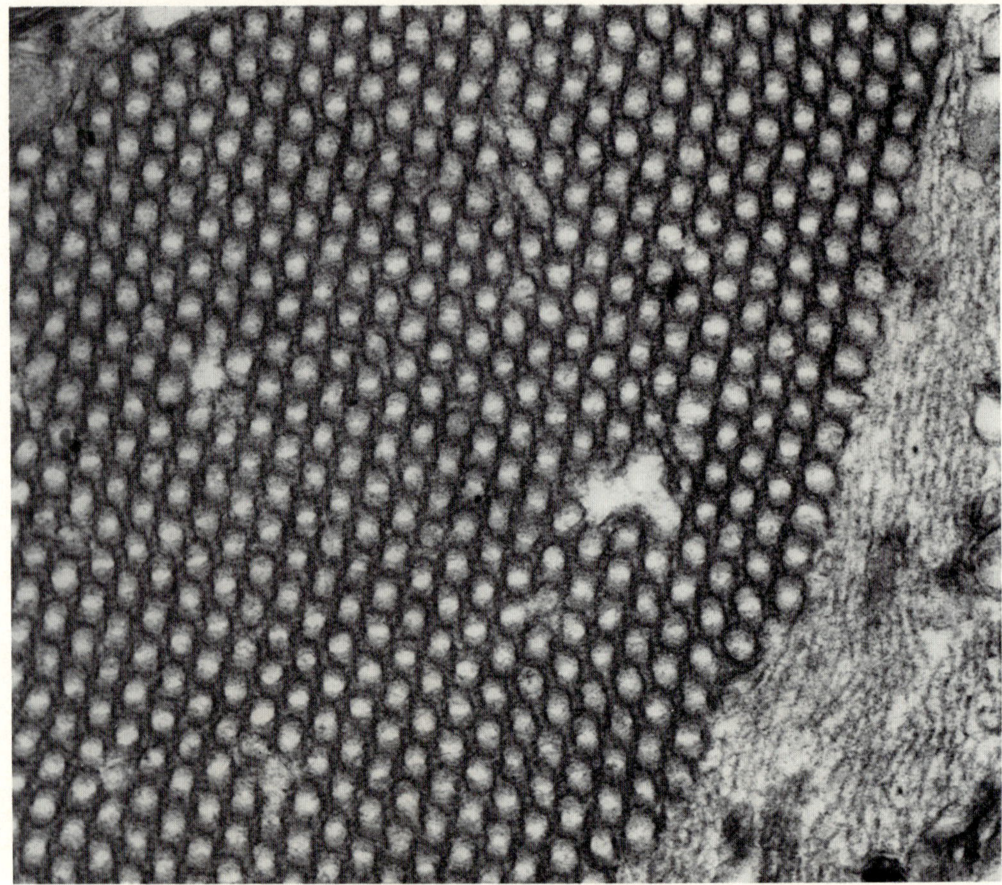

Fig. 175 Honeycomb-like structure in a myelinated axon of the cerebellar granule cell layer. × 64,000. (From Hirano, A. et al: Acta Neuropathol., 10: 17, 1968.)

Increase of Mitochondria, Vesicles and Dense Bodies (Figs. 176, 177)

Increases in these organelles are a common reaction to a variety of axonal insults. Best known among these is Wallerian degeneration. Webster (1962) has described the accumulation of mitochondria at the nodes of Ranvier in the initial stages of Wallerian degeneration. Implantation of foreign material into the white matter results in organelle accumulation in areas adjacent to the implant within one or two days after the operation.

Lampert (1967) has delineated four types of changes according to the phase and nature of the alteration accompanying various insults. The first is the *reactive change* which involves the segmental swelling of the axon associated with an increase in the number of mitochondria, vesicles and dense bodies. The second is the *degenerative phase* which is characterized by an increase in dense bodies associated with the accumulation of granular debris. *Regenerative changes* constitute the third phase which is associated with the formation of vesicular, tubular and filamentous elements as well as the change of dense bodies to residual bodies. The mitochondria tend to become smaller and assume a doughnut-shape

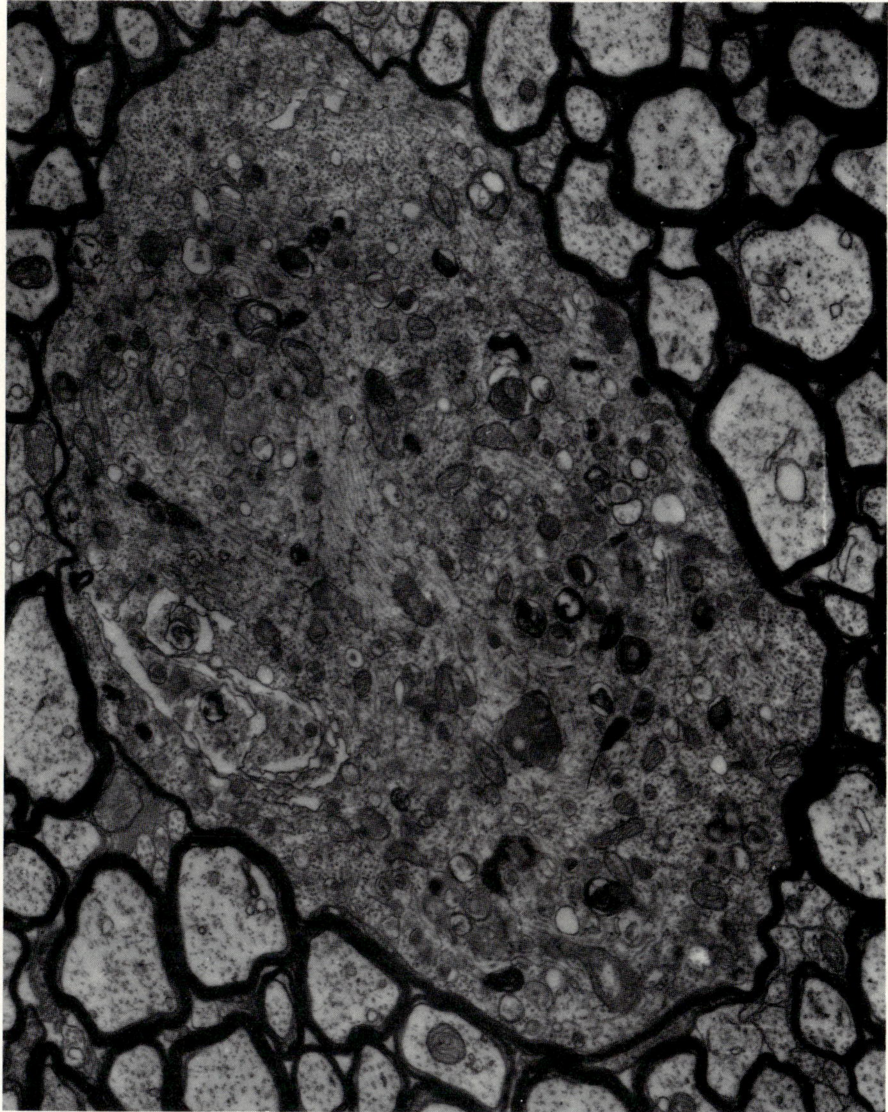

Fig. 176 A distended axon filled with numerous organelles in the cerebral white matter of an experimentally altered animal. × 20,000. (From Hirano, A.: Progress in Neuropathology. Vol.1, p. 1, Grune, & Stratton, 1971.)

configuration due to the paucity of cristae and the increased density of the matrix (Fig. 158). *Dystrophic axons* such as those seen in vitamin E-deficient rats or in human neuroaxonal dystrophy (Jellinger, 1973; Fujisawa and Shiraki, 1978) constitute the fourth category delineated by Lampert (1967). Under these conditions, in addition to all the changes of mitochondria, vesicles and dense bodies in the other categories described, there are also enormous accumulations of fibrils and the formation of the unusual membranous configurations of the endoplasmic reticulum discussed above.

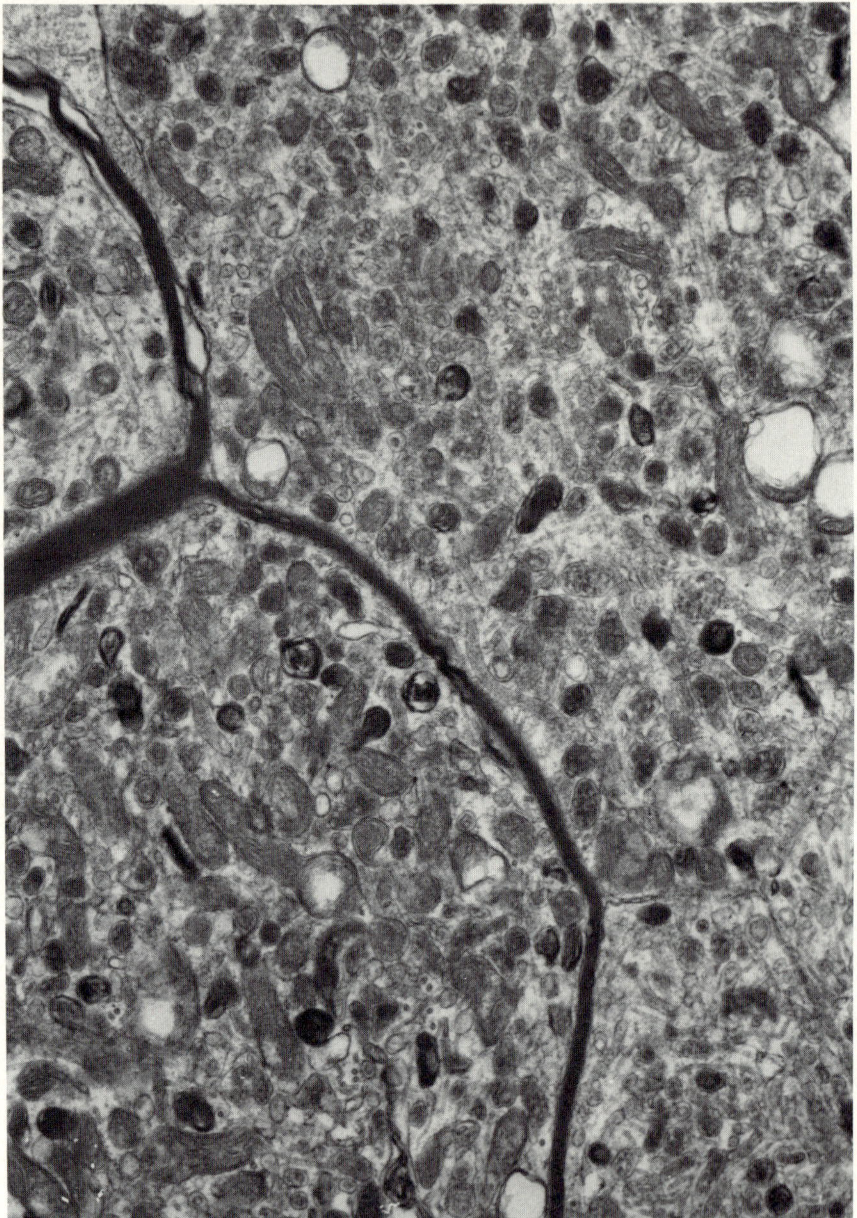

Fig. 177 Portions of axons showing numerous mitochondria, dense bodies, and other organelles in an experimentally altered animal. × 38,000. (From Hirano, A. et al.:J. Neuropathol. Exp. Neurol., 26: 200, 1967.)

Distension of axon terminals in the region of the nucleus gracilis is a conspicuous feature of the aging brain and of children with prolonged mucoviscidosis (cystic fibrosis of the pancreas) (Sung, 1964) or congenital biliary atresia (Sung and Stadlan, 1966).

REFERENCES

Webster, H. DeF.: Transient, focal accumulation of axonal mitochondria during the early stages of Wallerian degeneration. J. Cell Biol.,12: 361-377, 1962.

Sung, J.H.: Neuroaxonal dystrophy in mucoviscidosis. J. Neuropathol. Exp. Neurol., 23: 567-583, 1964.

Sung, J.H., & Stadlan, E.M.: Neuroaxonal dystrophy in congenital biliary atresia. J. Neuropathol. Exp. Neurol., 25: 341-361, 1966.

Lampert, P.: A comparative electron microscopic study of reactive, degenerative, regenerative and dystrophic axons. J. Neuropathol. Exp. Neurol., 26: 345-368, 1967.

Jellinger, K.: Neuroaxonal dystrophy: Its natural history and related disorders. *In* Progress in Neuropathology, Vol. 2, pp. 129-180, Zimmerman, H.M. (ed.) Grune & Stratton, New York, 1973.

Fujisawa, K., & Shiraki, H.: Study of axonal dystrophy. I. Pathology of the neuropil of the gracile and the cuneate nuclei in ageing and old rats. A stereological study. Neuropathol. Appl. Neurobiol., 4: 1-20, 1978.

Polyglucosan Bodies

Small numbers of polyglucosan bodies, which are virtually identical to Lafora bodies (see p. 161) may be found within axons of various patients over forty. This subject was recently summarized by Asbury and Johnson (1978). They are reported to be numerous in certain cases of progressive neurological diseases (Carpenter et al., 1978) where they were found throughout the central and peripheral nervous systems as well as in cardiac muscle.

REFERENCES

Hirano, A.: Some fine structural alterations of the central nervous system in aging. Proceedings of VIIth International Congress of Neuropathology, Vol. 2, pp. 83-90. Környey, St., Tariska, St., & Gosztonyi, G. (eds.), Excerpta Medica, Amsterdam, 1975.

Carpenter, S., & Karpati, G.: Intra-axonal polyglucosan bodies: An unusual lesion of peripheral nerves. Neurology, 26: 369 (abstract), 1976.

Carpenter, S., Karpati, G., Robitaille, Y., & Melmed, C.: Adult polyglucosan body axonopathy—A distinct chronic neurological disease. J. Neuropathol. Exp. Neurol. 37: 598 (abstract), 1978.

Asbury, A.K., & Johnson, P.C.: Pathology of Peripheral Nerve. W.B. Saunders Co., Philadelphia, 1978.

8. Synapses (Fig. 178)

NORMAL SYNAPSES

The morphological features of the synapses vary somewhat depending on the cell and its functional state. There is, however, a fundamental architecture common to all chemical synapses which differs from the electrical synapses seen in

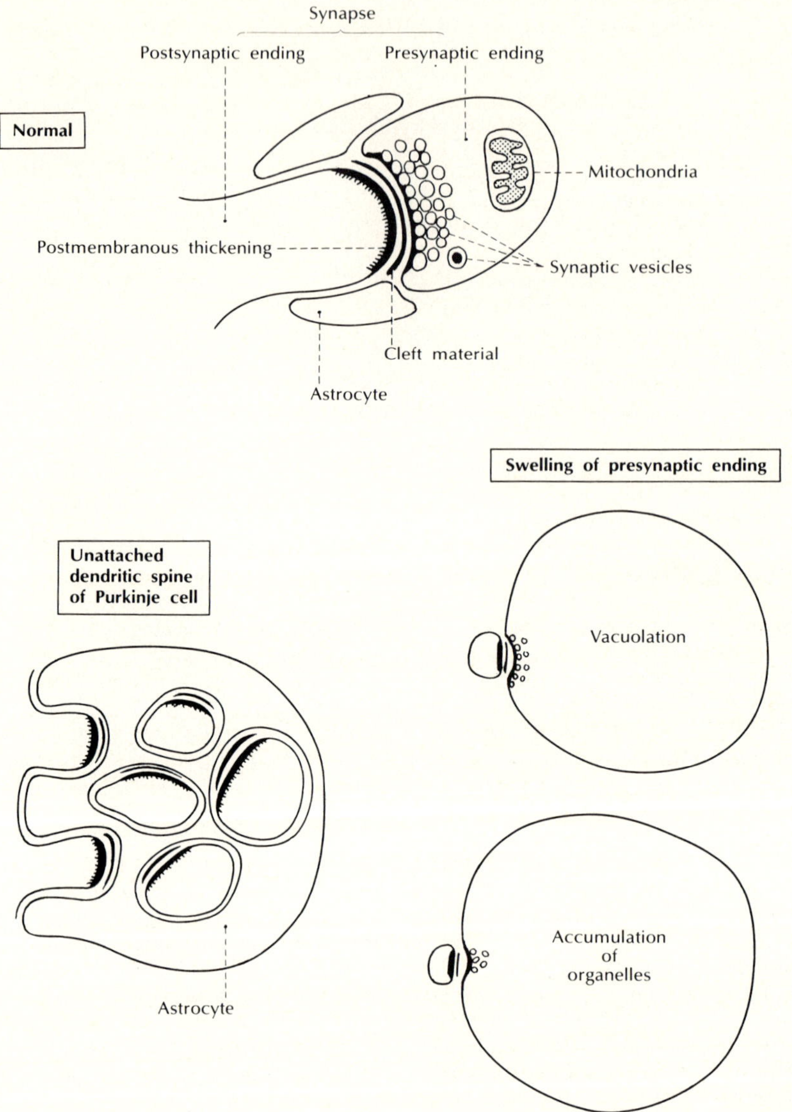

Fig. 178 Normal synapse and pathological variations.

invertebrates. The synapse is a highly specialized cell junction. It differs functionally from other junctions in that it is polarized allowing transmission in only one direction which is reflected in a fundamental morphological asymmetry. The synapse consists of two distinguishable elements; the presynaptic and the postsynaptic terminal separated by an extracellular space which contains an electron-dense cleft material.

The presynaptic element may be a protrusion of the axon which is frequently referred to as a "bouton" when it is widened, or it may be part of the relatively smooth area of the neuronal surface. In any event, it is characterized by the presence of membrane-bounded *synaptic vesicles*. Most of the vesicles in the central nervous system appear round and clear and are approximately 400Å in diameter. When processed by the ethanolic phosphotungstic acid or bismuth iodide technique a filamentous submembranous meshwork becomes apparent in which the vesicles are enmeshed. According to Uchizono (1975), when properly fixed, some clear synaptic vesicles are flattened or oval and these represent inhibitory synapses while the round ones are features of excitatory synapses. The overall applicability of this rule, however, is still to be clarified. Occasionally approximately 1,000Å diameter vesicles which contain dense cores are present. *Dense core vesicles* are more characteristic of the peripheral nervous system and certain hypothalamic nuclei.

The synaptic cleft consists of an extracellular space which may be increased to approximately 200Å depending on the interacting neurons. A dense cleft material is present, which is especially prominent in the wider synaptic clefts. The nature and function of this material is presently unknown.

The postsynaptic terminal may also be either at the surface of a protrusion or at a flat portion of the neuronal membrane. It is characterized by the presence of an osmiophilic submembranous density which is also stained by phosphotungstic acid or bismuth iodide. Small dendritic branchlets are common sites of postsynaptic terminals. These contain mitochondria and other organelles, especially microtubules, in addition to the submembranous density. In other cases, however, protrusions known as *spines*, which are devoid of any organelles except for fine filaments and occasional elements of the smooth endoplasmic reticulum, may bear the postsynaptic apparatus. In some of the pyramidal neurons of the cerebral cortex, the so-called "*spine apparatus*" is also present. The latter consists of ordered stacks of cisternae of smooth endoplasmic reticulum separated by a characteristic dense material. In other neurons, however, for example the cerebellar Purkinje cells, the dendritic spines are devoid of spine apparatus.

The presence of a synapse at a cell surface is usually regarded as the most reliable guide to the identification of a neuron. This is generally true, especially in the normal adult. It is worth pointing out, however, that during development, astrocytes can sometimes display submembranous specializations reminiscent of the postsynaptic element (Henrikson & Vaughn, 1974).

There are some well known instances in which a basal lamina is inserted between an axonal presynaptic ending and its target. The best known of these is the neuromuscular junction. In the *area postrema* and the *median eminence*, presynaptic terminals are found abutting a basal lamina surrounding the perivascular space of the fenestrated capillaries.

REFERENCES

Pappas, G.D., & Purpura, D.P.: Structure and Function of Synapses. Raven Press, New York, 1972.

Henrikson, C.K., & Vaughn, J.E.: Fine structural relationships between neurites and radial glial processes in developing mouse spinal cord. J. Neurocytol., 3: 659-675, 1974.

Uchizono, K.: Excitation and Inhibition Synaptic Morphology. Igaku Shoin Ltd., Tokyo, 1975.

ALTERATION OF SYNAPSES

Meaningful insights into the pathology of the synapse had to await the advent of the electron microscope. We are, therefore, still at the beginning of this undertaking and relatively little is known at this time.

Empty Swelling

Empty swelling of the synapse, like any other cell processes, is a common artifact encountered in poorly fixed nervous tissue. On the other hand, swelling of the presynaptic and/or the postsynaptic element may occur as the result of real pathological processes such as anoxia and hypoglycemia. It has also been induced experimentally by the application of ouabain, glutamate and methionine sulfoximine (Rizzuto and Gonatas, 1974). Lysis of the presynaptic terminal of the neuromuscular junction may be produced by spider venom (Gorio et al., 1978).

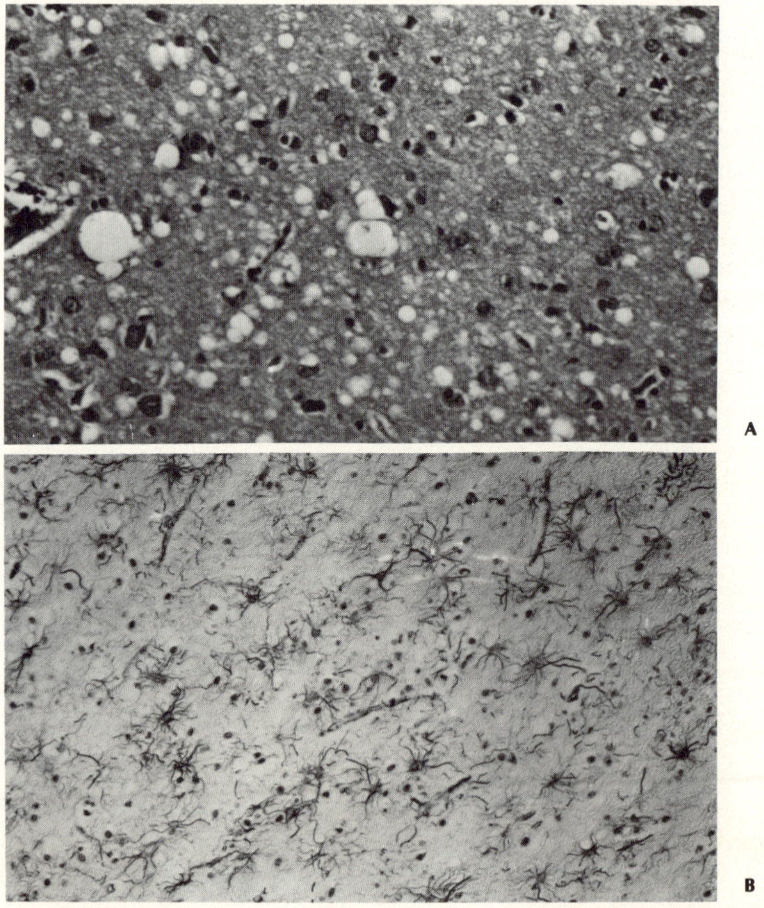

Fig. 179 Creutzfeldt-Jakob disease. A. Spongy state (H&E stain). B. Gliosis (Holzer stain). (Hirano, A. et al.: Arch. Neurol., 26: 530, 1972.)

If the swelling is pronounced enough and becomes generalized, the effect is visible in the optical microscope and a type of spongiform encephalopathy results (Figs. 179, 180). Among the most well known of these conditions are Creutzfeldt-Jakob and Kuru diseases in the human (Gajdusek et al., 1965). Scrapie and other slow virus infections in animals are other examples of spongiform encephalopathy. Sponginess is considered to result predominantly from the empty swelling of neuronal processes, especially synaptic terminals (Gonatas et al. 1965; Bignami and Forno, 1970; Lampert et al., 1972; Hirano et al., 1972).

REFERENCES

Gonatas, N.K., Terry, R.D., & Weiss, M.: Electron microscopical study in two cases of Jakob-Creutzfeldt disease. J. Neuropathol. Exp. Neurol., 24: 575-598, 1965.

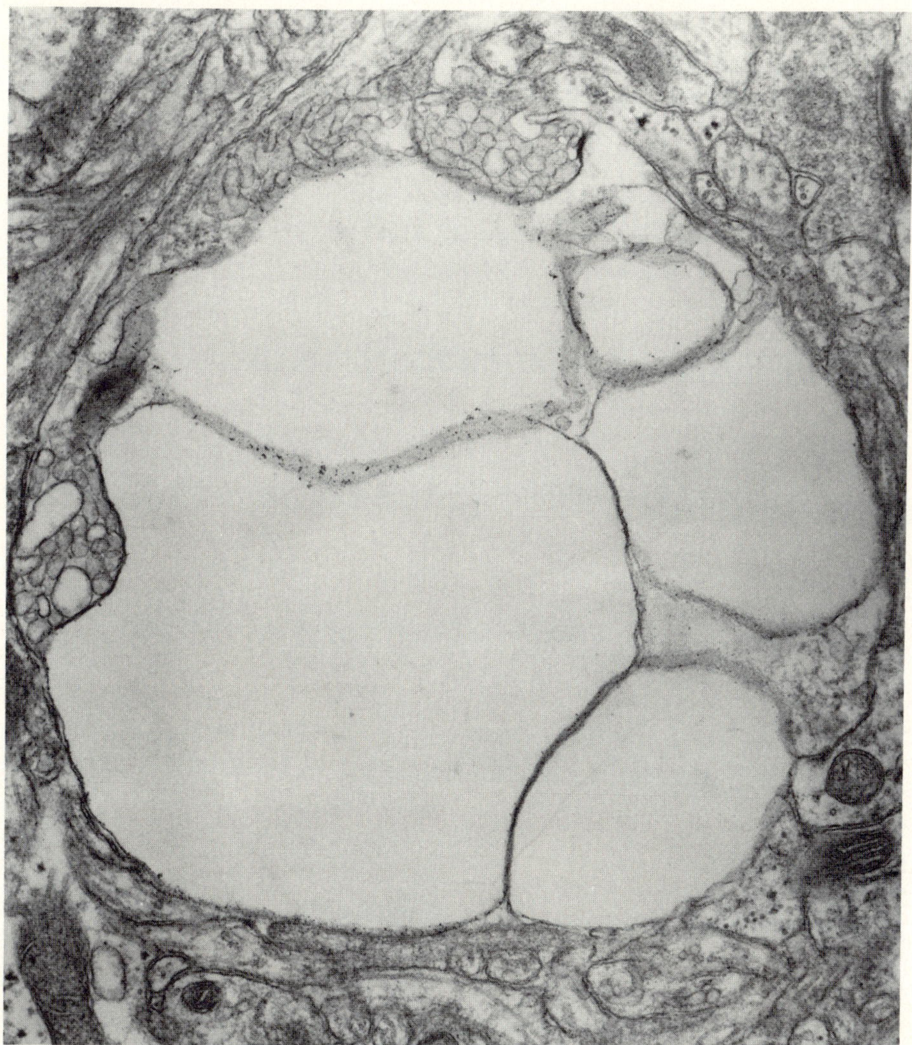

Fig. 180 Creutzfeldt-Jakob disease, Membrane bounded vacuoles in the neuropil. × 28,000. From Hirano, A. et al.: Arch. Neurol., 26: 530, 1972.)

Gajdusek, D.C., Gibbs, C.J. Jr., & Alpers, M. (eds.): Slow, Latent, and Temperate Virus Infections. NINDB Monograph No. 2, Washington, D.C., U.S. Department of Health, Education, and Welfare, 1965.
Bignami, A., & Forno, L.S.: Status spongiosus in Jakob-Creutzfeldt disease. Electron microscopic study of a cortical biopsy. Brain, 93: 89-94, 1970.
Lampert, P.W., Gajdusek, D.C., & Gibbs, C.J. Jr.: Subacute spongiform virus encephalopathies. Scrapie, Kuru and Creutzfeldt-Jakob disease: A review. Am J. Path., 66: 626-646, 1972.
Hirano, A., Ghatak, N.R., Johnson, A.B., Partnow, M.J., & Gomori, A.J.: Argentophilic plaques in Creutzfeldt-Jakob Disease. Arch. Neurol., 26:530-542, 1972.
Rizzuto, N., & Gonatas, N.K.: Ultrastructural study of effect of methionine sulfoximine on developing and adult rat cerebral cortex. J. Neuropathol. Exp. Neurol., 33: 237-250, 1974.
Gorio, A., Rubin, L.L., & Mauro, A.: Double mode of action of black widow spider venom on frog neuromuscular junction. J. Neurocytol., 7: 193-205, 1978.

Atrophy

Following axonal section or neuronal damage, the peripheral portions of the axon, including the synaptic terminals, degenerate. In some instances the degeneration of the presynaptic ending is accompanied by the abnormal accumulation of filaments so that they assume argentophilic properties. Eventually the presynaptic ending is removed by phagocytes. The reaction of the postsynaptic mate is variable. It is usually resorbed by the transsynaptic process but sometimes the postsynaptic ending is maintained for substantial periods of time. This effect is the subject of a number of interesting studies with regard to reinnervation and synaptogenesis.

REFERENCES

Gray, E.G.: Electron microscopy of experimental degeneration in the brain. *In* Head Injury Conference Proceedings. pp. 455-462, Caveness, W.F., & Walker, A.E. (eds.), Lippincott, Chicago, 1966.
Hirano, A., & Dembitzer, H.M.: Cerebellar alterations in the weaver mouse. J. Cell Biol., 56: 478-486, 1973.

Empty Presynaptic Bag

Occasionally, pathological areas may show alterations of synapses in which the presynaptic bag may be either devoid of synaptic vesicles or in which the few vesicles present are not attached to the presynaptic mesh. Other elements of the synapse, including the presynaptic mesh and the postsynaptic element are well developed and unremarkable. The interpretation of these phenomena requires further study.

Tubulovesicular Structures

Gonatas and his coworkers (1965) first described the tubulovesicular structure, very similar to that seen in axons in a variety of conditions (Fig. 173), in the distended presynaptic terminals of cortical neurons in an infant with convulsions, mental retardation and cortical blindness. Since that time it has been recognized as the most prominent alteration in several cases classified by light microscopy as infantile neuronal dystrophy (Seitelberger's disease). More recently, essentially the same findings were made in a family showing ALS accompanied by dementia. The tubulovesicular structure is seen in both presynaptic terminals and in axons in

Alzheimer's disease and in other conditions where it is associated with other changes as well.

REFERENCES

Gonatas, N.K., & Goldensohn, E.S.: Unusual neocortical presynaptic terminals in a patient with convulsions, mental retardation and cortical blindness. An electron microscopic study. J. Neuropathol. Exp. Neurol., 24: 539-562, 1965.

Sandbank, U.: Infantile neuroaxonal dystrophy. Arch. Neurol., 12: 155-159, 1965.

Hirano, A., & Zimmerman, H.M.: Aberrant synaptic development. Arch. Neurol., 28: 359-366, 1973.

Senile Plaques (Figs. 181-187)

Senile plaques are a well known aging change and are especially prominent in Alzheimer's disease. They are easily detectable after silver impregnation but are

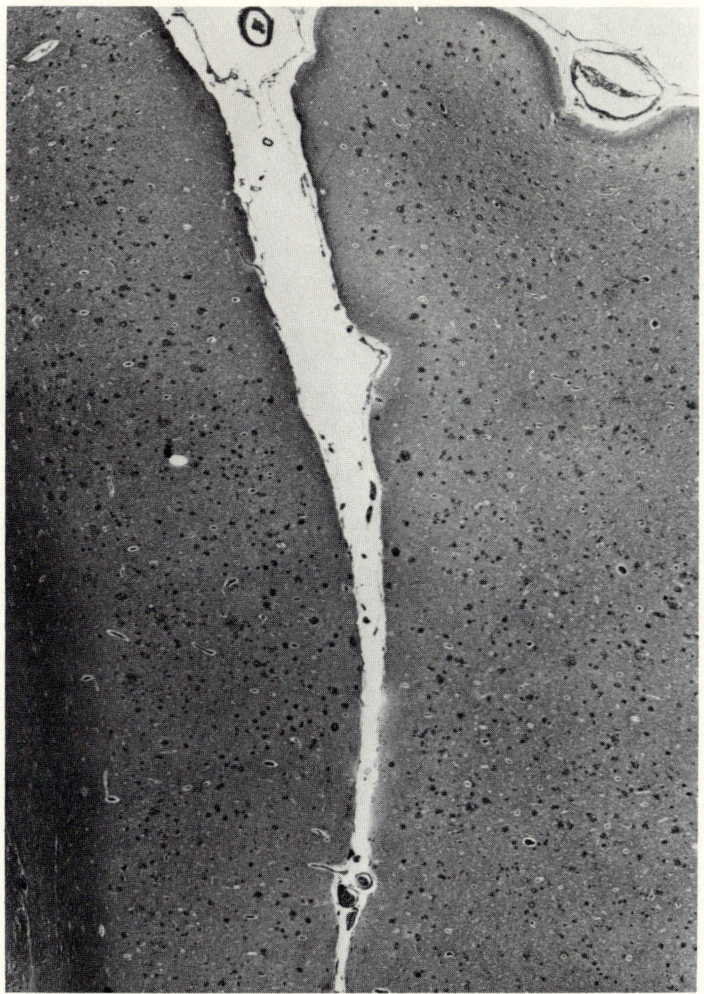

Fig. 181 Senile plaques in the cerebral cortex (silver stain).

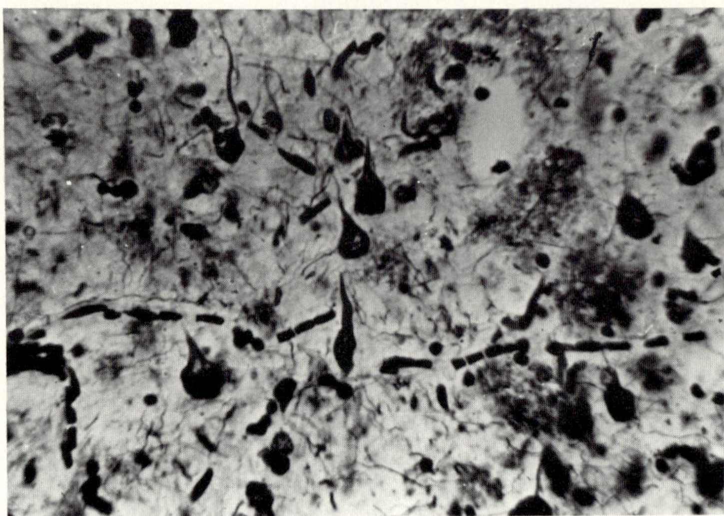

Fig. 182 Cerebral cortex in Alzheimer's disease (silver stain). Many Alzheimer neurofibrillary changes and senile plaques are visible.

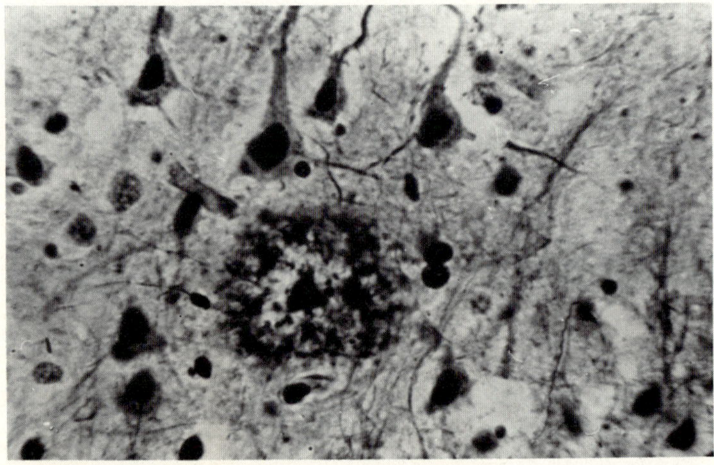

Fig. 183 Senile plaque (silver stain).

difficult to see in ordinary H&E preparations. The plaques are generally confined to the cerebral cortex but they may be seen in other areas of subcortical gray matter. They sometimes appear to be associated with the perivascular space (perivascular plaques). They consist of a spherical, argentophilic, amyloid-positive core surrounded by argentophilic material.

In the electron microscope the surrounding structures are found to consist of distorted neuronal processes often separated from the core by intervening astrocytic processes. Reactive astrocytes and microglia may be found at the periphery. The contents of the neuronal processes may include accumulations of neurofilaments, microtubules, mitochondria, dense bodies, synaptic vesicles, tubulo-vesicular structures, Alzheimer's neurofibrillary tangles and other abnormal organelles.

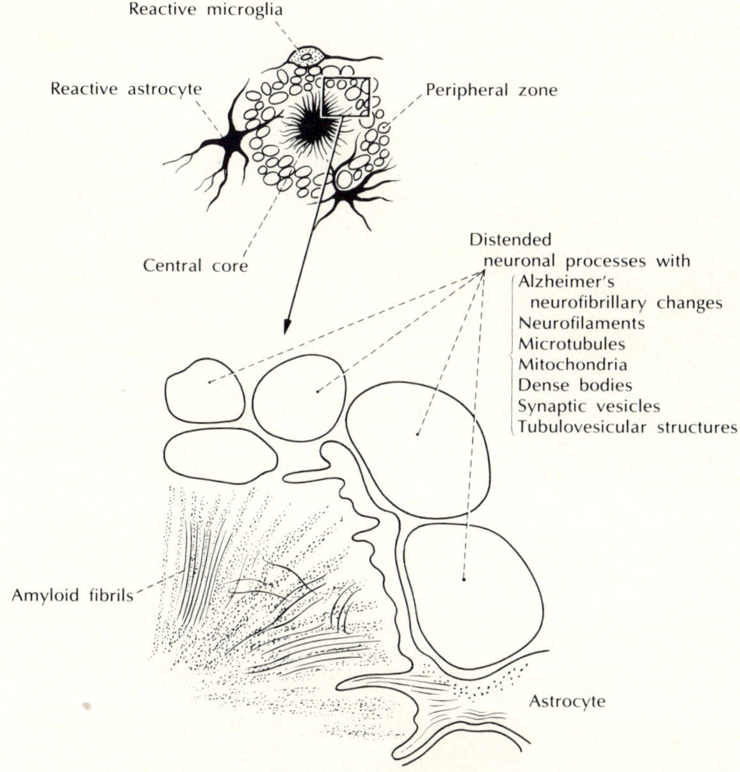

Fig. 184 Senile plaque.

The presence of these inclusions account for the positive histochemical reaction for oxidative enzymes and acid phosphatase as well as for their argentophilia.

The origin of senile plaques is still uncertain. They are found in man and in some other aged primates. Wiśniewski and Terry (1973) regard the neuronal changes to be primary and the amyloid deposits and glial changes to be secondary. On this basis they have proposed the use of the term "neuritic plaque" instead of "senile plaque", with neurite understood to refer to both dendrites and axons.

The origin of the amyloid in the senile plaque is also unclear but presumably derives from the blood stream. It apparently is identical to amyloid seen in any other organ outside the nervous system. There is, however, usually no correspondence between the presence of senile plaques and generalized amyloidosis.

The Alzheimer neurofibrillary tangle has been suggested as a primary change responsible for senile plaque formation. There are, however, at least four good reasons why this is probably not true. On Guam, patients with parkinsonism-dementia complex show numerous Alzheimer neurofibrillary tangles but are characteristically devoid of senile plaqes. Alzheimer neurofibrillary tangles may be seen in the brain stem, an area usually free of senile plaques. In some cases, senile plaques are abundant but neurofibrillary tangles are absent. Finally, in those non-human primates which show senile plaque formation the "paired helical filaments" of the Alzheimer neurofibrillary tangles are absent.

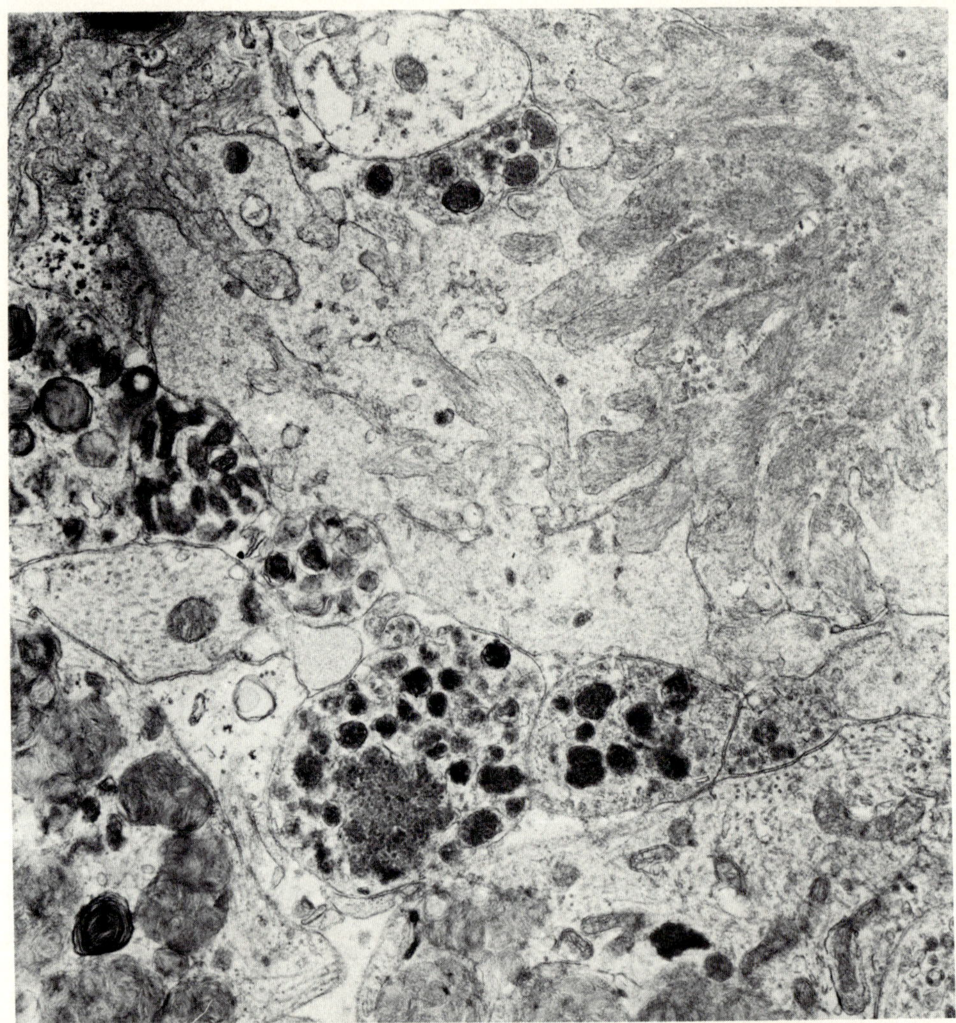

Fig. 185 Portion of a senile plaque. × 20,000. Amyloid deposits in the right upper corner are surrounded by many altered cell processes. (From Hirano, A. et al.: Arch. Neurol., 26: 530, 1972.)

REFERENCES

Terry, R.D., Gonatas, N.K., & Weiss, M.: Ultrastructural studies in Alzheimer's presenile dementia. Am. J. Pathol., 44: 269-297, 1964.

Gonatas, N.K., Anderson, W., & Evangelista, I.: The contribution of altered synapses in the senile plaque: An electron microscopic study in Alzheimer dementia. J. Neuropathol. Exp. Neurol., 26: 25-39, 1967.

Wiśniewski, H.M., & Terry, R.D.: Re-examination of the pathogenesis of the senile plaque. *In* Progress in Neuropathology, Vol 2, Zimmerman, H.M. (ed.), p. 1-26, Grune & Stratton, New York, 1973.

Katzman, R., Terry, R.D., & Bick, K.L. (eds.), Alzheimer's Disease: Senile Dementia and Related Disorders (Aging, Vol. 7), Raven Press, New York, 1978.

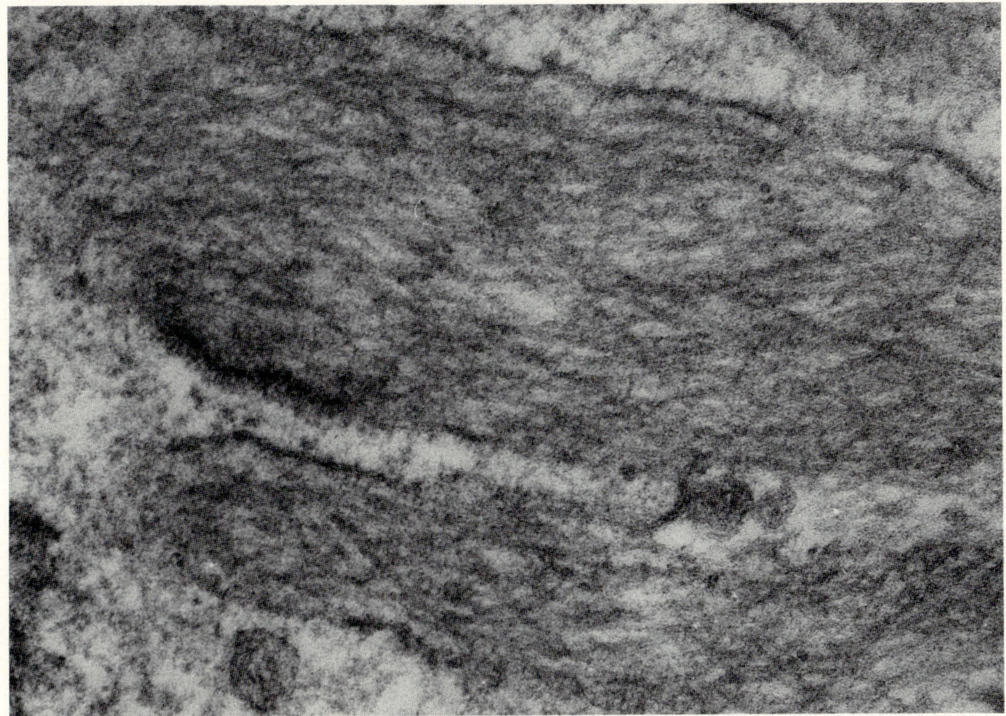

Fig. 186 Amyloid in a senile plaque. × 128,000.

Cerebral Congophilic (Amyloid) Angiopathy

A pathological alteration which may or may not be related to senile plaques is the accumulations of amyloid sometimes seen in and around blood vessels of the central nervous system. When such changes are present in the brain they are not prominent in other organs. Similarly, generalized amyloidosis, except for rare cases (Krücke, 1950), spares the brain.

Congophilic plaques in the brain are composed mainly of accumulations of amyloid filaments similar to those seen in other tissues. The amyloid filaments are found within the vascular walls and sometimes extend into the parenchyma (Schlote, 1965; Torack, 1975, 1978). Amyloid is currently believed to be immunoglobulin derived from the circulation (Glenner, 1978). Multiple, small cortical infarcts and hemorrhages were regularly observed in 23 autopsied cases of amyloid angiopathy by Okazaki et al. (1979).

REFERENCES

Krücke, W.: Das Zentralnervensystem bei generalisierter Paramyloidose. Arch. Psychiat. Nervenkr., 185: 165-192, 1950.

Schlote, W.: Die amyloid Natur der kongophilen drüsigen Entartung der Hirnarterien (Scholz) im Senium. Acta Neuropathol., 4: 449-468, 1965.

Torack, R.M.: Congophilic angiopathy complicated by surgery and massive hemorrhage. Am. J. Pathol., 81: 349-366, 1975.

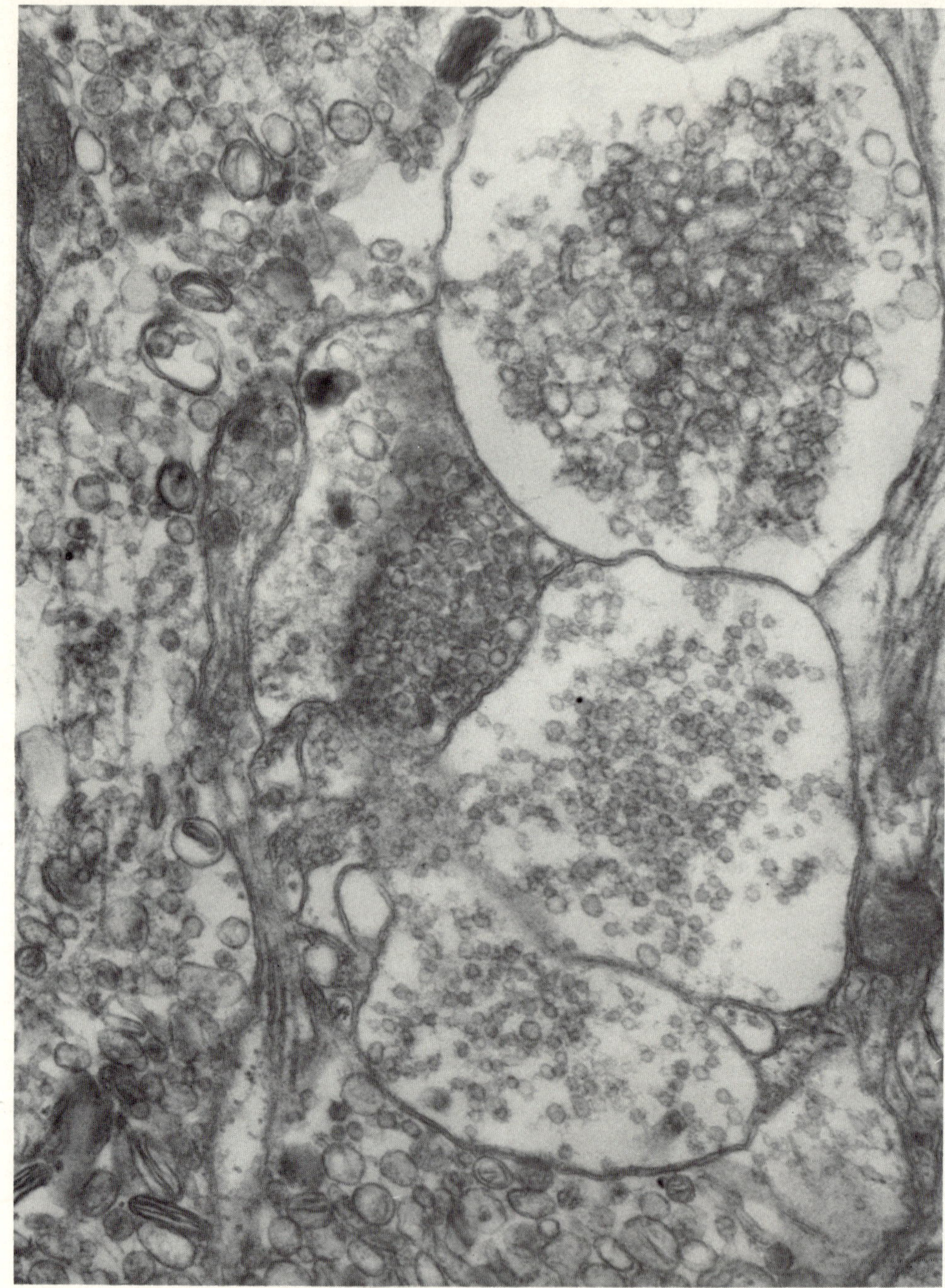

Fig. 187 Swollen synaptic terminals in a senile plaque. × 40,000.

Glenner, G.G.: Current knowledge of amyloid deposits as applied to senile plaques and congophilic angiopathy. *In* Alzheimer's Disease: Senile Dementia and Related Disorders. Aging Vol. 7, pp. 493-502, Katzman, R., Terry, R.D., & Bick, K.L., (eds.), Raven Press, New York, 1978.
Torack, R.M.: The Pathologic Physiology of Dementia with Indication for Diagnosis and Treatment. Monographien aus dem Gesamtgebiete der Psychiatrie. Vol. 20, Springer-Verlag, Berlin, 1978.
Okazaki, H., Reagan, T.J., & Campbell, R.J.: Clinicopathologic studies of primary cerebral amyloid angiopathy. Mayo Clin. Proc. 54: 22-31, 1979.

Kuru Plaques (Fig. 188)

Accumulations of amyloid-like material in the granule cell layer of the cerebellum are found in certain cases of kuru disease (Klatzo et al., 1959), a condition known to be transmitted by a slow virus (Gajdusek, 1977). They differ from senile plaques by the absence of any apparent involvement of neuronal elements and from the plaques of congophilic angiopathy by the absence of any obvious relationship to blood vessels. Although the electron microscope cannot distinguish between the filaments of kuru plaques and those of amyloid in senile plaques their staining properties show certain subtle differences.

Identical plaques have been identified in several cases of Creutzfeldt-Jacob disease (Chou and Martin, 1971). Creutzfeldt-Jakob disease, too, is known to be caused by slow virus infection and can be transmitted to primates. More recently, several cases of Creutzfeldt-Jacob disease were discovered among the Japanese which differ somewhat from previous cases. These were distinguished by prolonged clinical courses, severe involvement of the white matter and the presence of numerous Kuru-like plaques in the brain. Furthermore, these Japanese cases, unlike previous cases of Creutzfeldt-Jacob disease, could be transmitted to rats (Tateishi et al., 1978).

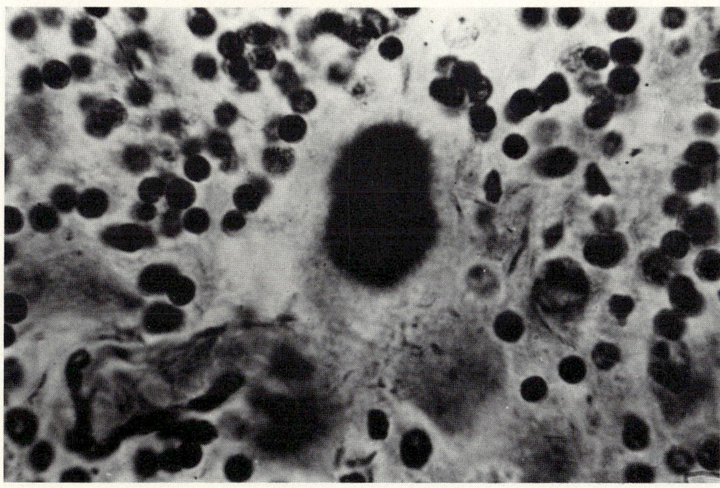

Fig. 188 Kuru plaque in the cerebellar granule cell layer (Silver impregnation).

Scrapie, another slow virus infection, originally affecting sheep is transmissible to certain strains of mice. These rodents, which display the usual spongiform changes seen in all slow virus infections, also show senile plaques (Bruce and Franser, 1975). The latter are identical to those found in humans, except for the absence of neurofibrillary tangles.

REFERENCES

Klatzo, I., Gajdusek, D.C., & Zigas, V.: Pathology of kuru. Lab. Invest., 8: 799-847, 1959.

Chou, S.M., & Martin, J.D.: Kuru plaques in a case of Creutzfeldt-Jacob disease. Acta Neuropathol., 17: 150-155, 1971.

Bruce, M.E., & Fraser: Amyloid plaques in the brain of mice infected with scrapie: Morphological variation and staining properties. Neuropathol. Appl. Neurobiol., 1: 189-202, 1975.

Tateishi, J., Ohta, M., & Kuroiwa, Y.: Subacute spongiform encephalopathy (SSE) with kuru plaques and its successful transmission to the small rodents. J. Neuropathol. Exp. Neurol., 37: 699, 1978 (Abstract).

Gajdusek, D.C.: Unconventional viruses and the origin and disappearance of kuru. Les Prix Nobel en 1976, pp. 167-216. Stockholm, Nobel Foundation, 1977.

Aberrant Synaptic Development

There are at least two pathological conditions leading to aberrant synaptic development of the Purkinje cells of the cerebellum in human. The first is the *granule cell type of cerebellar degeneration*, a congenital disorder in which dendritic arborization is depressed and bizarre compared to the normal (Fig. 189). In addition to apparently normal synapses, numerous examples of Purkinje cell dendritic spines are found on the large dendritic trunks (Hirano et al., 1973). These spines are unattached to their usual presynaptic mate, the parallel fiber of the granule cell. Instead, they are covered by voluminous astrocytic processes (Fig. 190). In all other respects, as far as can be told by histochemical and fine structural methods, the unattached dendritic spine is identical to its normal counterpart.

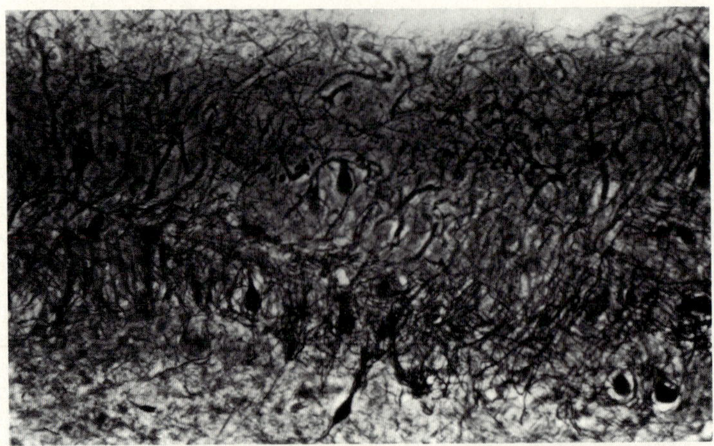

Fig. 189 Cerebellar degeneration (silver stain). Absence of granule cells and misaligned Purkinje cells (see Fig. 55).

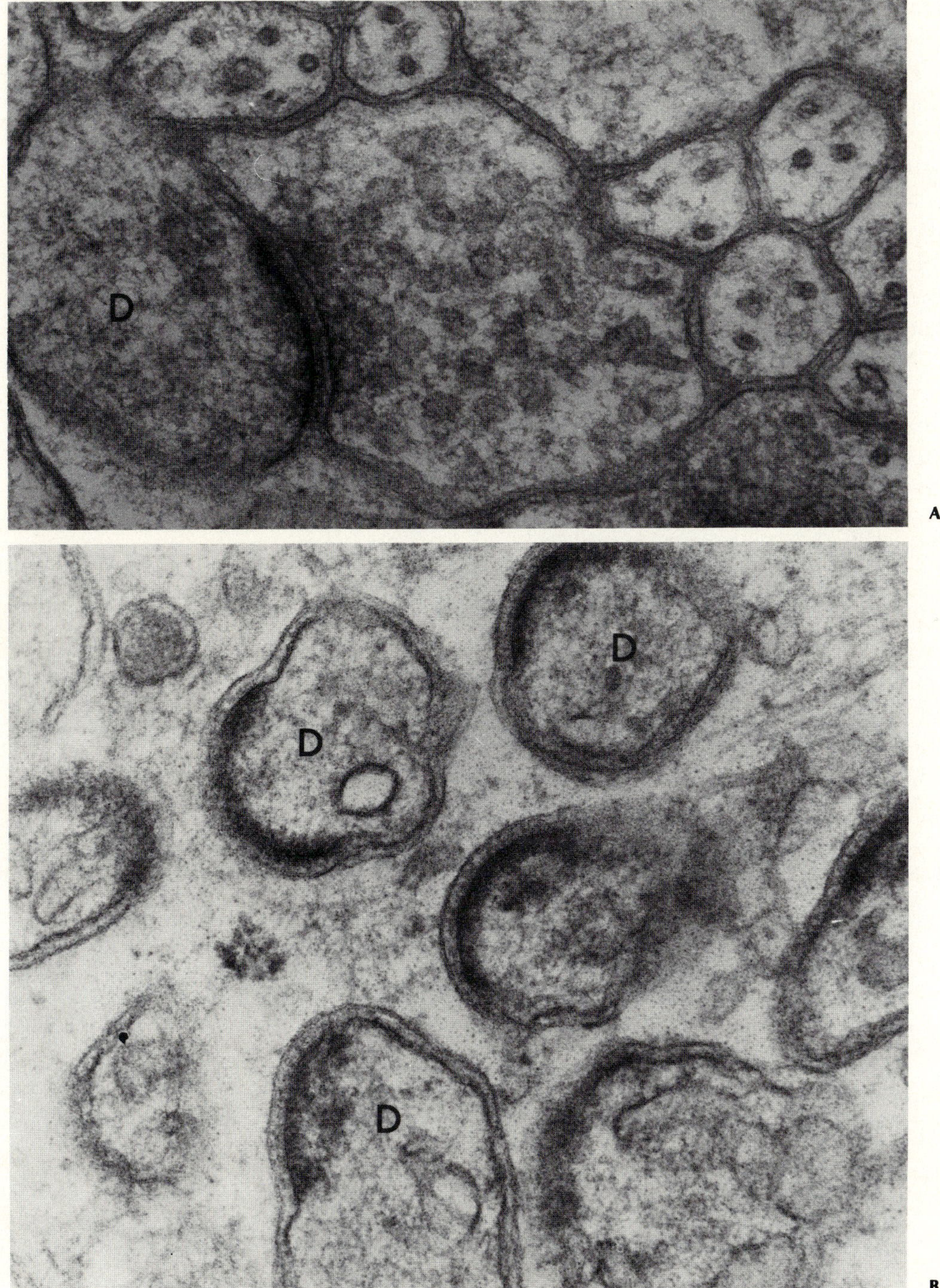

Fig. 190 A. Molecular layer of normal cerebellum in a mouse. × 90,000. B. Unattached dendritic spines (D) embedded in astrocytic cytoplasm. Cerebellum of a weaver mouse. × 90,000. (From Hirano, A.: Tokyo Igaku, 80: 438, 1973.)

Similar unattached Purkinje cell dendritic spines are found in another congenital anomaly, Menkes' kinky hair disease (Fig. 168) (Hirano et al., 1977a).

The origin of the unattached spine has been explored in several experimental model systems. Even in normal animals rare examples of unattached Purkinje cell dendritic spines may be found (Hirano et al., 1977b). When large numbers of granule cells are destroyed before their descent into the internal granule cell layer as the result of genetic defect (Hirano and Dembitzer, 1975: Hanna et al., 1976), intoxication (Hirano et al., 1972), infection or x-irradiation, the Purkinje cell is able to form dendritic spines without the one-to-one influence of a presynaptic element, but its tendency towards elaborate dendritic arborization is restricted and distorted. Often, the precise alignment of the Purkinje cells themselves is awry.

A similar ability for independent development of presynaptic terminals has been suggested in fine structural studies of neuroblastoma. (p. 203). In certain of these cases tumor cell processes were found complete with synaptic vesicles and submembranous densities virtually identical to young presynaptic terminals but with no postsynaptic element in the immediate vicinity (Hirano and Shin, 1979; Hirano, 1979). Similar findings have been suggested in certain experimental animals (Sotelo, 1973).

REFERENCES

Hirano, A., Dembitzer, H.M., & Jones, M.: An electron microscopic study of cycasin-induced cerebellar alterations. J. Neuropathol. Exp. Neurol., 31: 113-125, 1972.

Hirano, A., Dembitzer, H.M., Ghatak, N.R., Fan, K.-J., & Zimmerman, H.M.: On the relationship between human and experimental granule cell type cerebellar degeneration. J. Neuropathol. & Exp. Neurol., 32: 493-502, 1973.

Sotelo, C.: Permanence and fate of paramembranous synaptic specialization in 'mutant' and experimental animals. Brain Res., 62: 345-351, 1973.

Hirano, A., & Dembitzer, H.M.: Observations on the development of the weaver mouse cerebellum. J. Neuropathol. Exp. Neurol., 33: 354-364, 1974.

Hirano, A., & Dembitzer, H.M.: The fine structure of staggerer cerebellum. J. Neuropathol. Exp. Neurol., 34: 1-11, 1975.

Hanna, R.B., Hirano, A., & Pappas, G.D.: Membrane specializations of dendritic spines and glia in the weaver mouse cerebellum. A freeze fracture study. J. Cell Biol., 68: 403-410, 1976.

Hirano, A., Llena, J.F., French, J.H., & Ghatak, N.R.: Fine structure of the cerebellar cortex in Menkes' kinky hair disease. X-chromosome-linked copper malabsorption. Arch. Neurol., 34: 52-56, 1977a.

Hirano, A., Dembitzer, H.M., & Yoon, C.H.: Development of Purkinje cell somatic spines in the weaver mouse. Acta Neuropathol., 40: 85-90, 1977b.

Hirano, A., & Shin, Y.Y.: Unattached presynaptic terminals in a cerebellar neuroblastoma in the human. Neuropathol. Appl. Neurobiol., 5: 63-70, 1979.

Hirano, A.: On the independent development of the pre- and postsynaptic terminals. *In* Progress in Neuropathology, Vol. 4, pp. 79-99, Zimmerman, H.M. (ed.), Raven Press, New York, 1979.

9. Other Neuronal Changes (Fig. 191)

NEURONAL LOSS

Mature neurons are incapable of division so that once a neuron is lost it is not replaced. In certain cases, such as in Werdnig-Hoffmann disease, the former position of the degenerated neuron is recognizable as an "*empty cell bed*". Similarly, in cases of olivo-ponto-cerebellar degeneration the position of the Purkinje cell is marked by an "*empty basket.*" In other conditions, however, the former site of the neuron becomes obliterated by glial scar formation. Therefore,

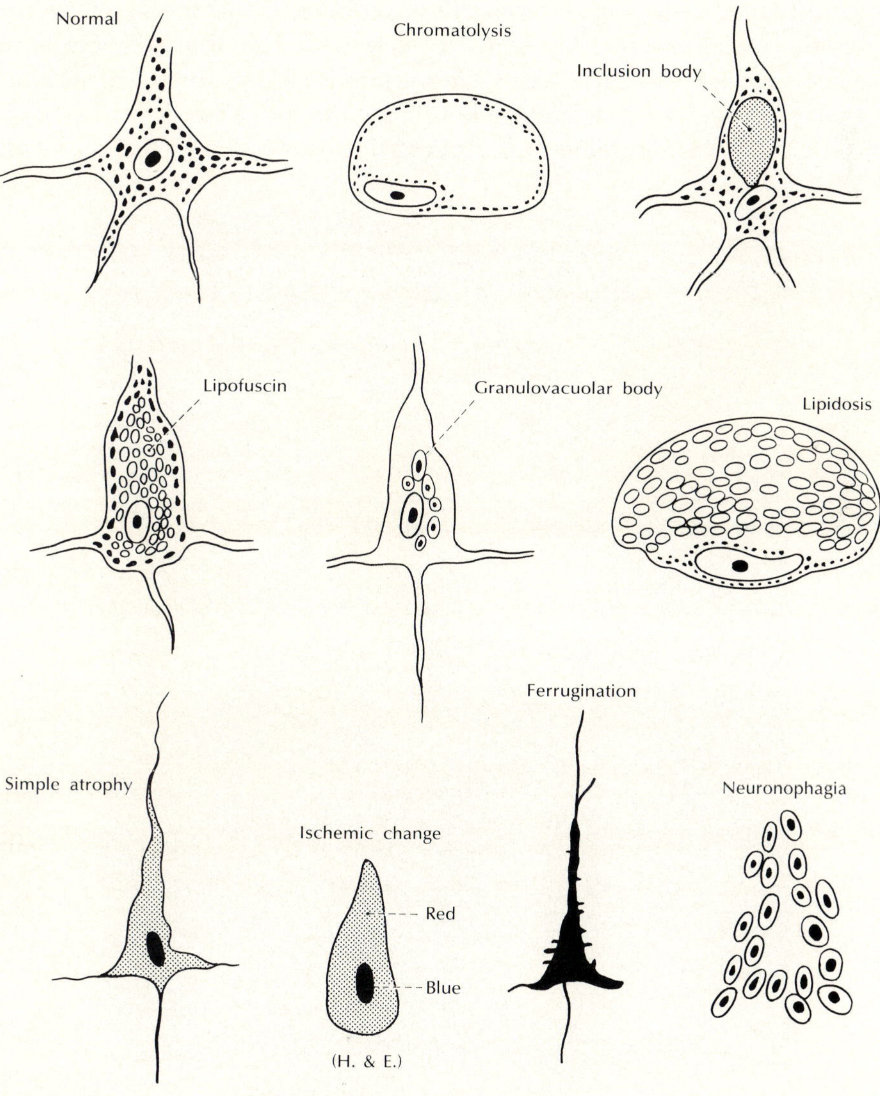

Fig. 191 Neuronal changes.

in order to fully appreciate the extent of neuronal cell loss in such areas as the substantia nigra in parkinsonism or the anterior horn in amyotrophic lateral sclerosis, one must either have available control sections in which the neuronal population is intact or have substantial experience in the normal histology.

The overall pattern of neuronal loss depends on the underlying pathology. In some conditions only certain systems of neurons are involved. For example, in motor neuron disease, large anterior horn cells seem to be selectively affected, leaving behind other cells and their processes. In other conditions, however, there is focal destruction of an entire region of the neuropil regardless of the nature of the cell or its process. Ischemic or inflammatory changes are good examples of this phenomenon. Similarly, in healed anterior poliomyelitis one may observe plaque-like loss of the entire involved neuropil.

Ferrugination is the process of mineral deposition at the site of a dead neuron. Blue-colored, fine, granular deposits are seen with iron stain, but a variety of minerals may, in fact, be deposited. Ferruginated neurons are easily seen in H & E preparations or after Nissl staining where they display a homogenous dark blue color. Ferrugination is an uncommon finding but has been observed in a variety of

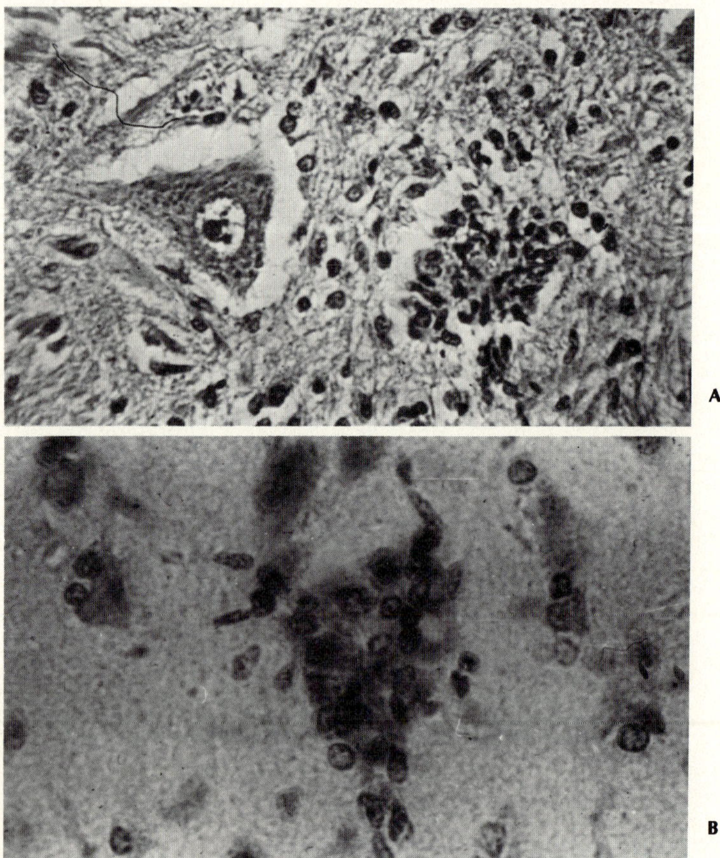

Fig. 192 Neuronophagia. A. Motoneuron in the hypoglossal nucleus (H&E stain). B. Betz cell (Nissl stain).

conditions including the after effects of Japanese B encephalitis, in old infarcts, etc.

In certain conditions such as acute poliomyelitis or Werdnig-Hoffmann disease, neuronal loss is often accompanied by the accumulation of small phagocytic cells at the site of the neuron (Fig. 192). In more chronic conditions involving neuronal loss such as amyotrophic lateral sclerosis, neuronophagia is a rather exceptional finding.

REFERENCES

Hirano, A.: Pathology of anterior horn cells. *In* Recent Advances in Myology, Bradley, W.G., Gardner-Medwin, D., & Walton, J.N. Excerpta Medica, Amsterdam, (eds.), pp. 537-541, 1975.

Iwata, M., & Hirano, A.: Neuropathological study of chronic healed anterior poliomyelitis. Neurol. Med. (Tokyo), 8: 157-166, 1978.

Iwata, M., & Hirano, A.: Current problems in the pathology of amyotrophic lateral sclerosis. *In* Progress in Neuropathology, Vol. 4, pp. 277-298, Zimmerman, H.M. (ed.), Raven Press, New York, 1979.

DARK AND SHRUNKEN NEURONS

In H & E or Nissl preparations of a number of chronic degenerative conditions such as Alzheimer's disease, amyotrophic lateral sclerosis and others which also result in neuronal loss, many neurons display a dark, hyperchromatic shrunken appearance. This phenomenon is sometimes referred to as "*simple neuronal atrophy*" or "*chronic nerve cell degeneration.*"

While these changes are more common in diseased areas of the central nervous system they may also be frequently found in apparently normal areas adjacent to a lesion such as a deep-seated brain tumor as well as in some poorly fixed tissue from experimental animals. In these cases, the dark neurons are usually regarded as artifacts of preparation. For some reason these changes are usually not seen in normal tissue from postmortem human specimens.

REFERENCE

Cammermeyer, J.: Nonspecific changes of the central nervous system in normal and experimental material. *In* The Structure and Function of Nervous Tissue. Vol. 4, pp. 131-251, Bourne, G.H. (ed.) Academic Press, New York, 1972.

ISCHEMIC CHANGES

A few days after systemic anoxia from whatever cause, characteristic ischemic changes occur in a number of neurons especially the pyramidal neurons of Sommer's sector or the Purkinje cells of the cerebellum. The cells become shrunken. In H&E the nucleus stains uniformly blue while the cytoplasm is red. Usually the perineuronal region becomes vacuolated due to the swelling of nearby cell processes. Similar changes occur in a more focal distribution a few days after circulatory disturbances such as occlusion.

BINUCLEATED NEURONS (Fig. 193)

Large neurons, apparently containing two nuclei, have been seen from time to time in a variety of conditions. They are known to be present in tuberous sclerosis or ganglioglioma. While they may appear as two separate nuclei in section, it is difficult to rule out the possibility that they are joined at some other level and actually represent a single deformed, lobulated nucleus.

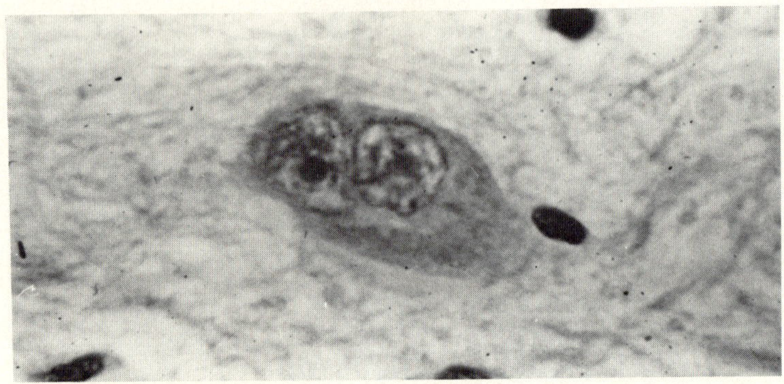

Fig. 193 Double nuclei in a neuron (H&E stain).

VACUOLATION

Vacuole formation in and around the neuronal perikarya leading to distention of the cell and accompanied by dendritic abnormalities is a characteristic change of neurons in the inferior olivary nucleus affected by lesions in the fibers of the central tegmental tract or in the dentate nucleus of the cerebellum. The vacuoles do not stain with H&E or in Nissl preparations.

Vacuole formation within the neuronal soma may be seen in anoxia, viral infection, and in certain degenerative disorders of unknown origin. Various slow virus infections have been recently shown to be associated with prominent vacuolization (see p. 182). They have also been observed in anterior horn cells in the murine mutant "wobbler".

It is important to note that developing neurons, such as those encountered in infant brain, tend to form halo-like vacuoles around the nuclei. This is considered to be artifactitious in nature. In general, because of the possibility of artifact, even in the adult, one must exercise caution in interpreting vacuolar changes.

REFERENCE

Hirano, A., & Iwata, M.: Pathology of motor neurons with special reference to amyotrophic lateral sclerosis and related diseases. *In* Amyotrophic Lateral Sclerosis, pp. 107-133, Tsubaki, T., & Toyokura Y. (ed.), University of Tokyo Press, Tokyo, 1979.

DEVELOPING NEURONS

During the postmortem examination of the brain of an infant it is not uncommon to encounter immature cells. They are especially common in the *subependymal area* at the angle of the lateral ventricles. They migrate from that region to the basal ganglia and to the cerebral cortex. Similar immature cells compose the *germinal granule cell layer* of the cerebellum. During the first year of life these cells complete their descent into the granule cell layer of the cerebellum. The age of the infant can be roughly estimated by the thickness of the remaining external layer. For the inexperienced, the migrating cells may sometimes be confused with inflammatory or neoplastic infiltrates. They are, of course, normal constituents of the brain.

As with most immature cells, the migrating cells show a relatively high nucleo:cytoplasmic ratio with numerous free ribosomes in the cytoplasm. Their cell processes are small and poorly developed and the extracellular spaces are relatively wide. Synapses and other cell junctions are few and immature.

DYING-BACK (DISTAL AXONOPATHY)

In some conditions changes occur in the distal portions of neuronal processes, especially the axon. These changes then progress back towards the soma which may appear completely intact during this process. Examples of such conditions include intoxication with triorthocresyl phosphate, acrylamide, n-hexane, methyl n-butyl ketone and 2,5-hexane dione. The same process is suspected in spinocerebellar degeneration, senile plaque formation, neuroaxonal dystrophy and subacute myelo-optico-neuropathy (SMON). (Japanese J. Med. Sci. Biol., 1975).

REFERENCES

Cavanagh, J.B.: The significance of the 'dying-back' process in experimental and human neurological disease. Rev. Exp. Pathol., 3: 219-267, 1964.

Prineas, J.: The pathogenesis of dying-back polyneuropathies. Parts I and II. J. Neuropathol. Exp. Neurol., 28: 571-621, 1969.

Japanese Journal of Medical Science and Biology. Vol. 28, supplement, pp. 1-293, National Institute of Health, Tokyo, 1975.

Spencer, P.S., & Schaumburg, H.H.: Central-peripheral distal axonopathy—The pathology of dying-back polyneuropathies. *In* Progress in Neuropathology, Vol. 3, pp. 253-295, Zimmerman, H.M., (ed.), Grune & Stratton, New York, 1976.

Spencer, P.S., & Schaumburg, H.H. (eds.): Experimental and Clinical Neurotoxicology. A Textbook of Environmental Neurobiology. The Williams & Wilkins Co., Baltimore, 1980.

TRANSNEURONAL DEGENERATION

Certain groups of neurons may become atrophied as a result of injury to the afferent neurons. This is called anterograde transneuronal transsynaptic degeneration. If degeneration follows the death of the target neuron it is referred to as retrograde transneuronal degeneration. Experimental studies in various animals indicates that transneuronal degeneration is apt to occur primarily in younger animals and after substantial deafferentation, after long postoperative survival and when there is a lack of other afferent neurons. This phenomenon differs a great deal according to the species of animal.

In humans this phenomenon is not well understood with the exception of the visual system, central tegmental tract-inferior olivary connection and limbic system, among others.

REFERENCES

Cowan, W.M.: Anterograde and retrograde transneuronal degeneration in the central and peripheral nervous system. *In* Contemporary Research Methods in Neuroanatomy, pp. 217-251, Nauta, W.J.H., and Ebbesson, S.O.E. (eds.), Springer, New York, 1970.

Ralston, H.J., III, & Chow, K.L.: Synaptic reorganization in the degenerating lateral geniculate nucleus of the rabbit. J. Comp. Neurol.,147: 321-349, 1973.

Ghetti, B., Horoupian, D.S., & Wiśniewski, H.M.: Acute and long-term transneuronal response of dendrites of lateral geniculate neurons following transection of the primary visual afferent pathway. Adv. Neurol., 12: 401-424, 1975.

Torch, W.C., Hirano, A., & Solomon, S.: Anterograde transneuronal degeneration in the limbic system: Clinical-anatomical correlation. Neurology, 27: 1157-1163, 1977.

SHAPE CHANGES

The fundamental shape of the neuron may be severely distorted during pathological change as mentioned previously (see p. 165). In addition, certain lipidoses as well as some other conditions result in the formation of the so-called "meganeurites" at the basal pole of the soma. These structures consist of enlargements filled with abnormal lipid accumulations and bear surface protrusions similar to somatic sprouts or dendritic cactus-like expansions (see p. 167). As described previously, various developmental or degenerative diseases result in the severe distortion of dendritic trees.

REFERENCES

Purpura, D.P., Hirano, A., & French, J.F.: Polydendritic Purkinje cells in X-chromosome-linked copper malabsorption: A Golgi Study. Brain Res., 117: 125-129, 1976.

Purpura, D.P.: Aberrant dendritic and synaptic development in immature human brain. J. Neuropathol. Exp. Neurol., 37: 578, 1978 (Abstract).

NEOPLASMS

Neoplasms of neuroblasts or neurons are extremely rare in the central nervous system. When they do occur they are often associated with gliomas (gangliogliomas). On the other hand, it is important to distinguish between gangliogliomas and those cases of gliomas which often entrap pre-existing neurons in the infiltrative process.

True neuronal neoplasms may be identified by the presence of synapses at the surface of the tumor cells. Interestingly, most of the synaptic vesicles so far reported in such cases are of the dense core variety similar to those seen in neuroblastomas of the peripheral nervous system.

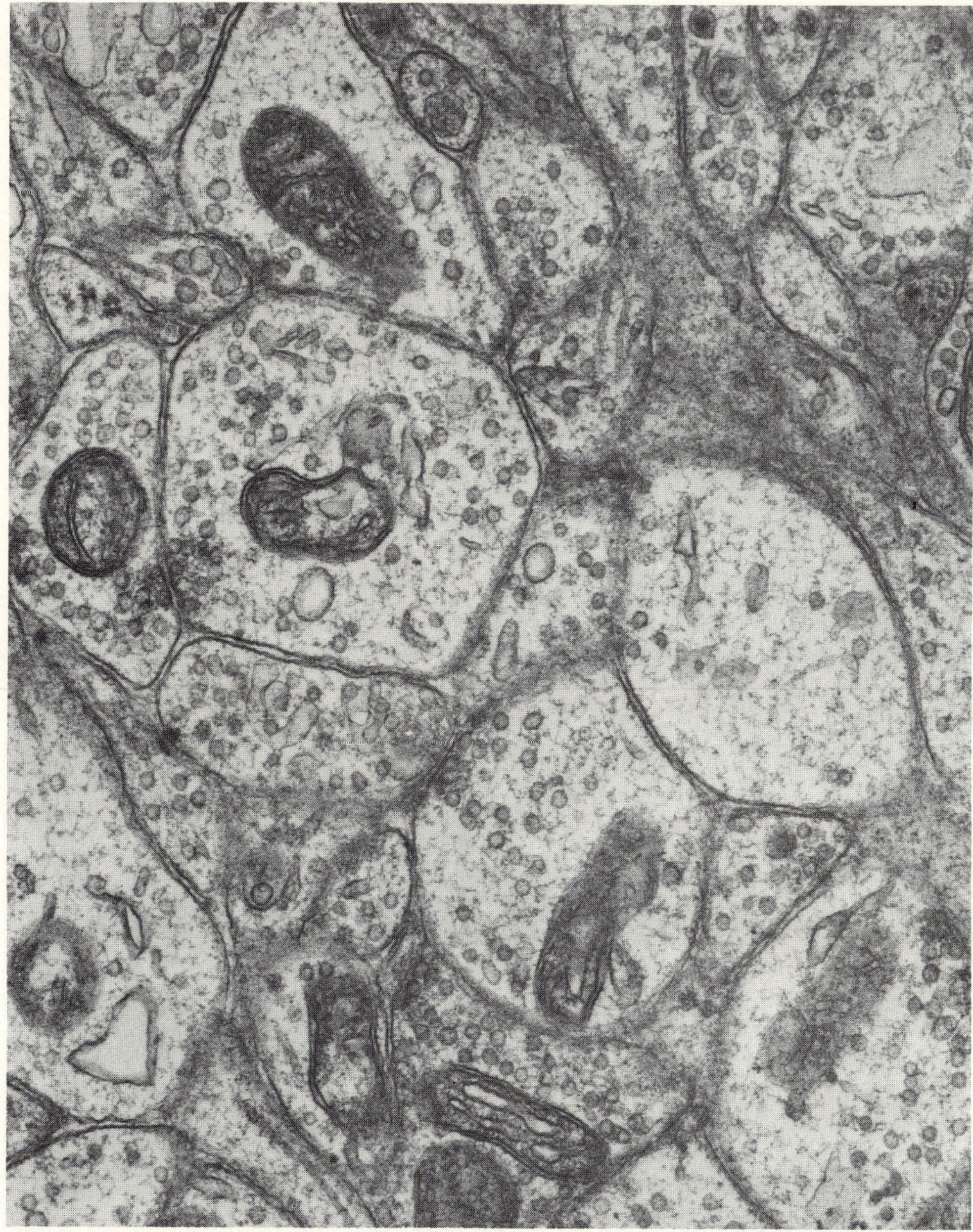

Fig. 194 Closely packed, circular processes in a cerebellar neuroblastoma. Numerous, clear synaptic vesicles may be seen in almost all of the processes. Some processes show peripheral aggregates of vesicles without a corresponding postsynaptic density. × 36,000. (From Hirano, A.: Acta Neuropathol. 43: 119, 1978.)

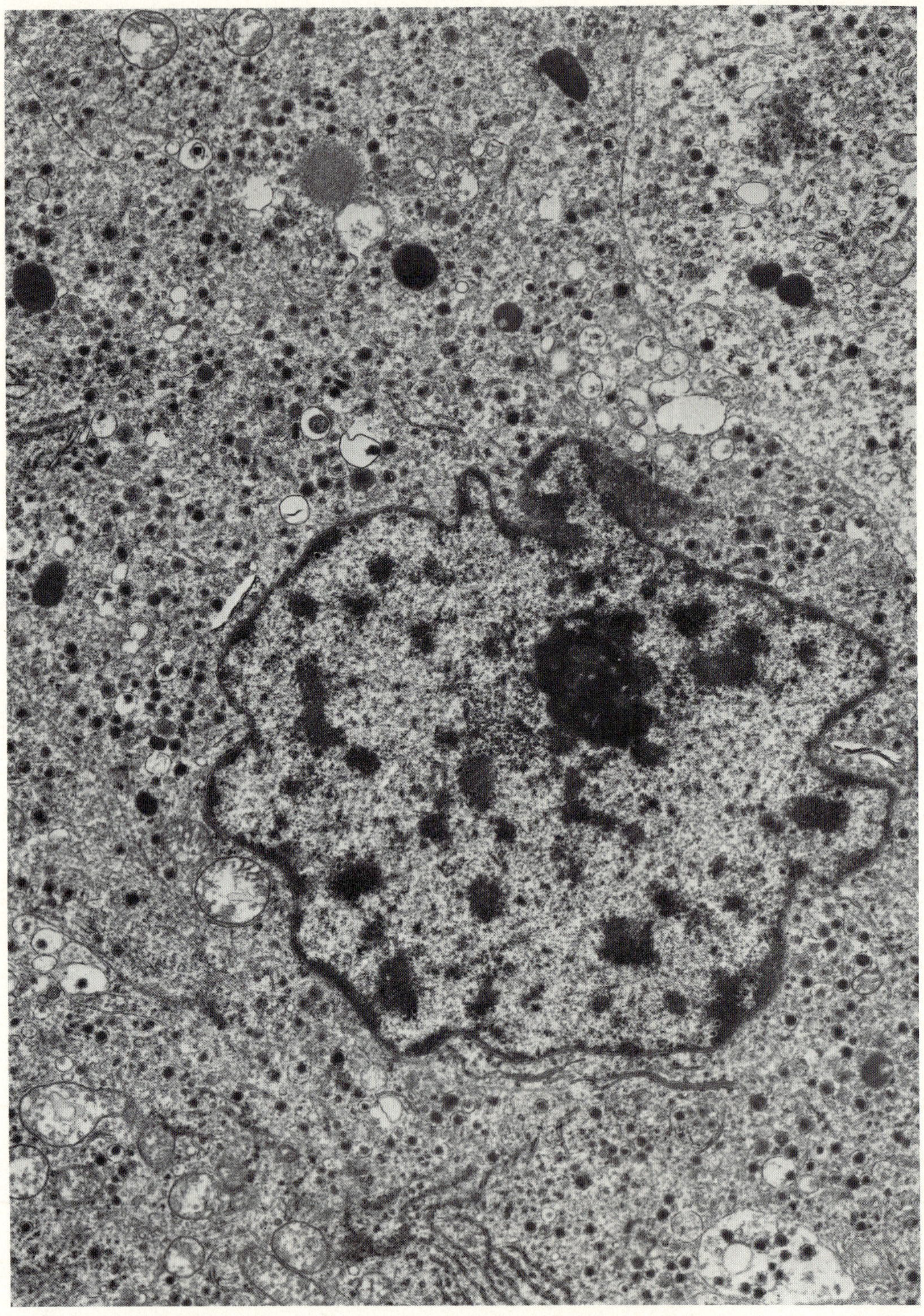

Fig. 195 Tumor cells in a paraganglioma in the cauda equina. Numerous dense core vesicles are visible. × 12,000. (From Hirano, A.: Acta Neuropathol. 43: 119, 1978.)

Recently, a case of cerebellar neuroblastoma was reported consisting entirely of neuronal elements devoid of any glial contributions (Shin et al., 1978). Synaptic terminals were frequent, but the vast majority of the vesicles were clear rather than dense. Interestingly, in this case, numerous examples of immature presynaptic terminals were seen apparently unattached to any postsynaptic element (Fig. 194).

Another neuronal neoplasm is the paraganglioma. While these, like neuroblastomas, are primarily tumors of the peripheral nervous system they have been observed within the area of the cauda equina where they are found in the subarachnoid space (Llena et al., 1979). Their morphology is indistinguishable from paragangliomas seen outside the central nervous system. The tumor cells are characterized by dense-core vesicles (Fig. 195) (Hirano, 1978). The blood vessels are fenestrated.

REFERENCES

Shin, W.-Y., Laufer, H., Lee, Y.-C., Aftalion, B., Hirano, A., & Zimmerman, H.M.: Fine structure of the cerebellar neuroblastoma. Acta Neuropathol., 42: 11-13, 1978.

Hirano, A.: Some contributions of electron microscopy to the diagnosis of brain tumors. Acta Neuropathol., 43: 119-128, 1978.

Llena, J.F., Hirano, A., & Rubin, R.C. Paraganglioma in the cauda equina region. Acta Neuropathol., 46: 235-237, 1979.

B. ASTROCYTES

1. Normal Astrocytes (Figs. 196, 197)

As may be inferred from its name several well-developed processes radiate from the perinuclear area of the astrocyte forming a fundamental star-like configuration. This pattern is subject to variation depending on the location of the cell. In the gray matter the processes of the so-called "protoplasmic astrocytes" contain fewer glial fibrils than their "*fibrillar*" counterparts in the white matter. Furthermore, the processes of certain specific astrocytes, such as those giving rise to the Bergmann fibers originating in the Purkinje cell layer of the cerebellum, may be oriented in predominantly one direction from the cell body rather than symmetrically.

In general, however, the astrocytes send cylindrical-shaped or sheet-like processes toward the periphery. At the target site the predominant shape of the astrocytic process is laminar or sheet-like. This configuration facilitates its ability to separate the central nervous system from the mesodermal tissue and to surround certain elements within the central nervous system. The sheet-like processes cover the outer aspects of the blood vessels as well as the inner aspects of the pial surface. At both of these sites, the astrocytic processes form a continuous layer joined by punctate adhesions and occasional gap junctions. A continuous basal lamina covers both the perivascular and subpial spaces.

Within the parenchyma, too, astrocytic processes serve as a covering layer for some neuronal cell surfaces. Both the dendritic and perikaryal surfaces of certain neurons are, except for synaptic sites, almost entirely covered by astrocytic sheets. Frequently, groups of, or individual synapses, are closely invested by astrocytic processes. In other cases, small bundles of neuronal processes are segregated by astrocytic sheet-like processes.

The function of the astrocyte is not clear. It has long been thought to play a skeletal role in the central nervous system. Because of its prominence around blood vessels it has also been suggested that the astrocyte may serve as a means of transport of nutrients between the blood vessels and neurons. Finally, because of its tendency to surround certain groups of synapses some workers have suggested that the astrocyte may serve as an isolator separating various functional types of synapses. On the other hand, astrocytes do not form a complete encapsulation of any synapses and, in fact, astrocytic insulation seems to be lacking in certain synapses. The effect of the astrocyte at neuronal surfaces may be to mediate the electrolyte balance, particularly potassium ions, as well as the concentration of certain transmitter substances in the microenvironment of the neuronal membranes.

Direct evidence for any of these hypotheses is lacking. Aside from the purely morphological observations the only other clue to the function of the astrocyte derives from tracer studies. The astrocyte does not seem to serve as a very effective

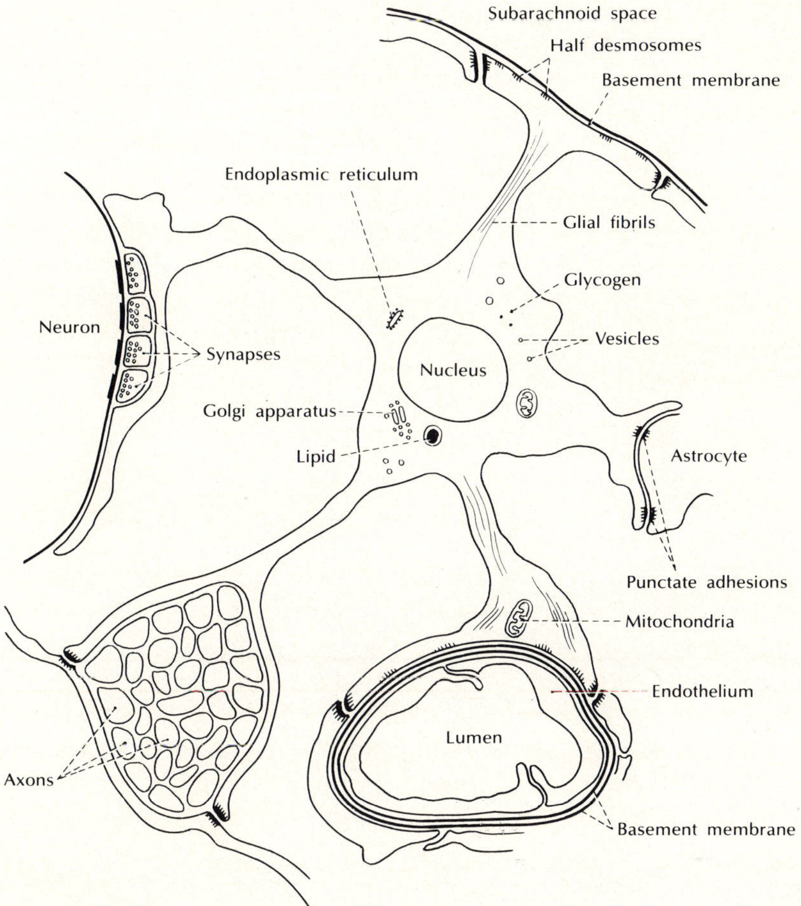

Fig. 196 A diagram of the possible configurations of the astrocytic processes.

barrier to the diffusion of large molecules. Horseradish peroxidase, for example, seems to be able to penetrate between astrocytic processes. Zonulae occludentes are not present either at mesodermal or neuronal surfaces.

The astrocytic nucleus is in the center of the cell and contains a small, inconspicuous nucleolus. The cytoplasm contains all the usual organelles. Mitochondria, rough endoplasmic reticulum, Golgi apparatus, vesicles, lipid droplets, lysosomes and glycogen are usually present but only in small amounts. Microtubules are seen in the developing or reactive astrocyte, but are inconspicuous in the mature cells. Glial fibrils and lipid droplets tend to increase in the astrocytes in aged brains, and sometimes corpora amylacea may be present.

The most characteristic cytoplasmic components are the glial fibrils, which are usually arranged in parallel bundles. These fibrils are especially prominent in the fibrous astrocytes of the white matter. They consist of 60-90Å filaments which, when seen in cross section, appear circular with a minute, clear center.

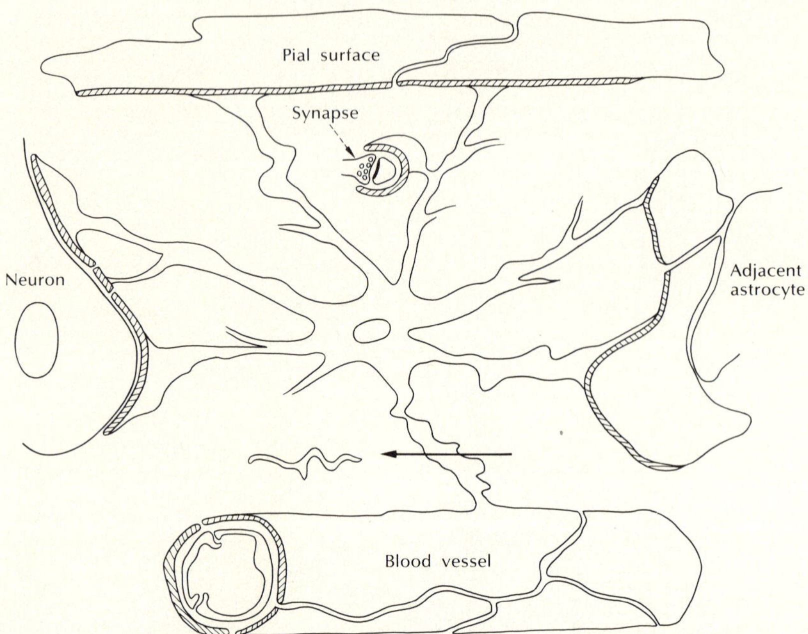

Fig. 197 A three dimensional representation of the distal, sheet-like expansions of the normal, protoplasmic astrocyte.

REFERENCES

Hirano, A.: Neuronal and glial processes in neuropathology. J. Neuropathol. Exp. Neurol., 37: 365-374, 1978.

Lasek, R.J. (Chairman) What do glia do? In Society for Neuroscience, 7th annual meeting. Summaries of Symposia. (BIS Conference Report #48 pp. 149-164). UCLA, Los Angeles, Brain Information Service/BRI Publication Office, 1978.

2. Pathology of Astrocytes

SWELLING (Figs. 198—200)

Astrocytic swelling is a well known change that occurs within 24 hours after hypoxic insult or other injuries. It may also occur as the result of improper fixation. Thus, one must be cautious in interpreting the significance of astrocytic swelling.

The swollen region within the cell appears clear and empty in the light microscope giving rise to a spongy appearance. In the electron microscope,

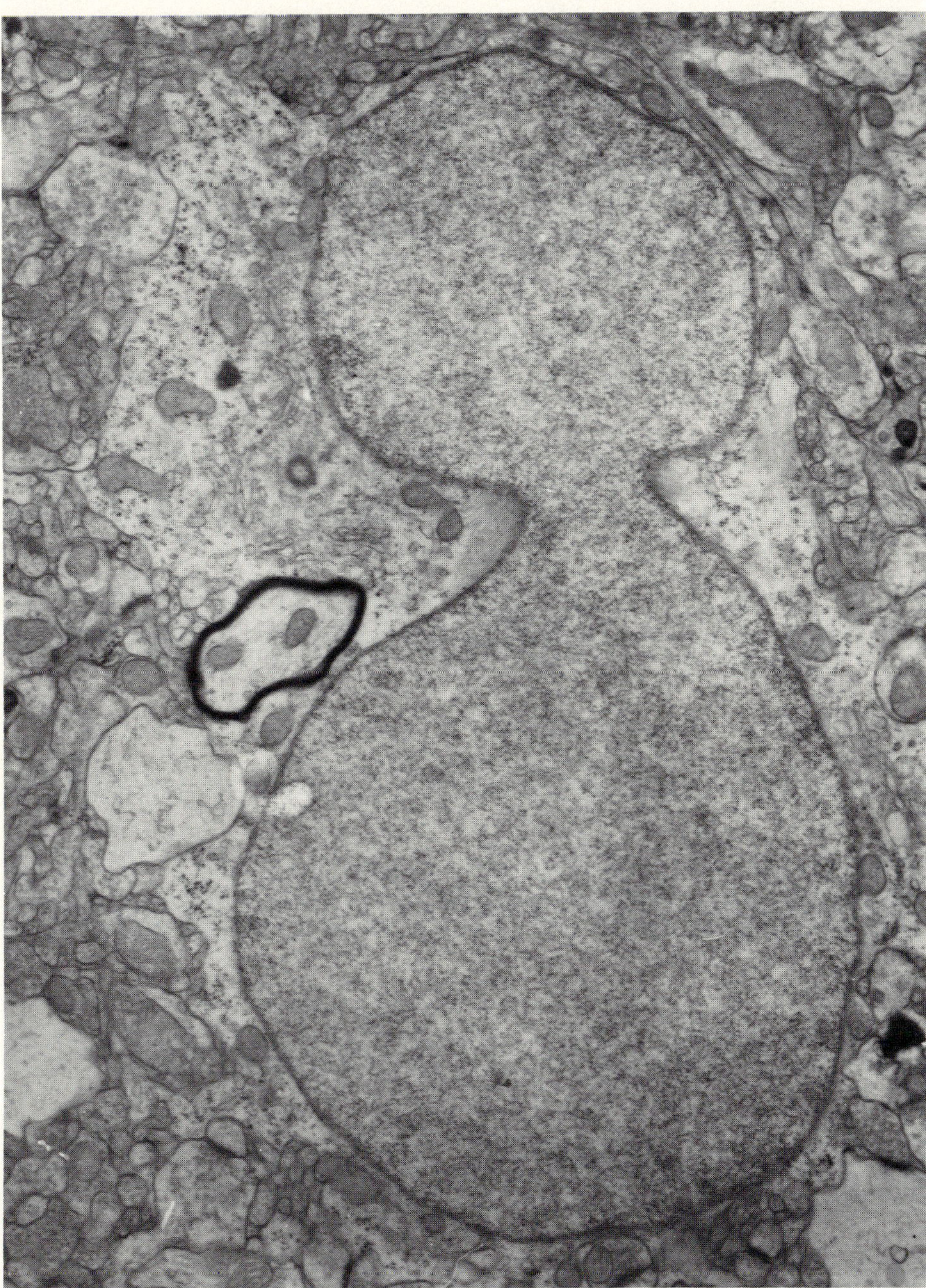

Fig. 198 A nucleus with an hour-glass shape in a reactive astrocyte. Very fine fibrillary material and scattered glycogen granules are distributed in the watery cytoplasm. × 17,000. (From Hirano, A.: J. Neuropathol. Exp. Neurol. 24: 386, 1965.)

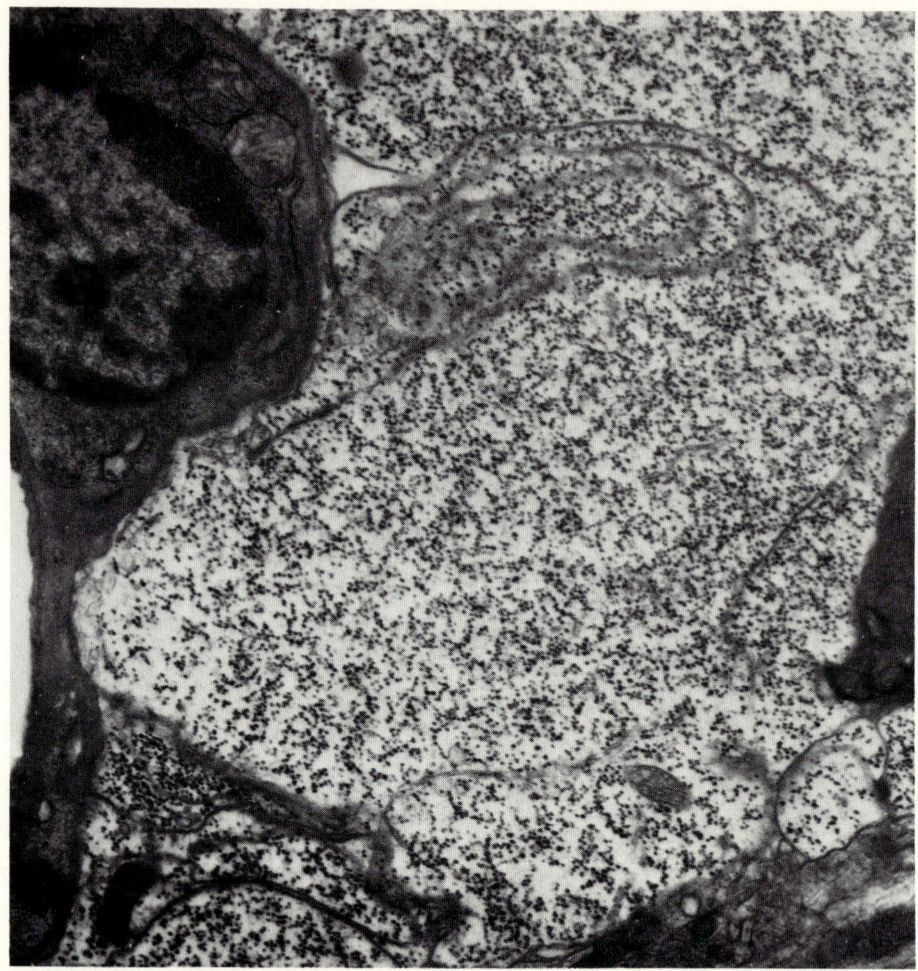

Fig. 199 Swollen perivascular glial processes are filled with numerous glycogen granules. A mononuclear cell is visible in the electron-dense edema fluid which fills the perivascular region. × 13,500. (From Hirano, A.: J. Neuropathol. Exp. Neurol. 24: 386, 1965.)

however, the swollen vacuole may be seen to contain fine filamentous material (Fig. 198) and, often, an accumulation of *glycogen* granules (Fig. 199). The nearby extracellular spaces are compressed.

REFERENCES

Hirano, A., Zimmerman, H.M., & Levine, S.: The fine structure of cerebral fluid accumulation. VII. Reactions of astrocytes to cryptococcal polysaccharide implantation. J. Neuropathol. Exp. Neurol., 24:386-397, 1965.

Lemkey-Johnson, N., & Reynolds, W.A.: Nature and extent of brain lesions in mice related to ingestion of monosodium glutamate. J. Neuropathol. Exp. Neurol., 33: 74-97, 1974.

Phelps, G.H.: An ultrastructural study of methionine sulphoximine-induced glycogen accumulation in astrocytes of the mouse cerebral cortex. J. Neurocytol., 4, 479-490, 1975.

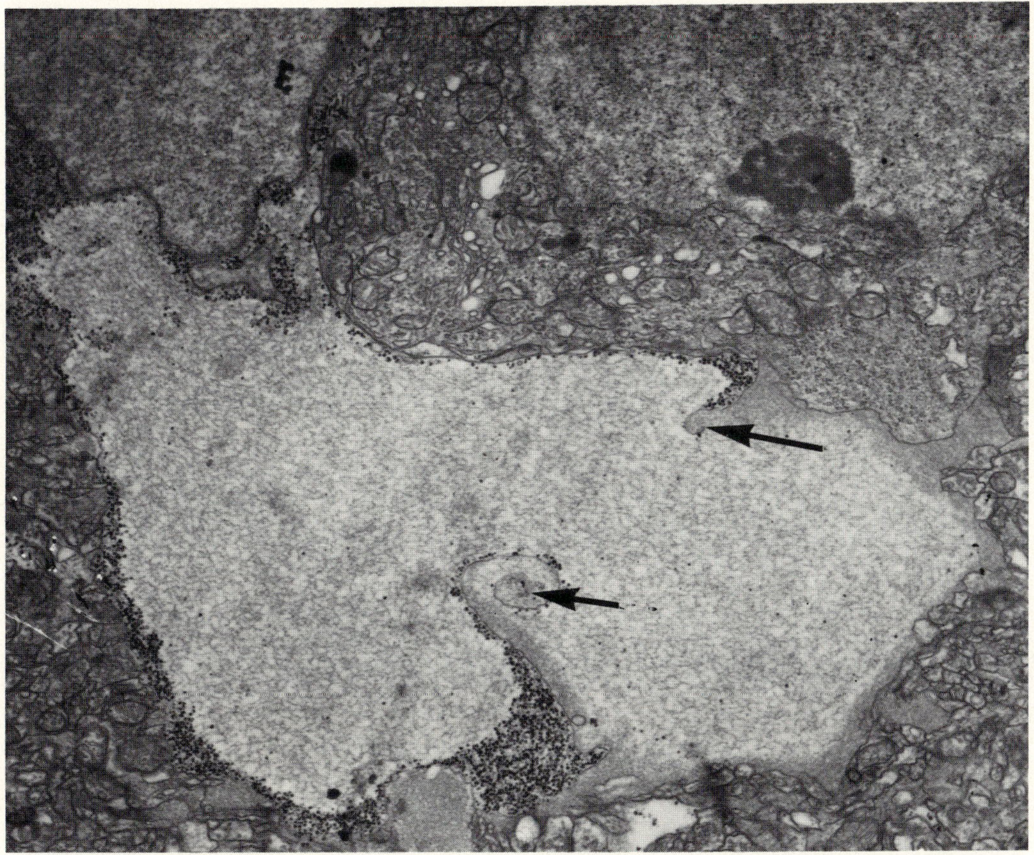

Fig. 200 Wide communication is evident between the extracellular space and the cytoplasm through the ruptured membrane (arrows) of an astrocyte. The edges of the ruptured membrane form a curled configuration illustrating the elastic nature of the plasma membrane during life. Glycogen granules are distributed in the periphery of the intracellular compartment, while fine, compact material is seen at the periphery of extracellular fluid. × 12,500. (From Hirano, A. et al.: Arch. Neurol. 11, 632, 1964.)

NUCLEAR CHANGES (Fig. 201)

Irregularly-shaped astrocytic nuclei are commonly seen after a variety of insults. When seen in thin sections such nuclei may appear to be multiple but are actually highly lobulated structures.

So-called "*nuclear bodies*" (Fig. 201B) consisting of spherical accumulations of filaments sometimes accompanied by granules have been seen in subacute sclerosing panencephalitis or astrocytoma. Similar nuclear bodies may be found after injury in a variety of cells such as endothelial cells and fibroblasts, etc. Other pathological intranuclear inclusions following infections or in tumors, among other conditions, consist of accumulations of filaments arranged in rod-shaped or crystalloid patterns (Fig. 201A).

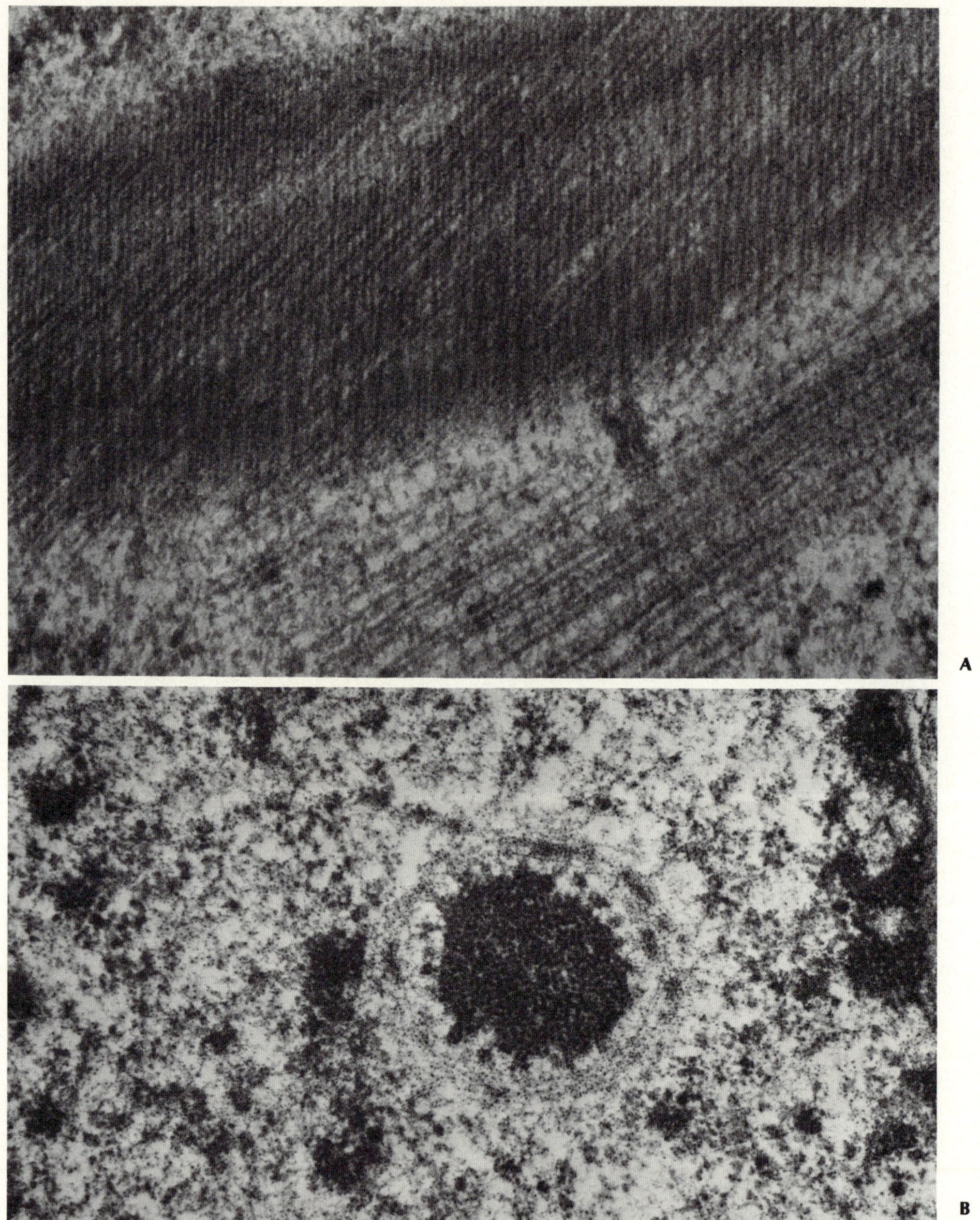

Fig. 201 Intranuclear inclusions in an astrocyte. A. Lattice-like fibrils. × 65,000. B. Nuclear body. × 25,000.

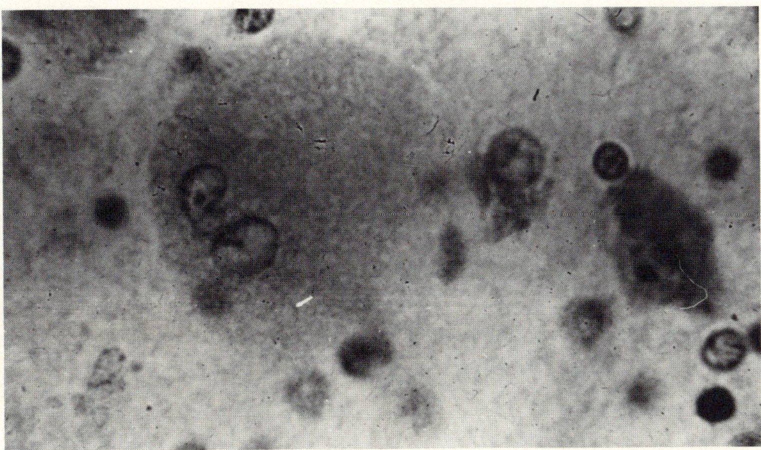

Fig. 202 Opalski cell (Nissl stain).

Eosinophilic intranuclear inclusions which have been shown to be viral particles within glia are characteristic features of progressive multifocal leucoencephalopathy and of subacute sclerosing panencephalitis, as well as of herpes encephalitis.

Other intranuclear inclusions within astrocytes are seen after experimental lead intoxication (Hirano and Kochen, 1976). These are similar to those found in renal and hepatic cells of patients with lead intoxication. Analysis of these intranuclear bodies has indicated that they contain measurable amounts of lead (Shirabe and Hirano, 1977).

Mitotic figures are generally not seen in astrocytes in post-mortem human material. Cavanagh (1970), however, has reported that astrocytes undergoing mitosis may be found in rat brain subjected to needle wounds if the tissue is fixed immediately after death. Abnormal mitosis of astrocytes has also been reported in anoxic encephalopathy (Diemer and Klinken, 1976).

Alzheimer type II glia, as found in Wilson's disease or in hepatic encephalopathy are astrocytes showing extraordinarily large, often kidney-shaped nuclei. They are most commonly seen in the globus pallidus, but are also present in the dentate nucleus of the cerebellum, the cerebral cortex and other areas. The nuclei are stained in both Nissl and H & E preparations in which they appear pale and swollen with a few chromatin and/or nucleoli-like granules scattered at the nuclear periphery. The cytoplasm is generally unstained except for a few pigment granules so that the phenomenon is sometimes referred to as "naked-nuclei gliosis". In *Alzheimer type I glia* the nuclei are also large and often lobulated, but the voluminous cytoplasm is also identifiable. Opalski cells (Fig. 202) may also be seen in Wilson's disease. The origin of this cell is unclear, but is considered to be derived either from neurons or from astrocytes.

Alzheimer type II glia were observed in experimental portocaval anastomosis in rats (Cavanagh and Kyu, 1971; Norenberg and Lapham, 1974). In addition, Diemer et al (1977) observed an increase in the number of astrocytic nuclei and a decrease in the number of oligodendrocytic nuclei in similar animals. These authors suggested that nuclei normally considered to be oligodendroglial were transformed into nuclei with the morphological characteristics of astrocytic nuclei.

REFERENCES

Cavanagh, J.B.: The proliferation of astrocytes around a needle wound in the rat brain. J. Anat., 106: 471-487, 1970.
Cavanagh, J.B., & Kyu, M.H.: Type II Alzheimer change experimentally produced in astrocytes in the rat. J. Neurol. Sci., 12: 63-75, 1971.
Diemer, N.H., & Klinken, L.: Astrocyte mitosis and Alzheimer type I and II astrocytes in anoxic encephalopathy. Neuropathol. Appl. Neurobiol., 2: 313-321, 1976.
Hirano, A., & Kochen, J.A.: Further observations on the effects of lead implantation in rat brains. Acta Neuropathol., 34: 87-92, 1976.
Diemer, N.H., Klee, J., Schröeder, H., & Klinken, L.: Glial and nerve cell changes in rats with porto-caval anastomosis. Acta Neuropathol., 39: 59-68, 1977.
Shirabe, T., & Hirano, A.: X-ray microanalytical studies of lead-implanted rat brains. Acta Neuropathol., 40: 184-192, 1977.
Hirano, A., & Iwata, M.: Neuropathology of lead intoxication. *In* Handbook of Clinical Neurology, Vol. 36, Intoxications of the Nervous System. Chap. 2, pp. 35-65, Vinken, P.J. & Bruyn, G.W. (eds.), North-Holland Pub. Co., Netherlands, 1978.

HYPERTROPHIC ASTROCYTES (Fig. 203)

In a number of subacute conditions resulting in glial reaction, large astrocytes are seen, usually with distinctly stained eosinophilic cytoplasm. In the electron microscope, the swollen cytoplasm appears crowded with the usual organelles such as mitochrondria, vesicles, endoplasmic reticulum, Golgi apparatus and lysosomes scattered in a background filled with fine glial fibrils. In addition, a number of lipid-like inclusions or phagocytosed material may be present.

The large, reactive astrocytes are a consistent feature after any insult including trauma, infarct, infection or tumor. Particularly large and bizarre, often multinucleated astrocytes are seen in progressive multifocal leucoencephalopathy (Richardson, 1965), and are associated with magnocellular glioblastoma. They are seen, but only rarely, in certain demyelinating diseases.

REFERENCES

Richardson, E.P. Jr.: Progressive multifocal leukoencephalopathy. *In* The Remote Effects of Cancer on the Nervous System: Contemporary Neurology Symposia, I, pp. 6-16, Brain, L., & Norris, F. Jr. (eds), Grune & Stratton, New York, 1965.
Hirano, A., & Zimmerman, H.M.: Some effects of vinblastine implantation in the cerebral white matter. Lab. Invest., 23: 358-367. 1970.

FIBRILLARY GLIOSIS (Figs. 204—206)

As lesions age and assume a chronic aspect, the glial fibrillary accumulations within the astrocyte virtually fill the cell. In the earlier stages, the perinuclear area as well as the cell processes are still large. Gradually, both areas shrink in size and eventually contain almost nothing but the glial fibrils. The cell processes usually lose their sheet-like configuration and often appear circular in cross-section. Large numbers of such astrocytes fill the site of the lesion and become recognizable as the well known "glial scar". In large lesions such as massive infarcts the astrocytes do not entirely fill the site but, instead, leave areas of extracellular space or cystic cavities.

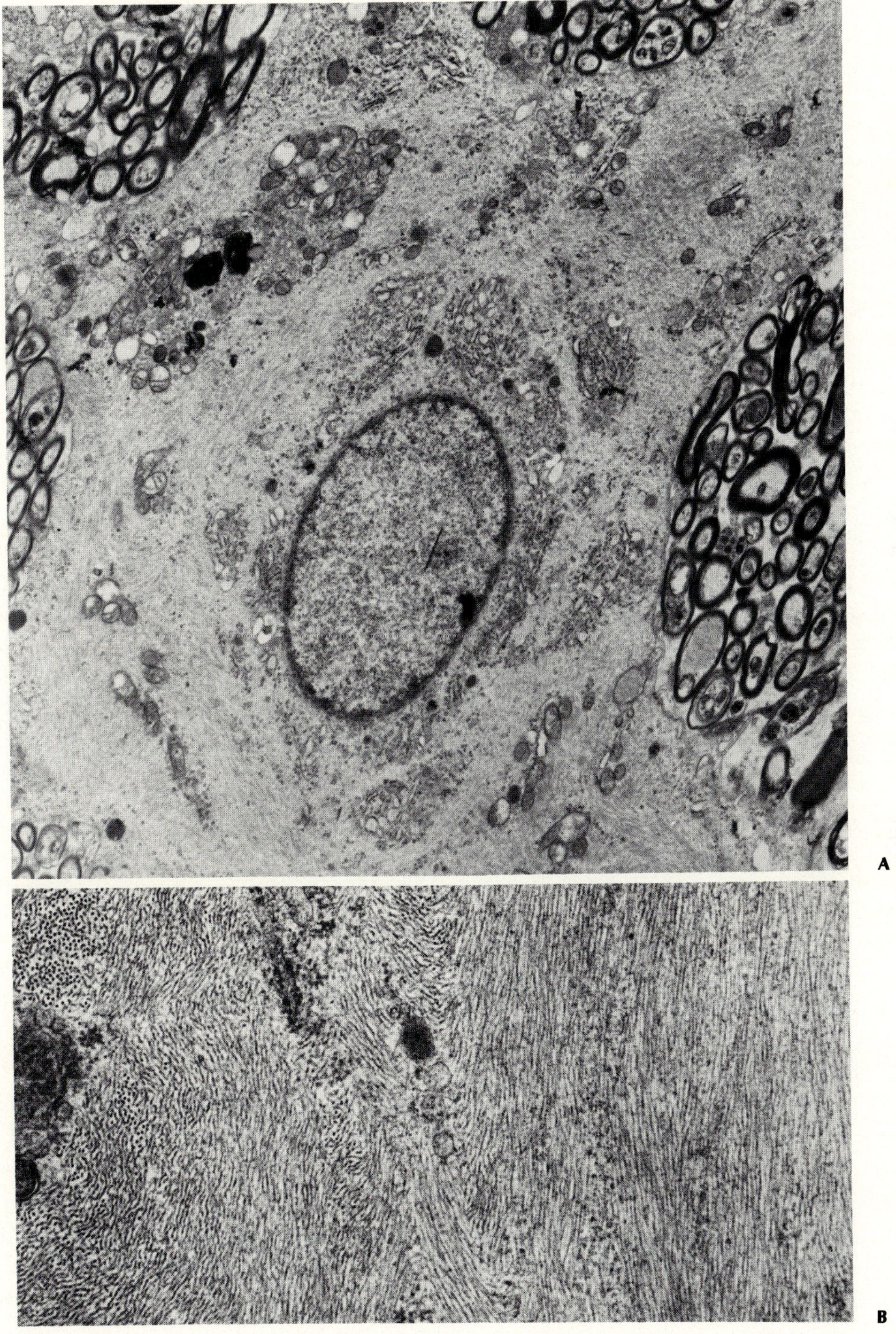

Fig. 203 Swollen astrocytes filled with numerous glial fibrils. A: × 6,000. B: × 25,000. (From Hirano, A., & Zimmerman, H.M.: Lab. Invest., 23: 358, 1970)

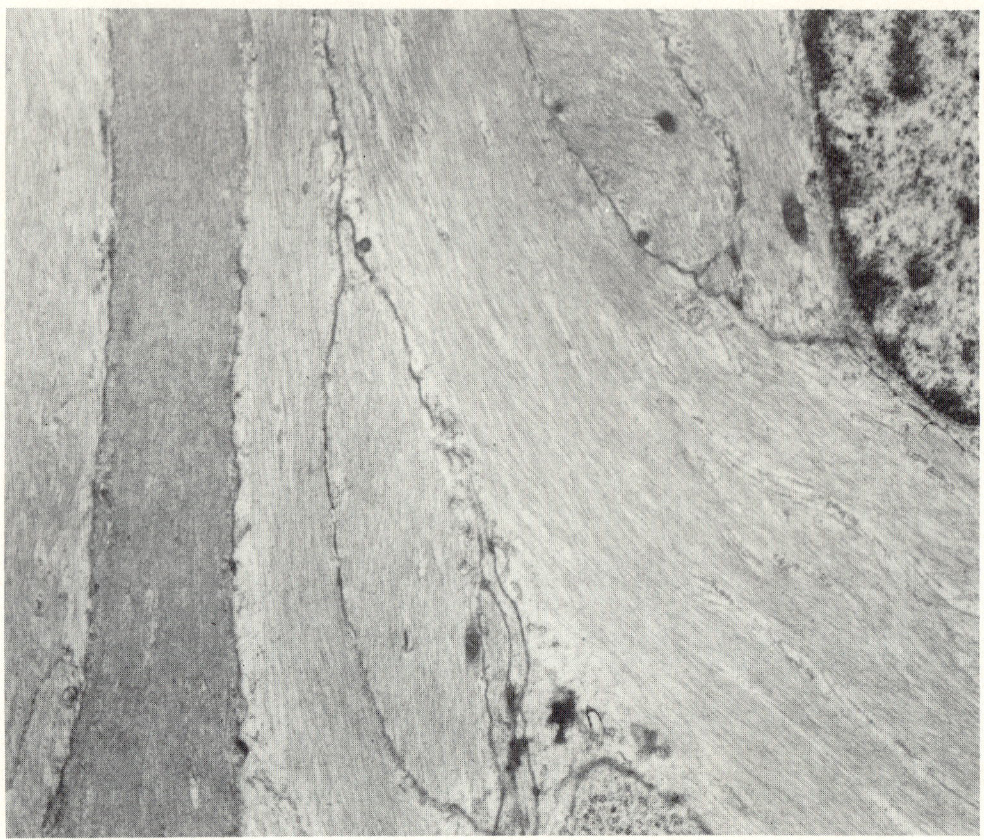

Fig. 204 Astrocytic gliosis. × 14,000. (From Hirano, A.: The Structure and Function of Nervous Tissue. Vol. 2, p. 69, Academic Press, 1969.)

The gliotic reaction is sometimes classified as either "*isomorphic*" or "*anisomorphic gliosis*". In the former the glial scar takes on the general pattern of the once-existing tissue. Gliosis seen in demyelinating plaques is a good example of isomorphic gliosis. In anisomorphic gliosis which follows focal destructive processes such as abscess, the scar forms no recognizable pattern.

The filaments forming the glial fibrils are morphologically indistinguishable from the filaments of the normal astrocytes (Fig. 205). Frequently, however, so-called "*Rosenthal fibers*" (Fig. 206) appear in long-standing lesions. These consist of electron dense granular material often permeated by condensed glial filaments. In the light microscope, the Rosenthal fibers and the glial fibrils are both eosinophilic. The conspicuous Rosenthal fibers, however, stain much more intensely and appear as a prominent homogenous mass assuming an elongated or circular configuration in the finer textured background. Rosenthal fibers are especially well known in Alexander's disease, but they are also found in various types of glial scars as well as in astrocytomas.

While visible in H & E preparations, the most effective stain for fibrillary gliosis is the Holzer stain or Mallory's phosphotungstic acid-hematoxylin stain in which

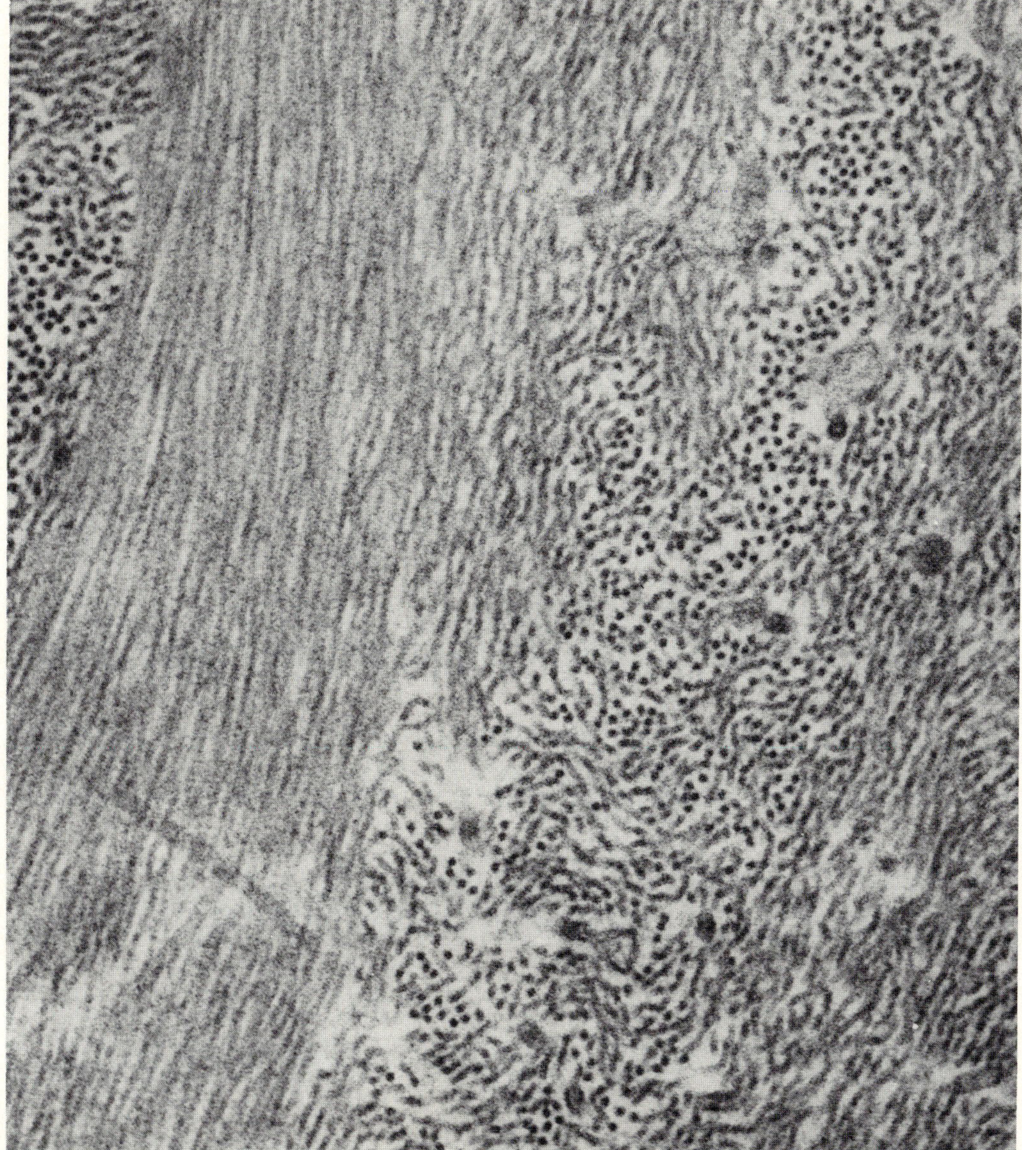

Fig. 205 Glial fibrils. × 111,000. (From Hirano, A.: Progress in Neuropathology. Vol. 1, p. 1, Grune & Stratton, 1971.)

the glial fibrils appear blue. Another elegant stain is Penfield's modification of the astroglial stain, which results in black fibrils. More recently, immunohistochemical methods have been utilized for the detection of glial fibrillary acidic protein in the glial cells (p. 114).

Increased glial fibrils in certain portions of the brain is a normal aging phenomenon. This is especially prominent in subpial and subependymal areas. The subependymal area overlying the caudate nucleus and the fornix and the floor of the fourth ventricle are particularly common sites of this change. The inferior olivary nucleus is another noteworthy area of gliosis.

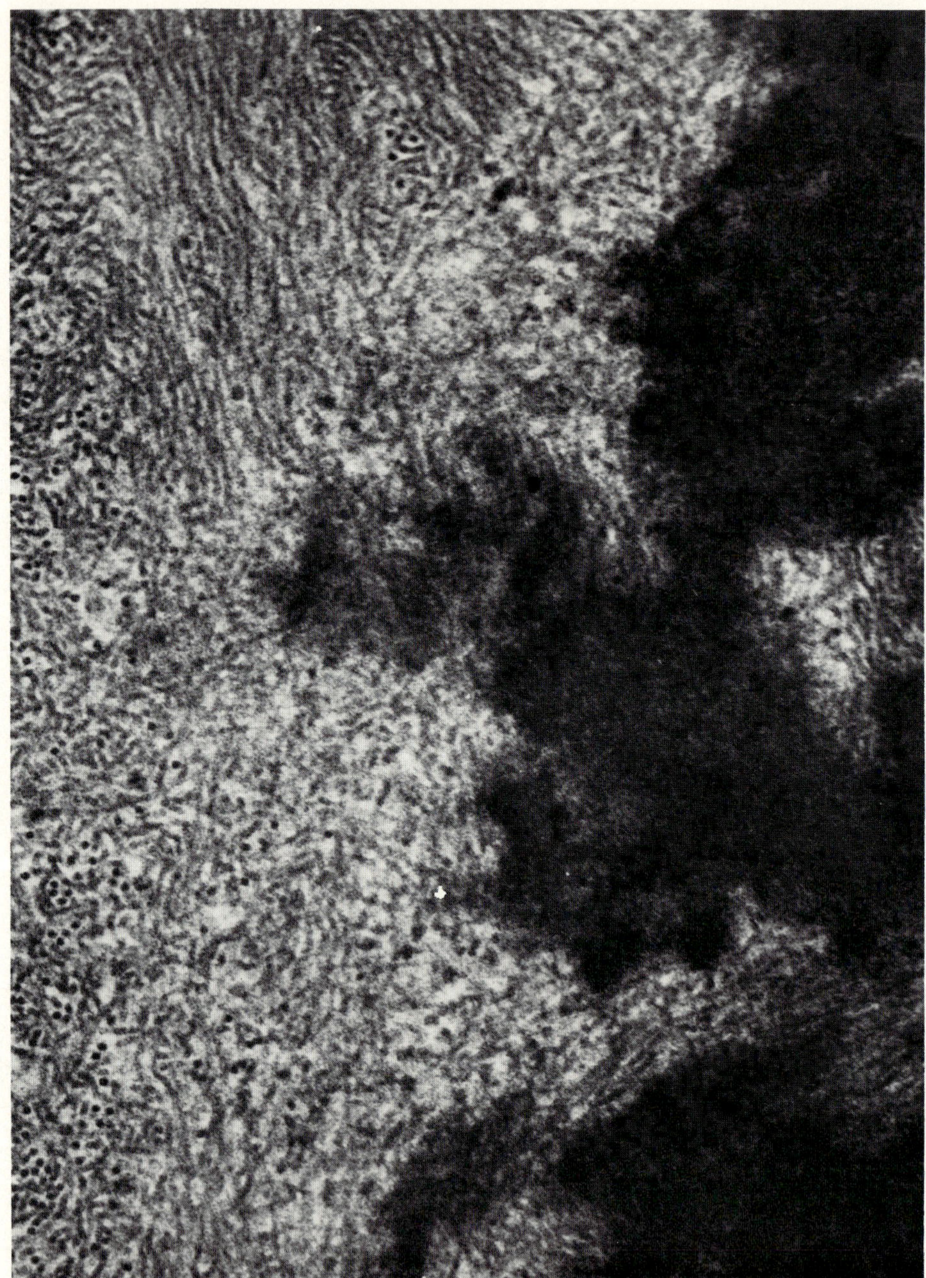

Fig. 206 High magnification of a Rosenthal fiber within a reactive astrocyte adjacent to a craniopharyngioma. Numerous glial fibrils are in close contact with the dense granular mass that constitutes the Rosenthal fiber. × 96,000.

REFERENCES

Tani, E., Hirano, A., & Zimmerman, H.M.: Glial cells with fibrillar structure in the optic nerve and the white matter. J. Neuropathol. Exp. Neurol., 23: 162, 1964 (abstract).

Schochet, S.S., Lampert, P.W., & Earle K.M.: Alexander's disease. A case report with electron microscopic observations. Neurology, 18: 543-549, 1968.

Glial Bundles

Glial bundles, consisting of large accumulations of filament-containing, astrocytic processes, were first reported in the spinal roots of patients with Werdnig-Hoffmann disease by Chou and Fakadej (1971). Since then, they have been seen in cases of healed poliomyelitis as well. Their formation and relationship to the disease process has been discussed (Iwata and Hirano, 1978).

REFERENCES

Chou S. M., & Fakadej, A.V.: Ultrastructure of chromatolytic motoneurons and anterior spinal roots in a case of Werdnig-Hoffmann disease. J. Neuropathol. Exp. Neurol., 30: 368:-379, 1971.

Iwata, M., & Hirano, A.: "Glial bundles" in spinal cord late after paralytic anterior poliomyelitis. Ann. Neurol., 4: 562-563, 1978.

ASTROCYTIC INCLUSIONS

Pigmented inclusions are fairly common in astrocytes in various conditions. Lipofuscin is the most common among these and it is seen especially in aged brains or after any chronic insult. Astrocytes display phagocytic activity and

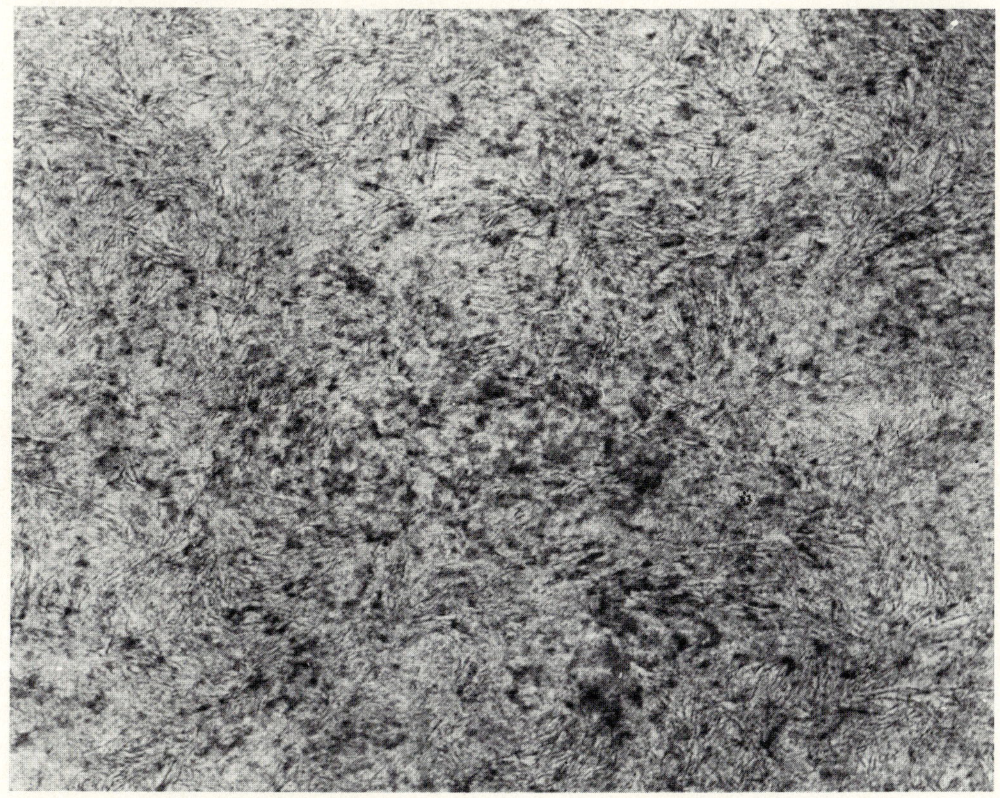

Fig. 207 Corpora amylacea. × 40,000. (From Hirano, A.: Progress in Neuropathology. Vol.1, p.1. Grune & Stratton, 1971.)

therefore, myelin debris will be found in them after demyelinating disease. Similarly, hemorrhage results in hemosiderin pigment inclusions in the astrocytes. So-called "marginal hemosiderosis" or "superficial siderosis" is the result of hemosiderin deposits in subpial astrocytes after subarachnoid hemorrhage. Lipids and other inclusions appear in astrocytes in association with various types of lipidoses. These often assume various characteristic configurations.

Corpora amylacea (Fig 207, 208) is probably the best known of astrocytic inclusions (Ramsey, 1965). It does not seem to be of any pathological significance, but is associated with aging (Takeya, 1970). It is apparently identical to the material composing the neuronal Lafora body. It is basophilic, argentophilic and PAS-positive. In astrocytes, it appears as variable-sized, 5-20 micron, spherical deposits usually in the process but sometimes in the soma. The inclusions tend to occur in subpial and subependymal astrocytes. They may also be expected in the median aspect of the lentiform nucleus, part of Ammon's horn and the posterior column of the spinal cord among other areas.

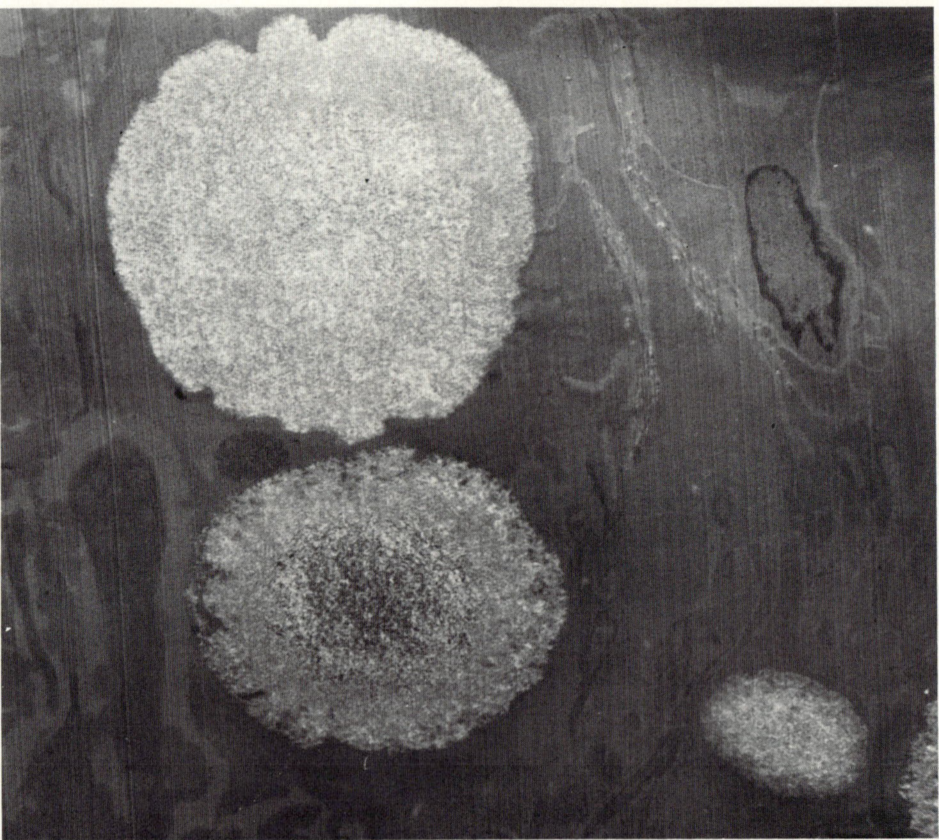

Fig. 208 Electron micrograph of corpora amylacea in white matter. The matrix of the bodies and myelin are negative for the ethanolic phosphotungstic acid stain applied to formalin-fixed tissue. × 6,000. (From Hirano, A. et al.: Acta Neuropathol. 26: 265, 1973.)

The significance of corpora amylacea in astrocytes is obscure. It is common in apparently normal aged brains and sometimes in adults with long-standing gliosis. Young children, even with chronic, severe gliotic conditions such as diffuse gliosis associated with leucodystrophy do not accumulate this material.

Other inclusions found in astrocytes are certain *dense core vesicles* seen in a variety of conditions including SSPE and are believed to be calcium deposits (Gambetti et al. 1975). Virus-like particles have also been detected in astrocytes in various conditions.

REFERENCES

Ramsey, H.J.: Ultrastructure of corpora amylacea. J. Neuropathol. Exp. Neurol., 24: 25-39, 1965.

Takeya, S.: Introduction to the General Neuropathology. Igaku Shoin Ltd., Tokyo, 1970 pp. 213-215.

Hirano, A., Dembitzer, H.M., & Zimmerman, H.M.: The fine structure of phosphotungstic acid stained neuropathologic tissue. Acta Neuropathol., 26: 265-273, 1973.

Gambetti, P., Erulkar, S.E., Somlyo, A.P., & Gonatas, N.K.: Calcium-containing structures in vertebrate glial cells. J. Cell. Biol., 64: 322-330, 1975.

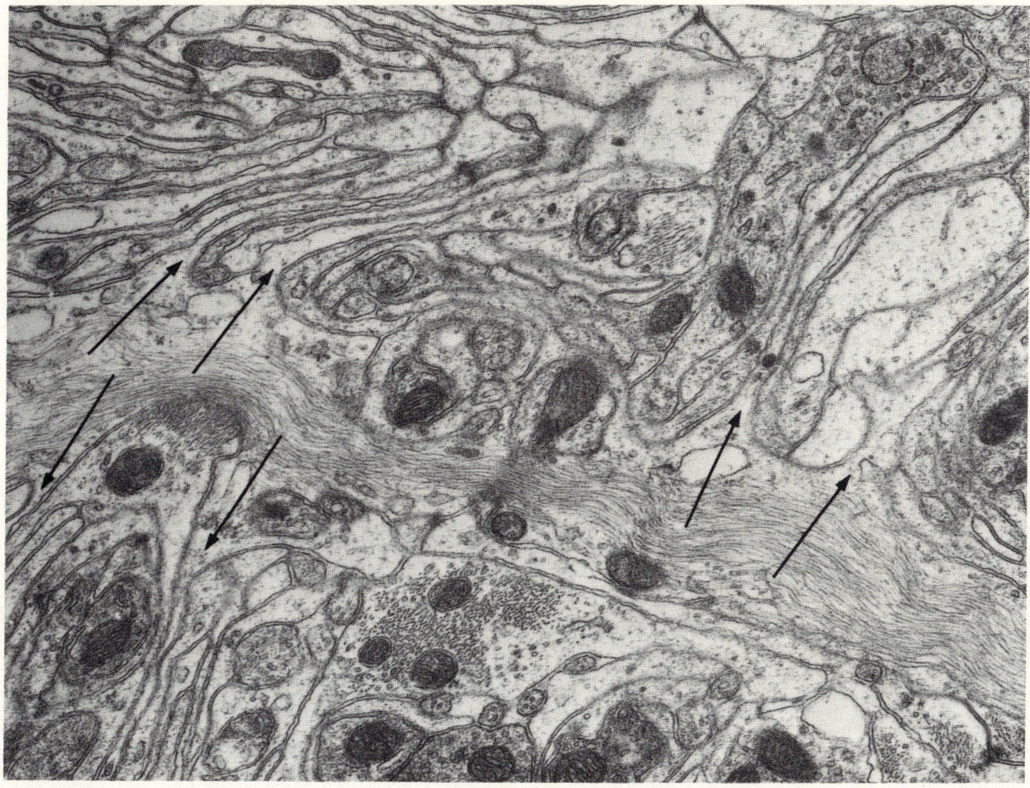

Fig. 209 Several sheet-like processes (arrows) arising from a filament-filled astrocytic trunk, in the cerebellum of an adult "staggerer" mouse. × 25,000. (From Hirano, A., & Dembitzer, H.M.: J. Neuropathol. Exp. Neurol. 35: 63, 1976.)

CHANGES IN THE SHAPE OF THE ASTROCYTE

The overall shape of the astrocytic process is subject to profound changes depending on the lesion. As already mentioned, the processes may become almost entirely cylindrical in glial scars. On the other hand, certain cases of substantial neuronal loss such as in granule cell type cerebellar degeneration or in the murine mutant, "weaver", astrocytic processes assume voluminous balloon-like shapes, often embedding the unattached dendritic spines of the Purkinje cells and filling the parenchymal spaces (Fig. 190B). In other conditions, such as the murine mutant "staggerer" and some areas of human gliosis, the tendency towards sheet-

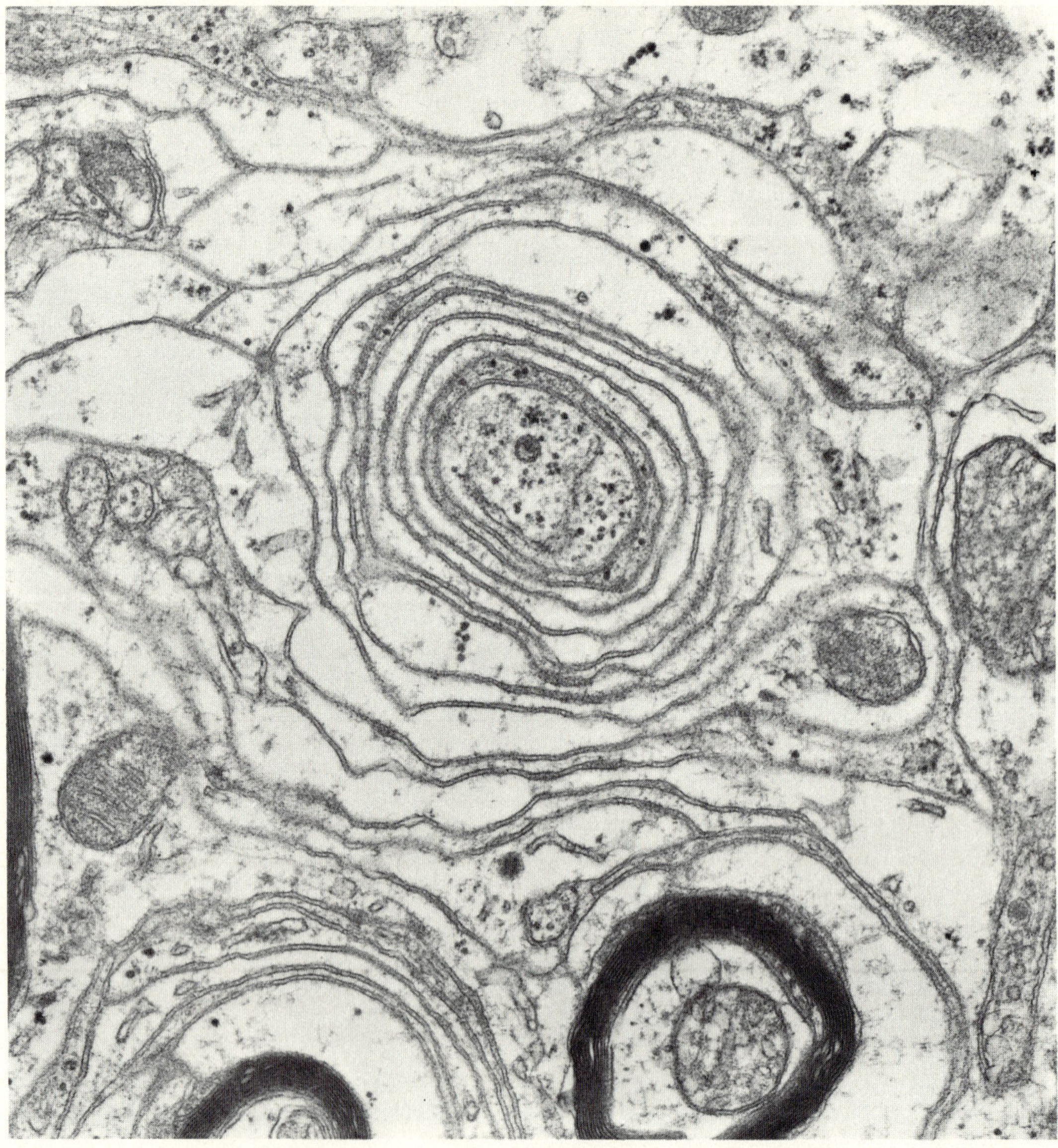

Fig. 210 Two myelinated fibers and a cell process are surrounded by sheet-like processes of reactive astrocytes in the cerebellum of an adult "staggerer" mouse. × 33,000. (From Hirano, A., & Dembitzer, H.M.: J. Neuropath. Exp. Neurol. 35: 63, 1976.)

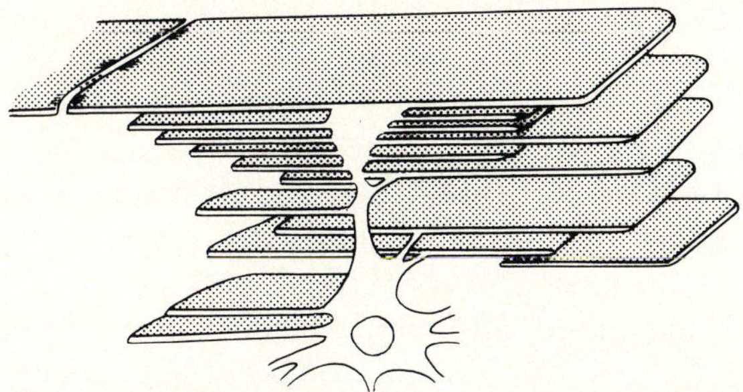

Fig. 211 A three dimensional representation of a reactive astrocyte in the cerebral cortex of an adult "staggerer" mouse showing the abnormal elaboration of distal, sheet-like expansions. (From Hirano, A.: *In*: Neurobiology of Neurons and Glia. Kyoritsu Pub. Co., Tokyo, p. 65, 1977.)

like elaboration of the astrocytic processes becomes exaggerated resulting in whorls composed of lamellae of flattened processes (Fig. 209-211). Finally, in astrocytic neoplasms or in newly reactive astrocytes the processes are relatively few in number and many are short and stubby resembling microvilli rather than elongated cell processes.

REFERENCES

Sax, D.S., Hirano, A., & Shofer, R.J.: Staggerer, a neurological murine mutant. An electron microscopic study of the cerebellar cortex in the adult. Neurology, 18: 1093-1100, 1968.

Hirano, A., & Dembitzer, H.M.: The fine structure of astrocytes in the adult staggerer. J. Neuropathol. Exp. Neurol., 35: 63-74, 1976.

Hirano, A.: Neuronal and glial processes in neuropathology. Presidential address to the American Association of neuropathologists. J. Neuropathol. Exp. Neurol., 37: 365-374, 1978.

Hirano, A.: Neuronal and glial processes. Form and function. *In* The Second Seminar for Neurobiology: Neurobiology of Neurons and Glia. Japan Medical Research Foundation, Modern Biology Series 32, pp. 65-87, Tsukada, Y. (ed.) Kyoritsu Shuppan, Tokyo, 1977.

NEOPLASMS

Astrocytomas (Fig. 212)

The tumor cells of astrocytomas show the basic features characteristic of non-neoplastic, reactive astrocytes or of immature astrocytes. Gliomas, in general, are infiltrative so that it is sometimes difficult to distinguish the truly neoplastic cell from adjacent non-neoplastic but reactive astrocytes. Most obvious are their star-like configurations, usually with many, long cell processes which contain glial fibrils and glycogen granules. Rosenthal fibers which consist of electron-dense granular material associated with marginal fibrillary accumulations, are characteristic, especially in the more benign tumors. In addition, fine vesicles, free ribosomes, occasional dense core vesicles, as well as punctuate adhesions and gap junctions, similar to those which may be found in normal and reactive astrocytes, are evident in the electron microscope. The extracellular space is often enlarged and microcyst formation is one of the characterisic features. Vascular feet are evident around blood vessels within the tumor. The tumors differ from normal tissue, or even from reactive tissue in that the cells form masses rather than their

more usual net-like arrangement in relation to the surrounding tissue. On the other hand, the characteristic relationship to the vessels and pial surface is generally maintained even in the tumor, although the intimate arrangements of the cell processes are often disturbed. The junctional apparatus is often poorly developed and areas of wide separation may be observed. The close relationship with neuronal elements is lost and the elaborate expansions of peripheral cell processes are generally markedly impaired (Kawamoto et al., 1978). Cross sections of the cell processes are more often circular in profile indicating cylindrical configurations rather than the laminar expansions seen in normal protoplasmic astrocytes. Cell bodies often display minute, short cell processes resembling filopodia or microvilli which are not features of the normal, mature astrocyte. A certain degree of pleomorphism is present, especially in more malignant tumors which also show frequent mitotic figures. In some cases, the nuclei may contain dense fibrillary material, nuclear bodies or other nuclear inclusions.
The blood vessels of the tumor show various changes, but they are rarely fenestrated.

REFERENCES

Poon, T.P., Hirano, A., & Zimmerman, H.M.: Electron Microscopic Atlas of Brain Tumors. Grune & Stratton, New York, 1971.

Miki, H., & Hirano, A.: Electron microscopic studies of optic nerve glioma in an 18-month old child Am. J. Ophthal., 79: 589-595, 1975.

Kawamoto, K., Hirano, A., & Matsui, T.: The fine structure of cell processes in astrocytoma. Neurol. Surg. (Tokyo), 6: 1173-1179, 1978.

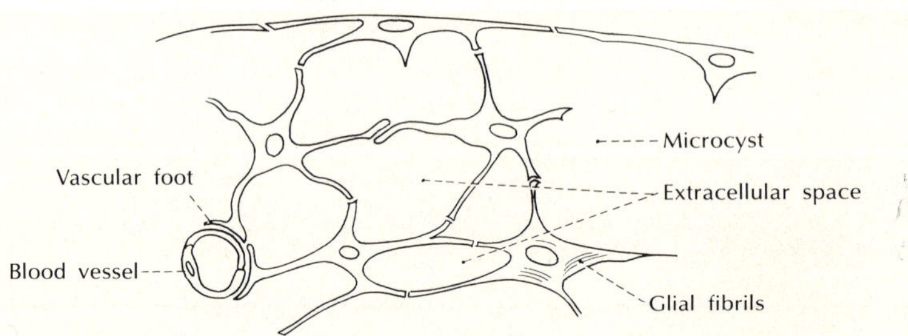

Fig. 212 Astrocytoma.

Glioblastoma Multiforme (Figs. 213-215)

This most malignant form of astrocytic neoplasm is histologically characterized by pleomorphism, pseudopalisading around necrotic areas, endothelial proliferation and lymphocytic cuffing (Fig. 213). The size and shape of the tumor cells vary considerably, and giant cells are often seen, some of which may be multinucleated (Fig. 215). Because of the pronounced irregularity of the nuclei, cytoplasmic invaginations may be misinterpreted as intranuclear inclusions. Palisading (Fig. 214), spindle-shaped, immature cells around necrotic areas are considered to be

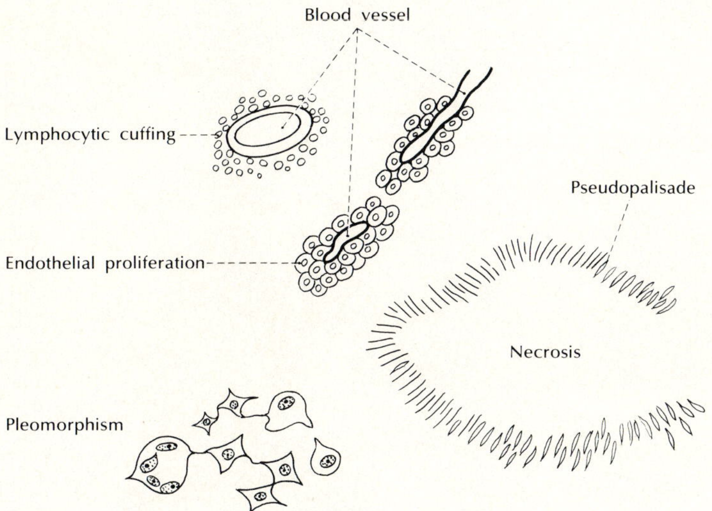

Fig. 213 Histology of glioblastoma.

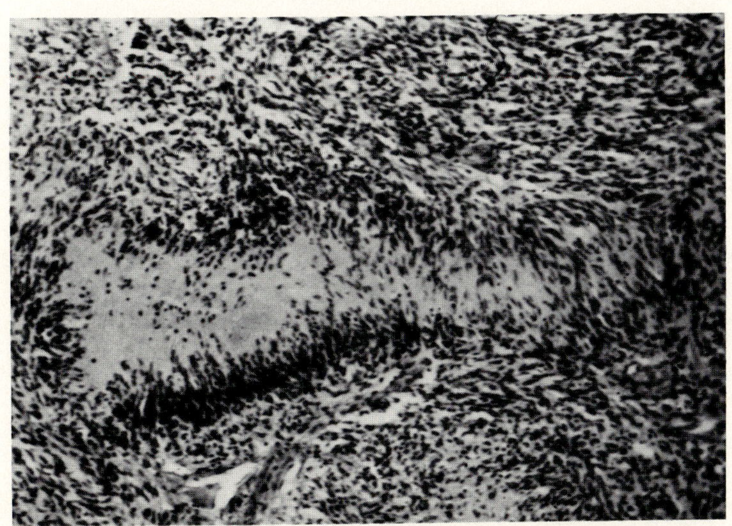

Fig. 214 Pseudopalisades of glioblastoma (H&E stain).

neoplastic cells migrating into the necrotic area. Other infiltrating cells are found in the adjacent white matter between the nerve cell processes. Endothelial proliferation is one of the characteristic features of malignant glioma, although it may also be seen in other malignant intracerebral neoplasms. Lymphocytic cuffing may be the result of an immune response of the host.

As might be expected, the fine structure of many of the tumor cells in glioblastoma show the morphological features characteristic of glial cells, especially astrocytes. Disarrangement and poor development of cell processes are, in general,

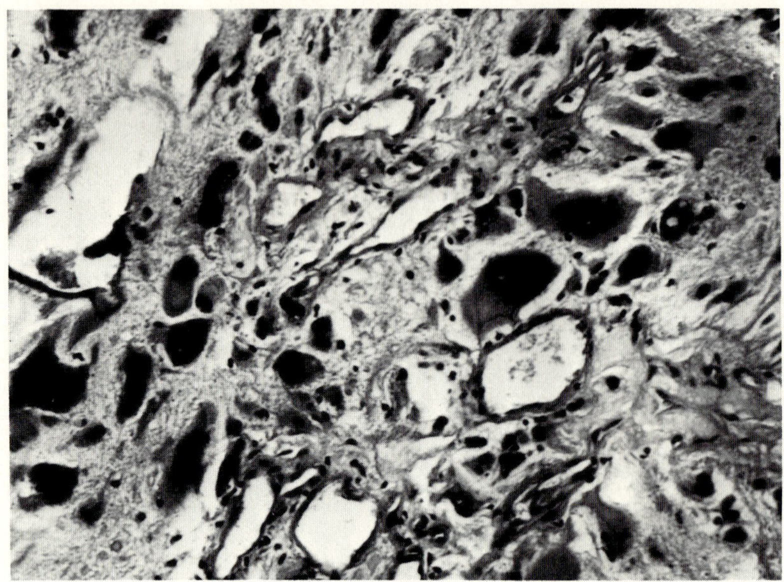

Fig. 215 Giant cell glioblastoma (H & E stain).

much more pronounced in this malignant form than in more benign astrocytomas. The extracellular space is not only filled with hematogenous edema fluid, but also often contains debris of necrotic tissue.

REFERENCES

Luse, S.A.: Electron microscopic studies of brain tumors. Neurology, 19: 881-905, 1960.

Robertson, D.M. & McLean, J.D.: Nuclear inclusions in malignant gliomas. Arch. Neurol., 13: 207-296, 1965.

Zülch, K.J. & Wechsler, W.: Pathology and classification of gliomas. *In* Progress in Neurological Surgery, Vol. 2, Krayenbuhl, H., Maspes, P.E., & Sweet, W.H. (eds.) pp. 1-84, Karger, Basel, 1968.

Tani, E., & Ametani, T.: Intercellular contacts of human gliomas. *In* Progress in Neuropathology, Vol. 1, Zimmerman, H.M. (ed.) pp. 218-232, Grune & Stratton, New York, 1971.

Golden, G.S., Ghatak, N.R., Hirano, A., & French, J.H.: Malignant glioma of the brain stem. A clinicopathologic analysis of 13 cases. J. Neurol. Neurosurg. Psychiat., 35: 732-738, 1972.

C. OLIGODENDROGLIA

1. Normal Oligodendroglia (Figs. 216-218)

The oligodendroglial cells are the myelin-forming cells of the central nervous system. For the most part, they are found deep within the white matter arranged in chains between the myelinated nerve fibers where they are referred to as the "*interfascicular oligodendroglia*". They are also normally present around certain neurons, especially the large pyramidal neurons in the deeper layers of the temporal cortex where they are known as "*satellite cells*".

Oligodendroglia appear as small dark cells in ordinary H & E preparations. The nucleo-cytoplasmic ratio is large and, in well preserved tissue, the cytoplasm forms a narrow rim around the round nucleus. More often, because of its location deep in the white matter, the oligodendroglial cells are not well-fixed and cytoplasmic autolysis leads to swelling of the cytoplasm and shrinking of the nucleus resulting in the so-called "fried egg" appearance in paraffin-embedded tissue.

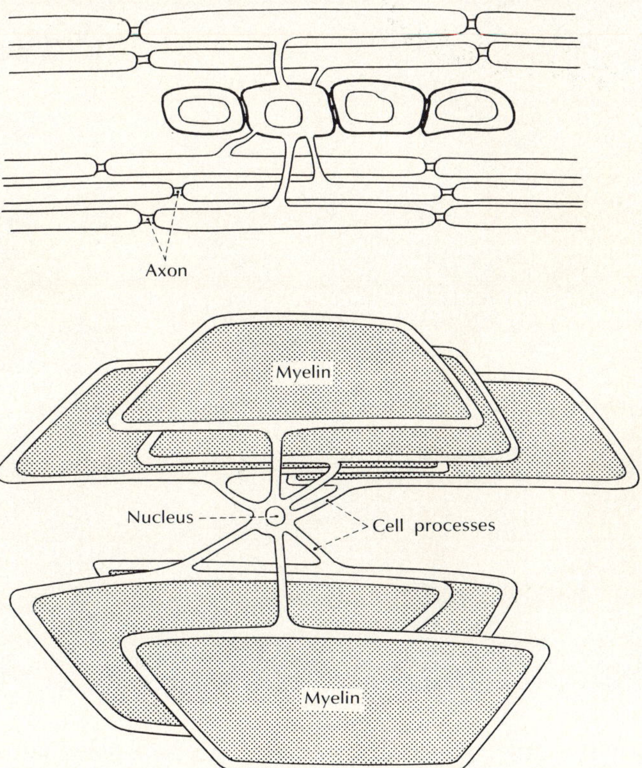

Fig. 216 Oligodendroglial processes and myelin. Upper: A diagram of the interfascicular oligodendroglia and their relationship to the myelin sheaths. Lower: Hypothetically unrolled myelin sheaths showing their connections to the oligodendroglia.

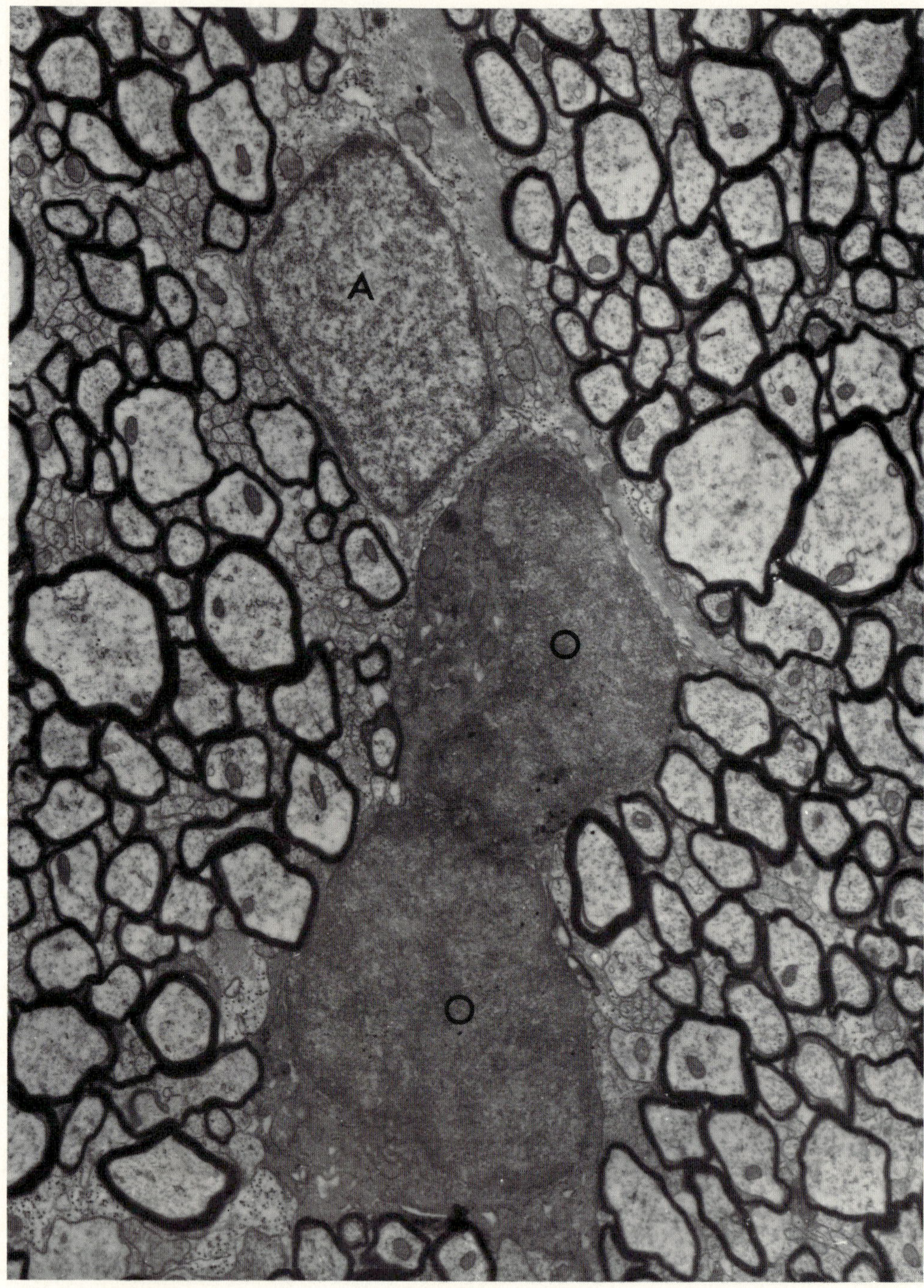

Fig. 217 Cerebral white matter. × 14,000. Two oligodendroglia (O), an astrocyte and many myelinated and unmyelinated cell processes are seen. (From Hirano, A. et al.: J. Neuropathol. Exp. Neurol., 24: 386, 1965.)

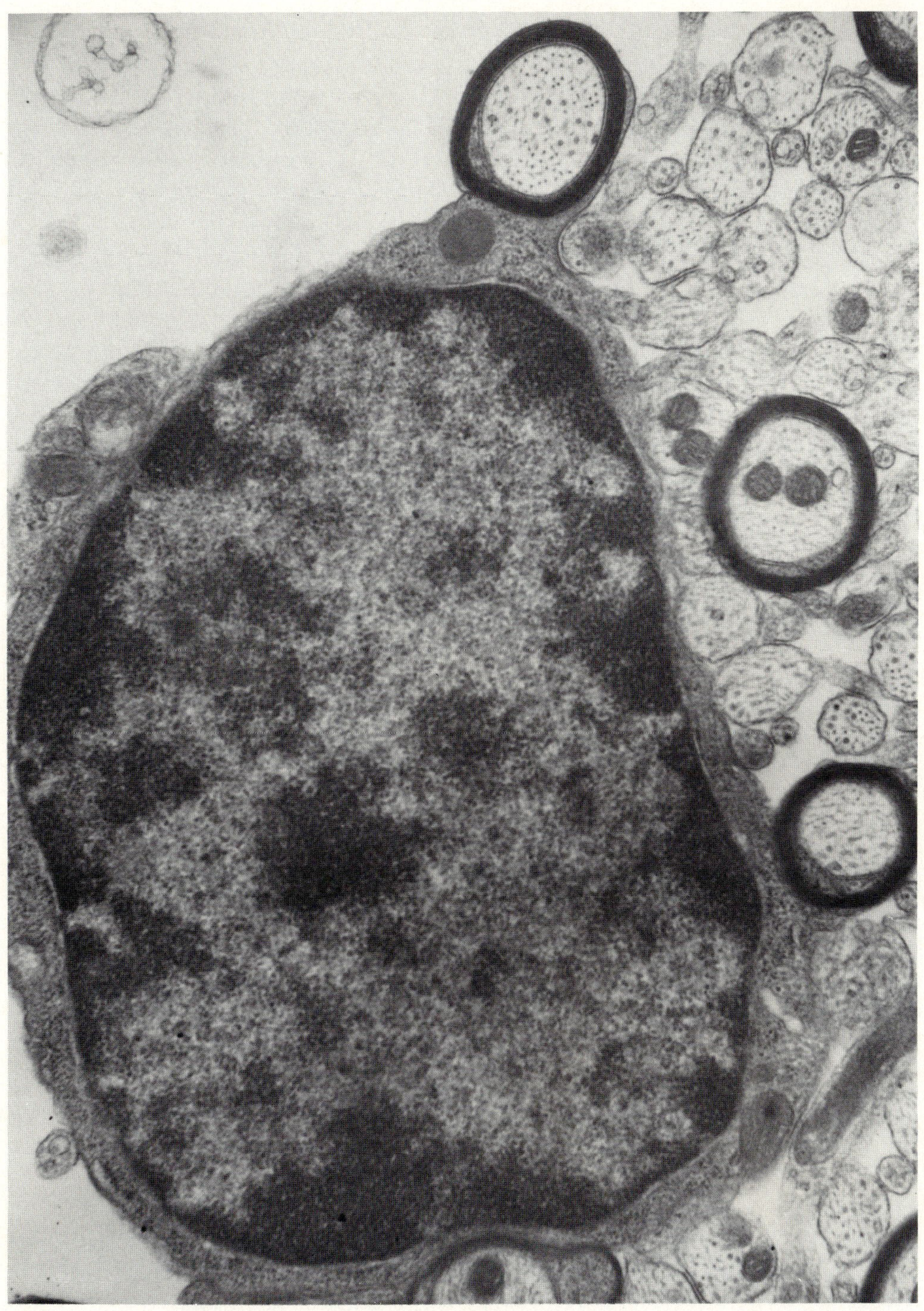

Fig. 218 An oligodendroglial cell. × 25,000. (From Hirano, A: J. Cell Biol., 38: 637, 1968.)

The cell processes usually require metallic impregnation methods for visualization. They are less prominent and fewer in number than in astrocytes.

In the electron microscope, the dense nucleus is surrounded by a narrow rim of cytoplasm around most of its periphery. The cytoplasm contains all the usual organelles including mitochondria, ribosomes, microtubules, and rough and smooth endoplasmic reticulum, including Golgi apparatus, but are devoid of glial filaments. Desmosome-like, as well as other cell junctions (Sotelo, 1973), are present between adjacent oligodendroglia in the interfascicular chain (Fig. 216). Astrocytes are sometimes interpolated in the chain and junctions may be found between them and oligodendroglia.

The oligodendroglial processes are attached to myelin sheaths but due to their length it is very difficult to trace a single process from its origin in the oligodendroglial cell body to the myelin sheath in normal, adult tissue. Direct continuities between the oligodendroglial cell body and the myelin sheath have, however, been illustrated in developing (Bunge et al., 1962; Peters, 1964), or remyelinating tissue (Hirano, 1968) (Fig. 218). The number of myelin-forming processes per oligodendroglial cell differs depending on the location of the cell. As many as 30-50 myelin-forming processes have been calculated to arise from a single oligodendroglia in the rat optic nerve.

The cytoplasmic elements of the myelin sheath are part of the oligodendroglial cytoplasm. Details of their fine structure will be described in a later section but it should be noted that the inner loop of the myelin sheath, which, as will be shown below, is continuous with the oligodendroglial cytoplasm, occasionally containing glial filaments (Hirano and Zimmerman, 1971).

REFERENCES

Bunge, M.B., Bunge, R.P., & Pappas, G.D.: Electron microscopic demonstration of connections between glia and myelin sheaths in the developing mammalian central nervous system. J. Cell Biol., 12: 448-453, 1962.

Hirano, A.: A confirmation of the oligodendroglial origin of myelin in the adult rat. J. Cell Biol., 38: 637-640, 1968.

Hirano, A., & Zimmerman, H.M.: Glial filaments in the myelin sheath after vinblastine implantation. J. Neuropathol. Exp. Neurol., 30: 63-67, 1971.

Peters, A.: Observations on the connexions between myelin sheaths and glial cells in the optic nerves of young rats. J. Anat., 98: 125-134, 1964.

Sotelo, C., & Angaut, P.: The fine structure of the cerebellar central nuclei in the cat. I. Neurons and neuroglial cells. Exp. Brain Res., 16: 410-430, 1973.

2. Pathological Changes of Oligodendroglia

Changes of the myelin sheaths are the most conspicuous effect of pathology of the oligodendroglia. This is easily understood, when one realizes that a single oligodendroglia forms numerous myelin segments. Changes of myelin will be discussed later. In the present section, we shall confine our discussion to changes in the oligodendroglial cell body.

Surprisingly, very little information is available concerning the pathology of the

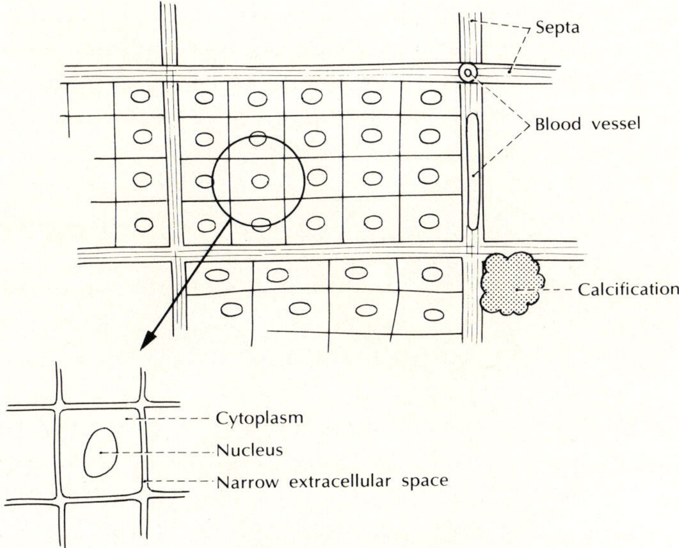

Fig. 219 Oligodendroglioma.

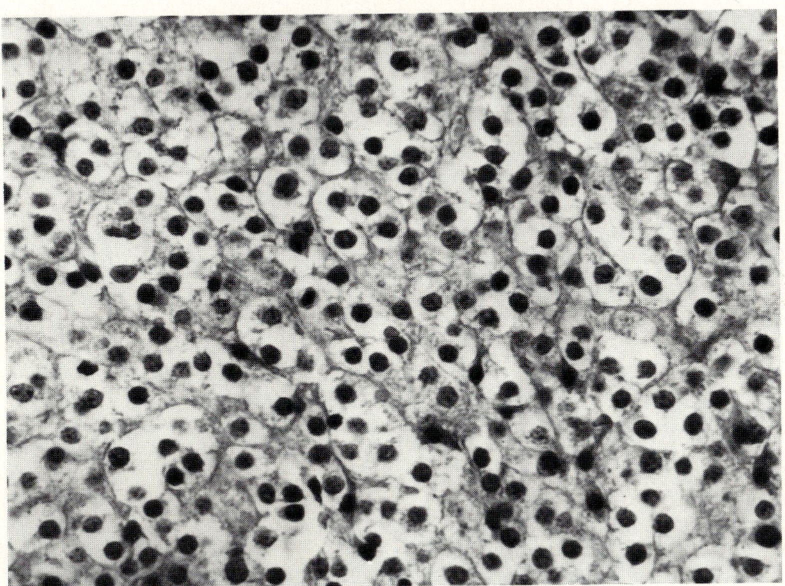

Fig. 220 Oligodendroglioma (H & E stain).

oligodendroglial soma. Artifactitious changes, due to poor preservation, are well known, resulting in the "*fried egg*" appearance described above. However, in certain instances the "*fried-egg*" appearance may be due to true pathological alteration namely anoxic changes following circulatory disturbances.

Grape-like vacuoles filled with endocytosed material can occur following experimental implantation of certain foreign material (Hirano et al., 1965). This phenomenon may correspond to the so-called "*mucoid degeneration*" of oligodendroglial cells described in traditional texts of neuropathology.

In cases of human metachromatic leucodystrophy the oligodendroglial cell body accumulates lipid-containing inclusions with characteristic structures. *Lipid inclusions* may also be found in some of the lipidoses or other leucodystrophies.

Recently, a number of reports have been published describing the effects of various experimental conditions on oligodendroglia (Suzuki and De Paul, 1971; Blakemore, 1972; Suzuki and Zagoren, 1973 and 1974; Meier and Bischoff, 1974; Ludwin, 1978; Yajima and Suzuki, 1979). These effects include dysmyelination often accompanied by the formation of various membranous inclusions within the oligodendroglial cytoplasm.

Viral particles have been observed in oligodendroglial nuclei in subacute sclerosing panencephalitis (Tellez-Nagel and Harter, 1966; Severs and Zeman, 1968; Oyanagi et al., 1971), and in progressive multifocal leucoencephalopathy (Zu Rhein and Chou, 1968; Weiner et al., 1973).

Oligodendrogliomas are tumors of the white matter, especially the cerebrum, in which the tumor cells are compartmentalized and divided by blood vessels and astrocytes. They frequently show calcification and the individual cells usually display a characteristic "fried-egg" appearance (Figs. 219, 220). Processes of tumor cells are poorly developed, but they may appear as a group between cell bodies (Plate 22, in Poon et al., 1971). Cross sections of cell processes are small and round. Intimate contacts with neurons, especially axons, are lacking and there is no myelin formation. In some cases, the tumor cells may contain limited numbers of eosinophilic lipid-like inclusions (Takei et al., 1976), which conceivably may represent abortive attempts of myelin formation and subsequent autophagia.

REFERENCES

Hirano, A., Zimmerman, H.M., & Levine, S.: Fine structure of cerebral fluid accumulation. VI. Intracellular accumulation of fluid and cryptococcal polysaccharide in oligodendroglia. Arch. Neurol., 12: 189-196, 1965.

Tellez-Nagel, I., & Harter, D.H.: Subacute sclerosing leukoencephalitis. I. Clinicopathological, electron microscopic and virological observations. J. Neuropathol. Exp. Neurol., 25: 560-581, 1966.

Severs, J.L., & Zeman. W. (eds.): Measles virus and subacute sclerosing panencephalitis. Neurology, Vol. 18, No. 1, Part 2, 1968.

ZuRhein, G.M., & Chou, S.M.: Papova virus in progressive multifocal leukoencephalopathy. *In* Infections of the Nervous System. ARNMD, Vol. 44, pp. 307-362. Zimmerman, H.M. (ed.), Williams & Wilkins, Baltimore, 1968.

Hirano, A., Sax, D.S., & Zimmerman, H.M.: The fine structure of the cerebella of Jimpy mice and their "normal" litter mates. J. Neuropathol. Exp. Neurol., 28: 388-400, 1969.

Poon, T.P., Hirano, A., & Zimmerman, H.M.: Electron Microscopic Atlas of Brain Tumors, pp. 44-49, Grune and Stratton, New York, 1971.

Suzuki, K., & DePaul, L.: Cellular degeneration in developing central nervous system of rats produced by hypocholesteremic drug AY 9944. Lab. Invest., 25: 546-555, 1971.

Oyanagi, S., Rorke, L.B., Katz, M., & Koprowski, H: Histopathology and electron microscopy of three cases of subacute sclerosing panencephalitis (SSPE). Acta Neuropathol., 18: 58-73, 1971.

Blakemore, W.F.: Observations on oligodendrocyte degeneration, the resolution of status spongiosus and remyelination in cuprizone intoxication in mice. J. Neurocytol., 1: 413-426, 1972.

Weiner, L.P., Johnson, R.T., & Herndon, R.M.: Viral infections and demyelinating diseases. New Eng. J. Med., 288: 1103-1110, 1973.

Suzuki, K., & Zagoren, J.C.: Effect of the hypocholesterolemic drug AY 9944 on developing central nervous system of rats: Alteration of endoplasmic reticulum in oligodendroglia. J. Neurocytol., 2: 369-381, 1973.

Suzuki, K., & Zagoren, J.C.: Degeneration of oligodendroglia in the central nervous system of rats treated with AY 9944 or triparanol. Lab. Invest., 31: 503-515, 1974.

Meier, C., & Bischoff, A.: Dysmyelination in "jimpy" mouse. Electron microscopic study. J. Neuropathol. Exp. Neurol., 33: 343-353, 1974.

Takei, Y., Mirra, S.S., & Miles, M.L.: Eosinophilic granular cells in oligodendrogliomas. Cancer, 38: 1968-1976, 1976.

Ludwin, S.K.: Central nervous system demyelination and remyelination in the mouse. An ultrastructural study of cuprizone toxicity. Lab. Invest., 39: 597-612, 1978.

Yajima, K., & Suzuki, K.: Oligodendroglia and myelin sheath changes following ethidium bromide injection. Neuropathol. Appl. Neurobiol., 5: 49-62, 1979.

D. MYELIN (Figs. 221-224)

At least two elements are required for the formation of the myelin sheath; the axon and the myelin forming cell. In the central nervous system, myelin is formed by the oligodendroglial cell while the Schwann cell serves this function in the peripheral nervous system. Despite fundamental similarities between the myelin sheaths of the central and peripheral nervous systems, certain differences exist. They will, therefore, be considered separately below.

REFERENCES

Morell, P. (ed.): Myelin. Plenum Press, New York, 1977.
Waxman, S.. (ed.): Physiology and Pathobiology of Axons. Raven Press, New York, 1978.

1. Normal Central Myelin

The myelin sheath consists of myelin segments arranged like beads on a string along the axon. Each segment is the product of a single oligodendroglial process which makes contact with the axon, and proceeds to wind around it in a spiral fashion (Fig. 221).

The anatomy of the sheath may, perhaps, best be understood by considering the effect of hypothetically unrolling a sheath from around the axon (Fig. 222). As can be seen, the myelin is a sheet-like membrane of compacted oligodendroglial plasma membrane surrounded by a continuous rim of glial cytoplasm.

In cross sections of the mature myelinated fiber the axon, at least 0.2 microns in diameter, is at the center and is separated from the myelin by a narrow *periaxonal space* (Fig. 221). The myelin itself is formed by a single spirally arranged membrane giving rise to a lamellated appearance with a periodicity of approximately 120Å. The innermost end of the myelin widens to form the *inner loop*, a tongue of oligodendroglial cytoplasm containing no organelles except for microtubules, occasional small vesicles and some glial filaments. There is a tight junction between the inner loop and the innermost lamella of myelin where some cytoplasm often remains.

It is the oligodendroglial plasma membrane which forms the myelin. The inner leaflets of the inner loop fuse and form the so-called "*major dense line*" of the myelin sheath which spirals around the axon dividing once again at the outer surface of the sheath to give rise to the inner leaflets of the *outer loop*. The latter is another tongue of oligodendroglial cytoplasm almost identical to the inner loop. The outer loop, too, is connected to the adjacent myelin lamella by means of a tight junction and a cytoplasmic area within the myelin may be present at that site as well. The outer leaflets of the succeeding lamellae of the myelin sheath are in close apposition virtually obliterating the extracellular space between the lamellae and forming the so-called "*intraperiod*" or "*minor dense line*".

When viewed in longitudinal section the segments are separated from one

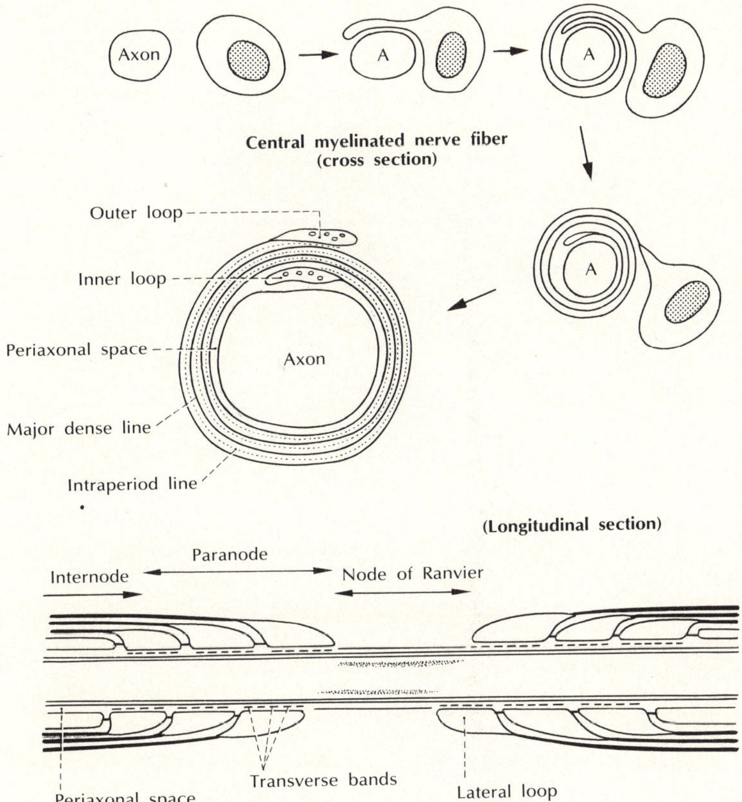

Fig. 221 Myelin formation.

another by the node of Ranvier where the axon surface is directly exposed to the extracellular space for a considerable distance (Fig. 221). The axoplasm subjacent to the exposed axolemma at the node of Ranvier contains the so-called "undercoating material" described previously. The most striking feature of the longitudinally sectioned myelin sheath is the parallel arrangement of the myelin lamellae on either side of the axon. Each lamella ends in another cytoplasmic tongue, the "*lateral loop*". The region of lateral loops is known as the *paranode* while the rest of the sheath is the *internode*. Each loop contacts the axon and a highly specialized junction is present at the interface. In well sectioned tissue, *transverse bands*, seen as regularly arranged separate densities, 150Å long, are present between the axolemma and the lateral loop (Figs. 221, 222, 224). Adjacent lateral loops are connected by tight junctions, but the spaces between the tight junction and the axolemma and between the transverse bands provide a means of limited access between the parenchymal extracellular spaces and the periaxonal space. The changes of the transverse bands in pathology have not been thoroughly investigated. It is known that they are either not present or only partially developed in the young animal and it may be that subtle changes involving the transverse bands are significant with regard to the function of the entire segment.

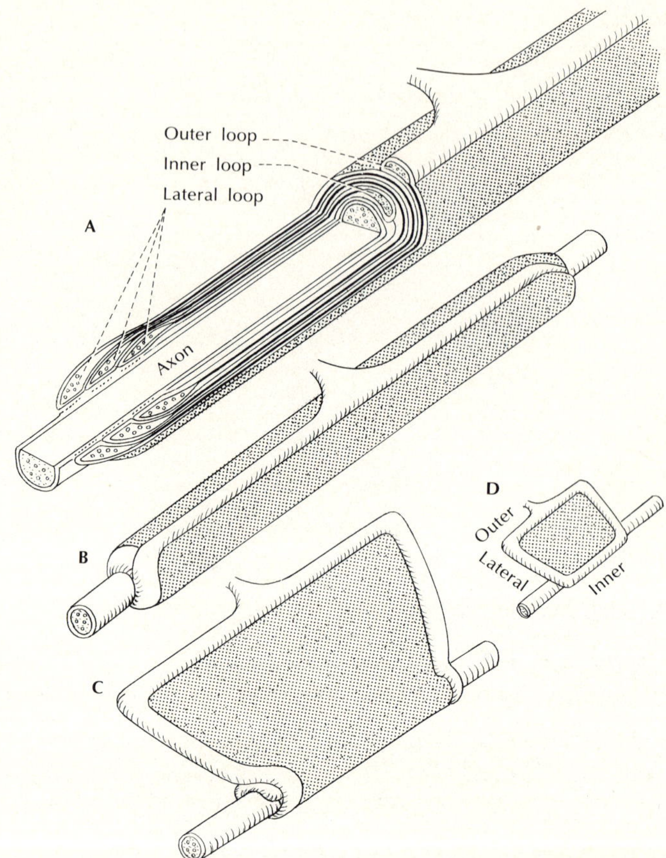

Fig. 222 Diagram of a myelinated axon and its relationship to the cytoplasmic regions of the hypothetically unrolled sheath.
A. Diagram of myelinated axon, modified after Bunge et al. (J. Biophys. Biochem. Cytol. 10: 67, 1961). Part of the myelin is cut away to show the relationship between the lateral loops and the lamellae as well as between the inner loops and the axon and between the outer loop and the connection to the myelin-forming cell. Note the periodic densities, representing sections through the transverse bands between the lateral loops and the axon.
B. Diagram of the intact myelin sheath around an axon.
C. Diagram of the results of partially unrolling the intact sheath from around the axon.
D. Diagram of a fully unrolled myelin sheath. The resulting shovel-shaped myelin sheet is bordered on four sides by a continuous thickened rim of cytoplasm. The outer rim, when seen in section, is represented by the outer loop, and is longer than the inner rim which is represented by the inner loop in cross section. The lateral rims are probably of equal length and are represented by the lateral loops in longitudinal sections through the nodes of Ranvier.
(From Hirano, A., & Dembitzer, H.M.: J. Cell. Biol., 34: 555, 1967.)

REFERENCES

Hirano, A., Zimmerman, H.M., & Levine, S.: Myelin in the central nervous system as observed in experimentally induced edema in the rat. J. Cell Biol., 30: 397-411, 1966.

Hirano, A., & Dembitzer, H.M.: A structural analysis of the myelin sheath in the central nervous system. J. Cell Biol., 34: 555-567, 1967.

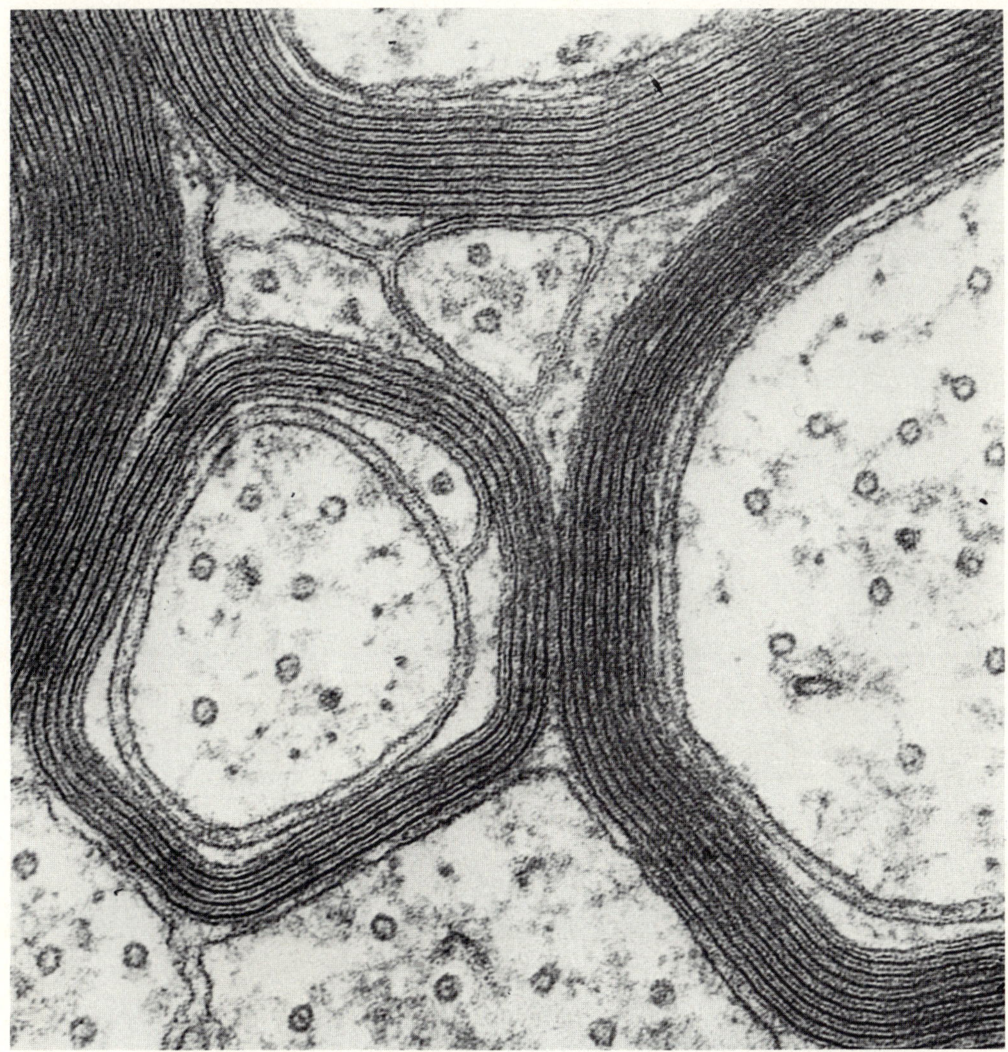

Fig. 223 Cross section of central myelinated nerve fibers. × 150,000.

Bunge, R.P.: Glial cells and the central myelin sheath. Physiol. Rev., 48: 197-251, 1968.

Hirano, A., Becker, N.H., & Zimmerman, H.M.: Isolation of the periaxonal space of the central myelinated nerve fiber with regard to the diffusion of peroxidase. J. Histochem. Cytochem., 17: 512-516, 1969.

Hirano, A., & Dembitzer, H.M.: The transverse bands as a means of access to the periaxonal space of the central myelinated nerve fiber. J. Ultrastruct. Res., 28: 141-149, 1969.

Peters, A., & Vaughn, J.E.: Morphology and development of the myelin sheath. *In* Myelination, pp. 3-79. Davison, A.N., & Peters, A. (eds.), Charles C Thomas, Springfield, Ill., 1970.

Bunge, R.P.: Structure and function of neuroglia: Some recent observations. *In* the Neurosciences Second Study Program, pp. 782-797. Schmitt, F.O. (ed.), Rockefeller University Press, New York, 1970.

Rosenbluth, J.: Intramembranous particle distribution at the node of Ranvier and adjacent axolemma in myelinated axons of the frog brain. J. Neurocytol., 5: 731-745, 1976.

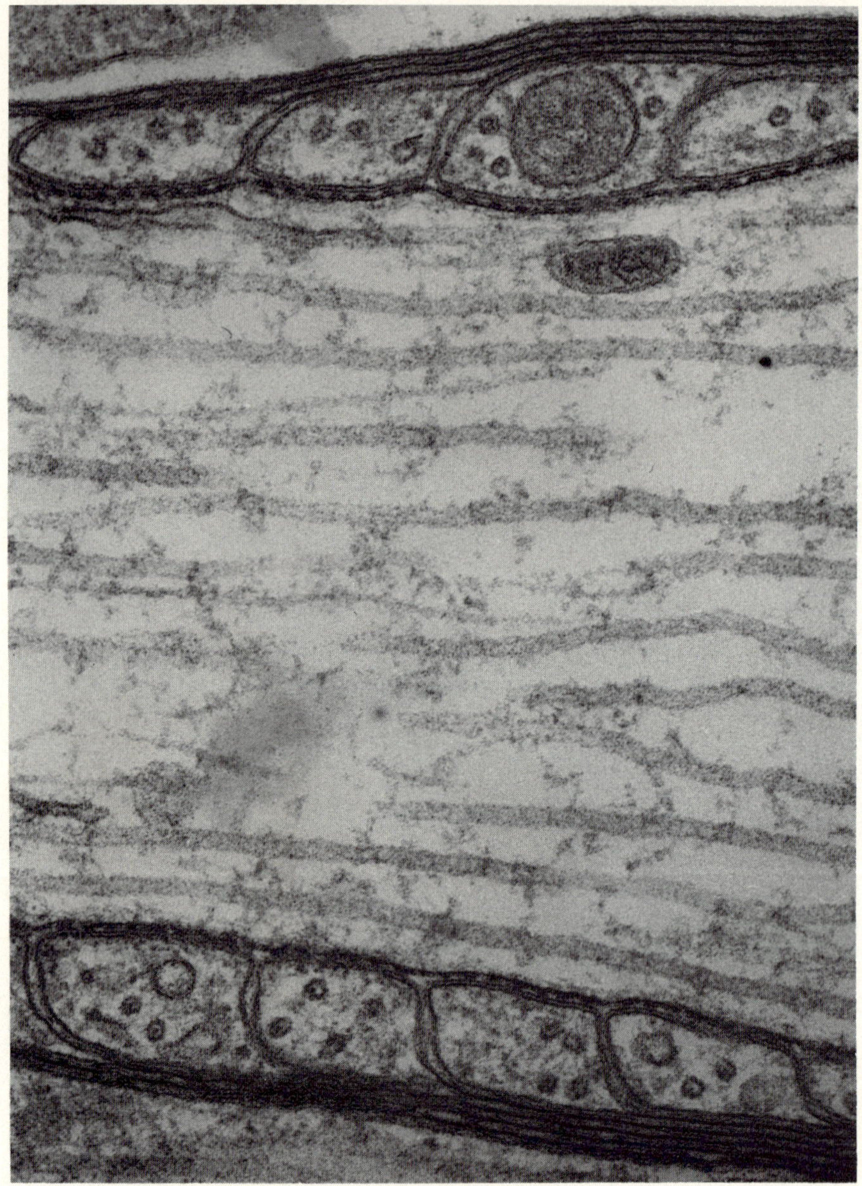

Fig. 224 Longitudinal section of the paranode of a central myelinated nerve fiber. × 110,000. (From Hirano, A., & Dembitzer, H.M.: J. Cell Biol., 35: 34, 1967.)

Hirano, A., & Dembitzer, H.M.: Fine structure of normal myelin. *In* International Encyclopedia of Neurol., Psychiatry, Psychoanalysis and Psychol., Vol 7, pp. 413-416, Wolman, B.B., (ed.), Van Nostrand, Reinhold, New York, 1977.

Raine, C.S.: Morphological aspects of myelin and myelination. *In* Myelin, pp. 1-49. Morell, P., (ed.), Plenum, New York, 1977.

Hirano, A., & Dembitzer, H. M.: Morphology of normal myelinated axon. *In* Physiology and Pathology of Axons, pp. 65-82. Waxman, S.G., (ed.), Raven Press, New York, 1978.

Sternberger, N.H., Itoyama, Y., Kies, M.W., & Webster, H. de F.: Immunocytochemical method to identify basic protein in myelin-forming oligodendrocytes of newborn rat C.N.S. J. Neurocytol., 7: 251-263, 1978.

2. Normal Peripheral Myelin (Fig. 225)

The myelin of the entire peripheral nervous system is composed of peripheral type myelin. Short segments of the roots, however, contain central type sheaths for variable distances from the neuroaxis. These include all the spinal roots as well as the roots of the third to twelfth cranial nerves. The lengths of these central type sheaths vary among the roots but, in general, those of the sensory roots are longer than the motor roots and the eighth nerve is longest of all (Tarlov, 1937).

Fundamentally, the architecture of the peripheral myelin sheath is the same as that of the central sheath. Indeed, the fine structure of the myelin sheath was first elucidated in peripheral nerve by Robertson (1955) and by Webster (1960, 1971) among others. Furthermore, the wrapping process of the myelin-forming cell around the axon was first described in peripheral nerve by Geren (1954). There are, however, several important differences between the central and peripheral myelin sheaths.

Most important is the fact that the peripheral sheath is formed by the Schwann cell rather than the oligodendroglial cell. Furthermore, each Schwann cell gives rise to only a single myelin internode so that both the Schwann cell body and an external collar of cytoplasm can often be found surrounding the myelin sheath (Fig. 225). The exterior of the Schwann cell cytoplasm is, itself, surrounded by a basal lamina. Longitudinal sections of the peripheral sheath reveal the presence of isolated islands of cytoplasm within the lamellae. These islands are in register with those of adjacent lamellae and form the Schmidt-Lanterman clefts. Unlike the central nervous system, the axolemma is not exposed at the nodes. Instead the collar of adjacent internodes covers the axon at these points.

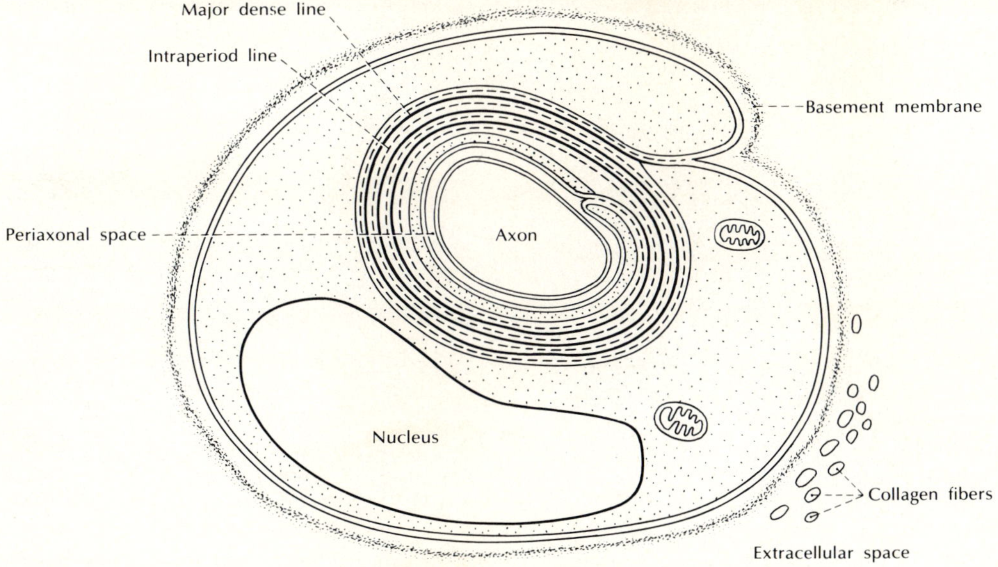

Fig. 225 A diagram of a peripheral myelinated nerve fiber.

A single basal lamina is continuous over the nodes. The periodicity of the individual lamellae of the peripheral sheath is approximately 10% wider than that of the central sheath.

The peripheral sheaths are generally much thicker than those of the central nervous system. This can be clearly seen in longitudinal sections through the exit

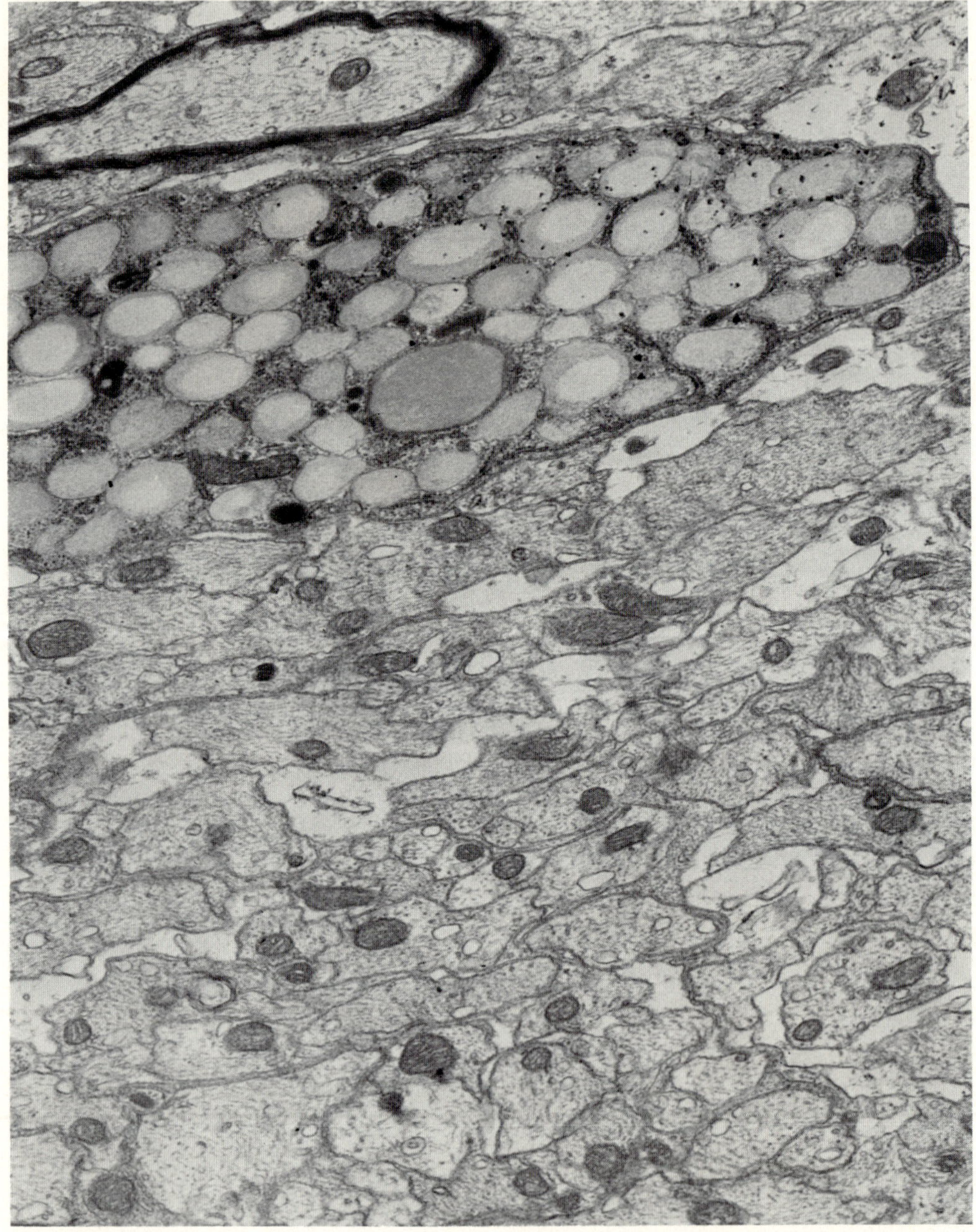

Fig. 226 White matter of the cerebellum of a jimpy mouse. A single myelinated axon is apparent adjacent to a macrophage filled with lipid granules. × 17,000. (From Hirano, A. et al.: J. Neuropathol. Exp. Neurol., 28: 388, 1969.)

zone of a root where the same axon may be covered by relatively thin sheaths within the central nervous system and by much thicker ones when it enters the peripheral nervous system.

The relationship between the Schwann cell and the axon is currently the subject of intense investigation. Noteworthy among these investigators are Aguayo and his associates who use the ingenious technique of transplantation of peripheral nerve derived from different sources (Aguayo 1976).

Peripheral nerves also differ from the white matter of the central nervous system by the presence of ample extracellular space, which usually contains collagen fibers, fibroblasts and small blood vessels. These capillaries show permeability characteristics similar to those of the central nervous system and impede the passage of large molecules. However, more recent studies indicate partial permeability of tracers across endoneurial vessel walls (Olsson and Kristenson, 1979). The individual fibers are grouped together into fascicles which are surrounded by a perineurium consisting of a number of thin layers of perineurial cells. Collagen fibers are interspersed in the intervening extracellular spaces. The perineurial cells are joined by various intercellular junctions including desmosomes and tight junctions. The latter prevent macromolecular tracer introduced into the surrounding tissue from gaining access to the myelinated fibers. The entire peripheral nerve is surrounded by a thick, collagenous epineurium.

The staining characteristics of peripheral sheaths differ from those of the central nervous system. After luxol fast blue-periodic acid-Schiff (LFB-PAS) staining of paraffin sections, the peripheral myelin appears purple rather than blue as in the central nervous system. This is due to the added red color provided by the PAS-positive peripheral myelin (Feigin & Cravioto, 1961). Woelcke staining is inconsistent for peripheral myelin whereas central myelin is always stained black by this method.

The reaction of peripheral sheaths to pathological processes or to genetic defects often varies from that of the central nervous system. Multiple sclerosis, for example, affects only central white matter with the only detectable changes in peripheral nerves being secondary complications and not the characteristic demyelinating plaques of the central nervous system. Certain genetic defects in mice known as "jimpy" and "quaking" affect the two systems differently. In jimpy, central myelin is virtually absent (Fig. 226) whereas the myelin of the peripheral nervous system is well-formed (p. 77). In the quaking mouse both types of sheaths are affected but the degree is many orders of magnitude greater in the central nervous system. In the "dystrophic" mouse, peripheral myelin is absent only in certain areas of spinal roots (Bradley & Jenkison, 1973).

REFERENCES

Tarlov, M.: Structure of the nerve root. II. Differentiation of sensory from motor roots; observations on identification of function in roots of mixed cranial nerves. Arch. Neurol. Psychiat., 37: 1338-1355, 1937.

Geren, B.B.: The formation from the Schwann cell surface of myelin in the peripheral nerves of chick embryos. Exptl. Cell Res., 7: 558-562, 1954.

Robertson, J.D.: The ultrastructure of adult vertebrate peripheral myelinated nerve fibers in relation to myelinogenesis. J. Biophys. Biochem. Cytol., 1: 271-278, 1955.

Webster, H. de F., & Spiro, D.: Phase and electron microscopic studies of experimental demyelination. I. Variations in myelin sheath contour in normal guinea pig sciatic nerve. J. Neuropathol Exp. Neurol., 19: 42-69, 1960.
Feigin, I., & Cravioto, H.: A histochemical study of myelin. A difference in the solubility of the glycolipid components in the central and peripheral nervous systems. J. Neuropathol. Exp. Neurol., 20: 245-254, 1961.
Hirano, A., Zimmerman, H.M., & Levine, S.: Electron microscopic observations of peripheral myelin in a central nervous system lesion. Acta Neuropathol., 13: 348-365, 1969.
Webster, H. de F.: The geometry of peripheral myelin sheaths during their formation and growth in rat sciatic nerves. J. Cell. Biol., 48: 348-367, 1971.
Ghatak, N.R., Hirano, A., Doron, Y., & Zimmerman, H.M.: Remyelination in multiple sclerosis with peripheral type myelin. Arch. Neurol., 29: 262-267, 1973.
Bradley, W.G., & Jenkison, M.: Abnormalities of peripheral nerves in murine muscular dystrophy. J. Neurol. Sci., 18: 227-247, 1973.
Aguayo, A.J., Epps, J., Charron, L., & Bray, G.M.: Multi-potentiality of Schwann cells in cross-anastomosed and grafted myelinated and unmyelinated nerves: Quantitative microscopy and radioautography. Brain Res., 104: 1-20, 1976.
Suzuki, K., & Zagoren, J.: Quaking mouse. An ultrastructural study of the peripheral nerves. J. Neurocytol., 6: 71-89, 1977.
Olsson, Y., & Kristensson, K.: Recent applications of tracer techniques to neuropathology, with particular reference to vascular permeability and axonal flow. *In* Recent Advances in Neuropathology, pp. 1-25, Smith, W.T., & Cavanagh, J.B. (eds.), Churchill Livingstone, Edinburgh, 1979.

3. Alteration of the Myelin Sheath

Myelin damage may be the result of either axonal pathology as in Wallerian degeneration, or it may be caused by changes of the myelin or the myelin-forming cell with apparent preservation of the axon such as in multiple sclerosis. According to convention, the term demyelination is reserved for those conditions in which the axon is spared.

DEMYELINATION

Theoretically, demyelination may be the result of damage to:
1) the soma of the myelin-forming cell
2) the myelin lamellae themselves, or
3) the inner loop.

REFERENCES

Lampert, P.W.: Fine structural changes of myelin sheaths in the central nervous system. *In* The Structure and Function of Nervous Tissue. Vol. 1, pp. 187-204. Bourne, G.H. (ed.), Academic Press, New York, 1968.
Hirano, A.: The pathology of the central myelinated axon. *In* The Structure and Function of Nervous Tissue. Vol 5, pp. 73-162, Bourne, G.H. (ed.), Academic Press, New York, 1972.
Hirano, A., & Llena, J.F.: Fine structural alterations of central myelin. *In* International Encyclopedia of Neurology, Psychiatry, Psychoanalysis and Psychology, Vol. 7, pp. 411-413, Wolman, B.B. (ed.), Van Nostrand, Reinhold, New York, 1977.
Lampert, P.W.: Oligodendroglia and myelin. J. Neuropathol. Exp. Neurol., 579, 1978 (abstract).

Pathology of Soma of Oligodendroglia

Destruction of an oligodendroglial cell body can be expected to result in the loss of all the processes of that cell including myelin sheaths formed by them. The cell body can be destroyed by a variety of insults including infarct, trauma, etc. Examples of the selective involvement of oligodendroglia are certain viral infections leading to subsequent demyelination as described by Lampert et al., (1973). Papova viruses have been observed in glial nuclei of patients with progressive multifocal leukoencephalopathy (Zu Rhein and Chou, 1968).

Genetic defects of the oligodendroglial cells may also lead to abnormal myelin formation. As described previously (p. 77) such lesions have been observed in "jimpy" mouse and in various leukodystrophies in the human and in experimental animals.

The Schwann cell body, too, may be affected. Demyelination due to diphtheria toxin is probably due to inhibition of the synthesis of myelin proteins by the Schwann cells (Pleasure et al., 1973). In tellurium intoxication of the young animal, Lampert (1971) reported that the Schwann cell becomes necrotic and demyelination follows. In leprosy, where peripheral neuropathy is prominent, Hansen's bacilli may be found in the Schwann cell. In metachromatic leukodystrophy, lipid inclusions are seen in the cytoplasm of the Schwann cell.

REFERENCES

Zu Rhein, G.M., & Chou, S.-M.: Papova virus in progressive multifocal leukoencephalopathy. *In* Infections of the Nervous System: Res. Publ. ass. nerv. ment. Dis., XLIV, pp. 307-362. Zimmerman, H.M. (ed.), Williams and Wilkins, Baltimore, 1968.

Pleasure, D.E., Feldman, B., & Prockop, D.J.: Diphtheria toxin inhibits the synthesis of myelin proteolipid and basic proteins by peripheral nerve in vitro. J. Neurochem., 20: 81-90, 1973.

Lampert, P.W., Sims, J.K., & Kniazeff, A.J.: Mechanism of demyelination in JHM virus encephalomyelitis. Electron microscopic studies. Acta Neuropathol., 24: 76-85, 1973.

Powell, H.C. & Lampert, P.W.: Oligodendrocytes and their myelin-plasma membrane connections in JHM mouse hepatitis virus encephalomyelitis. Lab. Invest., 33: 440-445, 1975.

Pathology of Myelin

In some forms of demyelination the myelin lamellae, themselves, are altered with no initial discernible changes in the oligodendroglial cell body. Later changes of the soma are interpreted as reactions to the more distal changes.

Intralamellar Split (Figs. 227, 228)

The intralamellar split of the myelin sheaths leading to the formation of large or small vacuole-like spaces in the white matter is one of the most common alterations of central and peripheral myelin. When extreme enough, these changes are apparent in the optical microscope as spongiform alterations of the white matter. They are seen in a variety of human diseases such as Canavan's disease (p. 76) where they are associated with other changes, in triethyltin intoxication and in hexachlorophene intoxication. They can be induced experimentally in almost pure form by various intoxications especially triethyltin, and isonicotinic acid hydrazide (INH) where they are found in the central nervous system only and by hexachlo-

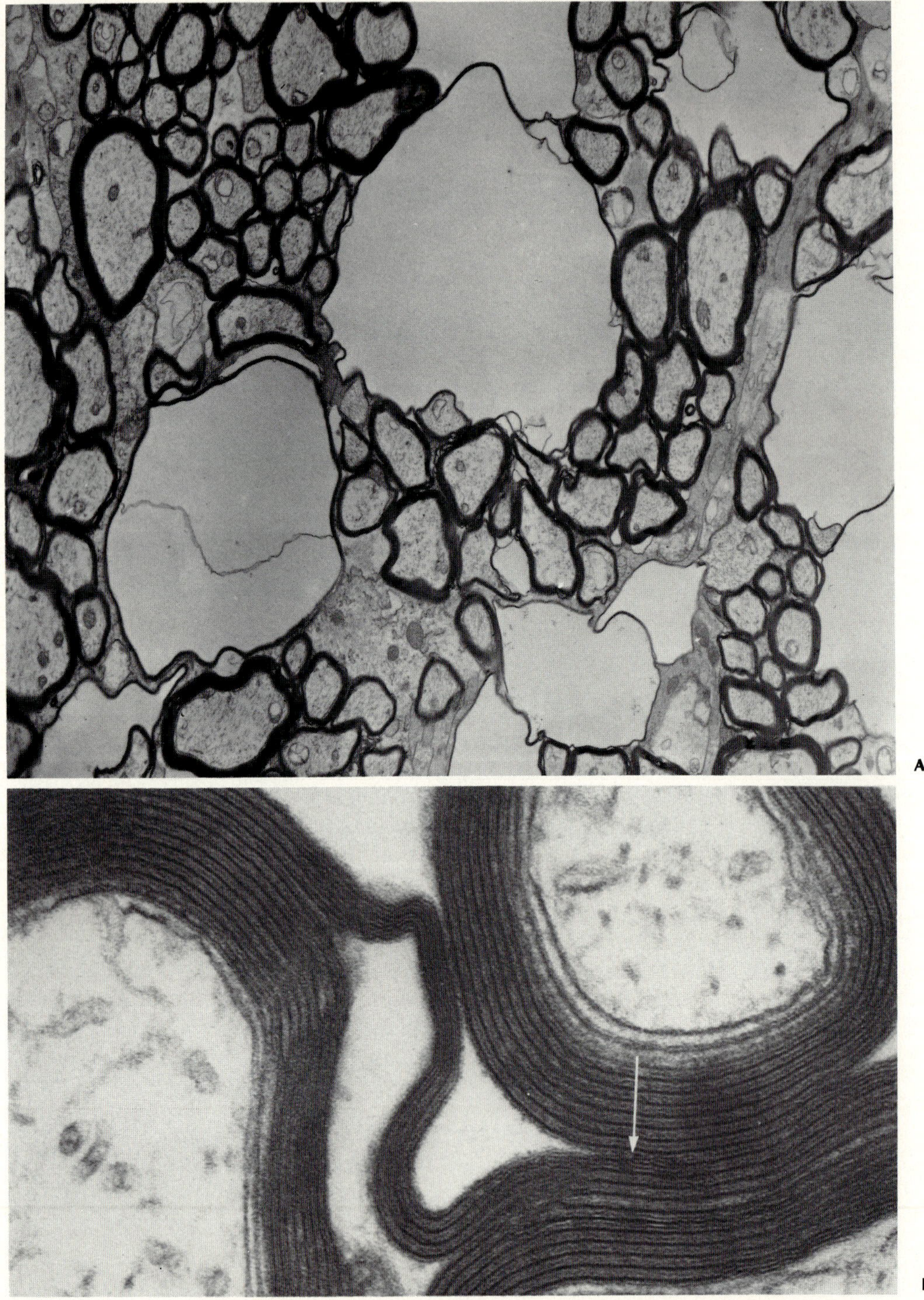

Fig. 227 Alterations of central myelin due to triethyltin intoxication. A. Vacuolar space in the white matter. × 6,000. B. Spaces are formed by a split of the intraperiod line (arrow). × 140,000. (From Hirano, A.: The Structure and Function of Nervous Tissue. Vol. 2, p. 69, Academic Press, 1969.)

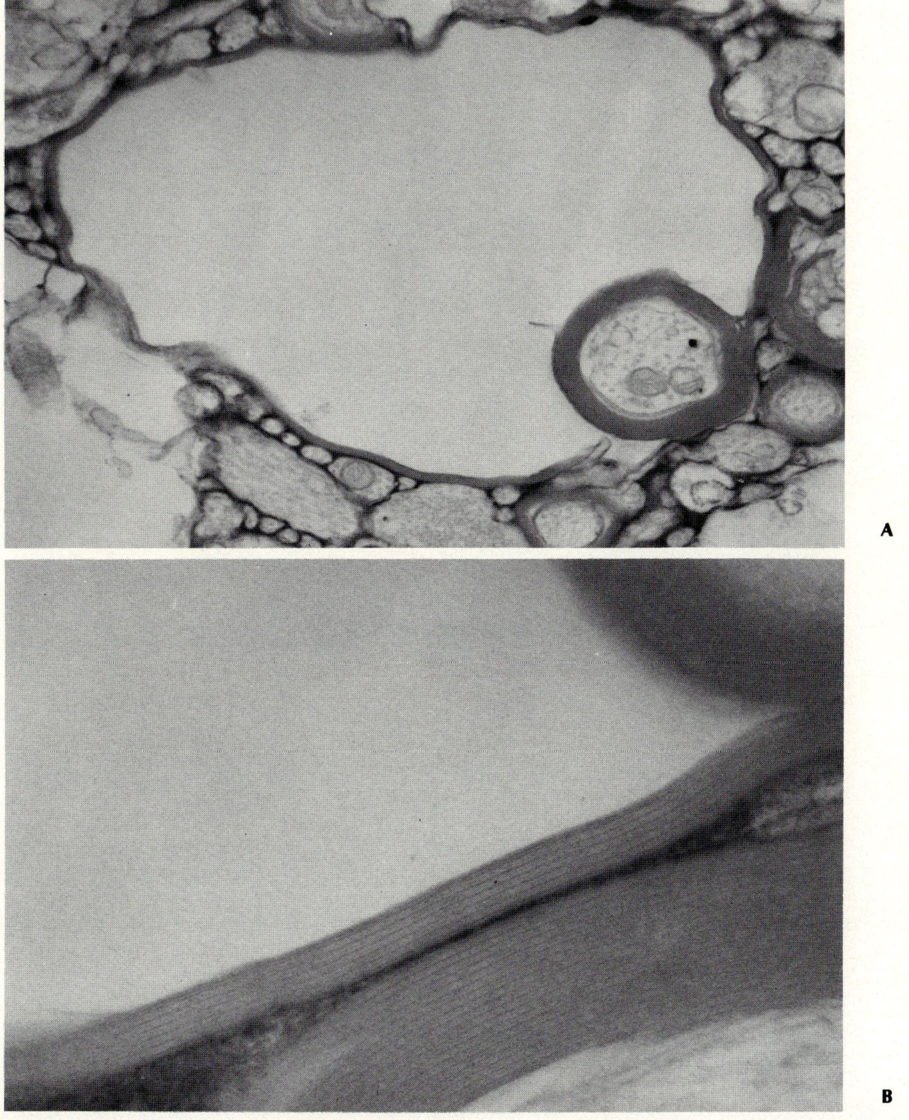

Fig. 228 Intramyelinic space is free of peroxidase. A. × 25,000. B. × 100,000. (From Hirano, A. et al.: J. Neuropathol. Exp. Neurol., 28: 507, 1969.)

rophene intoxication in the developing animal which affects peripheral myelin as well (Towfighi & Gonatas, 1973).

The fine structure of the lesion consists of both wide and narrow enlargements of the intralamellar space originating at a split in the intraperiod line. Theoretically this space is continuous with the extracellular space but the vacuoles are uniformly empty and devoid of interior structures. Electron-dense tracer introduced into the extra-cellular spaces do not, in general, penetrate into the vacuole (Fig. 228). Apparently the tight junctions at the periphery of the myelin sheet remain functional. Furthermore, tight junctions are apparently present at the edge of the split itself (Tabira et al., 1978). According to the chemists, the vacuolar spaces are associated with increased water and salt content in the white matter. The mechanism for the formation of the enlargements is unknown but it is assumed that the lamellae are able to slip past one another similar to the way in which a clock mainspring unwinds. It should be pointed out that other features such as the blood-brain barrier and the dimensions of the individual lamellae remain normal.

REFERENCES

Aleu, F.P., Katzman, R., & Terry, R.D.: Fine structure and electrolyte analysis of cerebral edema induced by alkyltin intoxication. J. Neuropathol. Exp. Neurol., 22: 403-413, 1963.

Hirano, A., Zimmerman, H.M., & Levine, S.: Intramyelinic and extracellular spaces in triethyltin intoxication. J. Neuropathol. Exp. Neurol., 27: 571-580, 1968.

Hirano, A., Dembitzer, H.M., Becker, N.H., & Zimmerman, H.M.: The distribution of peroxidase in the triethyltin intoxicated rat brain. J. Neuropathol. Exp. Neurol., 28: 507-511, 1969.

Towfighi, J., Gonatas, N.K., & McCree, L.: Hexachlorophene neuropathy in rats. Lab. Invest., 29: 428-436, 1973.

Tabira, T., Cullen, M.J., Reier, P.I., & Webster, H. de F.: An experimental analysis of interlamelar tight junctions in amphiibian and mammalian C.N.S. myelin. J. Neurocytol., 7: 489-503, 1978.

Regular Separation of the Intraperiod Line (Figs. 229-231)

This alteration has been seen in certain autoimmune diseases affecting either central (Lampert, 1965, 1967) (Fig. 229) or peripheral myelin (Hirano et al., 1971;

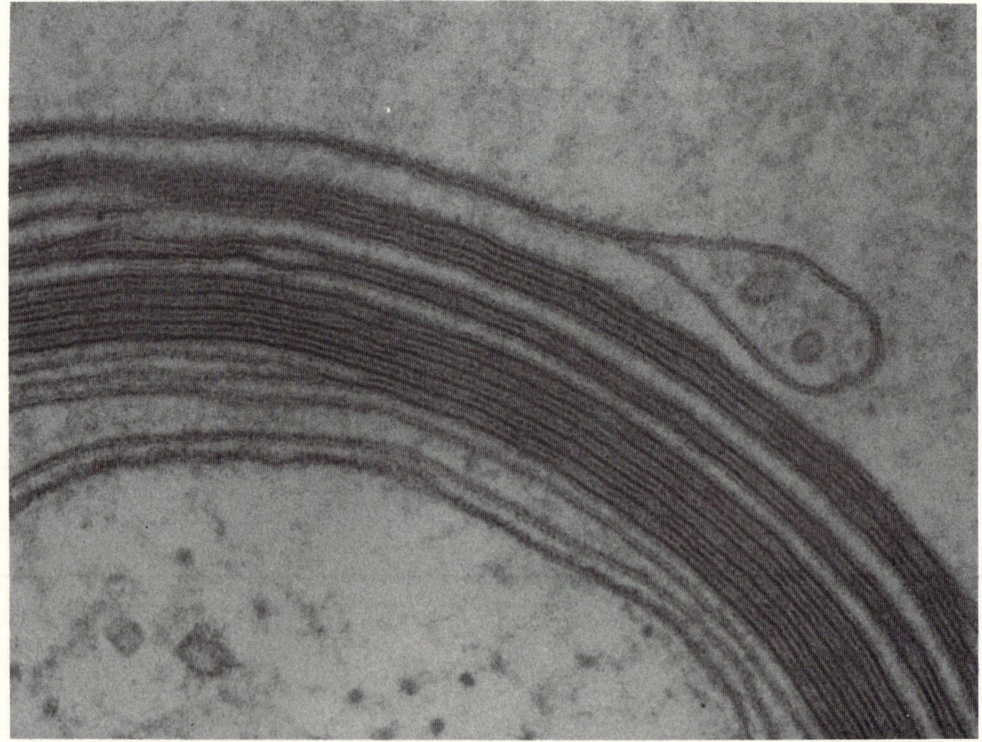

Fig. 229 Separation of the outer loop in a central myelin sheath. × 160,000. (From Hirano, A.: The Structure and Function of Nervous Tissue. Vol. 2, p. 69, Academic Press, 1969.)

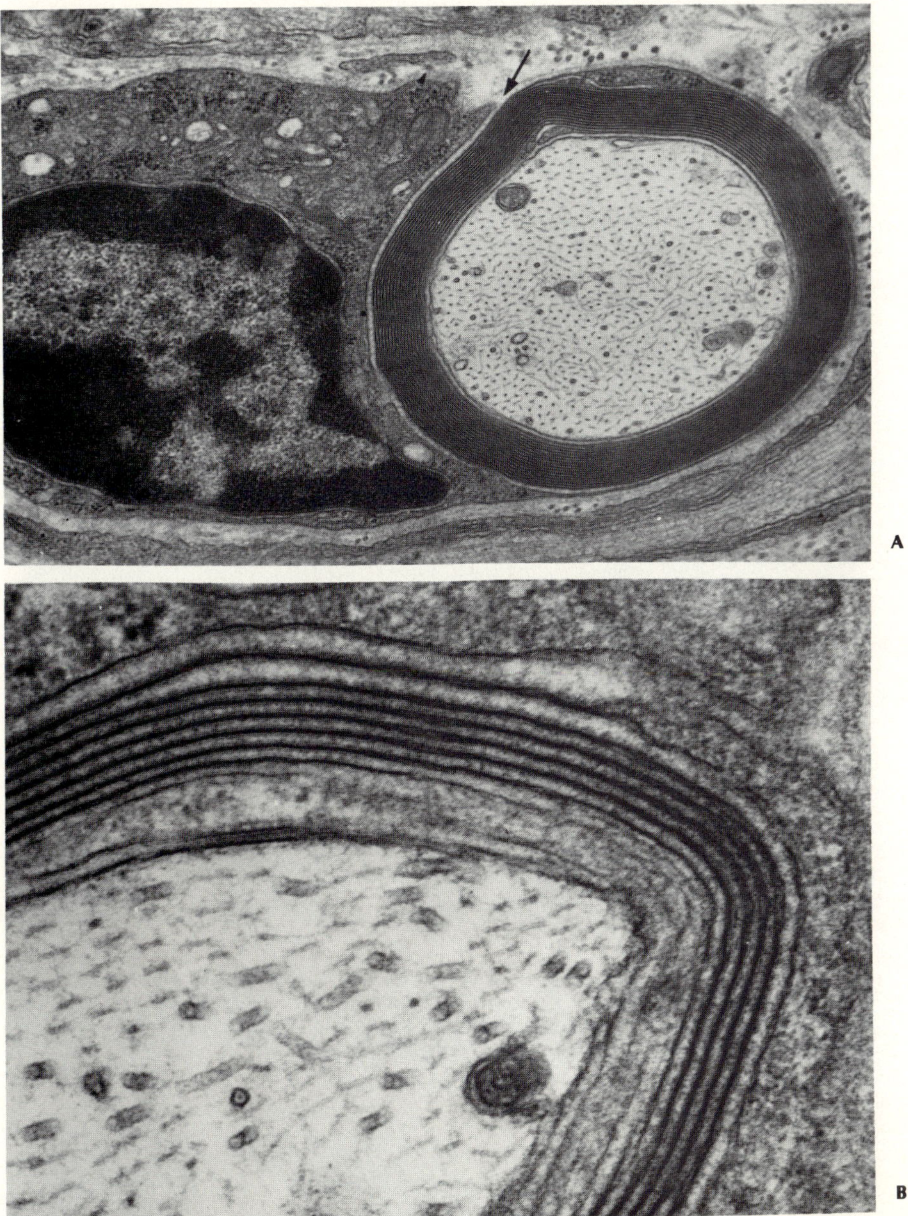

Fig. 230 Regular separation of the intraperiod line. A. A regular narrow space is evident between the Schwann cell and the outermost lamella of the myelin. × 24,000. B. Regular separation of the intraperiod line extending from the extracellular space to the periaxonal space. × 96,000 (From Hirano, A. et al.: J. Neuropathol. Exp. Neurol., 30: 249, 1971.)

Koeppen et al., 1971; Dropp, et al., 1975) (Fig. 230, 231). As in the intralamellar split described above, the essential change is an opening of the intraperiod line. In this case, however, the separation is continuous with the extracellular space so that extracellular fluid permeates the sheaths, usually, in a regular fashion between

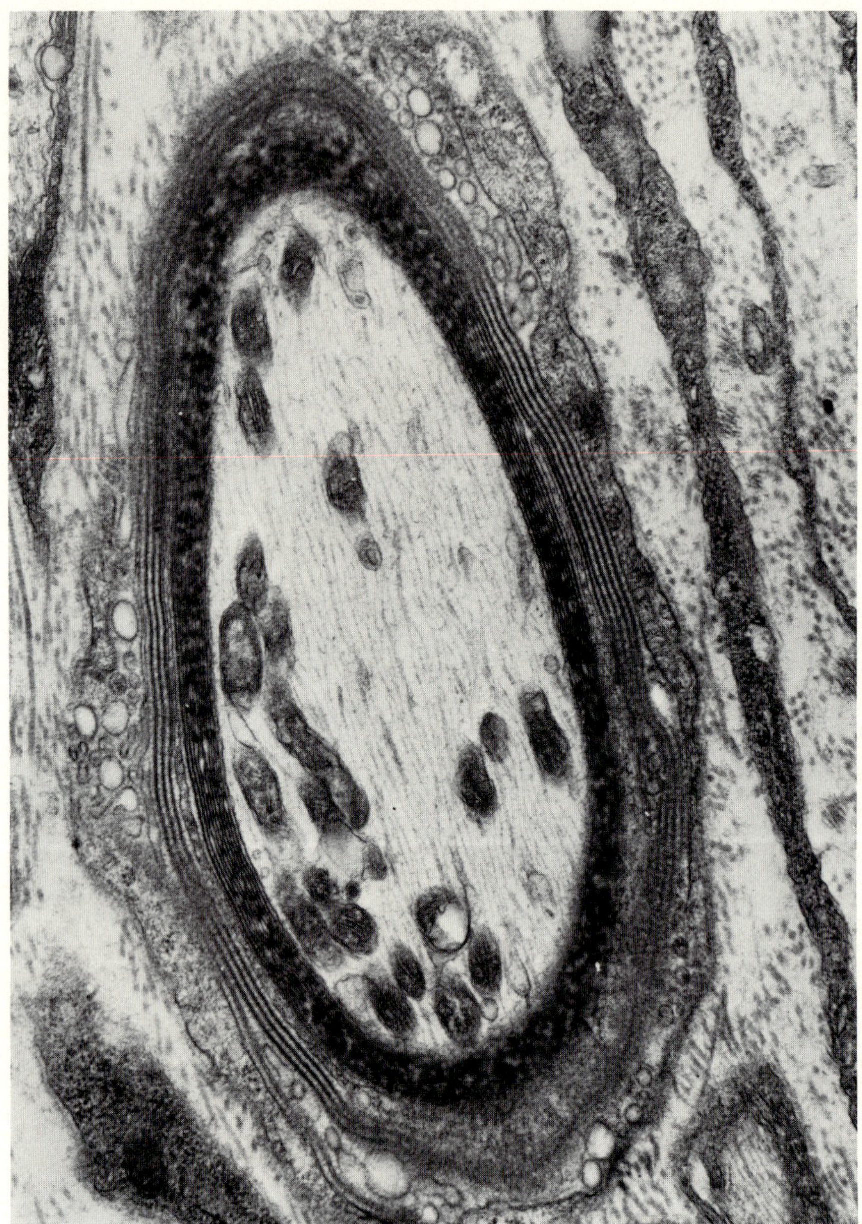

Fig. 231 Demyelination in a peripheral nerve. In contrast to the markedly altered myelin sheath, the axon is relatively well preserved. × 30,000. (From Hirano, A.: The Structure and Function of Nervous Tissue. Vol. 5, p. 73, Academic Press, 1972.)

adjacent lamellae beginning at the outer loop and finally penetrating to the periaxonal space.

The lesion may be best demonstrated in experimental allergic encephalomyelitis (Fig. 232) or neuritis, but similar changes have sometimes been seen, to a limited extent, in a variety of other experimental systems. The fundamental alterations

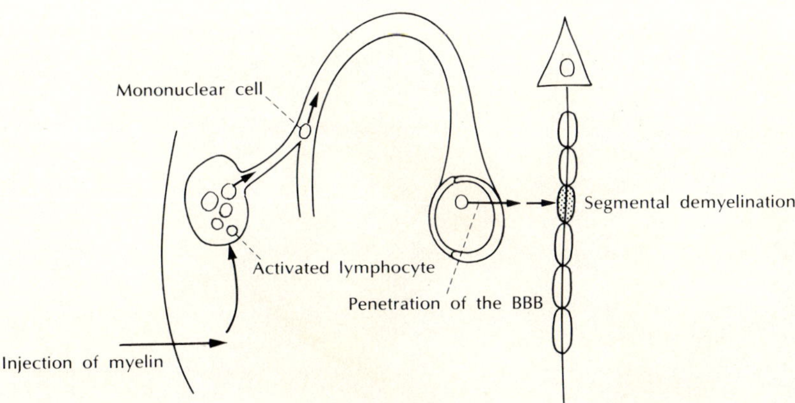

Fig. 232 Presumed mechanism of EAE.
Activated lymphocytes are produced in the lymph nodes by the systemic administration of suspensions of central nervous tissue, containing myelin, along with Freund's adjuvant (a mixture of killed tubercle bacilli and mineral oil designed to enhance immunological response). The lymphocytes enter the circulation and penetrate the BBB in the central nervous system where they exert their effects on individual segments of myelin causing demyelination.

seem to include a disruption of the tight junctions at the cytoplasmic areas surrounding the myelin sheet allowing the penetration of extracellular material as well as hematogenous cells (Mugaini and Schnapp, 1974). This condition is generally accompanied by disruption of the blood-brain barrier and eventually leads to demyelination. Similar effects on the intraperiod line have been described after experimental manipulation of cultured nervous tissue (Bornstein and Raine, 1976).

REFERENCES

Lampert, P.W.: Demyelination and remyelination in experimental allergic encephalomyelitis. J. Neuropathol. Exp. Neurol., 24: 371-385, 1965.

Lampert, P.W.: Electron microscopic studies on ordinary and hyperacute experimental allergic encephalomyelitis. Acta Neuropathol., 4: 99-126, 1967.

Hirano, A., Cook. S.D., Whitaker, J.N., Dowling, P.C., & Murray, M.R.: Fine structural aspects of demyelination in vitro. The effects of Guillain-Barré serum. J. Neuropathol. Exp. Neurol., 30: 249-265, 1971.

Mugnaini, E., & Schnapp, B.: Possible role of zonula occludens of the myelin sheath in demyelinating conditions. Nature, 251: 725-727, 1974.

Dropp, R.P., Means, E., Deibel, R., Sherer, .T., & Barron, K.: Waldenström's macroglobulinemia and neuropathy: Deposition of M-component on myelin sheaths. Neurology, 25: 980-988, 1975.

Bornstein, M.B., & Raine, C.: The initial structural lesion in serum-induced demyelination *in vitro*. Lab. Invest., 35: 391-401, 1976.

Vesicular Dissolution (Fig. 233)

This alteration is seen in a variety of conditions leading to the loss of myelin. It is most prominent in a certain type of experimental allergic encephalomyelitis (Saida et al., 1977), Guillain-Barré syndrome (Wiśniewski et al., 1969) and after the intracerebral implantation of diphtheria toxin (Wiśniewski, 1972). The fine structure of the lesion is characterized by the formation of honeycomb-like alterations most often near the outer layers of the sheath.

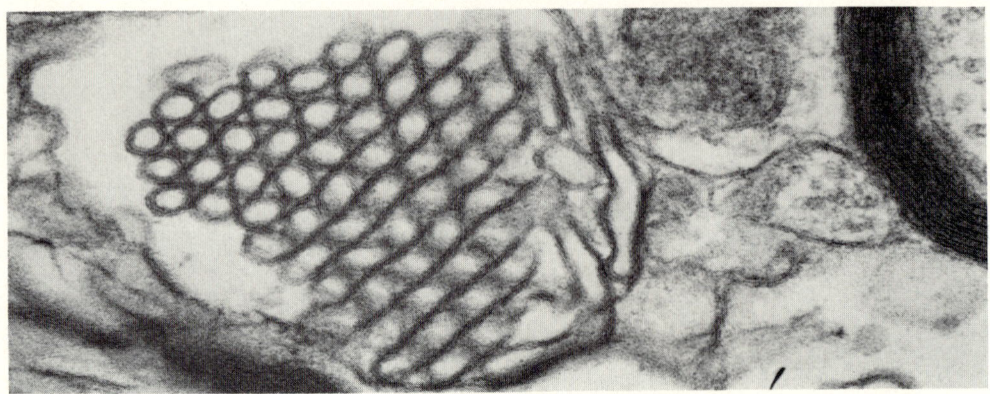

Fig. 233 Vesicular dissolution of central myelin. × 90,000. (From Hirano, A.: The Structure and Function of Nervous Tissue. Vol. 5, p. 73, Academic Press, 1972.)

REFERENCES

Wiśniewski, H., Terry, R.D., Whitaker, J.M., Cook, S.D., & Dowling, P.C.: Landry-Guillain-Barré Syndrome: A primary demyelinating disease. Arch. Neurol., 21: 269-276, 1969.

Wiśniewski, H.: Patterns of myelin damage resulting from inflammatory and toxin-induced lesions and their relationship to multiple sclerosis. *In* Multiple Sclerosis, Immunology, Virology and Ultrastructure, pp. 53-89. Wolfgram, F., Ellison, G.W., Stevens, J.G., & Andrews, J.A. (eds.), Academic Press, New York, 1972.

Saida K, Mendell Jr., & Sahenk Z.: Peripheral nerve changes induced by local application of bee venom. J. Neuropathol. Exp. Neurol., 36: 783-796, 1977.

Buscaino Bodies (Mucocytes)

In the light microscope these structures appear as focal, PAS-positive, scattered vacuoles in the white matter. When viewed in the electron microscope they appear as discrete, lytic, spherical disruptions within the myelin sheath. These are artifactitious in nature and do not signify pathological processes.

REFERENCES

Cancilla, P.A., & Berlow, R.M.: Morphologic abnormalities of myelin in Border disease of lambs. *In* Progress in Neuropathology, Vol. I., pp. 76-83, Zimmerman, H.M. (ed.), Grune & Stratton, New York, 1971.

Blackwood, W.: Normal structure and general pathology of nerve cell and neuroglia. *In* Greenfield's Neuropathology, pp. 18-20, Blackwood, W. & Corcellis, J.A.N. (eds.), Year Book Med. Pub. Inc., Chicago, 1976.

Invagination of Glio-axonal Membranes (Fig. 234)

Under certain conditions, both the glial and axonal plasma membranes can invaginate into the axoplasm. In its most simple form the invaginations appear as finger-like projections, but they may also form more complex interdigitations in advanced stages (Fig. 234). These configurations have been reported in both normal and various pathological conditions in the central and peripheral nervous system. In normal animals, they have been interpreted as representing a normal, intimate relationship between the axon and the Schwann cell facilitating the transfer of material from one to the other (Singer, 1968). Spencer and Thomas (1974), however, regard these configurations as the reflection of a phagocytic function of Schwann cells in the process of removing pathological portions of the axoplasm. It should be noted that they are most commonly observed at the edge of the internode adjacent to the paranodal region.

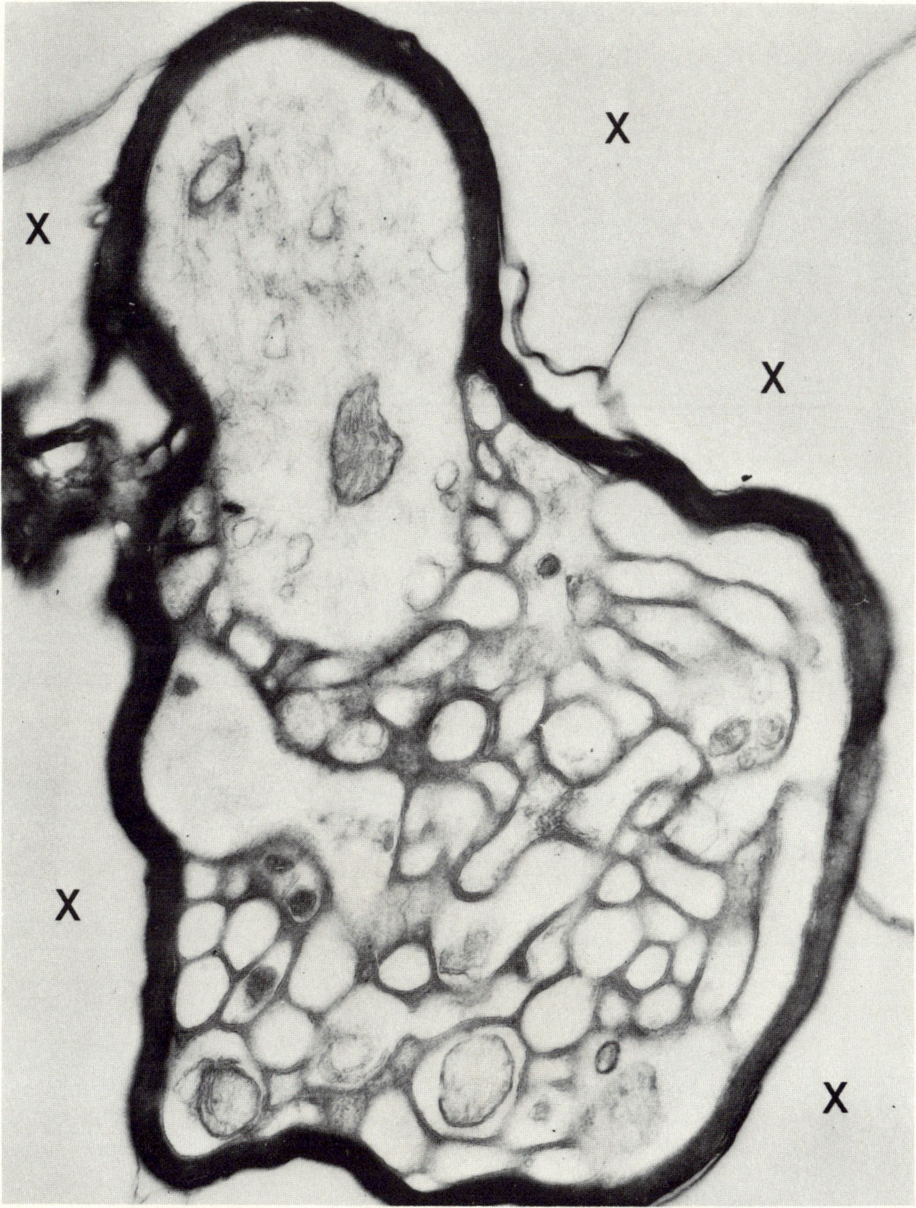

Fig. 234 A myelinated axon in the cerebral white matter of a rat subjected to systemic triethyltin intoxication. In addition to large intramyelinic splits (X), the apposed glio-axonal membranes have folded to form complicated configurations in the periaxonal space. × 30,000.

REFERENCES

Singer, M: Penetration of labelled amino acids into the peripheral nerve fibre from surrounding body fluids. *In* Growth of the Nervous System, pp. 200-215, Wolstenholme, G.E.W., & O'Connor, M., (eds.), Little Brown, Boston, 1968.

Spencer, P.S. & Thomas, P.K.: Ultrastructural studies of the dying-back process. II. The sequestration and removal by Schwann cells and oligodendrocytes of organelles from normal and diseased axons. J. Neurocytol., 3: 763-783, 1974.

Pathology of The Inner Loop (Figs. 235-238)

Demyelination resulting from changes in the inner loop has been observed in the peripheral neuropathy of mutant hamsters with hind leg paralysis. In these

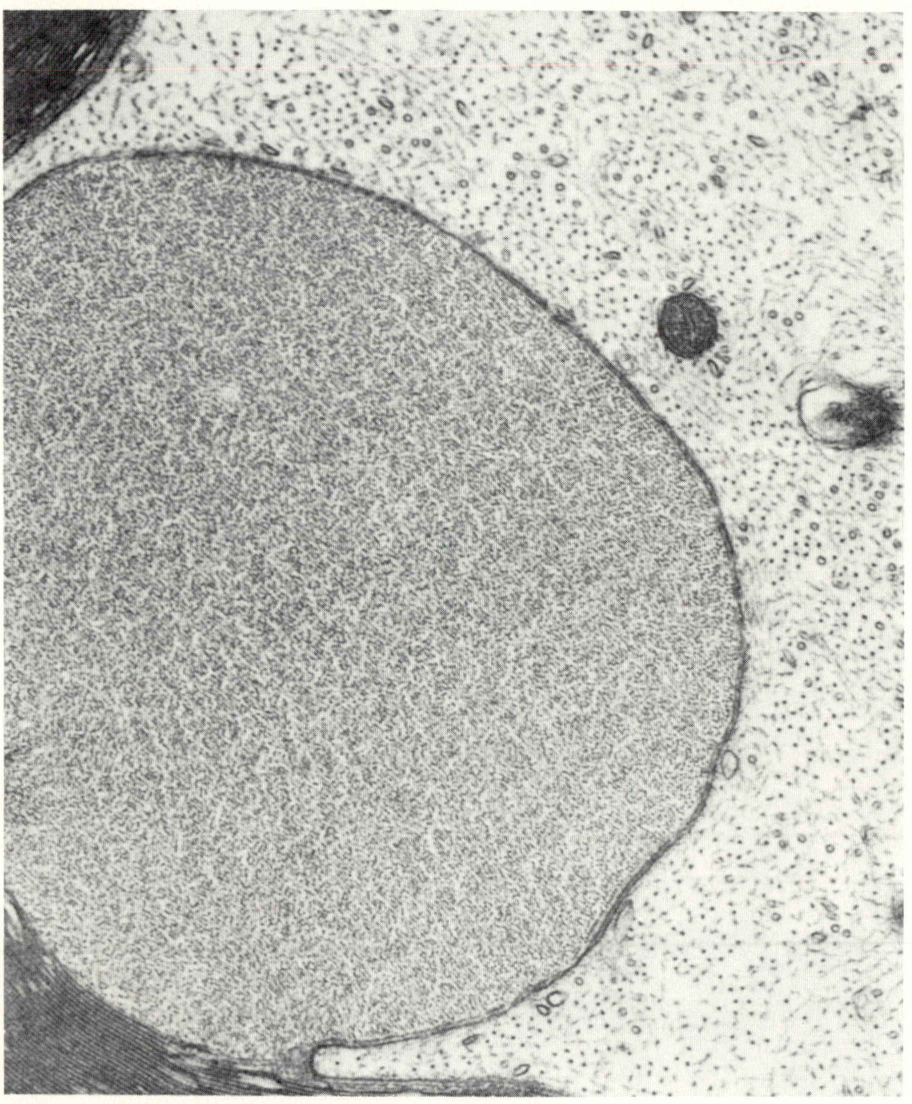

Fig. 235 A filament-filled inner loop of a myelin sheath in a mutant hamster. × 40,000. (From Hirano, A.: Lab. Invest., 38: 115, 1978.)

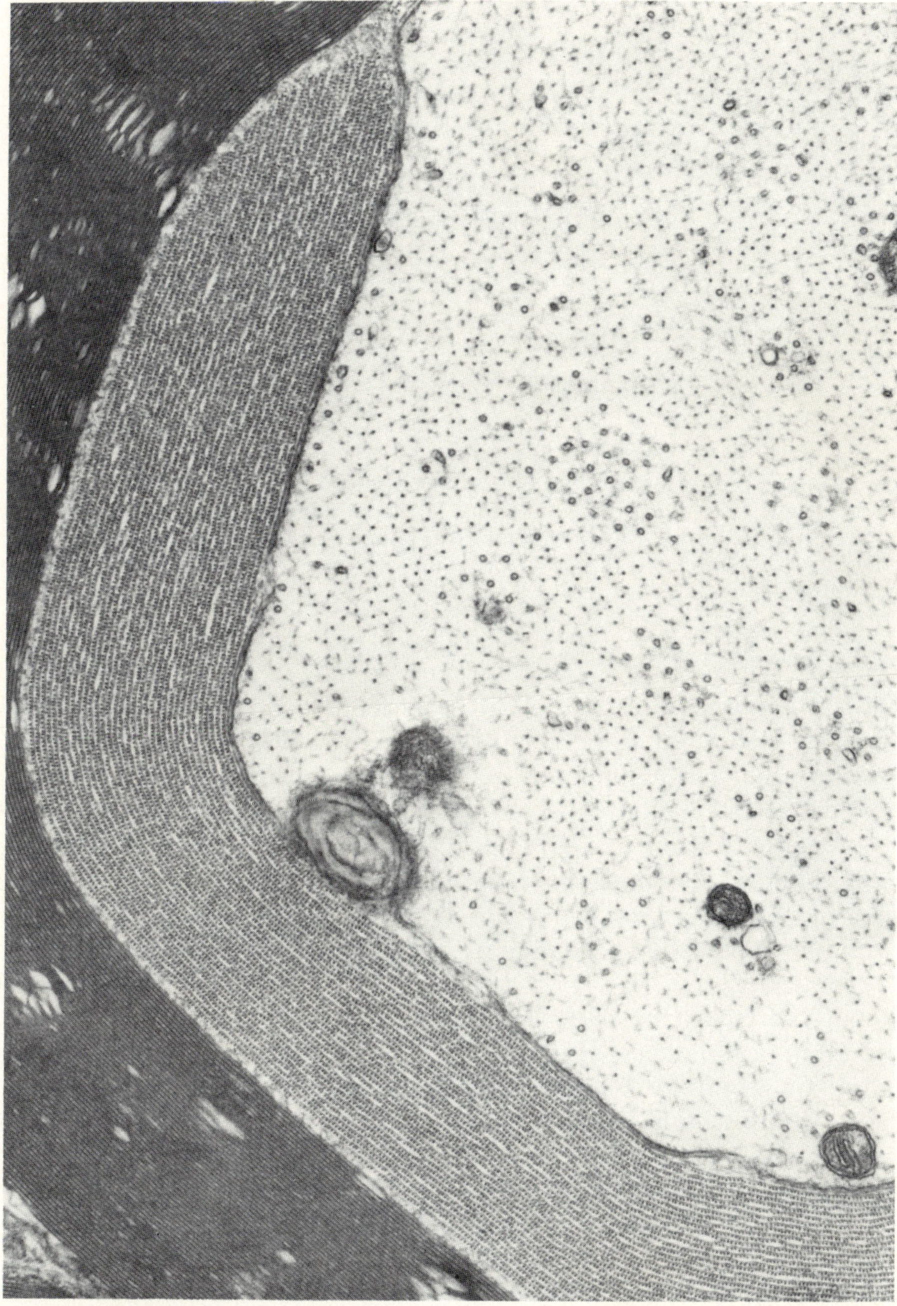

Fig. 236 A crystalloid, filamentous array in the inner loop of a myelinated fiber in a root of a mutant hamster with hind leg paralysis. The microtubules in the axoplasm are arranged in small groups. × 40,000. (From Hirano, A.: Acta Neuropathol., 39: 225, 1977.)

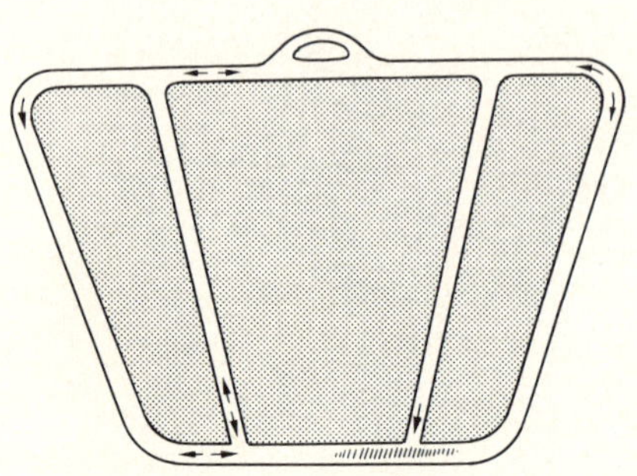

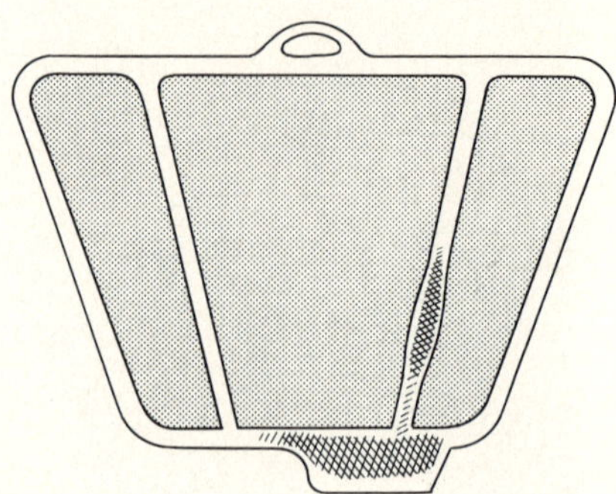

Fig. 237 Diagram of the hypothetically unrolled myelin sheath. On the left is the normal sheath with a few filaments in the inner rim. On the right the abnormal fibrillary accumulations are seen in the inner rim and distal portion of one of the Schmidt-Lanterman incisures where they may interfere with the flow of materials through the cytoplasmic pathways of the sheath. (From Hirano, A.: Lab. Invest., 38: 115, 1978.)

animals, fibrillary accumulations in the inner loop become conspicuous (Fig. 235), and often are associated with crystalloid formation (Fig. 236). These crystalloids correspond to the eosinophilic rod-like structure seen in the light microscope and are identical to the eosinophilic rod-like structures seen in Sommer's sector in various human conditions (p. 151). Demyelination of heavily myelinated peripheral nerve is followed by remyelination causing "onion bulb" formation (Fig. 238).

Similar fibrillary changes have been reported in the inner loops of oligodendroglia in experimental hepatic encephalopathy (Cavanagh et al., 1971).

It has been suggested that the mechanism of this type of demyelination actually constitutes a kind of dying-back phenomenon in which the most distal part of the myelin-forming cell is affected first. It is conceivable that this represents a special vulnerability of the inner loop due to its distance from the cell body similar to the distal axonopathy seen in various toxic neuropathies. On the other hand, it should be pointed out that these distal parts of the myelin-forming cell are the parts most intimately connected with the axon so that the changes seen may represent some change in the normal interaction between the two cell types.

REFERENCES

Cavanagh, J.B., Blakemore, W.F. & Kyu, M.H.: Fibrillary accumulations in oligodendroglial processes of rats subjected to portocaval anastomosis. J. Neurol. Sci., 14: 143-152, 1971.

Hirano, A.: Fine structural changes in the mutant hamster with hind leg paralysis. Acta Neuropathol., 39: 225-230, 1977.

Hirano, A.: A possible mechanism of demyelination in the Syrian hamster with hind leg paralysis. Lab. Invest., 38: 115-121, 1978.

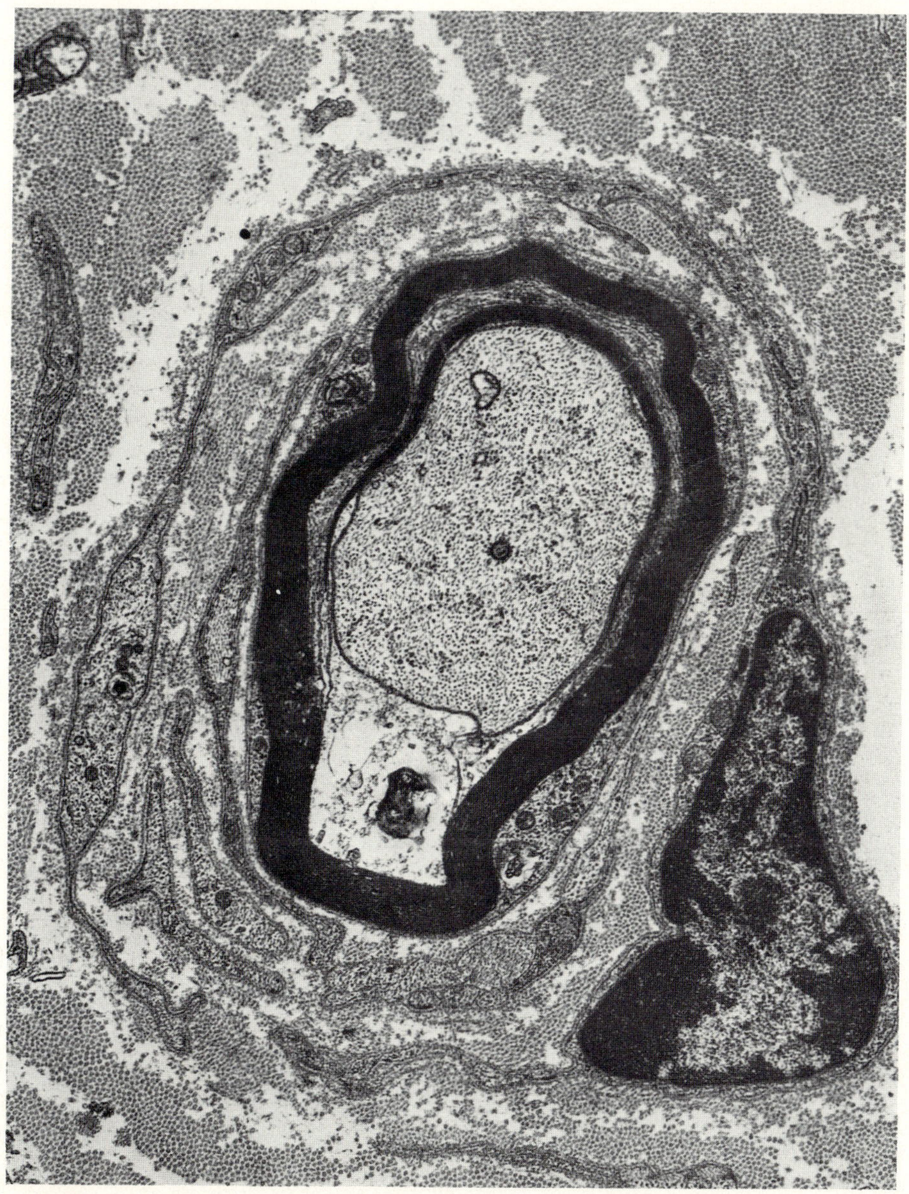

Fig. 238 "Onion bulb." × 12,000.

REMYELINATION (Figs. 239-243)

It was at one time believed that remyelination did not occur within the central nervous system. Electron microscopic evidence has shown that this is not the case

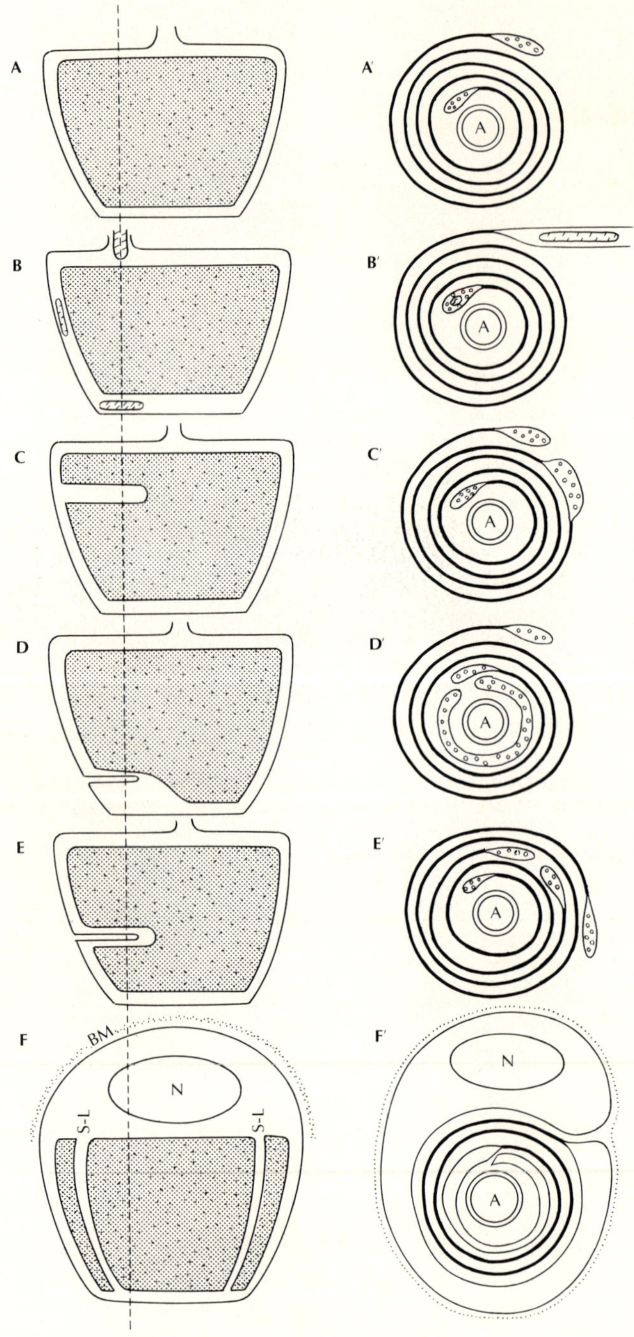

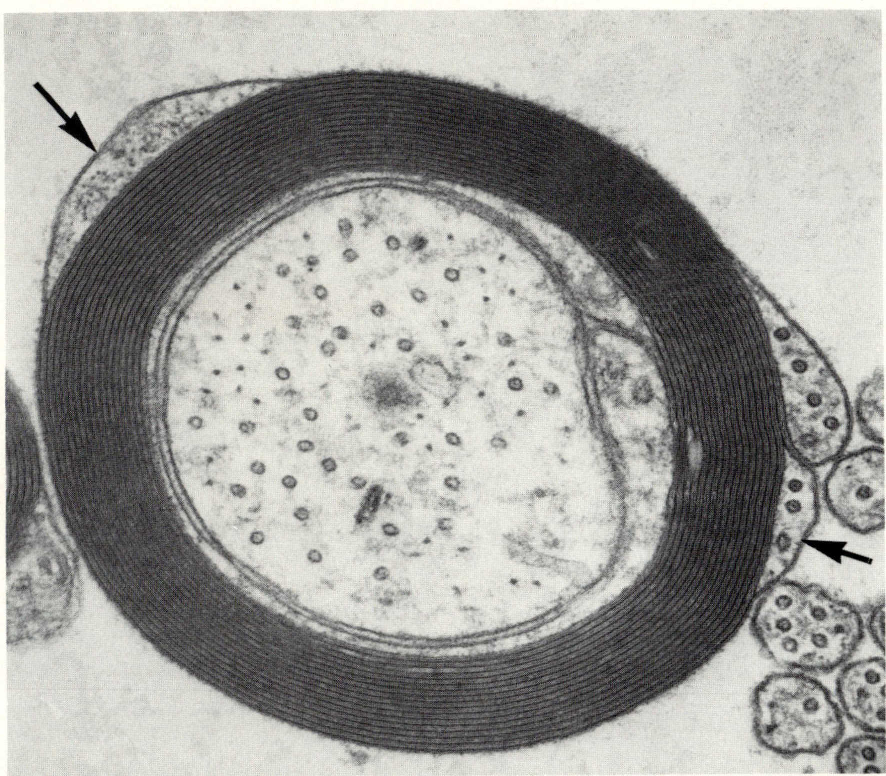

Fig. 240 A central myelinated axon. Two small cytoplasmic islands are indicated by the arrows. × 100,000. (From Hirano, A. et al.: J. Neuropathol. Exp. Neurol., 27: 234, 1968.)

← **Fig. 239** Various configurations of the myelin sheet predicted by the hypothetical unrolling of normal and certain abnormal myelin sheaths.
A. Type A myelin sheet. This is the usual form of the sheet. When rolled up around an axon and sectioned in the indicated plane, it results in the usual type A configuration diagrammed in A′. **B.** Type B myelin sheet. The continuous surrounding cytoplasmic rim contains formed organelles. When rolled up around an axon and sectioned in the indicated plane, it results in the type B configuration diagrammed in B′. **C.** Type C myelin sheet. An extension of the lateral cytoplasmic rim intrudes into the myelin sheet. When rolled up around an axon and sectioned in the indicated plane, it results in a type C configuration including an isolated cytoplasmic island as diagrammed in C′. **D.** Type D myelin sheet. The irregularly widened inner rim is indented by a cleft of extracellular space. When rolled up around an axon and sectioned in the indicated plane, it results in a type D configuration including an apparently unconnected cell process as diagrammed in D′. **E.** Type E myelin sheet. The lateral rim is folded into the myelin sheet. When rolled up around an axon and sectioned in the indicated plane, it results in a type E configuration including two complete concentric myelin sheaths both spiraling in the same direction as indicated in E′. **F.** A myelin sheet derived from the unrolling of a myelin sheath in the peripheral nervous system. The outer cytoplasmic rim is much wider than in the central nervous system and consists of the entire cell body of the Schwann cell, including the nucleus (N). Furthermore, two thickened, vertical cytoplasmic ridges, roughly parallel to the lateral rims, are present (S-L) which give rise to the incisures of Schmidt-Lanterman when seen in longitudinal section. The outer rim is covered by a basement membrane (BM). The inner and lateral rims, of course, are devoid of a basement membrane since, in the rolled up sheath, no basement membrane intervenes between the inner loop and the axon (A) or between adjacent lateral loops. When rolled up around an axon and sectioned in the indicated plane, it results in a typical peripheral myelin sheath as diagrammed in F′.

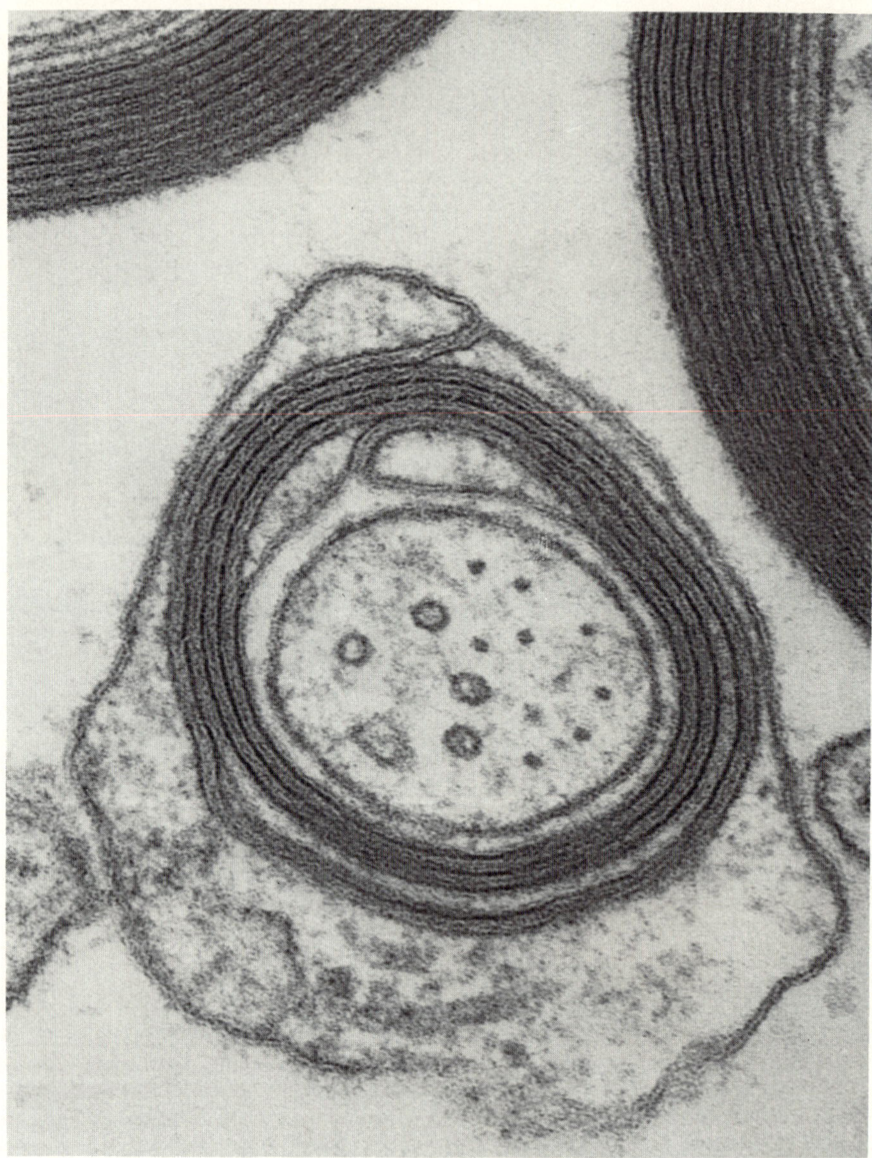

Fig. 241 A regenerating central myelinated axon. Several myelin lamellae are present as well as a large outer cytoplasmic area. × 180,000. (From Hirano, A. et al.: J. Neuropath. Exp. Neurol., 27: 234, 1968.)

and that remyelination can occur in the central nervous system, although it is generally very slow and limited compared to the peripheral nervous system. When it does occur in long-standing lesions of the white matter, it can be characterized by various alterations of the sheath representing stages in remyelination as illustrated in Fig. 239. These may be summarized as the occurrence of organelles

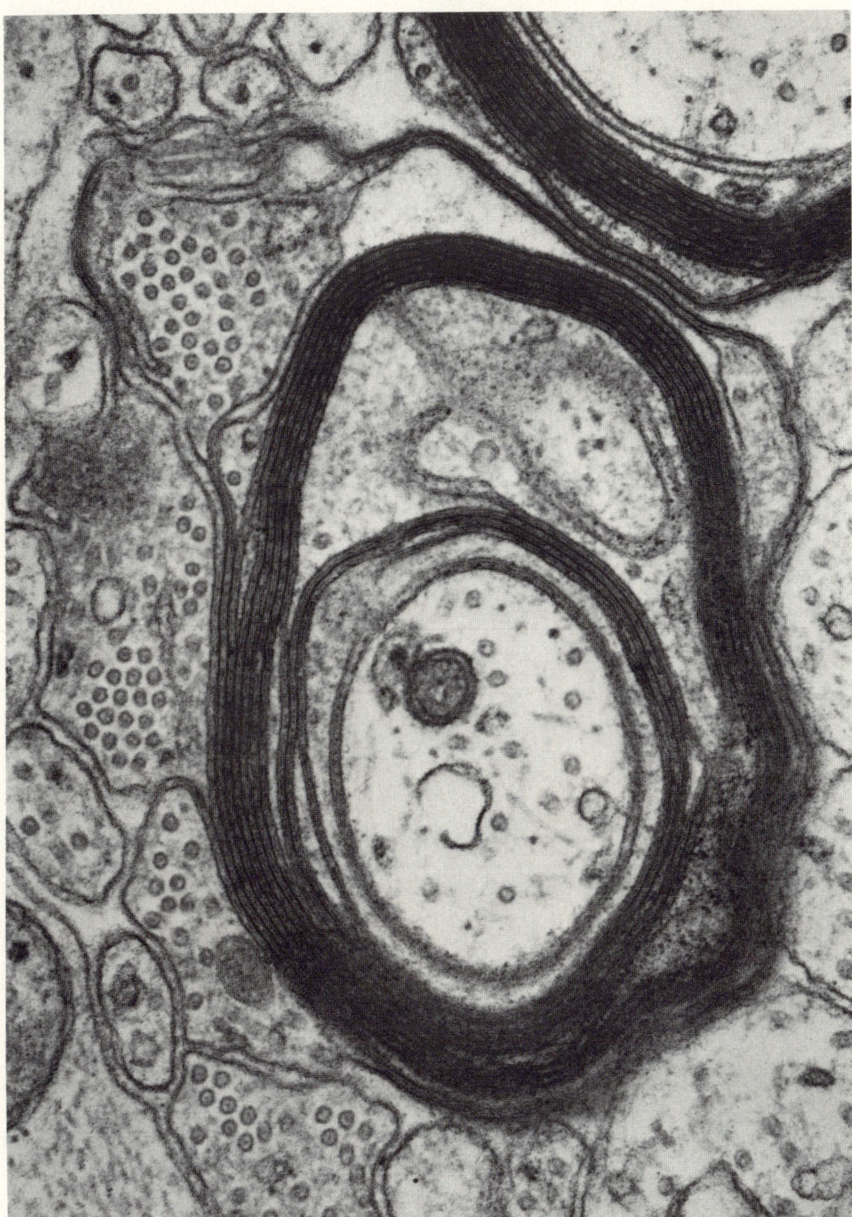

Fig. 242 A central myelinated axon. Large, cytoplasmic islands containing many microtubules are present within the sheath. × 96,000. (From Hirano, A.: The Structure and Function of Nervous Tissue. Vol. 5, p. 73, Academic Press, 1972.)

within the cytoplasmic area of the sheath, the presence of additional cytoplasmic areas (Fig. 240) and the apparent discontinuity of lamellae or the presence of two separate sheaths around a single axon.

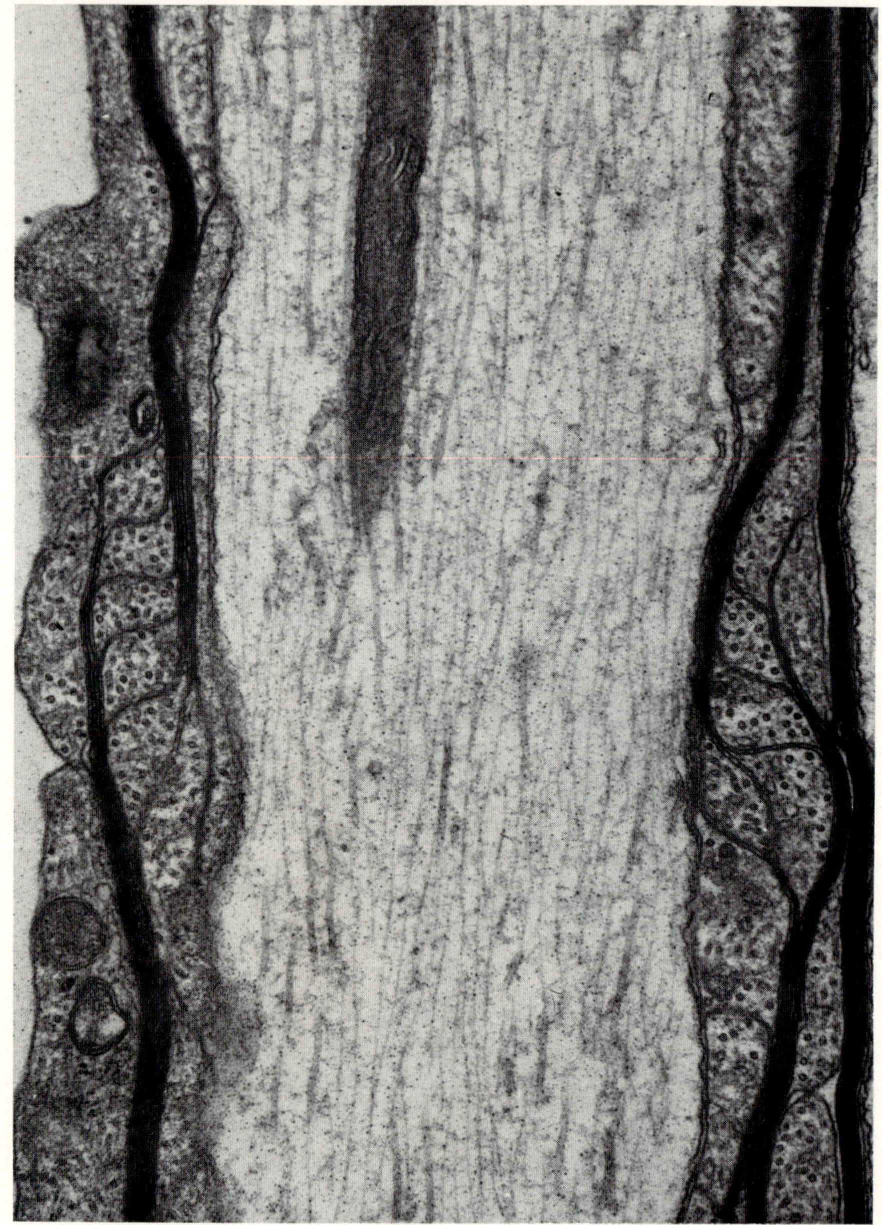

Fig. 243 A longitudinal section of a regenerating central myelinated axon. Regularly arranged cytoplasmic areas similar to Schmidt-Lanterman clefts are present × 36,000. (From Hirano, A. et al.: Acta Neuropath., 12: 348, 1969.)

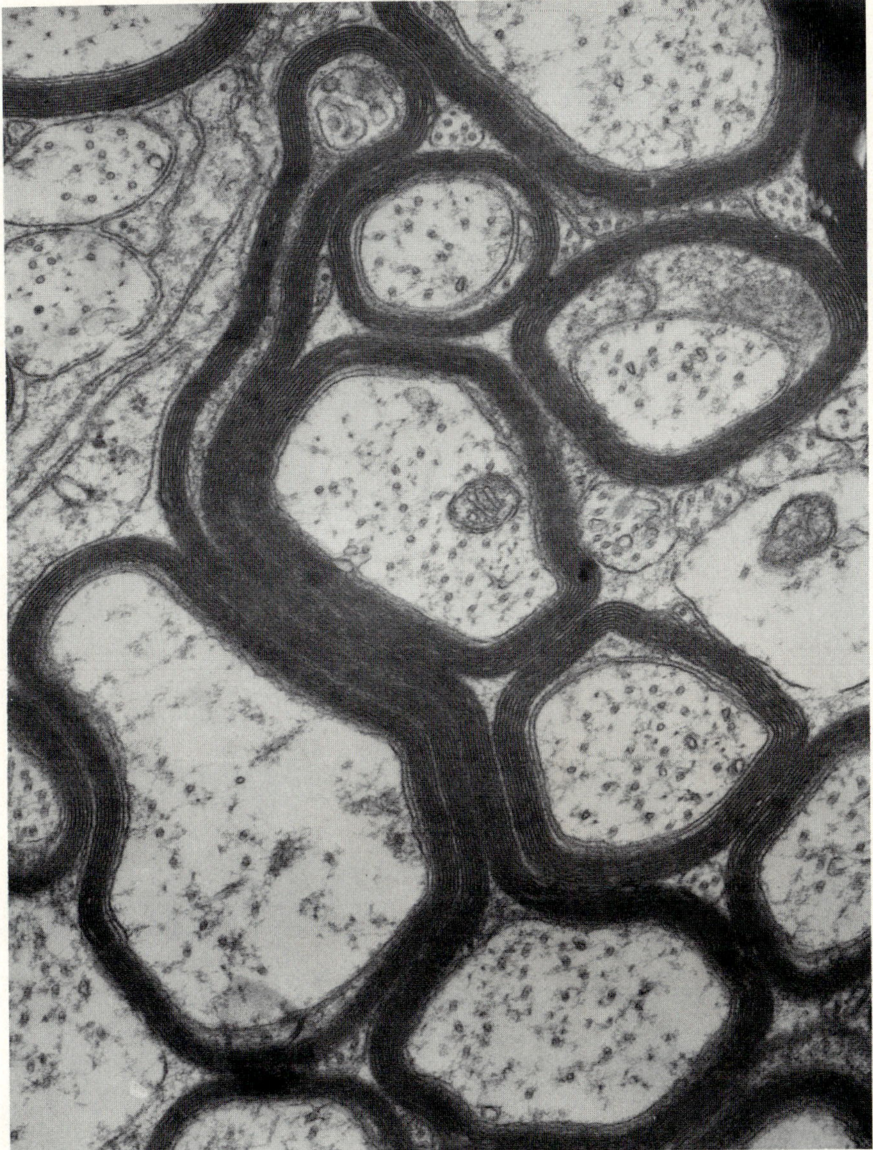

Fig. 244 Abnormal extension of the central myelin sheath. (From Hirano, A.: The Structure and Function of Nervous Tissue. Vol. 5, p. 73, Academic Press, 1972.)

Redundant Myelin Sheath

Usually after axonal loss or alteration, the myelin lamellae become distorted and can sometimes form bizarre configurations although the structures of the individual lamellae are well preserved (Figs. 244-246). Under these, as well as other conditions, myelin lamellae can sometimes be seen surrounding neuronal cell

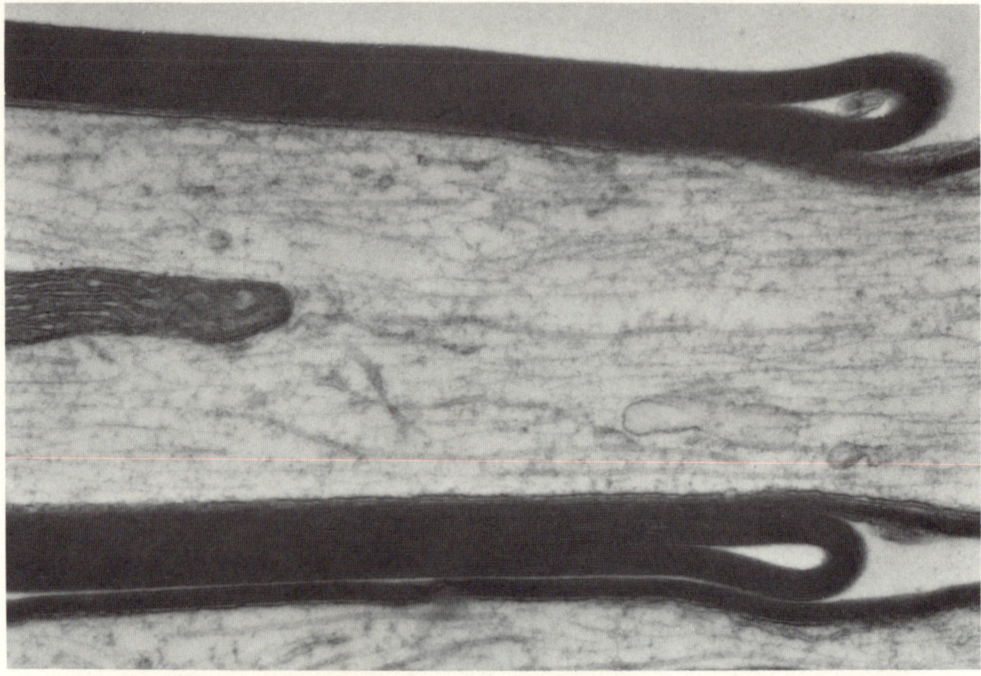

Fig. 245 Abnormal arrangement of a central myelin sheath. × 35,000. (From Hirano, A.: The Structure and Function of Nervous Tissue. Vol. 5, p. 73, Academic Press, 1972.)

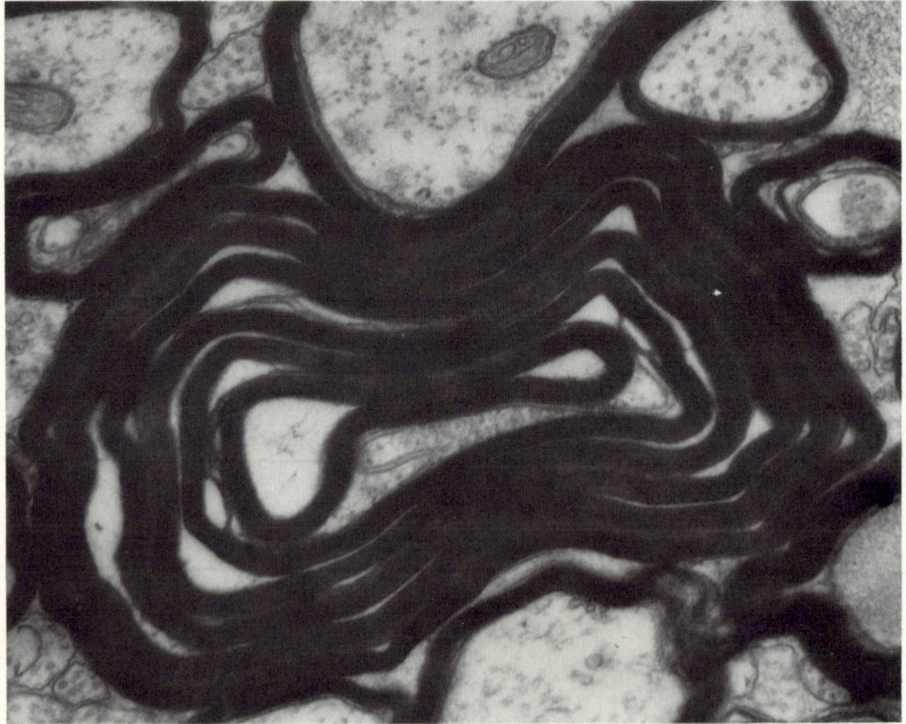

Fig. 246 Multiple invaginations of a degenerated central myelinated fiber. (From Hirano, A.: The Structure and Function of Nervous Tissue. Vol. 5, p. 73, Academic Press, 1972.)

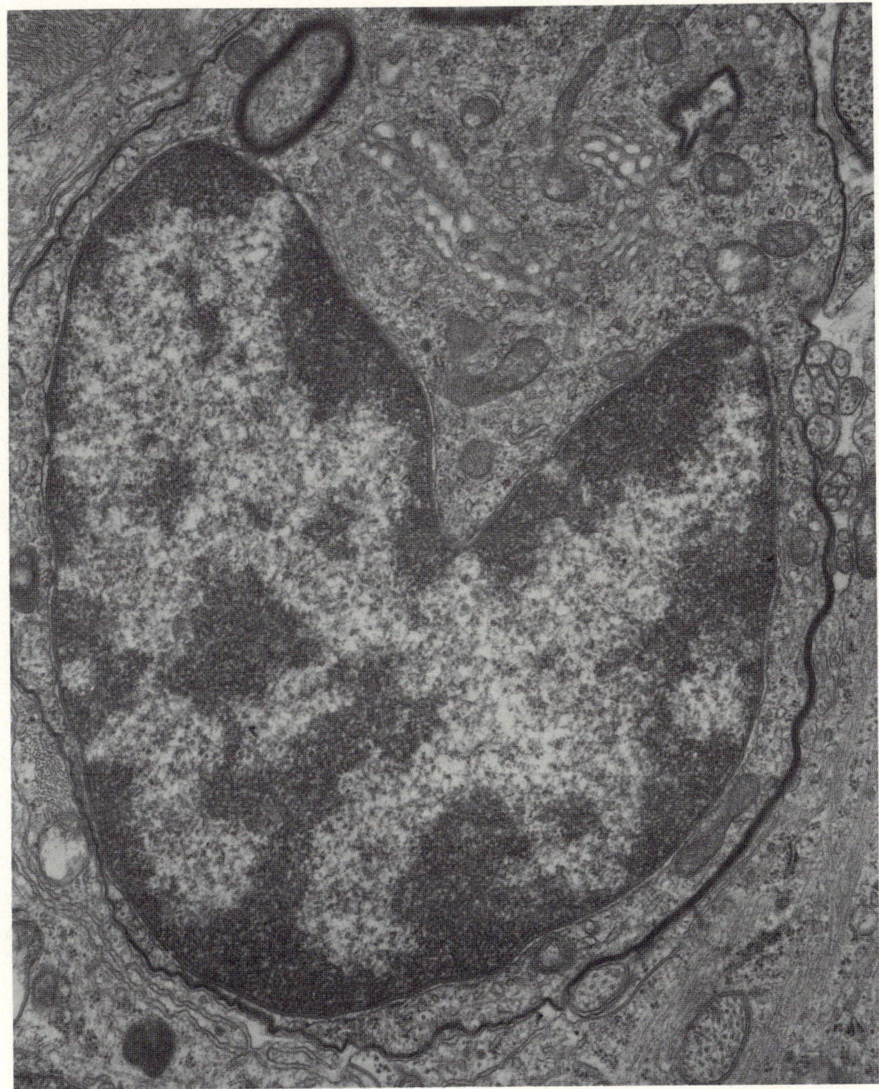

Fig. 247 An oligodendroglial cell surrounded by myelin lamellae. × 22,000. (From Hirano, A.: The Structure and Function of Nervous Tissue. Vol. 5, p. 73, Academic Press, 1972.)

bodies or glial cells (Fig. 247). These latter changes are sometimes associated with remyelination. The so-called myelin ovoids actually represent outpocketing of the myelin sheath into the Schwann cell cytoplasm (Fig. 248). These may be produced by both pathological and artifactitious alterations.

One important difference between the central and peripheral nervous system is the relatively great ability of the peripheral nerve to undergo remyelination (Fig. 249). A common pathological alteration after injury to the peripheral nerve is so-called traumatic neuroma which results from an excessive regeneration of all the elements of the peripheral nerve, especially the Schwann cell. Chronic, recurrent demyelinating phenomena followed by abortive attempts at remyelination results

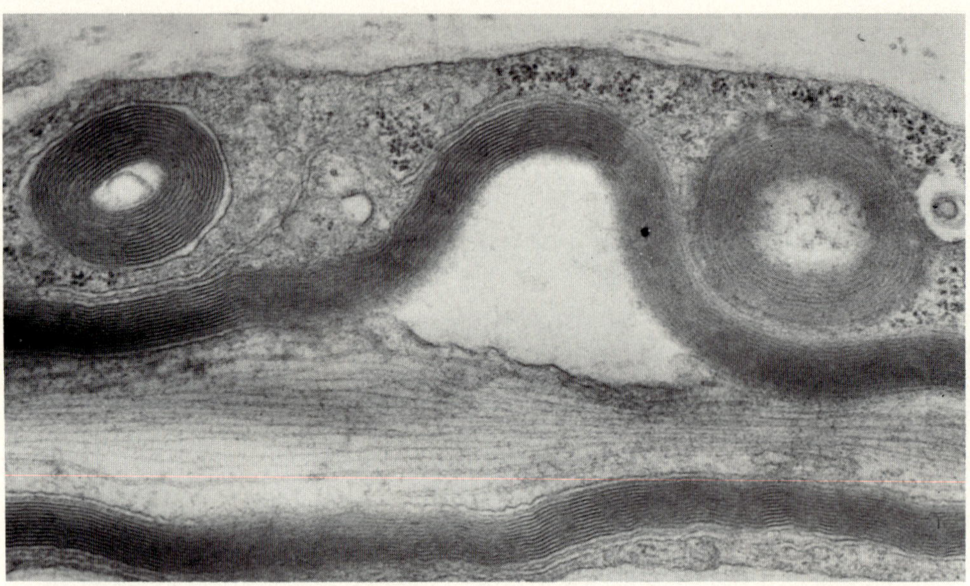

Fig. 248 A longitudinal section of a peripheral myelinated axon. Three myelin ovoids and a related outpocketing of the myelin sheath into the Schwan cell cytoplasm are visible. × 30,000. (From Hirano, A.: The Structure and Function of Nervous Tissue. Vol. 5, p. 73, Academic Press, 1972.)

in "*onion bulb*" formation (Figs. 238, 250) which consists of successive layers of Schwann cells separated by narrow, collagen-containing, extracellular spaces surrounding a single axon. Each layer presumably represents a single attempt at remyelination.

Because of the presence of abundant connective tissue, peripheral nerve is subject to alterations of these elements. Amyloid neuropathy is a good example of this effect characterized by the deposition of amyloid in the perivascular and the intercellular spaces of the peripheral nerve.

REFERENCES

Hirano, A., Levine, S., & Zimmerman, H.M.: Remyelination in the central nervous system after cyanide intoxication. J. Neuropathol. Exp. Neurol., 27: 234-245, 1968.

Hirano, A., Zimmerman, H.M., & Levine, S.: Electron microscopic observations of peripheral myelin in a central nervous system lesion. Acta Neuropathol., 12: 348-365, 1969.

Ghatak, N.R., Hirano, A., Doron, Y., & Zimmerman, H.M.: Remyelination in multiple sclerosis with peripheral type myelin. Arch. Neurol., 29: 262-267, 1973.

Krücke, W.: Pathologie der Peripheren Nerven. *In* Handbuch der Neurochirurgie, Bd. VII/3. pp. 1-267. Olivercrona, H., Tönnis, W., & Krenkel, W. (eds.), Springer-Verlag, Berlin, 1974.

Blakemore, W.F.: Invasion of Schwann cells into the spinal cord of the rat following local injections of lysolecithin. Neuropathol. Appl. Neurobiol., 2: 21-39, 1976.

Ludwin, S.K.: Central nervous system demyelination and remyelination in the mouse. An ultrastructural study of cuprizone toxicity. Lab. Invest., 39: 597-612, 1978.

Prineas, M.B., & Connell, B.S.: Remyelination in multiple sclerosis. Ann. Neurol., 5: 22-31, 1978.

Asbury, A.K., & Johnson, P.C.: Pathology of Peripheral Nerve: Vol. 9 in the Series, Major Problems in Pathology. W.B. Saunders Co., Philadelphia, 1978.

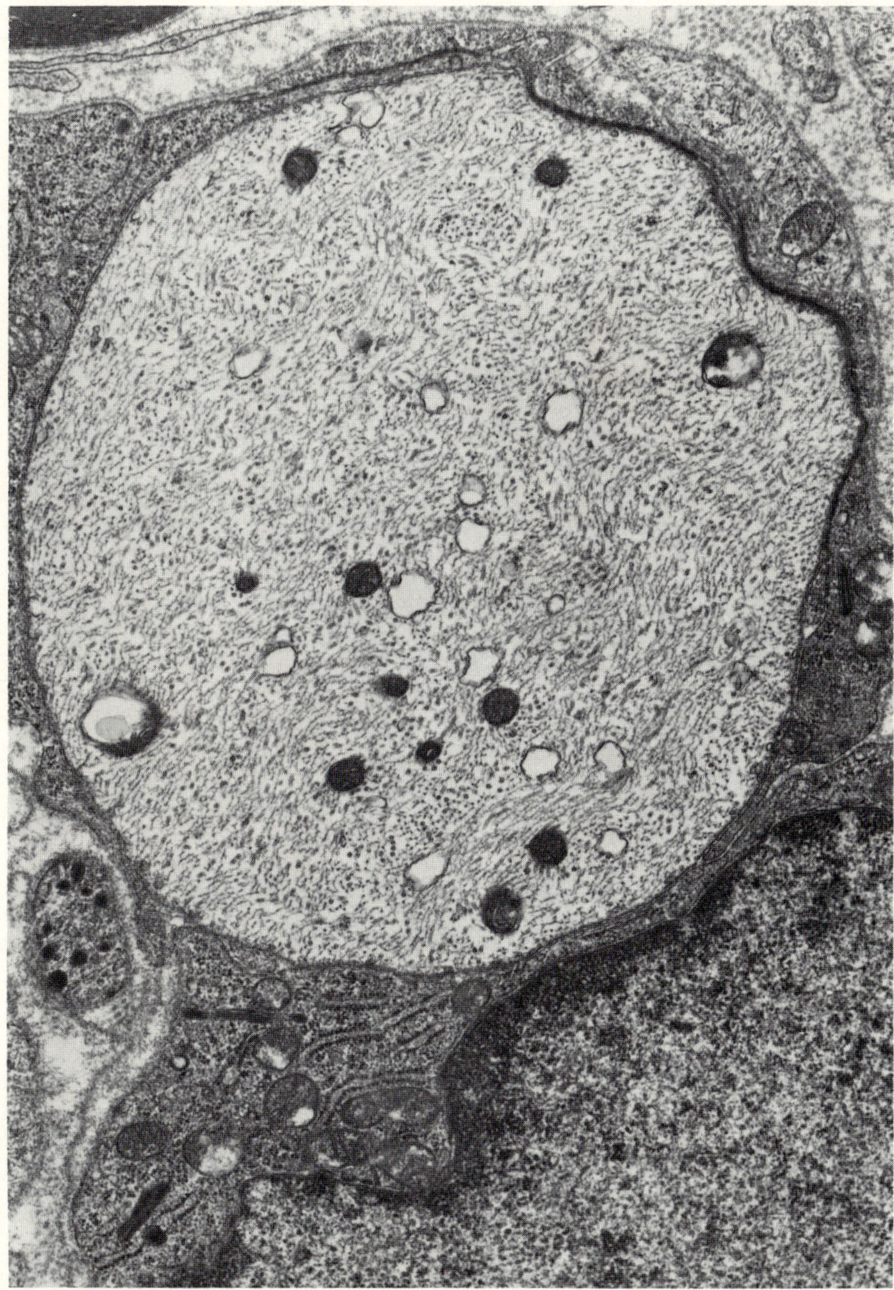

Fig. 249 A denuded axon surrounded by a Schwann cell in a mutant hamster. The beginning of remyelination is seen at the upper right quadrant of the axon. × 22,000.

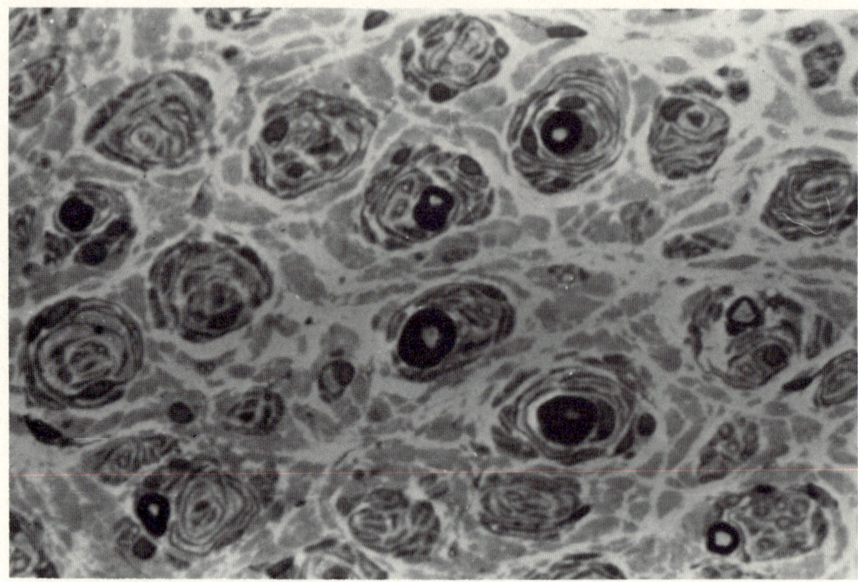

Fig. 250 "Onion bulb" formation in a peripheral nerve. This change is seen in Dejerine-Sottas disease, Refsum disease, Charcot-Marie-Tooth disease, etc.

ALTERATIONS OF THE TRANSVERSE BANDS

As described previously, transverse bands are characteristic components of the normal interface between the lateral loops of myelin-forming cells of the central or peripheral nervous system and the axon (Figs. 221, 224). Ordinarily, they apparently arise late in myelin development since their absence has been noted during remyelination and in the myelin sheaths of young experimental animals (Hirano and Zimmerman, 1971).

Under pathological conditions the transverse bands disappear when the lateral loops lose their connections with the axon (Hirano and Dembitzer, 1978). They can reappear under certain conditions when single, isolated lateral loops reattach to the axonal surface. More interestingly, transverse bands have been observed between Schwann cell cytoplasm and axons in certain dystrophic mice which are unable to form myelin in spinal roots (Rosenbluth, 1978). Similarly, transverse bands have been observed between oligodendroglial soma and denuded axons in patients with multiple sclerosis (Prineas, 1979).

REFERENCES

Hirano, A., & Zimmerman, H.M.: Some new pathological findings in the central myelinated axon. J. Neuropathol. Exp. Neurol., 30: 325-336, 1971.

Hirano, A., & Dembitzer, H.M.: Morphology of normal central myelinated axons, *In* Physiology and Pathobiology of Axons, pp. 65-82, Waxman, S.G. (ed.), Raven Press, New York, 1978.

Prineas, J.W., & Connel, F.: Remyelination in multiple sclerosis, Ann. Neurol., 5: 22-31, 1979.

Rosenbluth, J.: Freeze fracture studies of nerve fibers: Evidence that regional differentiation of the axolemma depends upon glial contact. *In* Current Topics in Nerve and Muscle Research, pp. 200-209, Aguayo, A.J. & Karpati, G. (eds.), Excerpta Medica, Amsterdam-Oxford, 1979.

4. Neoplasms of Peripheral Nerve (Figs. 251, 252)

The most common tumor among those involving the roots of the cranial and spinal nerves, is a benign, solitary neoplasm, usually referred to as schwannoma, neurilemmoma or neurinoma. It usually affects adults. Grossly, the tumor is encapsulated and spindle or spherical in shape. It is attached to the nerve root which traverses the capsule of the mass. The portion of the eighth cranial nerve at the cerebello-pontine angle is a region of special predilection.

Schwannomas are comprised of spindle-shaped cells with processes extending into relatively wide extracellular spaces, which contain collagen. The cell bodies contain the usual organelles around the nuclei. Each process may be covered by a basal lamina or may be grouped into small bundles which are themselves, surrounded by a basal lamina and within which the processes approach one another with no intervening basal lamina (Fig. 251). Luse bodies may be found among the collagen fibers. These spindle-shaped structures show a periodicity of 1,000-1,200Å and are found in various other conditions as well.

The blood vessels of the tumor are generally thin walled and often form large lumens (sinusoidal). The endothelium is characteristically fenestrated (Hirano et al., 1972). The vessels are often associated with hemosiderin-containing macrophages indicating old hemorrhages.

Histologically, two types of areas are often emphasized as characteristic features. The Antoni A type region consists of compactly arranged interlacing bundles of spindle-shaped cells sometimes forming a so-called palisading pattern. In Antoni B type regions the cells are more loosely arranged. Foamy cells are often seen which may contain sudanophilic lipids. Mast cells are also observed in schwannomas.

Although schwannomas are a benign neoplasm, a certain pleomorphism is a common feature. Axons are not observed within the tumor and myelin is not formed (Friede and Bischhausen, 1979). In general, elaborate, sheet-like expansions of normal mature Schwann cells or perineurial cells are not seen in these neoplasms.

In addition, there is a benign tumor of the peripheral nerve which presents certain distinctly different histological features. It is usually referred to as a neurofibroma to distinguish it from the more common above-mentioned schwannomas. Neurofibromas may be solitary, but more often they are multiple as in von Recklinghausen's disease. In this tumor, Schwann cells and occasional fibroblasts are loosely scattered within the large collagen-containing extracellular space. Mast cells and lymphocytes are sometimes encountered. Blood vessels are infrequent and unlike schwannomas they are not fenestrated. Again, differing from schwannomas, normal-appearing as well as degenerating myelinated and unmyelinated fibers are seen scattered throughout the tumor (Fig. 252).

Neurofibromas consist basically of a spindle-shaped expansion of the peripheral nerve whereas the schwannoma is a neoplastic growth with compression of the pre-existing nerve fibers at its periphery. "Onion bulb" formation resembling that seen in hypertrophic neuropathy was illustrated in multiple neurofibromatosis by

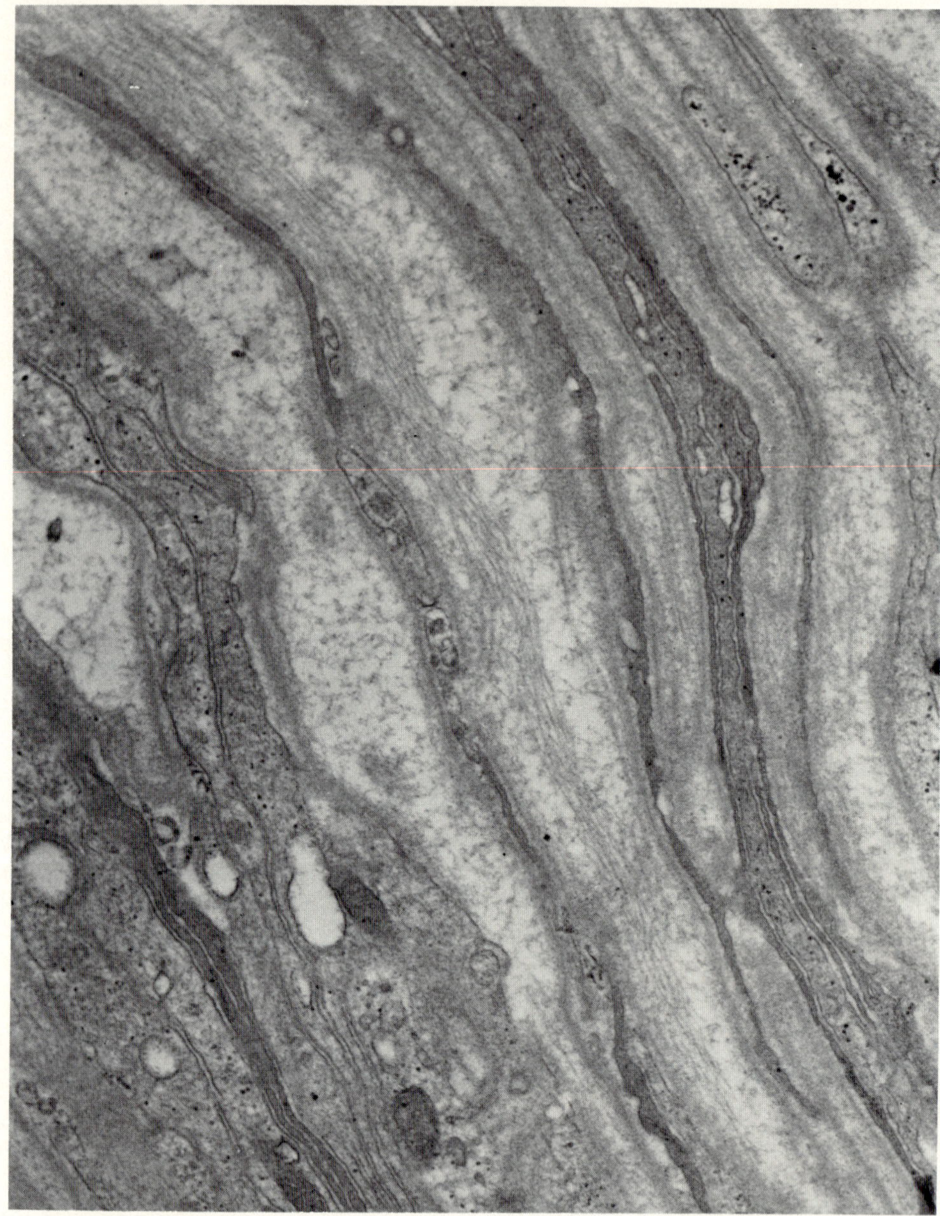

Fig. 251 Parallel arrangement of cell processes in a schwannoma. The surfaces of the processes exposed to the wide extracellular spaces are bounded by basal lamina. × 30,000.

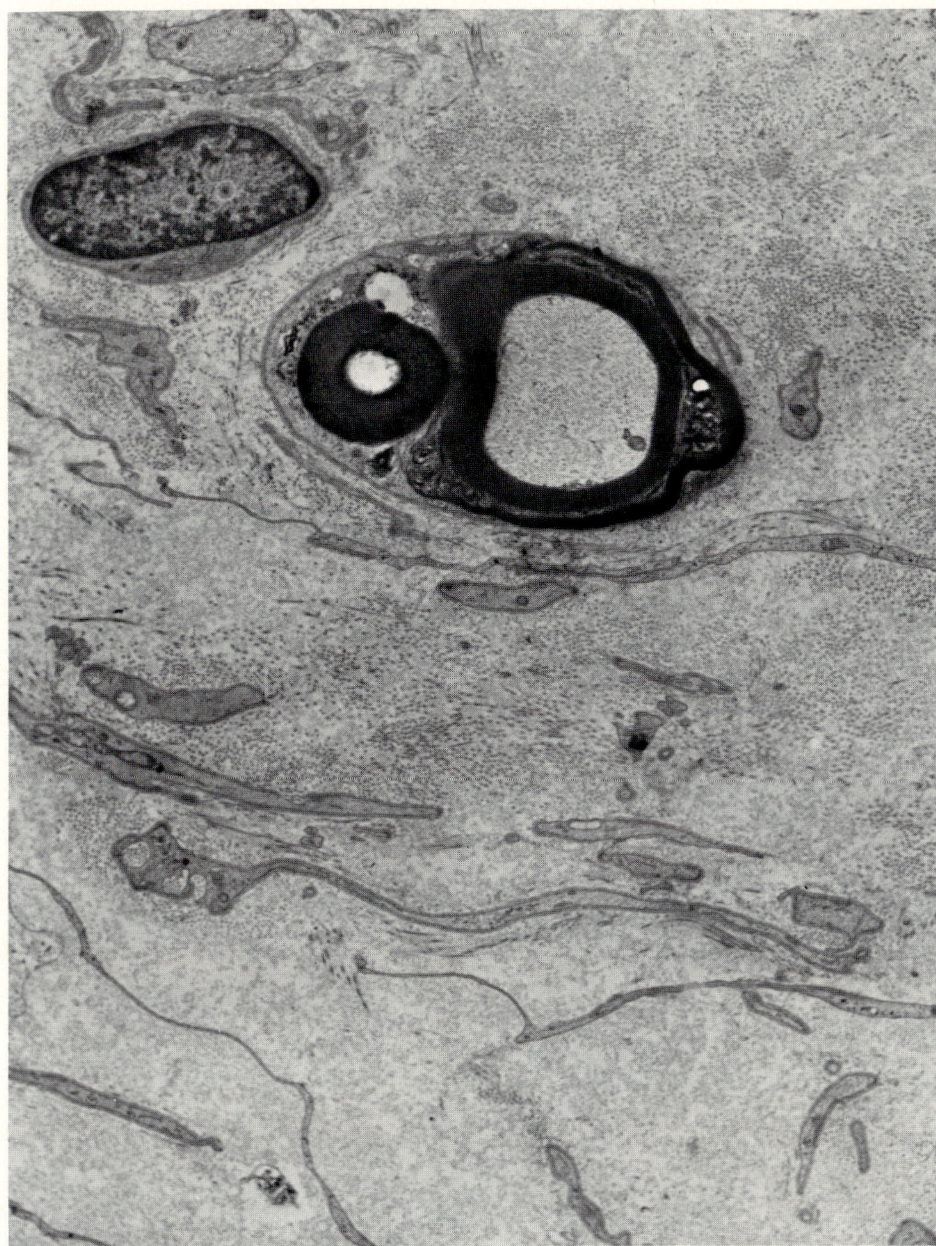

Fig. 252 Neurofibroma. A myelinated axon surrounded by a Schwann cell, is seen within the ample collagen-containing extracellular space. Another basement membrane-bounded Schwann cell is seen in the upper left. Various cell processes are present. × 6,000.

Asbury and Johnson (1978). Further information regarding tumors of peripheral nerves, including malignant schwannomas and nerve cell tumors is available in a number of excellent reviews (Harkin and Reed, 1969; Russel and Rubinstein, 1978, etc.).

REFERENCES

Harkin, J.C., & Reed, R.J.: Tumors of the Peripheral Nervous System. 2nd Series. Fascicle 3, Atlas of Tumor Pathology. Armed Forces Institute of Pathology, Washington, 1969.

Cravioto, H.: The ultrastructure of acoustic nerve tumors. Acta Neuropathol., 2: 116-160, 1969.

Hirano, A., Dembitzer, H.M., & Zimmerman, H.M.: Fenestrated blood vessels in neurilemmoma. Lab. Invest., 27: 305-309, 1972.

Russell, D.S., & Rubinstein, L.J.: Pathology of Tumours of the Nervous System. 4th Ed. Edward Arnold Ltd., London, 1977.

Asbury, A.K., & Johnson, P.C.: Pathology of Peripheral Nerve. Vol. 9 in the series Major Problems in Pathology. Bennington, J.L. (ed.), W.B. Saunders, Philadelphia, 1978.

Friede, R.L., & Bischhausen, R.: Production of myelin by neoplastic cells. Acta Neuropathol., 45: 241-245, 1979.

E. MACROPHAGES, INFLAMMATION AND CONNECTIVE TISSUE (Figs. 253-261)

As in any other organ, macrophages displaying active phagocytic properties may be found in the central nervous system following various injuries (Figs. 253-255). In most transient lesions, such as vascular occlusion or trauma, these cells appear within 48 hours and are prominent from five or six days up to approximately four or five weeks. Occasional macrophages may persist for well over several months.

The nature of the phagocytosed material depends on the location and etiology of the lesion as well as on the stage of the pathological process. On occasion, infectious organisms or other foreign material may be found within the phagocytes. Tissue debris is a common inclusion and, in white matter lesions, fragments of myelin as well as products of its degradation form lipid inclusions (Fig. 255). All of these inclusions become part of the lysosome system of the macrophages.

The question of the origin of the macrophages has been controversial. Hortega

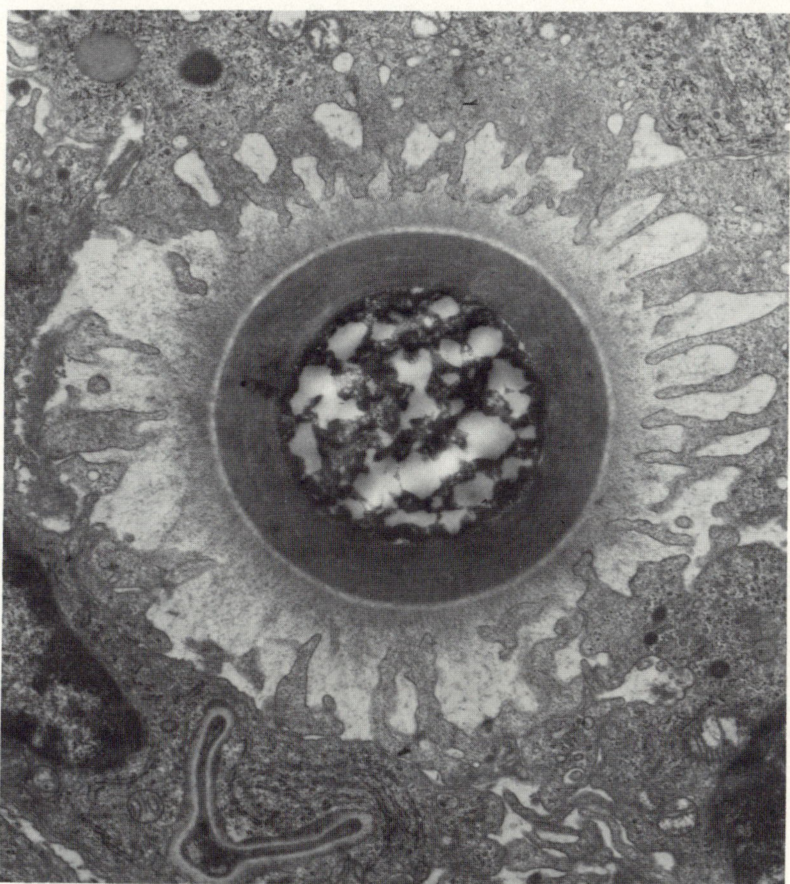

Fig. 253 A cryptococcal cell is surrounded by several macrophages. Many pseudopods have contacted the capsule, but none have penetrated it. × 10,000. (From Levine, S. et al.: Infections of the Nervous System. ARNMD, Vol. 44, p. 393, 1968.)

originally suggested that macrophages were derived from the so-called "resting *microglia*" visible after silver impregnation and which were considered to be normal residents of the central nervous system. These cells were considered to be of mesodermal origin which entered the brain during embryonic vascularization. Fujita and his co-workers (1976), however, have concluded that the resting microglia are neuroectodermal in origin and are not the precursors of macrophages. While some electron microscopists have found it difficult to easily differentiate these cells from oligodendroglia under normal conditions, others have described them as elongated, with marginated chromatin in the nucleus (Vaughn and Skoff, 1972). They are reported to contain dense bodies and a few stacks of well-developed rough endoplasmic reticulum. In contrast to oligodendroglia, microtubules are inconspicuous.

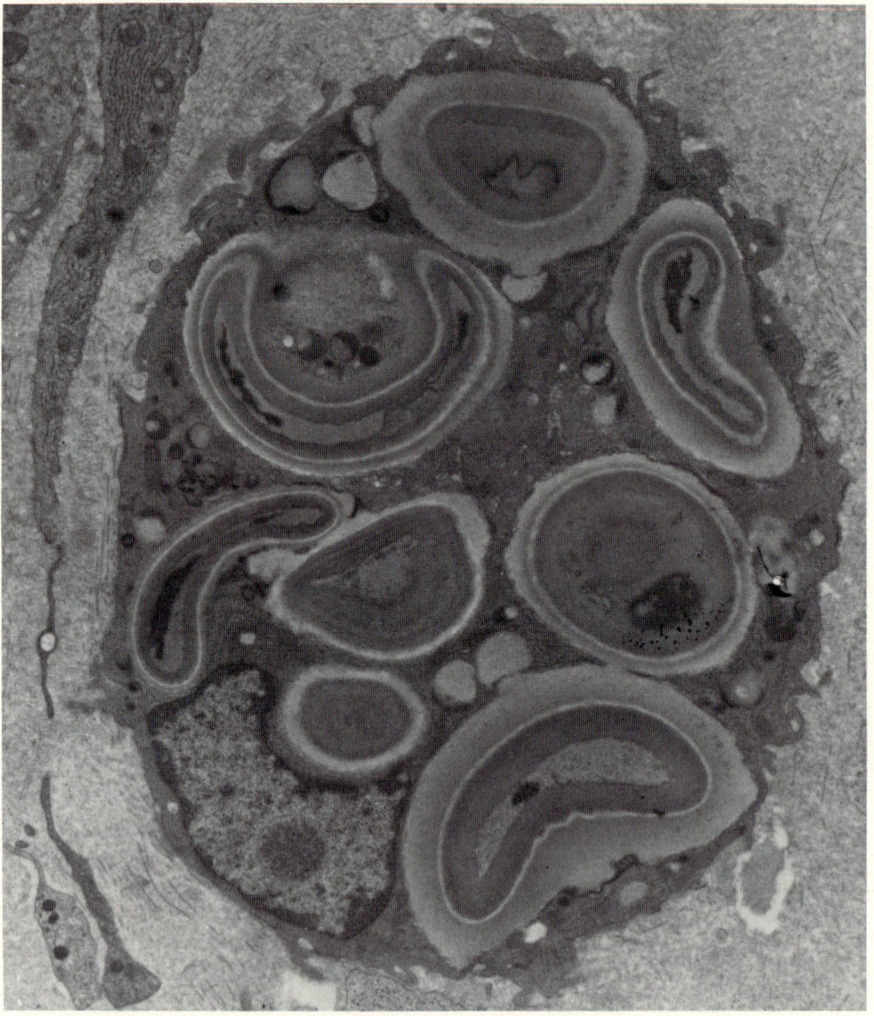

Fig. 254 A phagocyte with eight engulfed cryptoccal cells. × 9,000. (From Levine, S. et al.: Infections of the Nervous System. ARNMD, Vol. 44, p. 393, 1968.)

Pericytes have also been considered as precursors of macrophages. It is known that pericytes can, indeed, act as phagocytes in response to tracer substances such as peroxidase when these materials are introduced into the perivascular space (Cancilla et al., 1972).

In any event, many of the macrophages found in the parenchyma of pathological

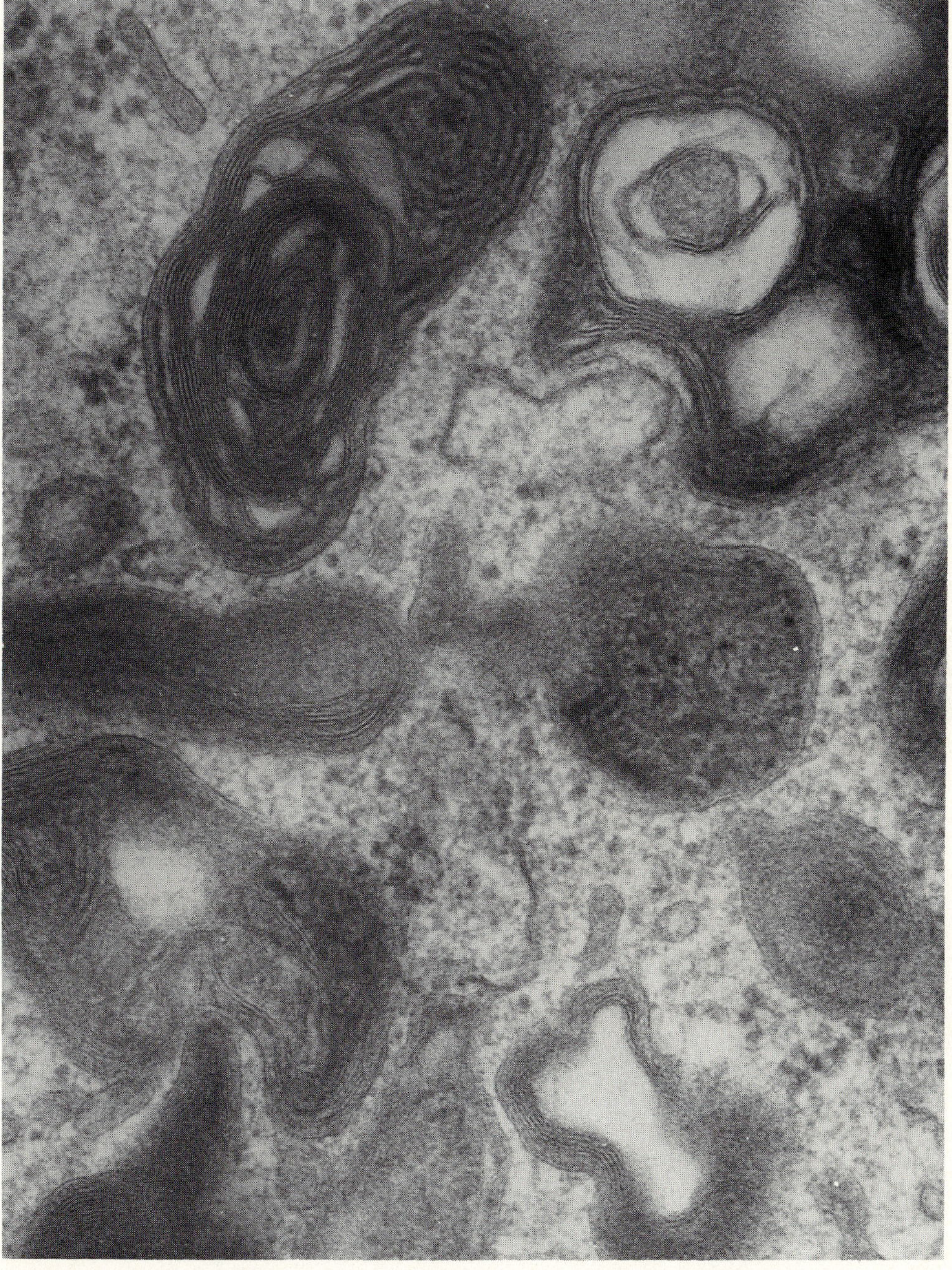

Fig. 255 Laminated bodies in a macrophage in a necrotic area of rat white matter. × 112,000.

tissue are known to be derived from the blood stream. In autoradiographic studies of experimental stab wound or experimental allergic encephalomyelitis it was demonstrated that the vast majority of the macrophages were hematogenous in origin (Konigsmark and Sidman, 1963).

Other hematogenous cells, too, enter the brain during inflammatory processes. During the acute phase polymorphonuclear leucocytes are seen in the lesion. In more chronic stages both lymphocytes and plasma cells are characteristic (Fig. 256).

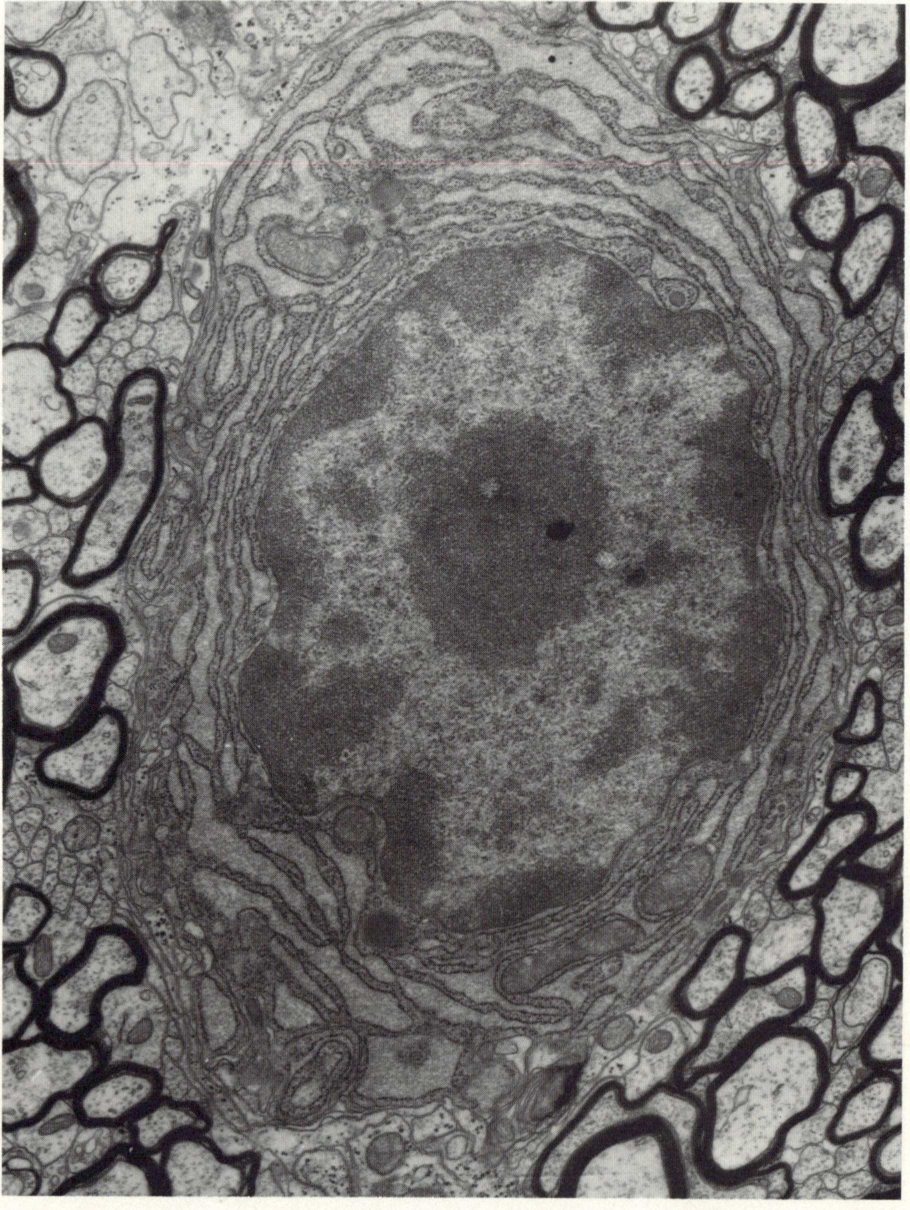

Fig. 256 A plasma cell in the white matter after brain injury. × 16,000. (From Hirano, A.: *In* Progress in Neuropathology. Vol. 1, p. 1, Grune & Stratton, 1971.)

Ordinarily, except for the meninges and the perivascular space of the larger vessels, connective tissue is not present in the central nervous system. After chronic inflammation, however, as well as some other pathological processes, connective

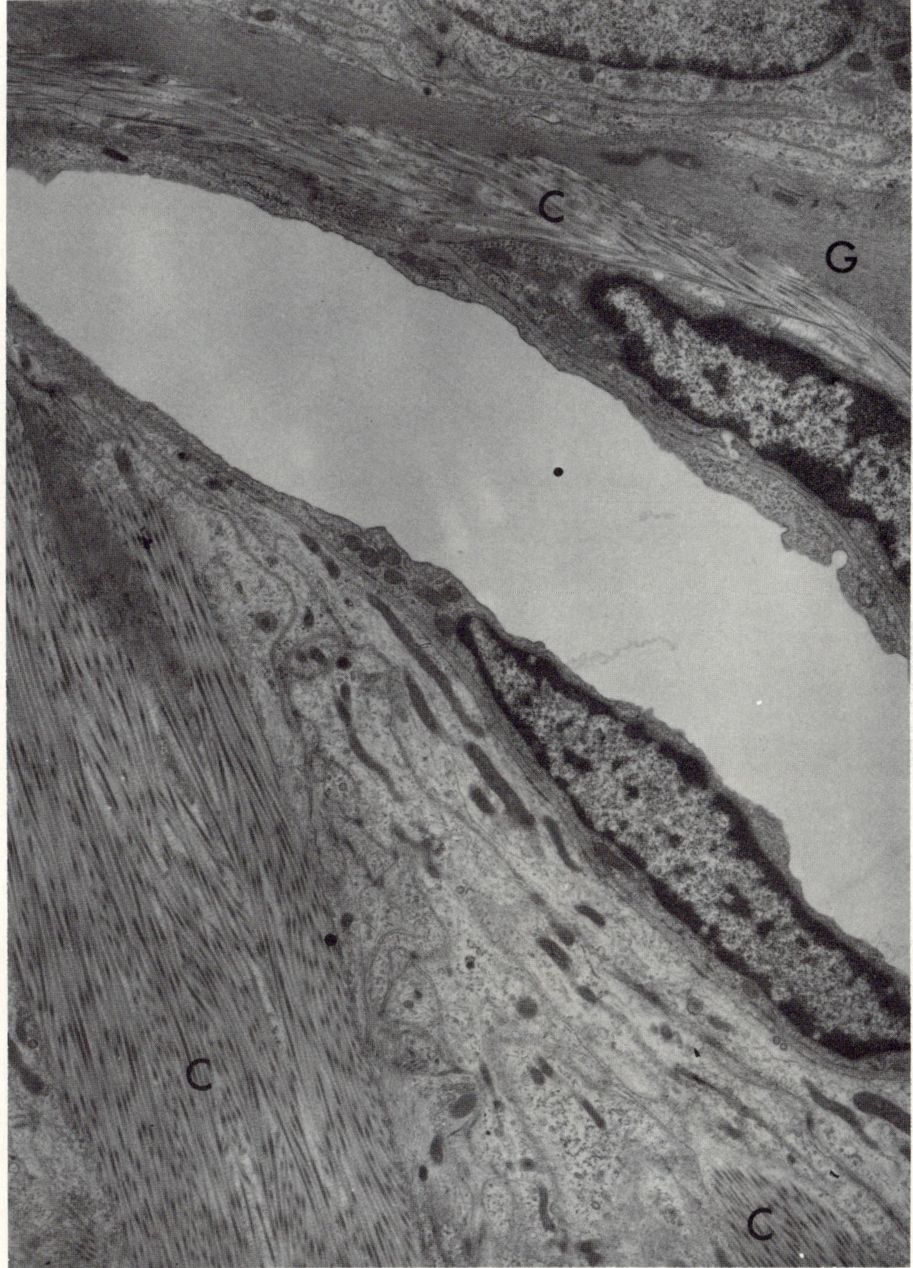

Fig. 257 A perivascular region in the wall of a well-encapsulated brain abscess. Glial fibrils (G) and collagen fibrils (C) are visible. × 18,000. (From Hirano, A.: *In* Progress in Neuropathology. Vol. 1, p. 1, Grune & Stratton, 1971.)

tissue elements such as fibroblasts and collagen fibers may be found (Figs. 257, 258).

Brain abscesses provide a good example of this phenomenon (Fig. 259). The first step in the formation of a brain abscess is infection either by the direct route, i.e. from surrounding bone and other tissue after otitis or sinusitis, etc., or via the

Fig. 258 Collagen fibers × 30,000.

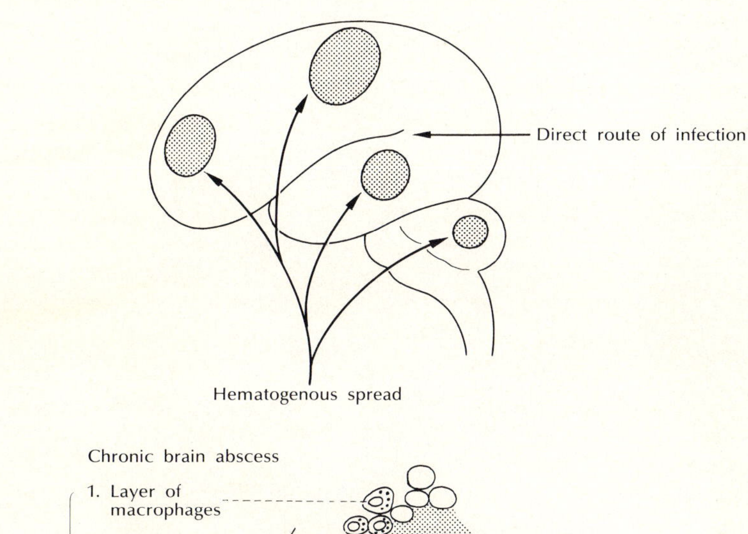

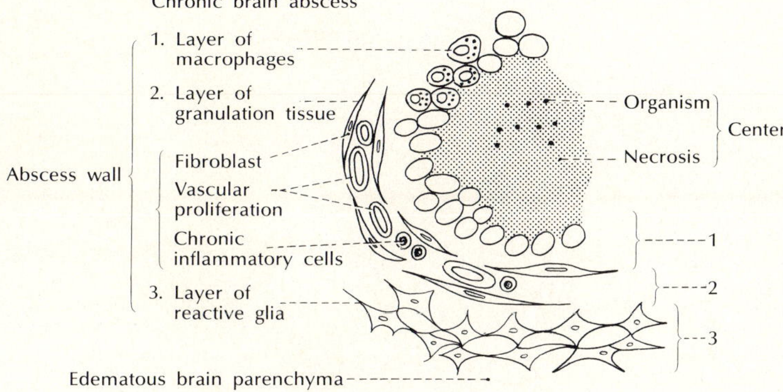

Fig. 259 Brain abscess.

blood stream, usually after bronchiectasis, lung abscess or endocarditis. The organisms most likely to cause infection are Staphylococcus, Streptococcus, or E. (Escherichia) coli which cause necrosis of the brain tissue. The second step consists of an inflammatory reaction to the necrosis in the form of a vascular exudate and intrusion of macrophages associated with a glial reaction. In the chronic stage, the infected and necrotic area is encapsulated by the abscess wall which consists of an inner layer of macrophages surrounded by fibroblasts and proliferated blood vessels. Hematogenous leucocytes infiltrate the abscess wall. The connective tissue is further surrounded by layers of reactive glial cells. The surrounding brain parenchyma becomes edematous.

The histology of viral encephalitis (Fig. 260) is considerably different from that of bacterial infection. Regardless of the specific virus the light microscopic view of acute viral encephalitides are all essentially similar although certain characteristic topographic distributions are seen. Perivascular lymphocytic cuffing is visible in the Virchow-Robin's space and in the subarachnoid space. Mononuclear cells infiltrate into the brain parenchyma along with edema fluid and pervade the neuropil. The neurons in the involved areas display a spectrum of changes ranging from completely normal-looking, despite the presence of viral particles within the cell, to complete cell loss. Between these two extremes one may find satellitosis,

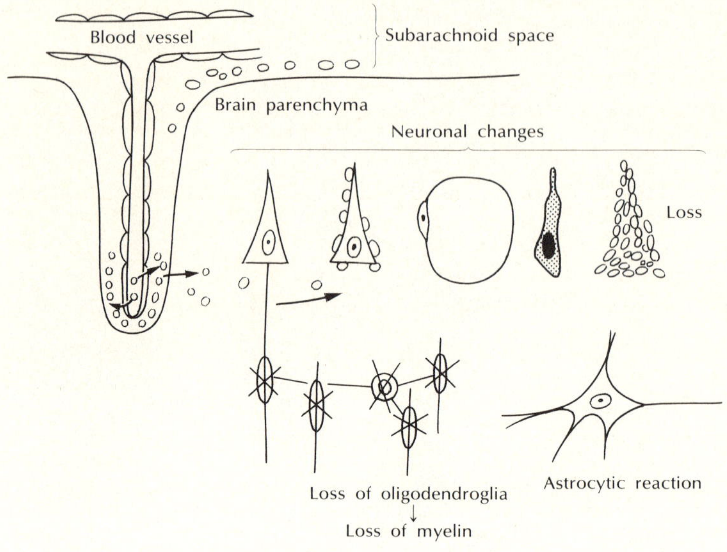

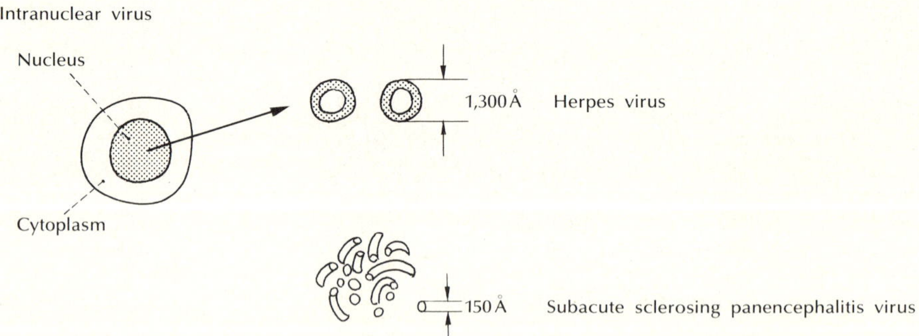

Fig. 260 Viral encephalitis.

chromatolysis, pyknotic changes and neuronophagia. The glial cells, too, react to the presence of the viral infection. Reactive astrocytes are common features and loss of myelin and oligodendroglia may also be present.

In certain viral diseases such as herpes encephalitis and subacute sclerosing panencephalitis, intranuclear eosinophilic inclusions within parenchymal cells constitute diagnostic features. Individual viral particles can be visualized with the electron microscope. Herpes virus appears doughnut-like and approximately 1300Å in diameter (Fig. 261). In subacute sclerosing panencephalitis virus appears as a coiled tube approximately 150Å in diameter. Immunohistochemical methods are also useful for identification of the virus. (Kumanishi and In, 1979).

REFERENCES

Konigsmark, B.K., & Sidman, R.L.: Origin of brain macrophages in the mouse. J. Neuropathol. Exp. Neurol., 22: 327-328, 643-676, 1963.

Hirano, A., Zimmerman, H.M., & Levine, S.: Fine structure of cerebral fluid accumulation. V.

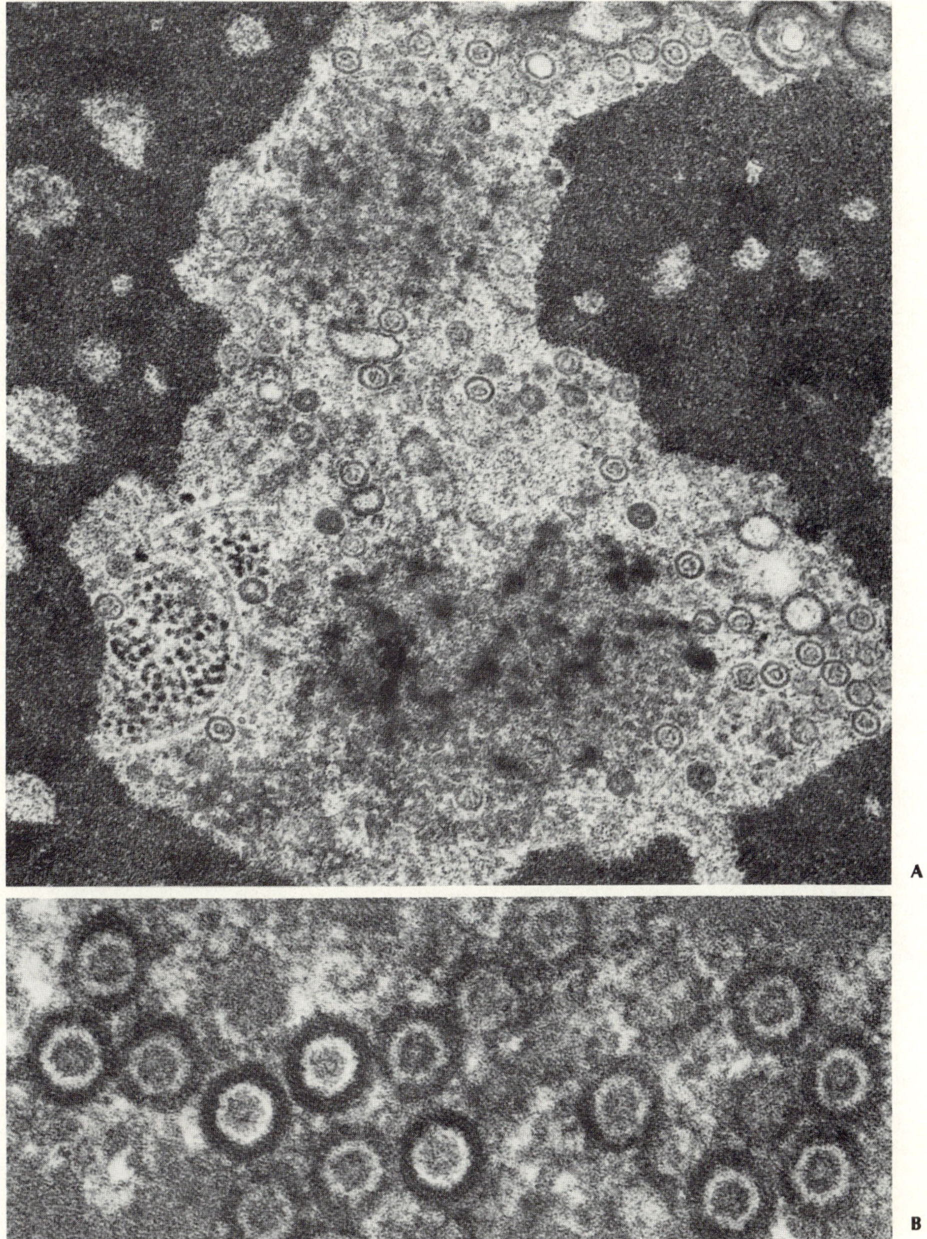

Fig. 261. Herpes encephalitis. A. Virus particles in the nucleus. × 40,000. B. Higher magnification. × 106,000.

Transfer of fluid from extracellular to intracellular compartments in acute phase of cryptococcal polysaccharide lesions. Arch. Neurol., 11: 632-641, 1964.

Levine, S., Hirano, A., & Zimmerman, H.M.: Hyperacute allergic encephalomyelitis. Electron microscopic observations. Am. J. Pathol., 47: 209-221, 1965.

Levine, S., Hirano, A., & Zimmerman, H.M.: The reaction of the nervous system to cryptococcal infection: An experimental study with light and electron microscopy, *In* Infections of the Nervous System: Proceedings of the Association for Research in Nervous and Mental Disease, pp. 393-423, Zimmerman, H.M. (ed.). The Williams & Wilkins Co., Baltimore, 1968.

Cancilla, P.A., Baker, R.N., Pollock, P.S. & Frommes, S.P.: The reaction of pericytes of the central nervous system to exogenous protein. Lab. Invest., 26: 376-383, 1972.

Vaughn, J.E., & Skoff, R.P.: Neuroglia in experimentally altered central nervous system. *In* The Structure and Function of Nervous Tissue. Vol. 5, pp. 39-72, Bourne, G.H. (ed.), Academic Press, New York, 1972.

Kitamura, T., Hattori, H., & Fujita, S.: Autoradiographic studies on histogenesis of brain macrophages in the mouse. J. Neuropathol. Exp. Neurol., 31: 502-518, 1972.

Llena, J.F., Chung, H.D., Hirano, A., Feiring, E.H., & Zimmerman, H.M.: Intracerebellar "fibroma" A case report. J. Neurosurgery, 43: 98-101, 1975.

Hirano, A., Llena, J.F., & Chung, H.D.: Fine structure of a cerebellar "fibroma." Acta Neuropathol., 32: 175-186, 1975.

Fujita, S., & Kitamura, T.: Origin of brain macrophages and the nature of microglia. *In* Progress in Neuropathology. Vol. 3, pp. 1-50. Zimmerman, H.M. (ed.), Grune & Stratton, New York, 1976.

Kitamura, T., Tsuchihashi, Y., Tatebe, A., & Fujita, S.: Electron microscopic features of the resting microglia in the rabbit hippocampus, identified by silver carbonate staining. Acta Neuropathol., 38: 195-201, 1977.

Kumanishi, T., & In, S.: SSPE: Immunohistochemical demonstration of measles virus antigen(s) in paraffin sections. Acta Neuropathol., 48:161-163, 1979.

F. EPENDYMA (Figs. 262, 263)

1. Normal Ependyma

Ependymal cells line almost the entire surface of the ventricles and the central canal of the spinal cord. They are cuboidal in shape and display three well-defined surfaces. The luminal surface is characterized by the presence of cilia with a typical 9+2 arrangement of tubules and by short, stubby microvilli devoid of any coating material such as that seen on the epithelium of the digestive or respiratory tracts. The lateral surfaces display well developed junctional complexes including zonulae and maculae adhaerentes as well as gap junctions and interdigitation of apposing plasma membranes. Tight junctions are absent so that macromolecular tracers such as horseradish peroxidase are free to penetrate the ependymal layer. The basal surface most often abuts directly on the neuronal and glial processes of the neuropil with no intervening basal lamina. On the other hand, when an ependymal cell is in contact with either a perivascular space or the subarachnoid space of the lamina terminalis at the end of the spinal cord, a basal lamina is interposed and hemidesmosomes are present.

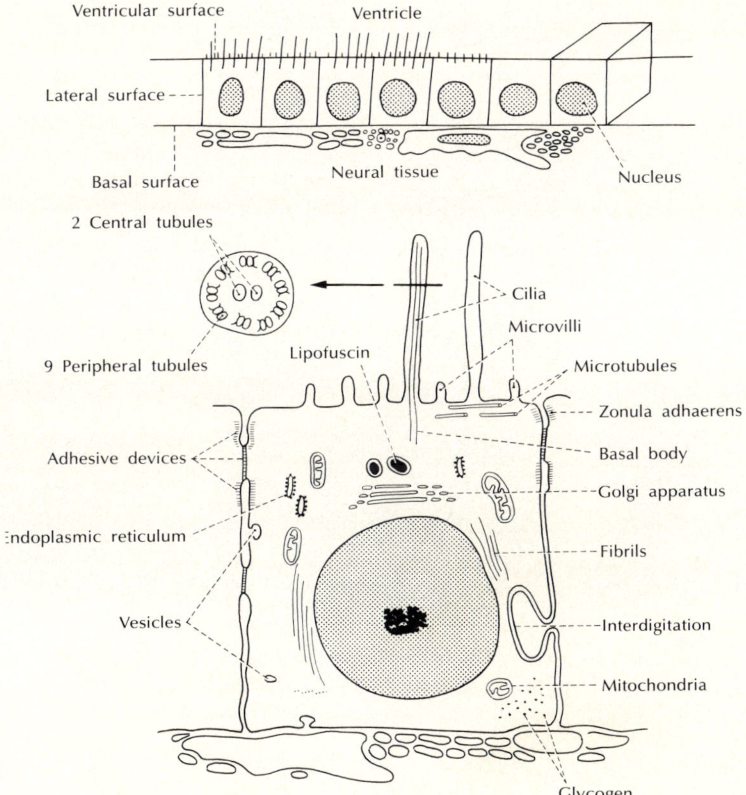

Fig. 262 Ependyma.

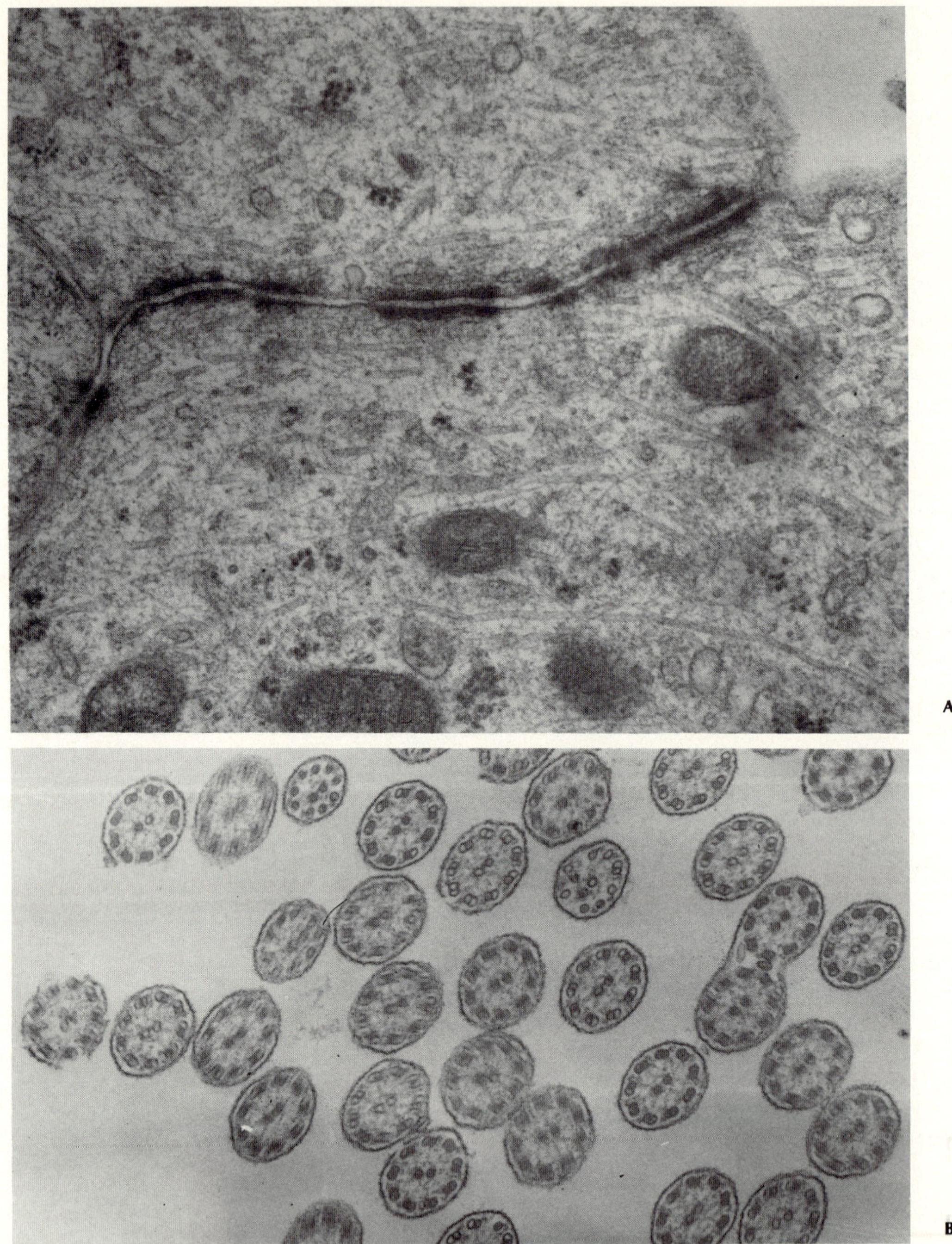

Fig. 263 Ependyma. A. Junctional complex and microtubules. × 175,000. B. Cilia. × 110,000. (From Hirano, A. & Zimmerman, H.M.: Anat. Rec., 158: 293, 1967.)

The ependymal cell body contains all the usual organelles. A Golgi apparatus is present in the apical portion of the cell where dense bodies are also more often found. Microtubules are not common and are confined to the region just below the apical surface; a region which also contains the blepharoplasts or basal bodies of the cilia. Fine filaments, similar to those seen in astrocytes, are present as are a small number of glycogen granules.

A variant of the ependymal cell is the *tanicyte* which is found lining parts of the third ventricle. These cells are typically ependymal at the luminal surface where they provide a cilia-bearing lining. Their lateral surfaces attach to adjacent ependymal cells in the manner described above. Rather than cuboidal, however, the tanicyte cell body is elongated and the basal end of the cell abuts on blood vessels relatively deep in the parenchyma and assumes the features of an astrocytic foot process.

Although the ependyma normally provides an almost continuous lining for the ventricles and the central canal of the spinal cord, the lining of the third ventricle as well as the central canal of the spinal cord contain occasional neuronal processes. These cell processes protrude into the lumen between ependymal cells and are in direct contact with the cerebrospinal fluid (Vigh et al., 1973). One type of cell process which forms cell junctions with adjacent ependymal cells, has cilia with a characteristically 9+0 arrangement of tubules. A second type of process contains both clear and dense core synaptic vesicles. Some workers consider the former receptors for changes in the cerebrospinal fluid, while the latter may serve as secretors of neuroamines. The significance of these neurons is still obscure.

REFERENCES

Brightman, M.W., & Palay, S.L.: The fine structure of ependyma in the brain of the rat. J. Cell Biol., 19: 419-439, 1963.

Hirano, A., & Zimmerman, H.M.: Some new cytological observations of the normal rat ependymal cell. Anat. Rec., 158: 293-302, 1967.

Vigh, B., & Vigh - Teichmann, I.: Comparative ultrastructure of the cerebrospinal fluid-contacting neurons. Internat. Rev., Cytol., 35: 189-251, 1973.

Roy, S., Hirano, A., & Zimmerman, H.M.: Ultrastructual demonstration of cilia in the adult human ependyma. Anat. Rec., 180: 547-550, 1974.

Hirano, A., Matsui, T., & Zimmerman, H.M.: Electron microscopic observations of ependyma. Neurol. Surg. (Tokyo), 3: 237-244, 1975.

2. Pathological Alterations of the Ependyma

REACTIVE CHANGES

Under pathological conditions the ependymal cells display a number of reactions similar to those of astrocytes. After a variety of insults they swell and accumulate large numbers of glycogen granules and fine filaments.

The cell shape can become deformed in other ways as well. In hydrocephalus, for example, the ependyma becomes flattened and stretched. The lateral extracellular spaces become swollen and large pockets form between the desmosomes.

As a result of conditions which lead to the loss of ependymal cells such as ventriculitis, the astrocytic processes of the subependyma proliferate and form a lining for the ventricle. This can lead to glial scars which may protrude into the lumen in the form of irregular nodular protrusions. These are especially prominent in syphilis, tuberous sclerosis and other conditions. When found in the aqueduct they may cause stenosis or obstruction resulting in obstructive hydrocephalus.

REFERENCES

Hirano, A., Zimmerman, H.M., & Levine S.: The fine structure of cerebral fluid accumulation: Reaction of ependyma to implantation of cryptococcal polysaccharide. J. Pathol. Bacteriol., 91: 149-155, 1966.

Weller, R.O., Wisniewski, H., Shulman, K. & Terry, R.D.: Experimental hydrocephalus in young dogs: Histological and ultrastructural study of the brain tissue damage. J. Neuropathol. Exp. Neurol., 30: 613-626, 1971.

Matthews, M.A., St. Onge, M.F., & Faciane, C.L.: An electron microscopic analysis of abnormal ependymal cell proliferation and envelopment of sprouting axons following spinal cord transection in the rat. Acta Neuropathol., 45: 27-36, 1979.

Page, R.B., Rosenstein, J.M., Dovey, B.J., & Leure-du Press, A.E.: Ependymal changes in experimental hydrocephalus. Anat. Rec., 194: 83-104, 1979.

EPENDYMOMA (Figs. 264, 265)

Ependymomas differ from normal ependyma by the loss of the precise, regular arrangement of a single layer lining the ventricular system. Instead, they form large masses of cells showing ependymal rosettes (Fig. 264) and perivascular pseudorosette configuration in some areas. The rosettes consist of small groups of tumor cells arranged around a small lumen reminiscent of a central canal. These cells retain some of their normal fine structural features such as microvilli, cilia on the luminal surface and junctional specializations at their lateral borders. Usually the lumens are obliterated and the miniscule space is filled with microvilli and cilia (Fig. 265). The perivascular pseudorosettes are formed by tumor cells

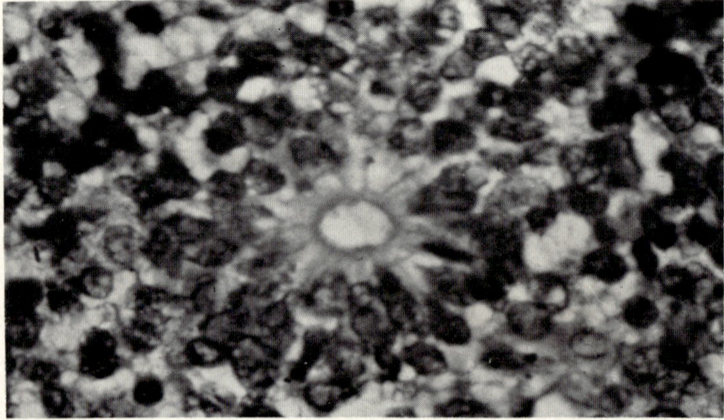

Fig. 264 Ependymal rosettes seen in an ependymal tumor (H&E stain.).

Fig. 265 Ependymoma.
A. Aggregate of microvilli, basal bodies and junctional complexes. × 20,000. B. High magnification of microvilli and a junctional complex. × 64,000. (From Hirano, A.: *In* Progress in Neuropathology. Vol. 1, p. 1, Grune & Stratton, 1971.) ▶

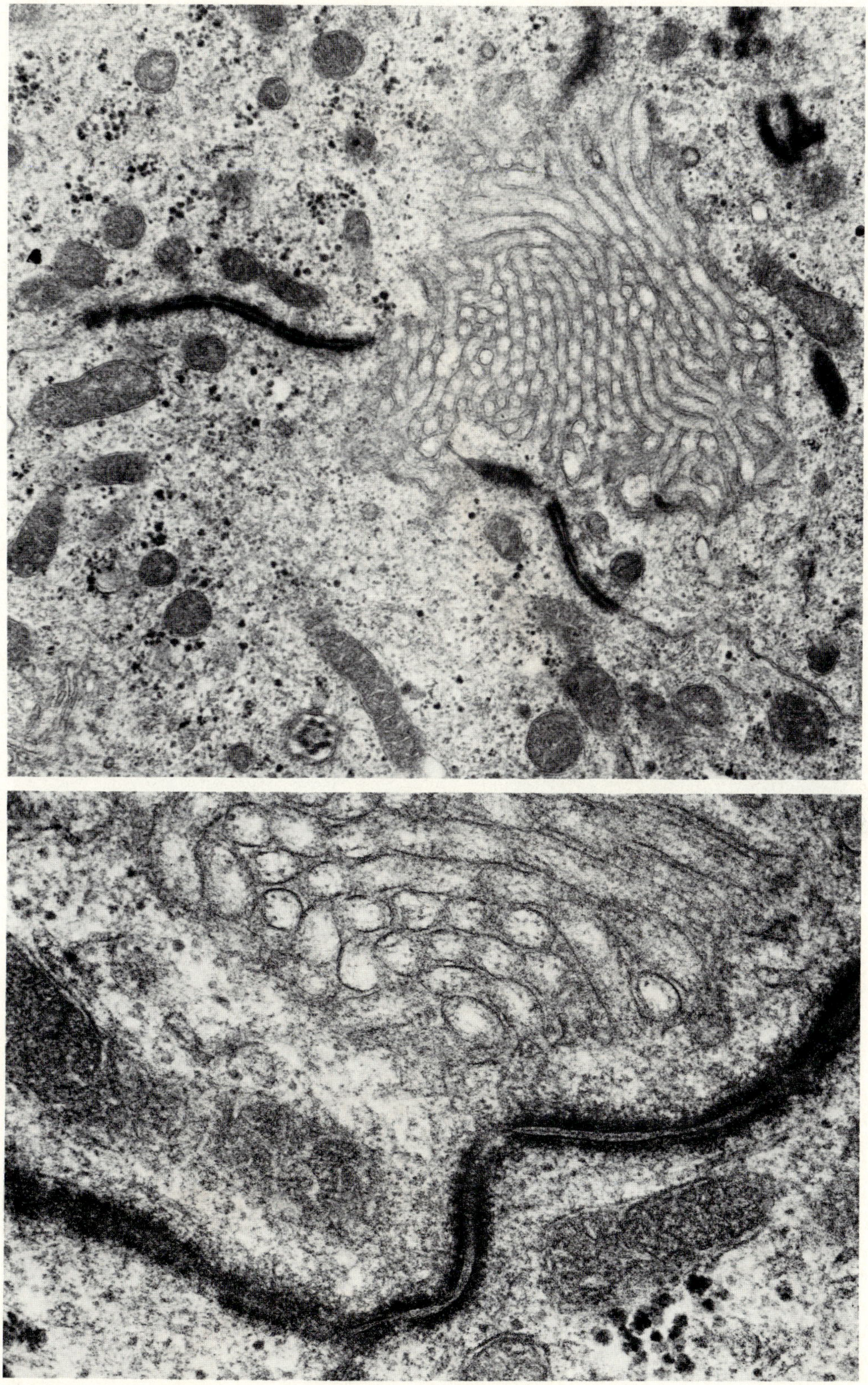

A

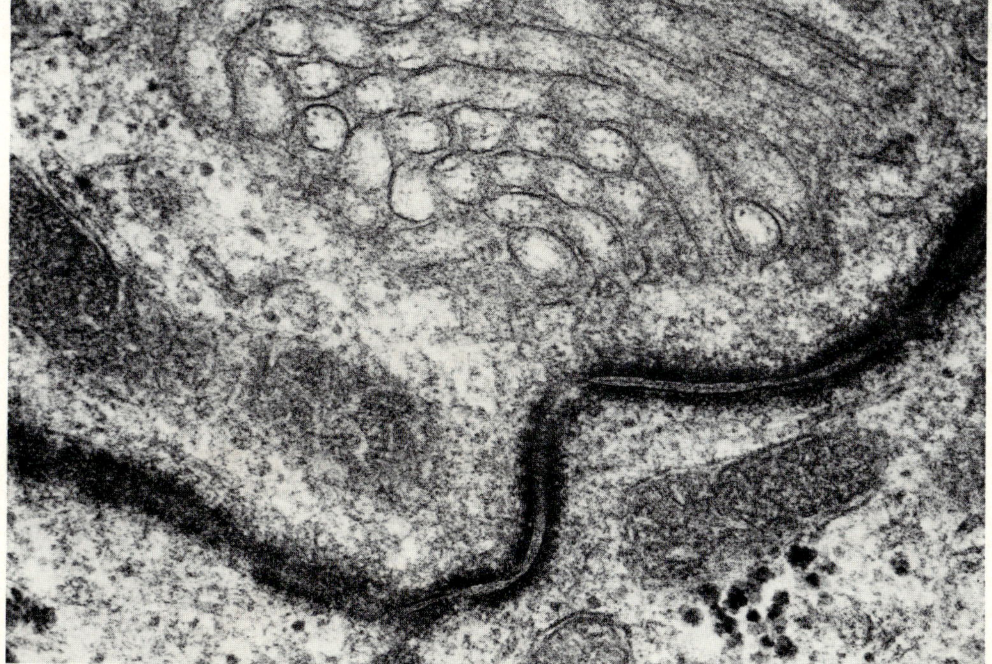

B

arranged around blood vessels. Other fine structural details of the tumor cells differ from those of the normal ependymal cell. Microtubules may be found scattered throughout the cytoplasm in contrast to their confinement to the apical region of normal ependyma. The tumor cells may also show abnormally large numbers of glial fibrils.

REFERENCE

Hirano, A., Matsui, T., & Zimmerman, H.M.: The fine structure of ependymoma. Neurol. Surge. (Tokyo), 3: 557-563, 1975.

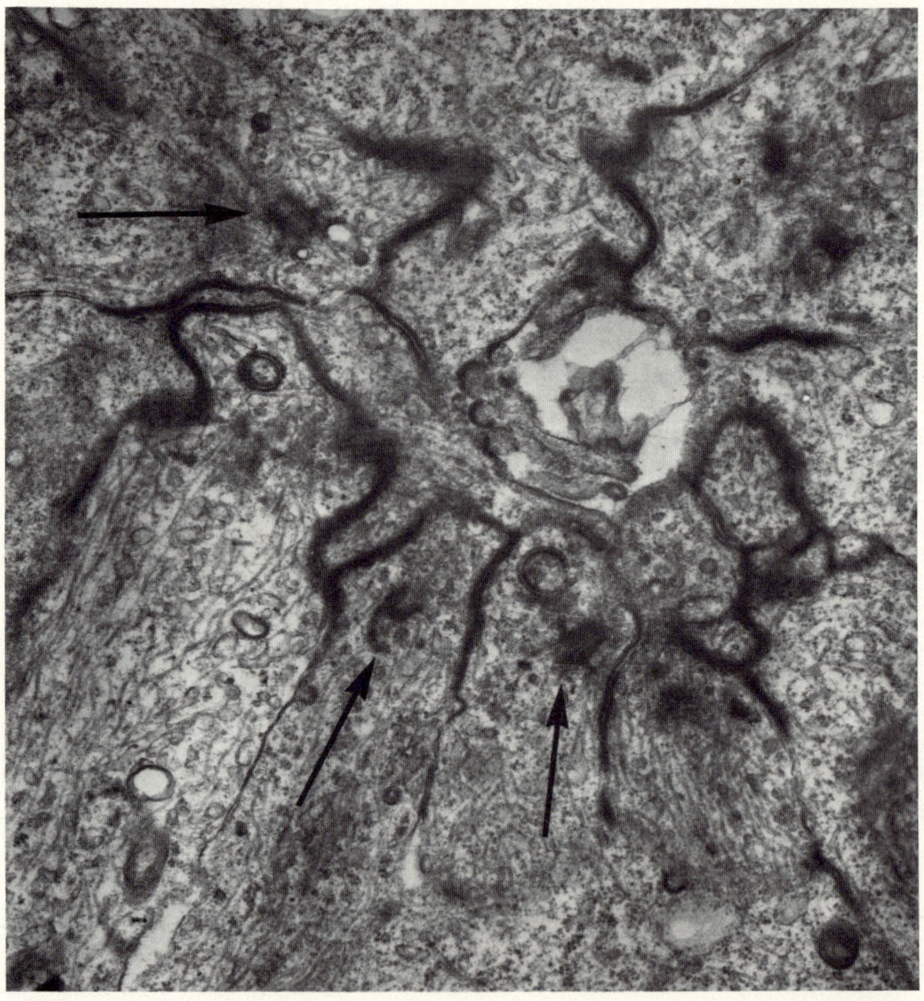

Fig. 266 Rosette-like structure in an ependymoblastoma in the cerebellar vermis. Radially oriented tumor cell processes are arranged around a lumen and are knit together by a network of junctional devices. Each process contains numerous radially arranged microtubules and one or two basal bodies (arrows). × 200. (From Hirano, A. et al.: J. Neuropathol. Exp. Neurol., 32: 144, 1973.)

Myxopapillary Ependymoma

Ependymomas in the filum terminale may display characteristic histological features somewhat different from ependymomas elsewhere. This is due to the accumulation of mucicarmine-positive, hyaline substance in the connective tissue stroma between cuboidal tumor cells and small vessels. Loosely arranged collagen fibers are observed between the basal laminae of the ependymoma cells and of the endothelium.

REFERENCE

Rawlinson, D.C., Herman, M.M., & Rubinstein, L.J.: The fine structure of myxopapillary ependymoma of the filum terminale. Acta Neuropathol., 25: 1-13, 1973.

Subependymal Piloid Astrocytoma (Subependymoma) (Fig. 94)

As its name indicates, this benign, solid, well-defined tumor is found in the subependymal region; often protruding into the ventricle. Abundant, fine, glial fibrillary processes of spindle-shaped cells form diagnostic histological features.

Ependymoblastoma

This is a less differentiated ependymoma and resembles medulloblastoma to a great extent. The presence of occasional ependymal rosettes (Fig. 264) and fine structural features similar to those of developing ependymal cells provide diagnostic clues. Tumor cells are compactly arranged and the ventricular lumen is almost obliterated. Radially oriented cells have only a limited ventricular surface (Fig. 266). Cilia and microvilli, characteristic of ependyma are not formed, but one or two basal bodies may be seen in the apical portion of the cytoplasm. Prominent junctional apparatus is evident between tumor cells at the lateral surfaces.

REFERENCE

Hirano, A., Ghatak, N.R., & Zimmerman, H.M.: The fine structure of ependymoblastoma. J. Neuropathol. Exp. Neurol., 32: 144-152, 1973.

Medulloblastoma (Figs. 267, 268)

Medulloblastomas are malignant tumors predominantly affecting the region of the vermis of the cerebellum in children. The characteristic clinical features are rapidly progressive cerebellar dysfunction and signs of obstructive hydrocephalus. The infiltrating tumor cells tend to seed into the meninges and ventricles spreading over the surface of the neuroaxis. The cells are compactly arranged and show a uniform pattern throughout the tumor. The nuclei are generally hyperchromatic and round and are surrounded by only scanty cytoplasm. Mitosis is common. Rosettes are usually described as characteristic features. This tumor is radiosensitive.

Fine structural examination reveals poorly differentiated cells with a high nucleo-cytoplasmic ratio (Fig. 267). All the usual organelles, including free ribosomes, microtubules, mitochondria and Golgi apparatus are present. Both rough and smooth endoplasmic reticulum are present, but only in small amounts. In one unusual form of the tumor, however, the cells appear spongy due to a marked proliferation of the endoplasmic reticulum (Fig. 268) (Llena et al., 1978). Focal accumulations of 60-90Å fibrils may be found in occasional cells. The cells are compactly arranged with very little extracellular space and occasional punctate adhesions are found between adjacent cells. The background density of the

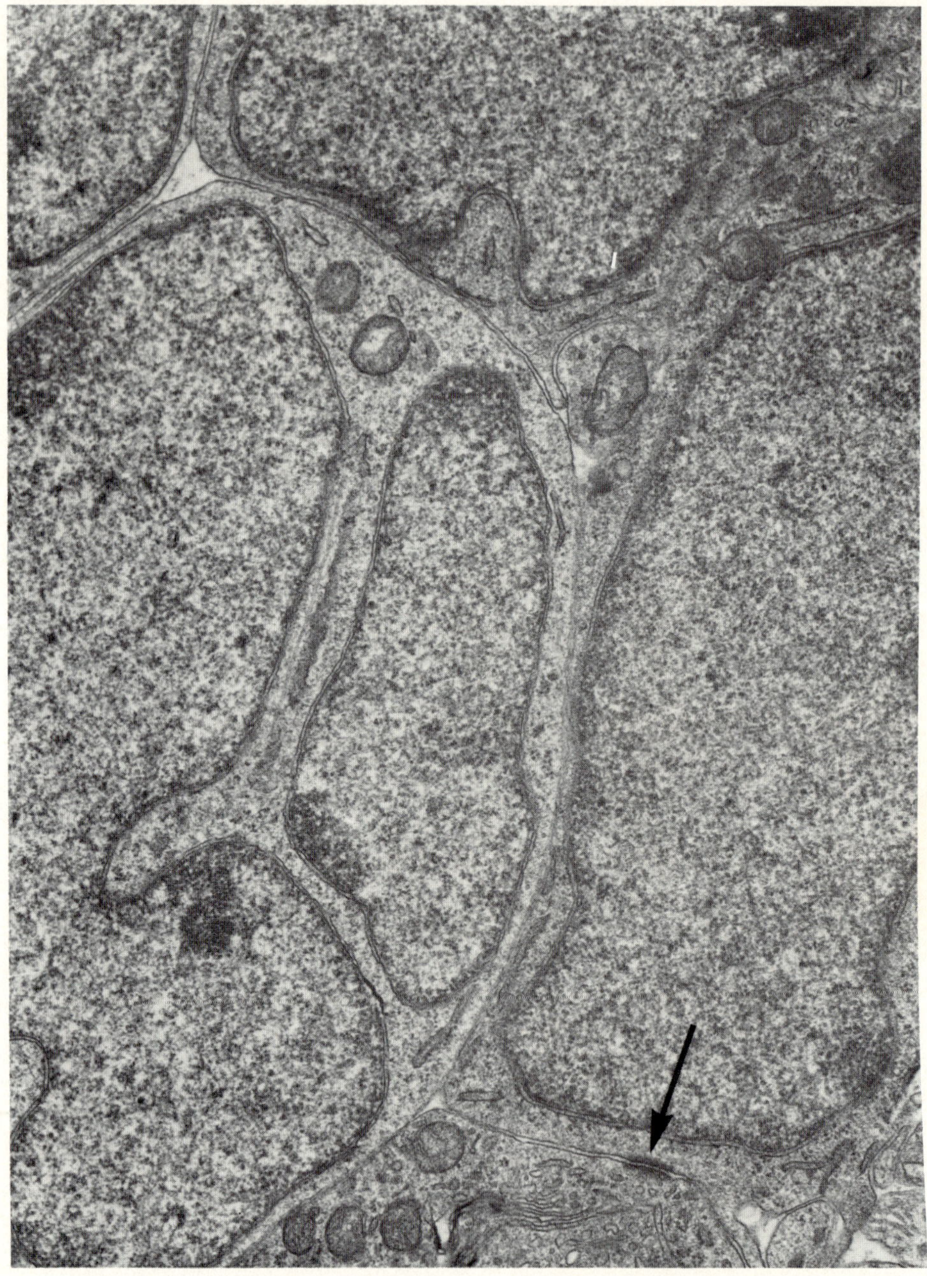

Fig. 267 Medulloblastoma. The arrow indicates a junction. × 26,000.

cytoplasm may vary between cells. The blood vessels within the tumor mass are usually not fenestrated (Hirano et al., 1975).

The origin of medulloblastoma is unclear. The argument centers around the presence of glial-like fibrils and/or microtubules. On these bases various authors have suggested a number of different origins, including neuroblasts, glioblasts or some other more primitive cell which gave rise to both of the above. Other workers

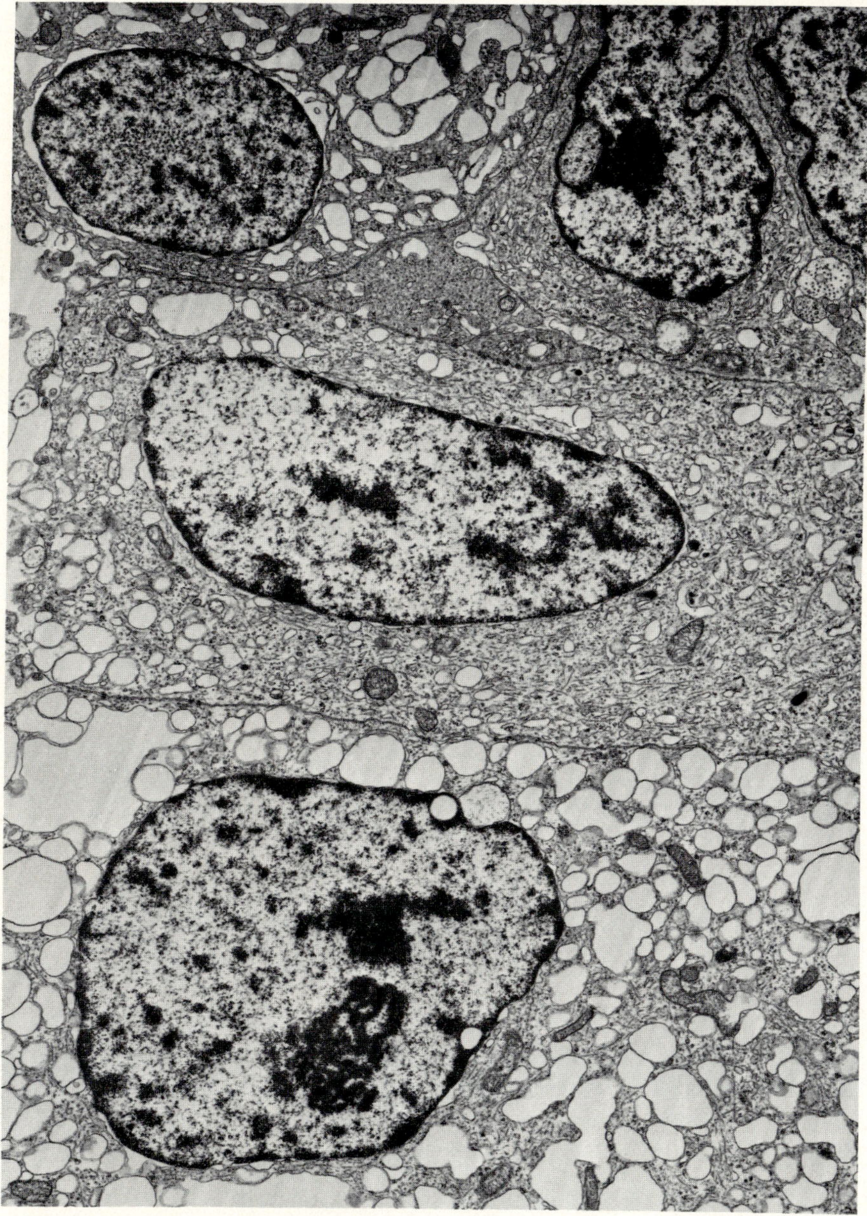

Fig. 268 Tumor cells with various degrees of distension of the smooth endoplasmic reticulum in a spongy variant of medulloblastoma. × 4,500. (From Llena, et al.: Acta Neuropathol., 44: 83, 1978.)

consider a mixed origin for medulloblastoma. The reason for the uncertainty is probably based on the fact that all of the fine structural criteria used are generally nonspecific in nature. Furthermore, one must keep in mind that, due to its infiltrative nature, medulloblastomas are likely to entrap nonneoplastic cells within it giving rise to confusing observations. It is worth pointing out that, except for a single case reported by Ermel and Brucher (1974), synapses have not been described in medulloblastomas. Reports of smooth muscle filaments within the tumor cells of certain variations of medulloblastoma raise additional possibilities concerning the origin of medulloblastoma (Misugi and Liss, 1971; Stahlberger and Friede, 1977).

REFERENCES

Misugi, K., & Liss, L.: Medulloblastoma with cross-striated muscle. Cancer, 25: 1279-1285, 1970.

Ermel, A.E., & Brucher, J.M.: Arguments ultrastructuraux en faveur de l'appartenance du medulloblastome a la lignée neuronale. Acta Neurol. Belg., 74: 208-220, 1974.

Hassoun, J., Hirano, A., & Zimmerman, H.M.: Fine structure of intercellular junctions and blood vessels in medulloblastomas. Acta Neuropathol., 33: 67-78, 1975.

Malamud, N., & Hirano, A.: Atlas of Neuropathology, 2nd ed., University of California Press, Berkeley, 1974. pp. 242-243.

Stahlberger, R., & Friede, R.L.: Fine structure of myomedulloblastoma. Acta Neuropathol., 37: 43-48, 1977.

Llena, J.F., Hirano, A., & Wisoff, H.S.: Fine structure of an unusual spongy variant of medulloblastoma. Acta Neuropathol., 44: 83-84, 1978.

G. CHOROID PLEXUS (Figs. 269-271)

The choroid plexus consists of an epithelium-covered, convoluted extension of the subarachnoid space into the body and temporal horns of the lateral ventricle, the third ventricle and the posterior half of the fourth ventricle. It is the major source of cerebrospinal fluid.

The single layered cuboidal epithelial surface is continuous with the ependymal lining but the cells differ in certain important respects. The choroidal cells are larger than those of the ependyma. All the usual organelles are present and they are more abundant than in ependymal cells. Mitochondria, Golgi apparatus and rough endoplasmic reticulum as well as free ribosomes and vesicles crowd the cytoplasm. The luminal surfaces are much more heavily populated by microvilli, which are larger than those of the ependyma and which are club-shaped rather than short and stubby. Cilia are absent except for those cells at the border of the choroid plexus. The lateral surfaces show tight junctions at the luminal shoulder which prevent the passage of macromolecules, such as horseradish peroxidase between the lumen and the interstitial spaces. Desmosomes are also present and interdigitation is particularly well developed, especially along the basal third or quarter of the lateral surfaces. The basal surface is separated from the underlying connective tissue by a basal lamina. The numerous blood vessels of the choroid plexus have lumens larger than most intracerebral capillaries and, unlike almost any other vessel in the central nervous system, they are lined by a heavily fenestrated endothelium.

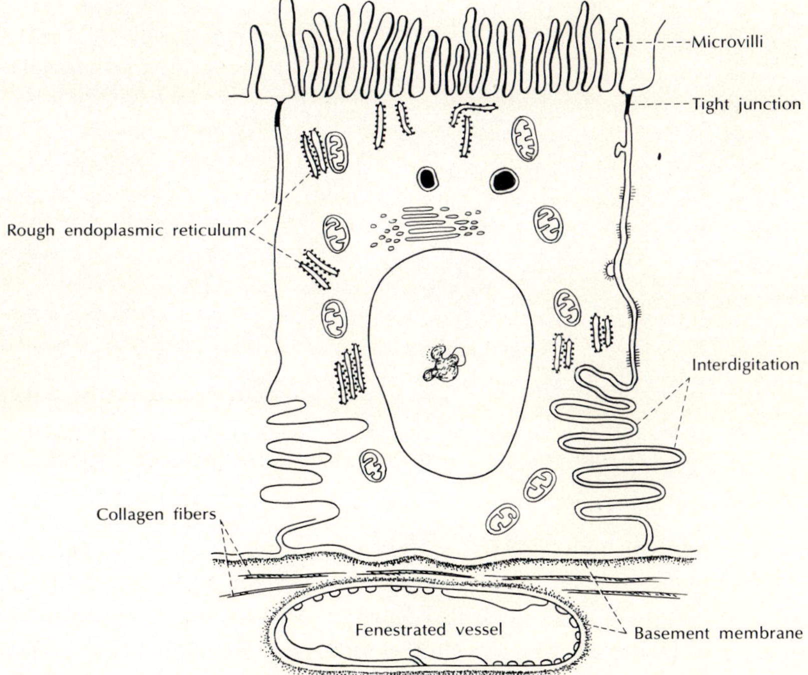

Fig. 269 Choroid plexus.

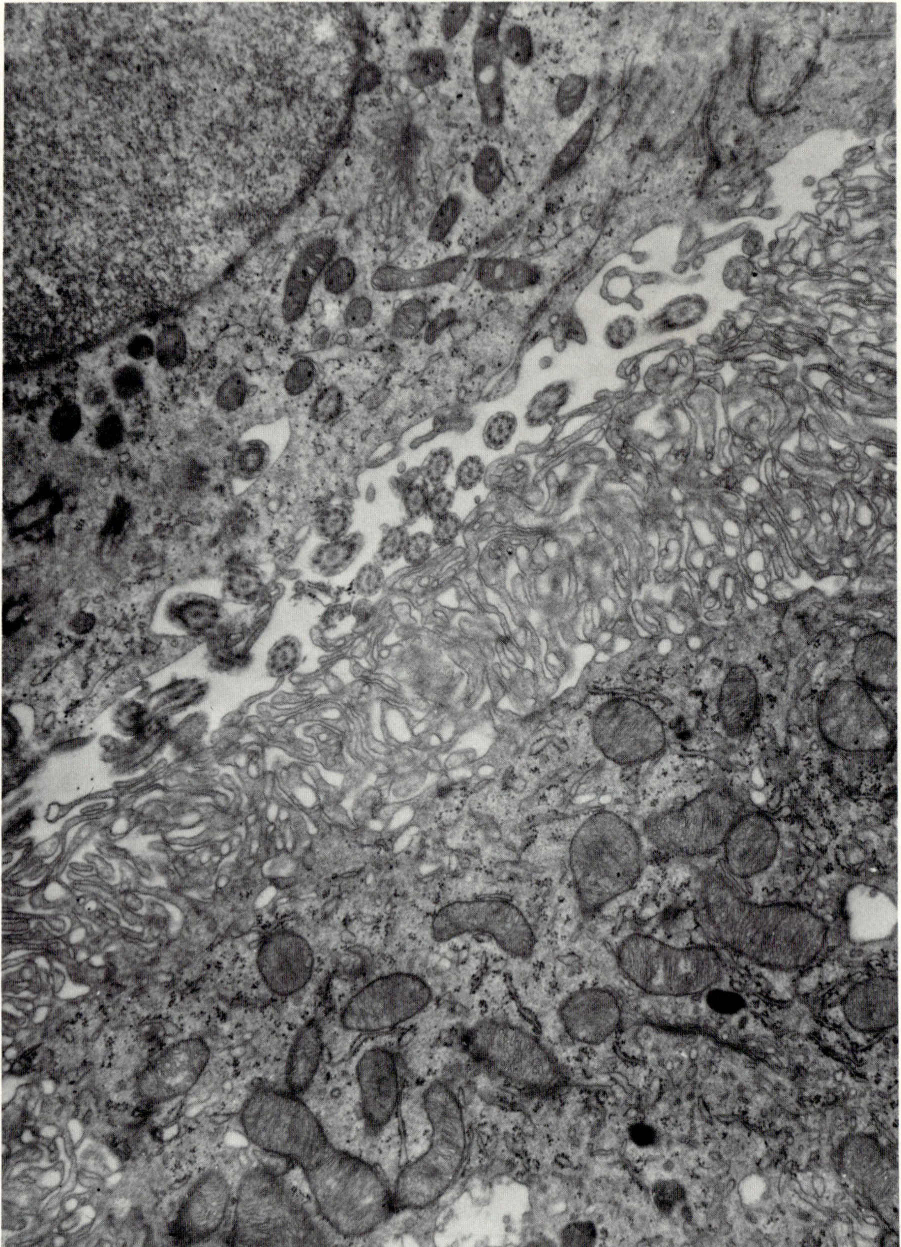

Fig. 270 Portion of ependyma (upper left) and choroid plexus (lower right) in the rat. Compare the shape of the villi and size of the mitochondria between the two cell types. × 20,000.

Aging often results in characteristic changes of the choroid plexus especially at the choroid glomus which is a protrusion of the choroid plexus at the junction of the body, temporal horn and occipital horn of the lateral ventricle. Connective tissue fiber accumulation occurs, associated with proliferation of granulation tissue, cyst formation, cholesterol deposition, and hyaline degeneration (multiloculated xanthogranuloma). Psammoma bodies are often found in these regions which become visible in plain skull x-rays.

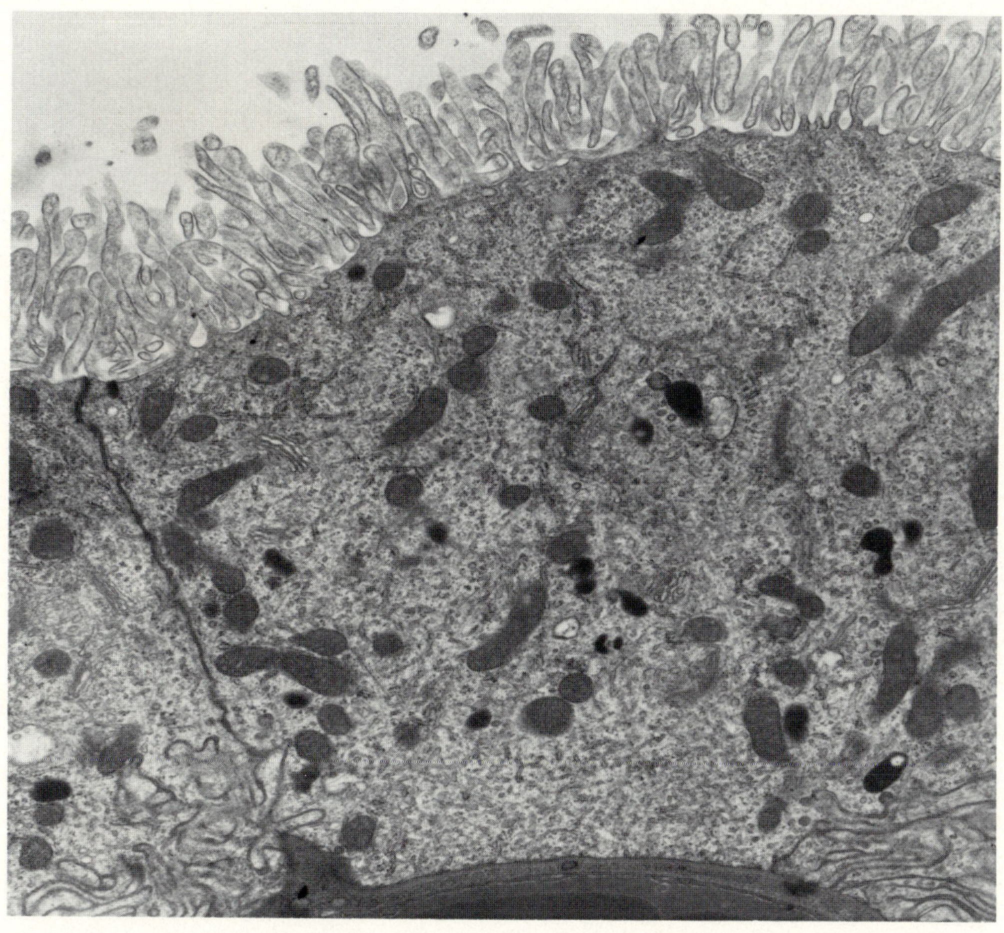

Fig. 271 Choroid plexus. × 14,000.

Pathological changes include *choroid plexus papilloma* which is usually seen in neonates (Ghatak and McWhorter, 1976). The accompanying overproduction of cerebrospinal fluid results in hydrocephalus. Vacuolar disintegration confined to the choroid plexus epithelium has been induced in experimental animals by the systemic administration of some tertiary amines (Levine, 1977; Wenk et al., 1979).

REFERENCES

Hoenig, E.M., Ghatak, N.R., Hirano, A., & Zimmerman, H.M.: Multiloculated cystic tumor of the fourth ventricle choroid plexus. Report of a case. J. Neurosurg., 27: 574-579, 1967.

Netsky, M.G., & Shuangshoti, S.: The Choroid Plexus in Health and Disease. University Press of Virginia, Charlottesville, Va., 1975.

Ghatak, N.R., & McWhorter, J.M.: Ultrastructural evidence for CSF production by a choroid plexus papilloma. J. Neurosurg., 45: 409-415, 1976.

Levine, S: Degeneration of choroid plexus epithelium induced by some tertiary amines. *In* Neurotoxicology, pp. 419-425, Roizin, L., Shiraki, H., Grcevic, N., (eds.), Raven Press, New York, 1977.

Wenk, E.J., Levine, S., & Hoenig, E.M.: Fine structure of contrasting choroid plexus lesions caused by tertiary amines or cyclophosphamide. J. Neuropathol. Exp. Neurol., 38: 1-9, 1979.

H. MENINGES

1. Dura Mater

The dura mater is divided into internal and external layers each composed, for the most part, of a sheet of tightly packed, parallel collagen fibers and occasional fibroblasts. The orientation of the fibers within each layer is roughly at right angles to the other. Most blood vessels, including the venous sinuses lie between the layers along with lymphatics and some nerves.

Hematomas, both epidural and subdural, are among the most common pathological changes associated with the dura mater. The pathogenesis of these changes have been described in the legends to Figs. 8 and 9.

2. Leptomeninges

NORMAL ANATOMY

The leptomeninges are situated between the dura and the brain parenchyma. They are constituted of the arachnoid membrane and the pia mater which are connected by numerous trabeculae.

The brain parenchyma is covered by a continuous layer of astrocytic processes connected by punctate adhesions known as the glial limiting membrane. These processes are separated from the pia mater by a basal lamina. The pial cells form a loosely arranged layer of cells which underlie the subarachnoid space and which are joined by occasional junctions, but in which zonulae occludentes are not present. The outer surface of the subarachnoid space is covered by several layers of closely arranged cells joined by tight junctions, which form the arachnoid membrane. Extensions of the arachnoid cells reach through the subarachnoid space where they join processes from the pial cells and form the trabeculae of the subarachnoid space. The cells of the trabeculae are joined by gap junctions and puncture adhesions (Nabeshima et al., 1975). Fibroblasts and collagen fibers may be found among them. Blood vessels, mostly arteries and veins, permeate the trabeculae and course through the subarachnoid space. Although rare under normal conditions, some capillaries are present (Hirano et al., 1976; Ohsugi and Hirano, 1976). The permeability characteristics of the endothelium of the blood vessels of the subarachnoid space are similar to those of the cerebrum providing a blood-cerebrospinal fluid barrier in the subarachnoid space. On the other hand, vesicular transport of horseradish peroxidase has been shown to occur across some arteriolar endothelium in limited regions of the subarachnoid space of the mouse brain (Westergaard and Brightman, 1973).

The arachnoid membrane forms a permeability barrier between the subdural space and the central nervous system. Tracer substances such as horseradish peroxidase, when introduced into the subarachnoid space penetrate to the pia mater and find their way into the brain parenchyma, but are excluded from the subdural space.

Movement of cerebrospinal fluid between the subarachnoid space and the venous sinuses of the dura mater is mediated by the arachnoid villi. These consist of a column of arachnoid cells which penetrate the collagen of the internal layer of the dura mater and form an endothelial-covered protrusion into the sinus lumen (Shabo and Maxwell, 1968)

REFERENCES

Shabo, A.L., & Maxwell, D.S.: The morphology of the arachnoid villi: A light and electron microscopic study in the monkey. J. Neurosurg., 29: 451-463, 1968.

Westergaard, E., & Brightman, M.W.: Transport of proteins across normal cerebral arterioles. J. Comp. Neurol., 152: 17-44, 1973.

Nabeshima, S., Reese, T.S., Landis, D., & Brightman, M.W.: Junctions in the meninges and marginal glia. J. Comp. Neurol., 164: 127-170, 1975.

Hirano, A., Cervós-Navarro, J., & Ohsugi, T.: Capillaries in the subarachnoid space. Acta Neuropathol., 34: 81-85, 1976.

Ohsugi, T., & Hirano, A.: Are there capillaries in the subarachnoid space? Neurol. Med. (Tokyo), 4: 233-241, 1976.

PATHOLOGICAL ALTERATIONS OF THE LEPTOMENINGES

Meningitis (Fig. 272)

Meningitis is most often due to bacterial infection which reaches the brain either via the bloodstream or directly as the result of inflammation in adjacent tissues, especially the bones. Mastoiditis due to otitis media and subsequent thrombophlebitis, nasal sinusitis and fracture, are common sources of infection. The organisms most often responsible for acute purulent meningitis are meningococcus, pneumococcus and hemophilus influenzae. Staphylococcus, streptococcus and Escherichia coli are less common, but are more likely to result in brain abcess.

During acute stages of infection edema fluid, polymorphonuclear leukocytes, red blood cells and fibrin accumulate within the leptomeninges. In the chronic stages lymphocytes, plasma cells and macrophages are seen. Pronounced proliferation of connective tissues and meningeal cells occurs which may result in obstructive hydrocephalus.

Infection by the tubercle bacillus or the syphilitic spirochete can result in chronic granulomatous meningitis with the formation of tuberculoma characterized by caseous necrosis or of gumma in the case of syphilis. These changes are most pronounced in the basal aspects of the brain and are referred to as basal meningitis.

In addition to bacteria, certain fungal infections may also result in meningitis. Cryptococcus is the most well known among these. Other fungal infections are actinomycosis, coccidiomycosis, blastomycosis, mucormycosis, candidiosis (moniliasis), nocardiosis and aspergillosis.

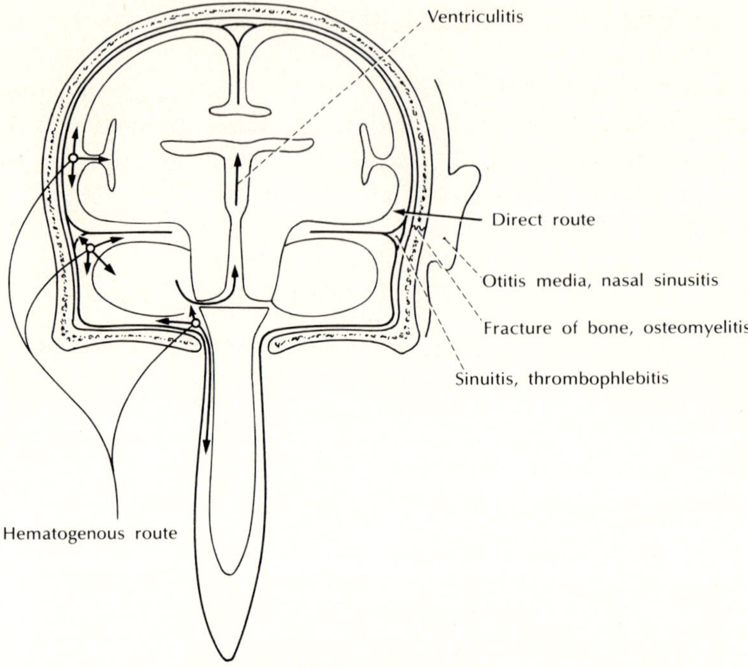

Fig. 272 Meningitis.

Meningioma (Figs. 273-275)

The principal element of meningioma is the neoplastic arachnoid cell. Whorl formation and the presence of psammoma bodies constitute the characteristic features at the light microscopic level (Fig. 273).

Fine structural study reveals that one of the most prominent features of meningioma cells is the highly irregular cell surface characterized by the interdigitation of numerous narrow sheet-like cell processes (Fig. 274). Many desmosomes are evident along the cell borders so that, for the most part, the extracellular space is quite narrow. Normal arachnoidal cells also display elongated cell processes which are connected to one another by cell junctions including desmosomes, gap and tight junctions (Tani et al., 1974). In contrast to meningiomas, however, the normal leptomeninges are characterized by an ample extracellular space, that is, the subarachnoid space. On the other hand, some areas within meningiomas contain large extracellular spaces which may include large numbers of collagen fibers, some of which appear much wider than normal. Often, calcium deposits are present in the same areas, around which collagen and tumor cells arrange themselves in a concentric fashion. The tumor cells themselves contain the usual organelles but are often marked by highly irregular nuclei so that, sometimes, extensions of cytoplasm appear within the nucleus (Fig. 275). These are the nuclear inclusions described by light microscopy. In addition, some glycogen is occasionally seen, but more prominent is the frequent presence of filaments which sometimes accumulate in large numbers.

The blood vessels of meningiomas are fenestrated (Cervós-Navarro, 1971) unlike those of the normal meninges. Some of the psammoma bodies originate from degenerated blood vessels. Thus, in addition to the usual round configuration, some of the psammoma bodies appear cylindrical and may form branches (Gonatas and Besen, 1963).

REFERENCES

Gonatas, N.K., & Besen, M.: An electron microscopic study of three human psammomatous meningiomas. J. Neuropathol. Exp. Neurol., 22: 263-273, 1963.

Poon, T.P., Hirano, A., & Zimmerman, H.M.: Electron Microscopic Atlas of Brain Tumors. Grune & Stratton, New York, 1971.

Cervós-Navarro, J.: Electronenmikroskopie der Hemangioblastoma des ZNS und der angioblastischen Meningiome. Acta Neuropathol., 19: 184-207, 1971.

Tani, E., Ikeda, K., Yamagata, S., Nishiura, M., & Higashi, N.: Specialized junctional complexes in human meningioma. Acta Neuropathol., 28: 305-315, 1974.

Kawamoto, K., Herz, F., Kajikawa, H., & Hirano, A.: An ultrastructural study of cultured human meningioma cells. Acta Neuropathol., 46: 11-15, 1979.

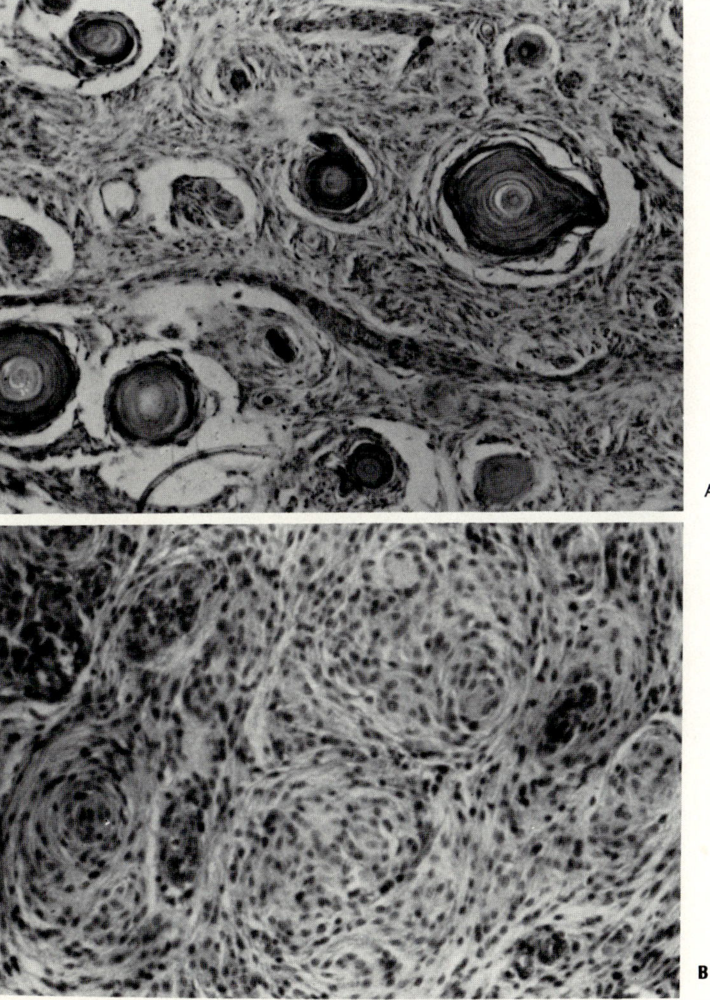

Fig. 273 Meningioma (H&E). A. Psammoma bodies. B. Whorls.

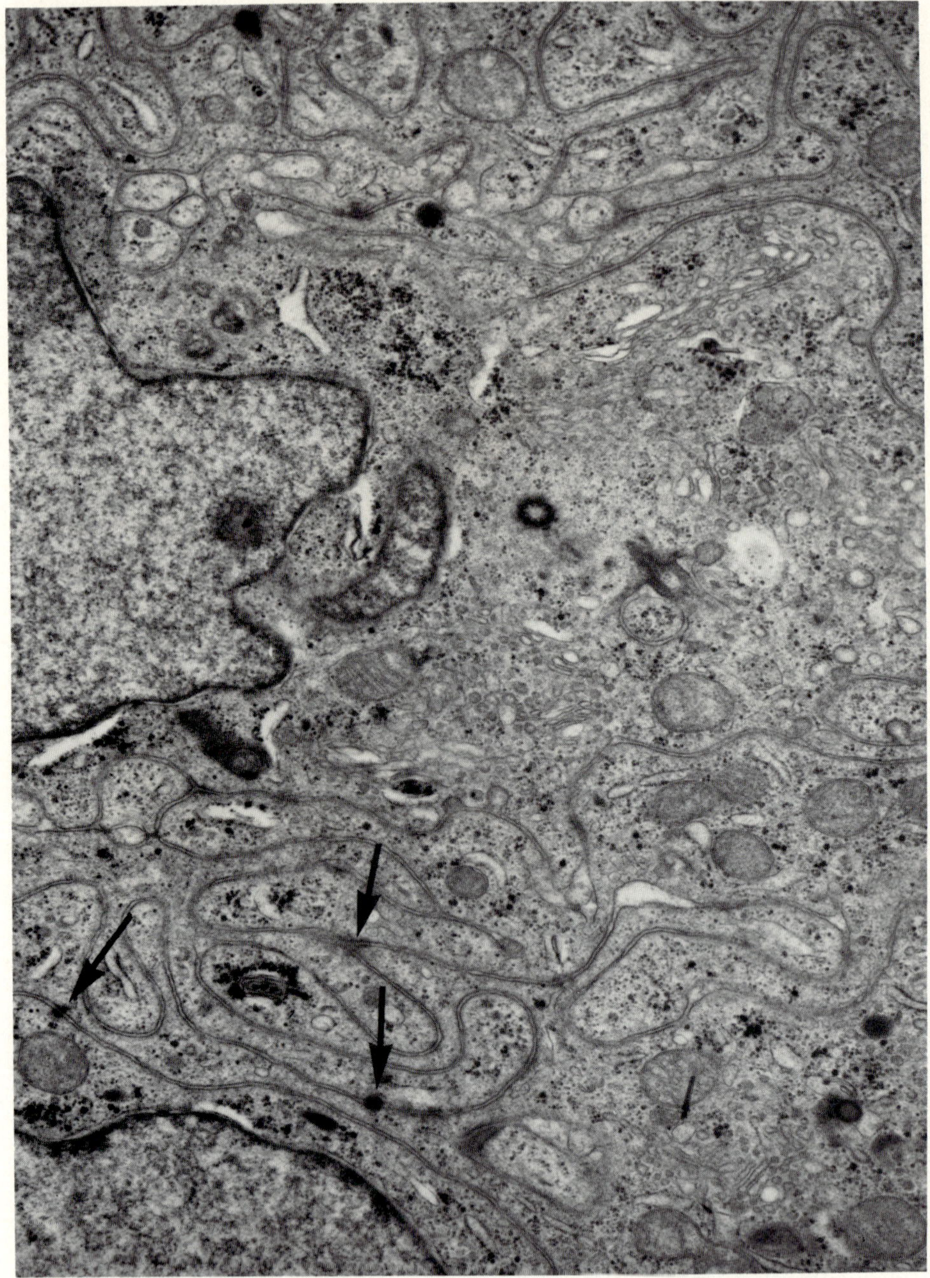

Fig. 274 Meningioma. Arrows indicate desmosomes. × 25,000. (From Hirano, A.: Progress in Neuropathology. Vol.1, p.1, Grune & Stratton, 1971.)

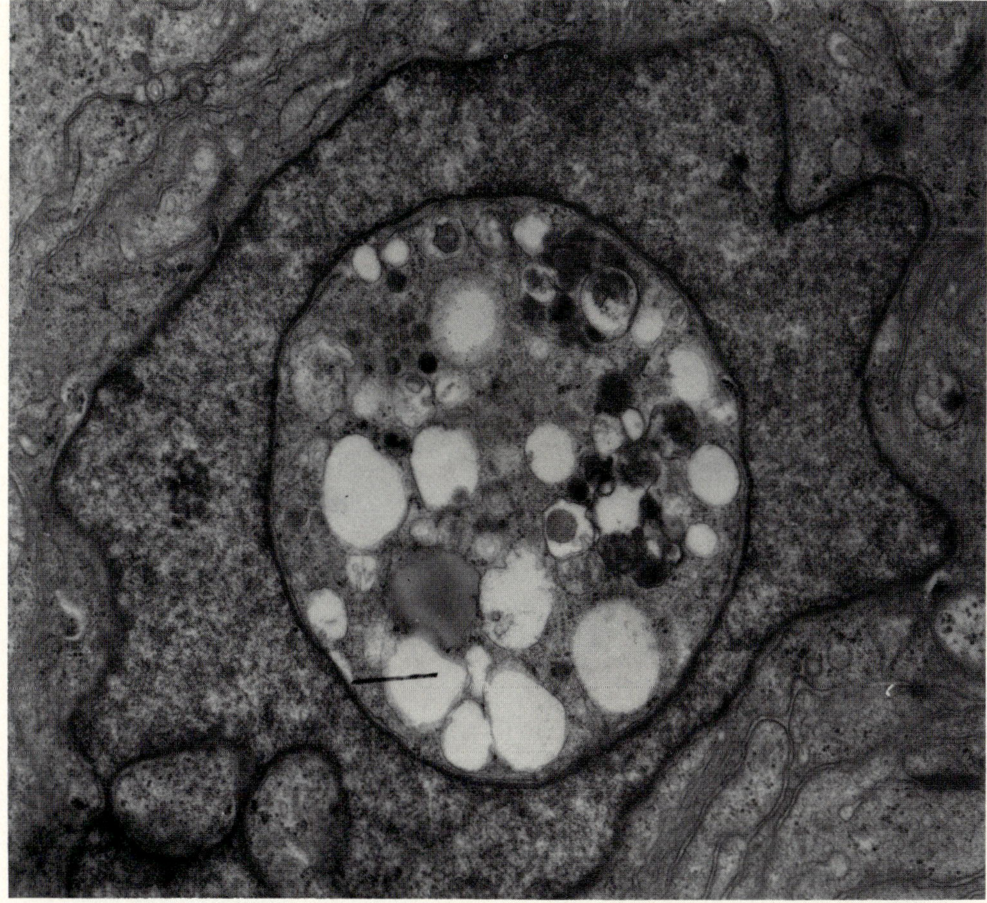

Fig. 275 Meningioma. Invagination of cytoplasm into the nucleus corresponding to an intranuclear eosinophilic inclusion. × 22,000.

Hemangiopericytoma

Although meningiomas are, in general, benign neoplasms, occasional malignant tumors may also be seen. One such tumor is the hemangiopericytoma, which is also referred to as angioblastic meningioma by some authors. The histological features are similar to those of hemangiopericytomas seen elsewhere in the body. Unlike other meningiomas they lack whorl formation or psammoma bodies. Immature tumor cells are compactly arranged between the rich vascular network. Some of the tumor cells are partially or completely surrounded by basal laminae, while others are in close contact with one another via various junctions. Glycogen granules and fibrils may be seen in addition to the usual cell organelles. The fibrils may occasionally form bundles and there may be marginal accumulation of vesicles; features reminiscent of smooth muscle. The origin of the tumor cells is still a matter of controversy. It is important to differentiate between this type of tumor and the usual benign meningioma because it may not only recur rapidly, but the same tumors may also be found outside the central nervous system.

I. THE VASCULATURE (Fig. 276)

During embryonic development the blood vessels of the leptomeninges penetrate the growing parenchyma and are the source of all the blood vessels of the central nervous system. The endothelial cells are the first to develop; forming a solid column of cells which later form an interior lumen. A basal lamina appears

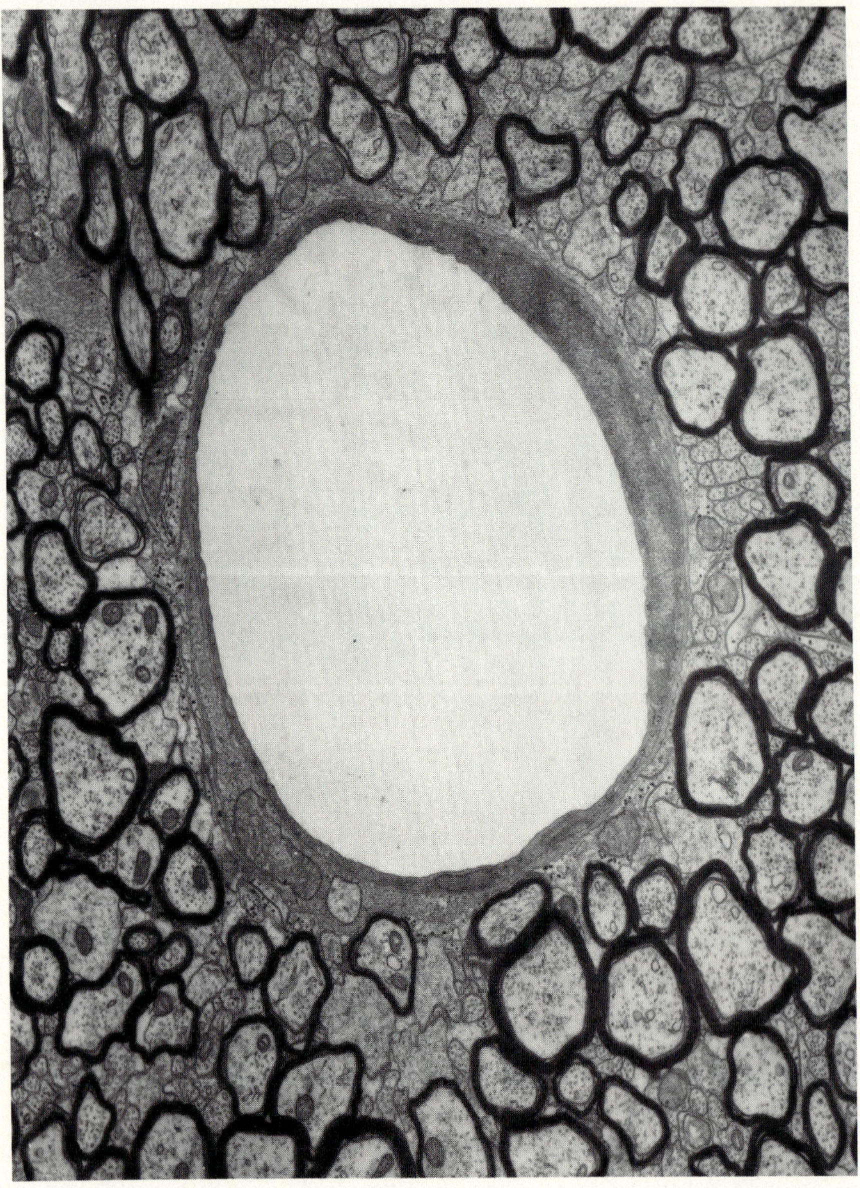

Fig. 276 A blood vessel in the white matter of a rat. The lumen of the vessel is empty and distended due to perfusion fixation. × 16,000. (From Hirano, A.: The Structure and Function of Nervous Tissue. Vol. 2, p. 69, Academic Press, 1969.)

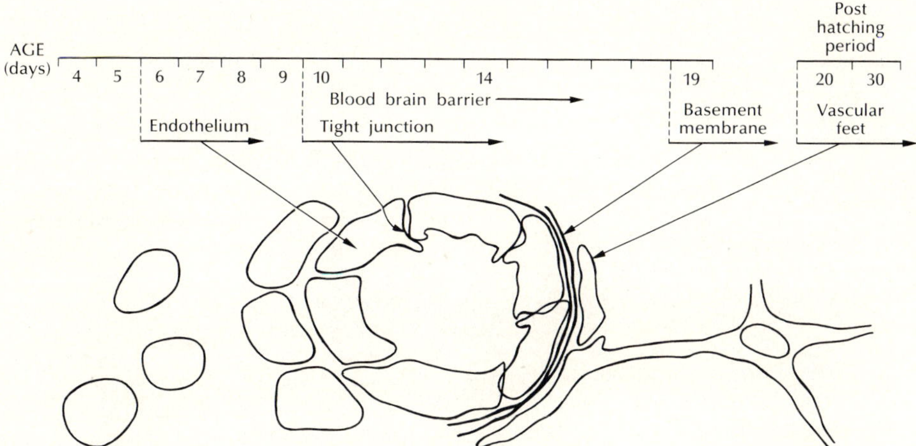

Fig. 277 A diagram of blood vessel development in the chick brain. (From Hirano, A.: Lab. Invest., 29: 659, 1973.)

surrounding the endothelium and, in the case of capillaries, astrocytes from the parenchyma eventually extend their vascular feet and surround the perivascular space (Fig. 277).

1. Arteries

NORMAL ARTERIES (Fig. 278)

The fundamental architecture of the intracranial arteries is similar to those of other organs. There is an intima consisting of endothelial cells whose cell bodies and nuclei are oriented longitudinally and which are covered by a basal lamina. Beneath the endothelium there is a narrow connective tissue space which is inconspicuous in the light microscope under normal circumstances. Between the intima and the media is a prominent, wavy, internal elastic lamina. The latter is easily recognized and is rendered black by the elastic van Gieson stain. The media is the thickest of all the layers and is composed of smooth muscle cells. These are spindle-shaped cells filled with numerous myofilaments. They are characterized by a single row of numerous vesicles at the periphery and a basal lamina which surrounds them except for the occasional junctions which link the cells. Sometimes, smooth muscle cells penetrate the internal elastic lamina and form myoendothelial junctions. The adventitia is composed of loose connective tissue, occasional nerve endings and their axons which are associated with Schwann cells.

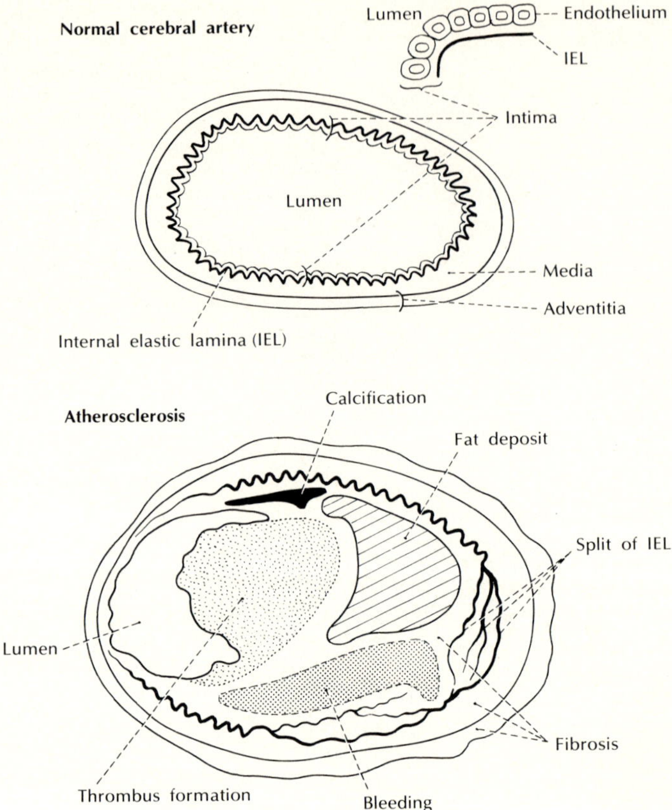

Fig. 278 Normal and atherosclerotic intracranial arteries.

PATHOLOGICAL ALTERATIONS OF ARTERIES

Atherosclerosis (Figs. 27, 278)

Pathological changes of the sclerotic artery are usually most pronounced in the intima which may show marked fibrous thickening. The intimal fibrosis is often associated with fat deposits and calcification. The internal elastic lamina is often split or discontinuous. Additionally, thrombi can often be found occluding the lumen and endothelial cells are frequently missing. Thrombi or emboli are, in due time, organized by granulation tissue, and followed by the formation of new, small, vascular channels (recanalization).

The pathogenesis of arteriosclerosis in the aorta has recently been elucidated. The process apparently begins by a primary injury which somehow results in the loss of endothelium. This results in thrombus formation and migration of the smooth muscle cells through the internal elastic lamina. Chronic insult, including persistent hypercholesterolemia, leads to formation of the typical sclerotic plaques (Ross and Glomset, 1976).

REFERENCE

Ross, R., & Glomset, J.A.: The pathogenesis of atherosclerosis. New England J. Med., 293: 369-376, 420-425, 1976.

Occlusion and Rupture of the Arteries

See pages 25 and 81.

Aneurysms

See page 26.

Vascular Malformations

See page 22.

2. Veins

The veins of the central nervous system are characterized by their large lumens and relatively thin walls. The endothelium is surrounded by a thin layer of connective tissue. There is no internal elastic lamina and the smooth muscle layer is relatively inconspicuous.

3. Capillaries

NORMAL CAPILLARIES (Fig. 279)

The numerous capillaries of the central nervous system differ from those of most other organs with respect to the permeability of the endothelium which constitutes the anatomical basis of the *blood-brain barrier*. If a macromolecular tracer such as horseradish peroxidase is introduced into the blood stream, it will, in most tissues, find its way into the perivascular space and into the parenchyma. The tracer can penetrate between endothelial cells, through fenestrae in the cells and/or by means of *plasmalemmal (pinocytotic) vesicles*. In muscle, for example, pinocytotic vesicles occupy approximately one third of the area of the endothelium under normal conditions. In most parts of the central nervous system, however, despite their especially attenuated nature, often as narrow as 0.1 micron thick, the endothelial cells provide a remarkably effective barrier to the movement of the tracer. Adjacent endothelial cells are joined by *zonulae occludentes* preventing penetration of the tracer substance between the cells. Plasmalemmal vesicles, about 700Å in diameter, are rare and those with tracer are confined to the luminal surface. *Fenestrae*, except for areas of the brain devoid of a blood-brain barrier are not present in cerebral vessels. Areas containing fenestrated blood vessels include the choroid plexus, the pineal and pituitary glands, area postrema, tuber cinereum and the median eminence.

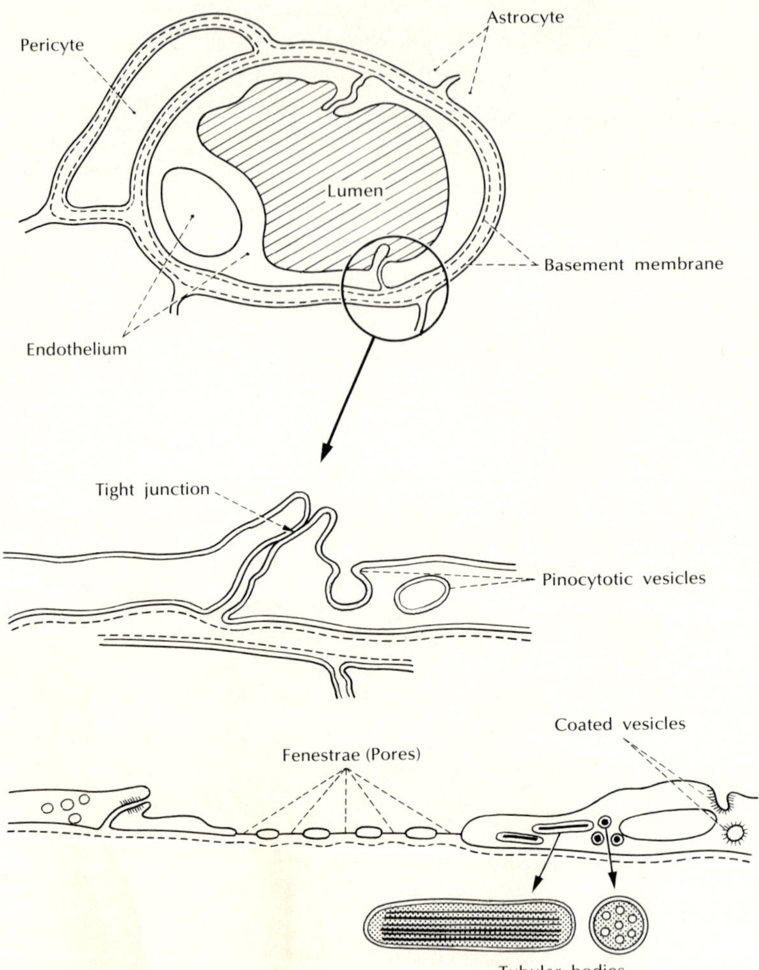

Fig. 279 Endothelium.

Except for the gray matter of the spinal cord, the *perivascular space* of the capillaries of the central nervous system is very narrow and devoid of any connective tissue elements. It is bordered on one side by the basal lamina of the endothelial cell and on the other by the basal lamina of the astrocytic foot processes. In some instances the perivascular space is virtually obliterated and the two basal laminae form a single moderately dense, homogenous structure. In the gray matter of the spinal cord, the majority of the capillaries are surrounded by a perivascular space of relatively wide dimensions sometimes containing small amounts of connective tissue.

Occasional *pericytes* are found outside the endothelial cells of capillaries and venules. The origin and function of these cells are obscure. They are completely surrounded by a basal lamina and show certain fine structural characteristics reminiscent of smooth muscle. Some workers consider them to have a phagocytic function and to be part of the reticulo-endothelial system.

The endothelial cells of the central nervous system contain all the usual organelles including mitochrondria, Golgi apparatus, some rough endoplasmic reticulum, free ribosomes, fibrils, multi-vesicular bodies, occasional microtubules and centrioles. On the other hand, the *tubular body* (*Weibel-Palade body*), a conspicuous organelle in the endothelium of many organs is relatively rare in the central nervous system of experimental animals. These structures, considered to be specific markers of endothelial cells were first described by Weibel and Palade in the endothelium of aortae and other vessels. They are membrane-bounded organelles about 0.1 micron wide and up to about three microns long. The mature organelle contains 6-20 closely packed tubules, about 150-200Å wide, embedded in a dense matrix. The immature organelle, often found associated with the Golgi apparatus has a less dense matrix. Sometimes the limiting membrane of the coated vesicles of the Golgi apparatus are found to be continuous with that of the tubular body itself.

Tubular bodies are commonly seen in the endothelium of large vessels and even in capillaries of many organs outside the central nervous system. Within the central nervous system, however, they are unusual in most capillaries although they have been observed in the capillaries and venules of normal aged human brain (Herringer et al, 1974). Within the central nervous system of normal experimental animals they seem to be limited to the endothelium of large vessels such as the internal carotid artery and to those fenestrated capillaries found in limited areas of the central nervous system.

REFERENCES

Weibel, E.R., & Palade, G.E.: New cytoplasmic cmponents in arterial endothelia. J. Cell Biol., 23: 101-112, 1964.

Reese, T.S., & Karnovsky, M.J.: The structural localization of a brain barrier to exogenous peroxidase. J. Cell Biol., 34: 207-217, 1967.

Herringer, H., Anzil, A.P., Blinzinger, K., & Kronski, D.: Endothelial microtubular bodies in human brain capillaries and venules. J. Anat., 118: 205-209, 1974.

PATHOLOGICAL ALTERATIONS OF CAPILLARIES AND OTHER SMALL VESSELS (Fig. 279)

Most of the changes of the capillaries and venules associated with pathological processes in the central nervous system may be directly related to the changes in permeability, i.e. the breakdown of the blood-brain barrier that almost always accompanies pathological alteration.

REFERENCES

Stehbens, W.E.: Pathology of Cerebral Blood Vessels. C.V. Mosby, St. Louis, 1972.

Cervós-Navarro, J. (ed.): Pathology of Cerebral Microcirculation. Walter de Gruyter, New York, 1974.

Hirano, A., & Matsui, T.: Vascular structure in brain tumors. Human Path., 6: 611-621, 1975.

McCormick, W.F. & Schochet, S.S. Jr.: Atlas of Cerebrovascular Disease. W.B. Saunders Co., Philadelphia, 1976.

Cervós-Navarro, J., & Matakas, F. (eds.): The Cerebral Vessel Wall. Raven Press, New York, 1976.

Cervós-Navarro, J., Betz, E., Ebhardt, G., Ferszt, R., & Wüllenweber, R.: Advances in Neurology. Vol. 20: Pathology of Cerebrospinal Microcirculation. Raven Press, New York, 1978.

Fenestrations (Figs. 279-281)

Probably the most obvious of these changes is the formation of fenestrae, or pores, through the abnormally attenuated endothelial cell. These pores are apparently identical to those seen in limited areas of the brain under normal circumstances. The pores are formed by circular 500Å diameter areas of fusion of the luminal and basal plasma membranes. The fused region forms a continuous diaphragm about 50Å thick apparently sealing the pore itself. Tracer substances seem to penetrate the walls of fenestrated vessels quite freely.

Fenestrated capillaries may be found in any part of the central nervous system in a variety of both neoplastic and non-neoplastic pathological conditions (Hirano and Kochen, 1975; Snyder et al., 1975). Unlike normal conditions, fenestrae may even appear in abnormally large caliber, thin walled vessels which are seen in pathological conditions such as in certain neoplasms or after radiation necrosis, etc. The source of these vessels is not always clear. In some instances, they may be derived from the proliferation of pre-existing fenestrated vessels. For example, the fenestrated capillaries of chromophobe adenoma may be derived from the normally fenestrated vessels of the pituitary gland (Hirano et al., 1972). One might similarly explain the origin of the fenestrated capillaries of choroid plexus papilloma. On the other hand, we cannot rule out the possibility that, at least in some circumstances, fenestrated capillaries may be formed by the alteration of previously non-fenestrated vessels. Schwannomas of the subarachnoid space of spinal roots contain numerous fenestrated blood vessels (Hirano et al., 1972 a, b) but under normal circumstances the blood vessels of those areas are not fenestrated. While unusual, some gliomas also may show vessels with small numbers of fenestrae. It has been shown that metastatic renal carcinoma in the brain contains fenestrated vessels similar to those seen in the normal kidney (Hirano and Zimmerman, 1972) and it has been suggested that the tumor cell, at least in this case, may induce otherwise non-fenestrated vessels to become fenestrated.

REFERENCES

Hirano, A., Dembitzer, H.M., & Zimmerman, H.M.: Fenestrated blood vessels in neurilemmoma. Lab. Invest., 27: 305-309, 1972, a.

Hirano, A., Tomiyasu, U., & Zimmerman, H.M.: The fine structure of blood vessels in chromophobe adenoma. Acta Neuropathol., 22: 200-207, 1972.

Hirano, A., Hasson, J., & Zimmerman, H.M.: Some new fine structural observations of ethylnitrosourea-induced nerve tumors in rat. Lab. Invest., 27: 555-560, 1972b.

Hirano, A., & Zimmerman, H.M: Fenestrated blood vessels in a metastatic renal carcinoma in the brain. Lab. Invest., 26: 465-468, 1972a.

Hirano, A., Ghatak, N.R., Becker, N.H., & Zimmerman, H.M.: A comparison of the fine

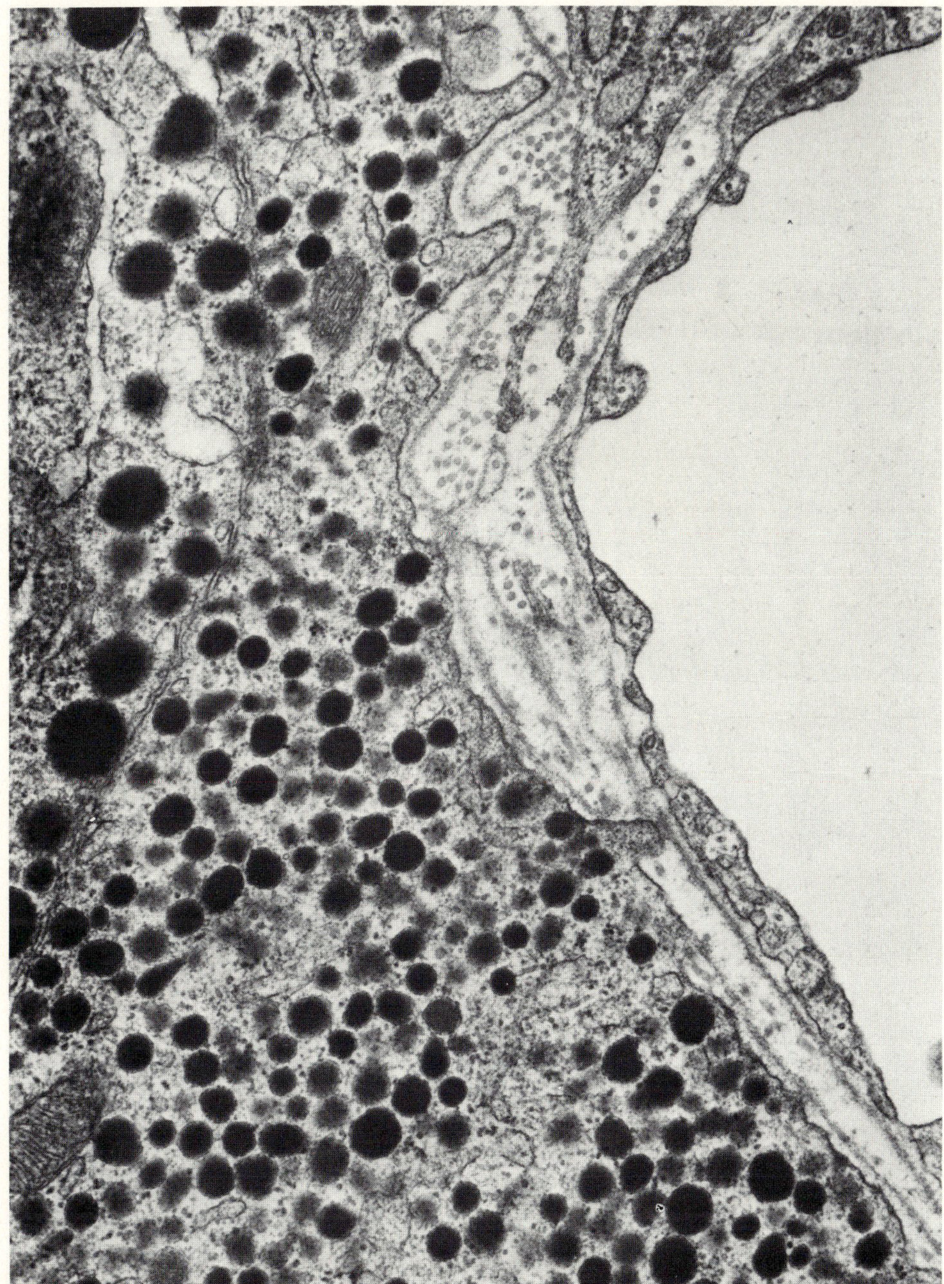

Fig. 280 Pituitary gland in the normal rat. Pituitary cells with dense secretory granules and fenestrated endothelial cells are visible. × 25,000.

structure of small blood vessels in intracranial and retroperitoneal malignant lymphoma. Acta Neuropathol., 27: 93-104, 1974.

Hirano, A., & Kochen, J.A.: Some effects of intracerebral lead implantation in the rat. Acta Neuropathol., 33: 307-315, 1975.

Snyder, D.H., Hirano, A., & Raine, C.S.: Fenestrated CNS blood vessels in chronic experimental allergic encephalomyelitis. Brain Res., 100: 645-649, 1975.

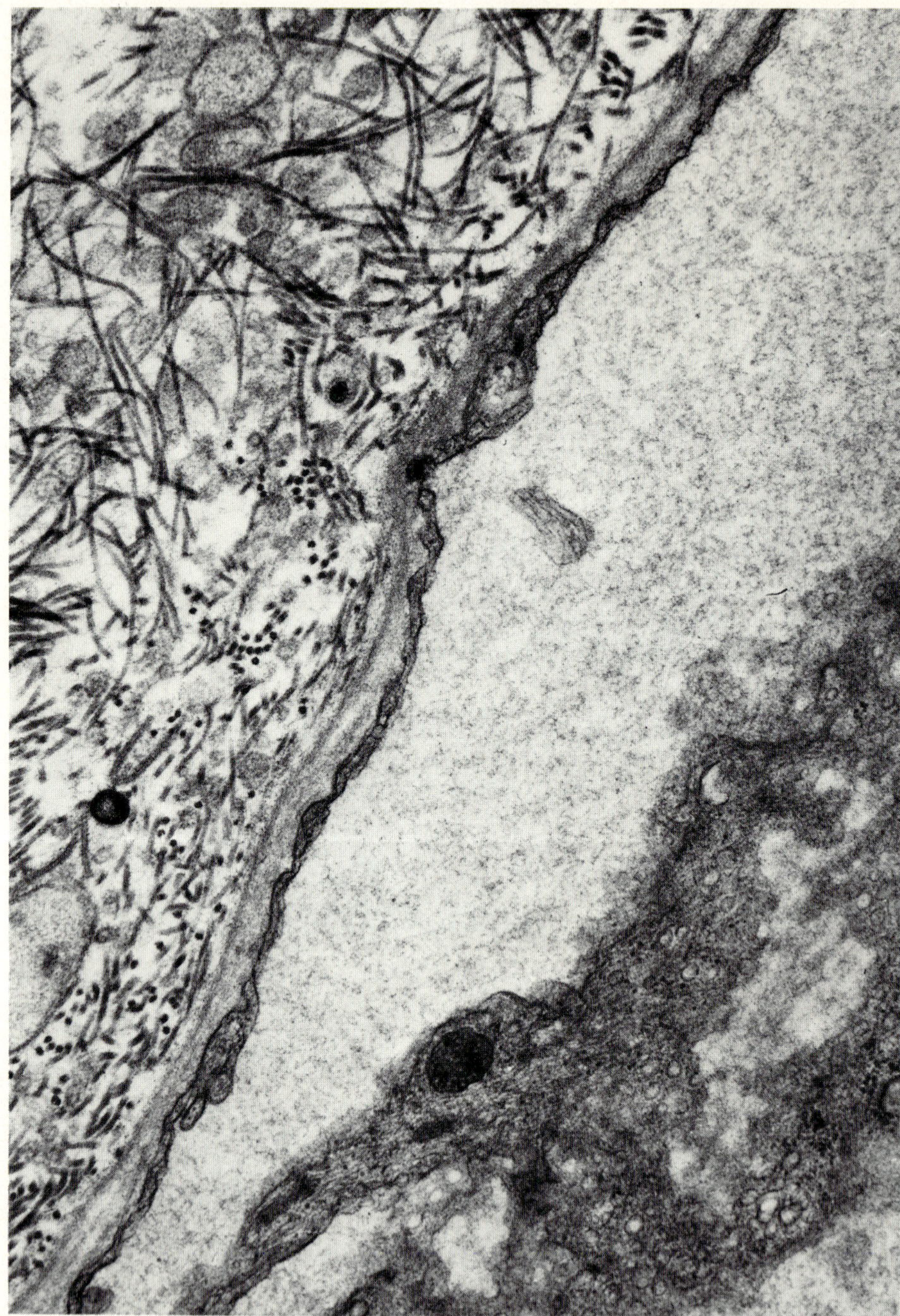

Fig. 281 A blood vessel within a schwannoma. Collagen fibers fill the ample perivascular space. The endothelial cells are fenestraed. × 110,000. (From Hirano, A.: *In* Pathology of Cerebral Microcirculation. p. 203, Walter de Gruyter, Berlin, 1974.)

Intercellular Junctions (Figs. 282-284)

Without the use of tracers it is difficult to detect changes in the thin sections of tight junctions that normally join adjacent endothelial cells in most parts of the brain. Such studies have been performed in experimental animals and while the results are not always clear it seems reasonable to suspect that the tight junctions are broken in a variety of pathological conditions. Indeed, it is known that certain hematogenous cells can penetrate between endothelial cells during the inflammatory process (Fig. 285B). Fluid components of the blood have also been observed to penetrate the endothelial barrier between adjacent cells under pathological conditions. It is difficult to believe that some of these separations were present during life since their dimensions would have resulted in frank hemorrhage which was not present. It seems reasonable, therefore that the wide separation represents an artifactitious exaggeration of a real, underlying change.

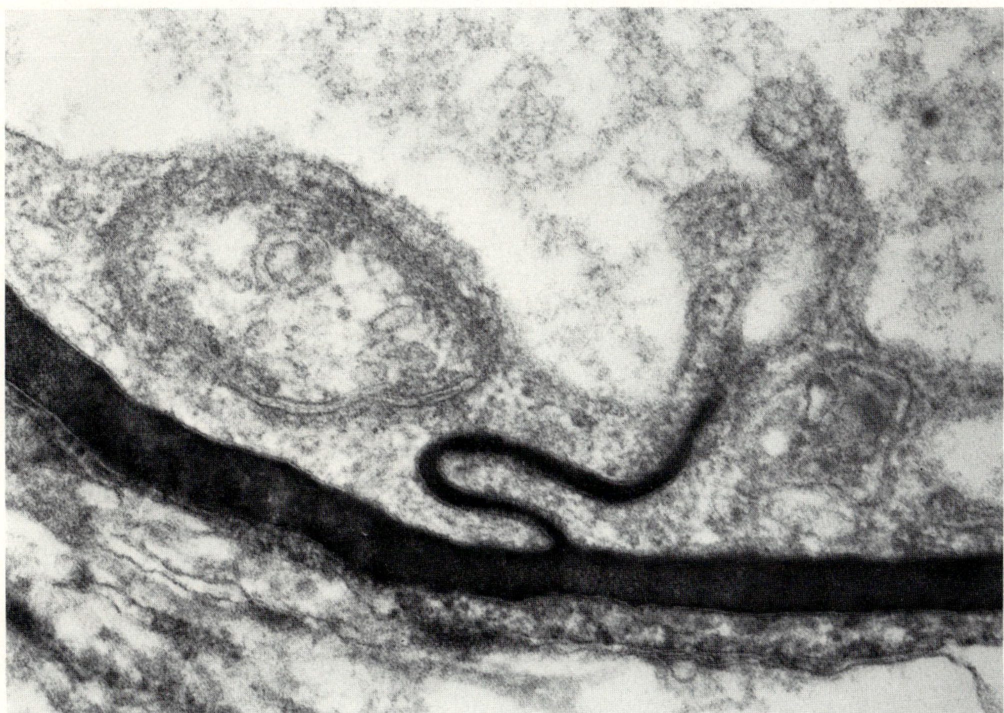

Fig. 282 A junction between two endothelial cells in the brain of a rat implanted with lanthanum nitrate illustrating the impenetrability of the intact tight junction between the cells. (From Hirano, A.: *In* Pathology of Cerebral Microcirculation. p. 203, Walter de Gruyter, Berlin, 1974.)

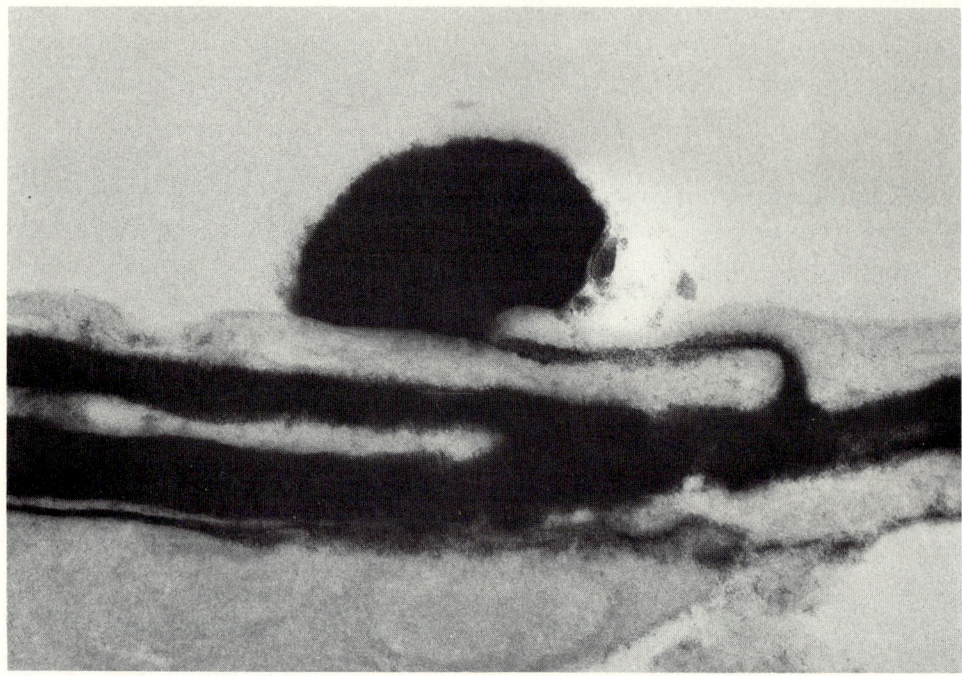

Fig. 283 An unstained section of an area similar to that illustrated in Figure 282. A bolus of tracer protrudes into the lumen of the vessel illustrating the occasional patency of the intercellular space presumably due to the pathological changes induced by the implantation of the lanthanum. (From Hirano, A.: *In* Pathology of Cerebral Microcirculation. p. 203, Walter de Gruyter, Berlin, 1974.)

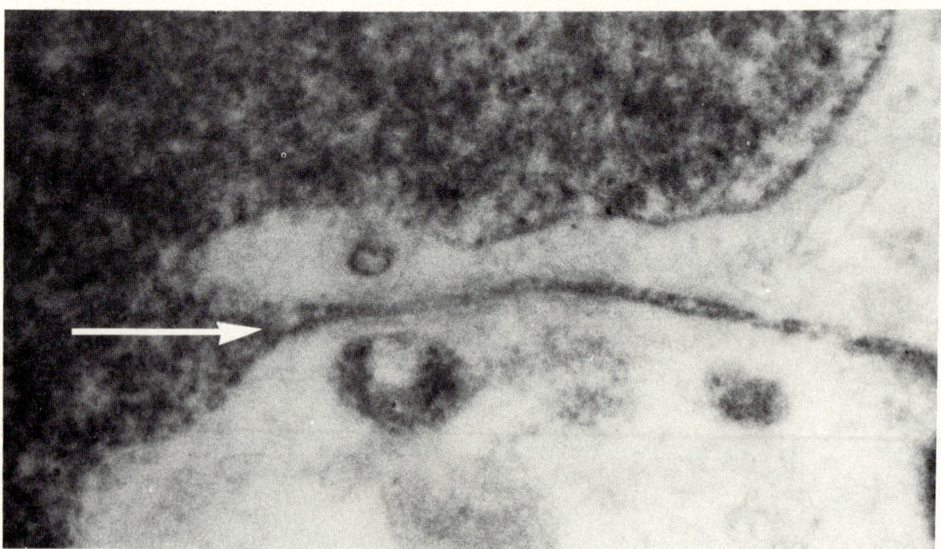

Fig. 284 Infiltration of electron dense peroxidase between two endothelial cells (arrow) in the cerebrum of a rat subjected to stab wound injury. × 96,000. (From Hirano, A. et al.: J. Neurol. Sci., 10: 205, 1970.)

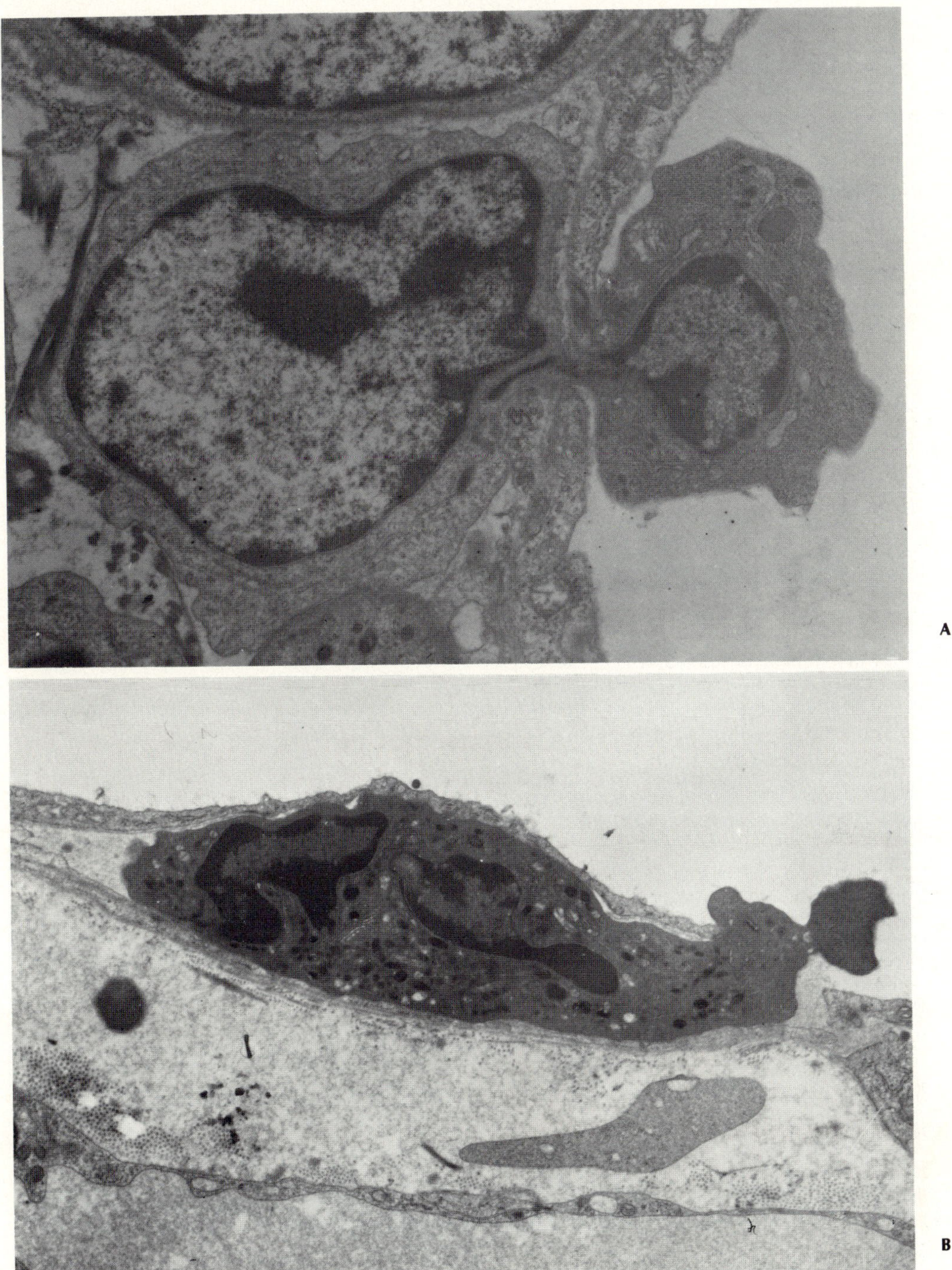

Fig. 285 Leukocyte penetrating the vascular wall during inflammation. A. × 13,000. B. × 8,500. (From Hirano, A. et al.: Am. J. Path., 47: 209, 1965.)

REFERENCES

Hirano, A., Dembitzer, H.M., Becker, N.H., Levine, S., & Zimmerman, H.M.: Fine structural alterations of the blood-brain barrier in experimental allergic encephalomyelitis. J. Neuropathol. Exp. Neurol., 29: 432-440, 1970.

Brightman, M.W., Hori, M., Rapoport, S.I., Reese, T.S. & Westergaard, E.: Osmotic opening of tight junctions in cerebral endothelium. J. Comp. Neurol., 152: 317-325, 1973.

Hirano, A.: Fine structural alterations of small vessels in the nervous system. *In* International Symposium on the Pathology of Cerebral Microcirculation. pp. 203-217, Cervós-Navarro, J. (ed.), Walter de Gruyter & Co., Berlin, 1974.

Plasmalemmal (Pinocytotic) Vesicles (Fig. 286)

As pointed out previously, plasmalemmal vesicles often increase in number under pathological conditions. Where tracer substances are used in experimental animals tracer-filled vesicles are found at both the luminal and basal portions of the cell. These vesicles are considered by some to be the principal mechanism of fluid transfer under some conditions. Rows of plasmalemmal vesicles forming a chain across an endothelial cell can form a channel through the cell which may serve as a direct route of fluid transfer.

REFERENCES

Hirano, A., Becker, N.H., & Zimmerman, H.M.: Pathological alterations in the cerebral endothelial cell barrier to peroxidase. Arch. Neurol., 20: 300-308, 1969.

Hirano, A., Becker, N.H., & Zimmerman, H.M.: The use of peroxidase as a tracer in studies of alterations in the blood-brain barrier. J. Neurol. Sci., 10: 205-213, 1970.

Westergaard, E.: The blood-brain barrier to horseradish peroxidase under normal and experimental conditions. Acta Neuropathol., 39: 181-187, 1977.

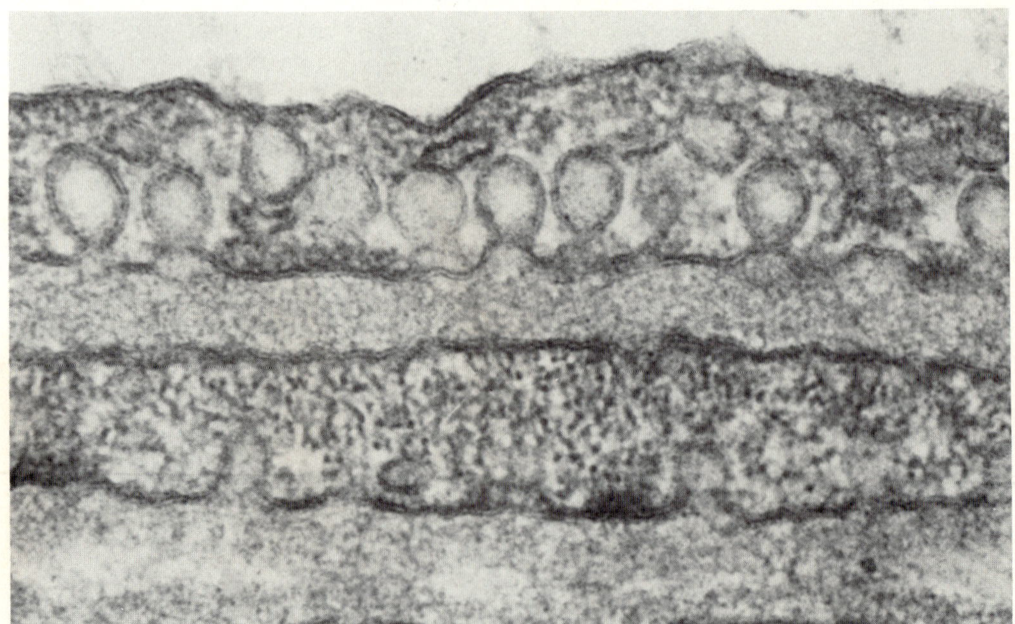

Fig. 286 Numerous pinocytotic vesicles in the endothelial cells of the brain of a rat with experimental brain edema. × 130,000. (From Hirano, A.: *In* Pathology of Cerebral Microcirculation. p. 203, Walter de Gruyter, Berlin, 1974.)

Surface Modulation

Another possible mechanism of channel formation through endothelial cells may be the result of extensive infoldings of the surfaces of the endothelial cells. Under a variety of conditions both the luminal and basal endothelial surfaces may become very irregular showing pronounced infolding of the plasma membrane. This often results in the formation of large pockets (Fig. 287) which may penetrate completely through the cell and form ephemeral channels allowing the massive transfer of fluid between the blood and the parenchyma.

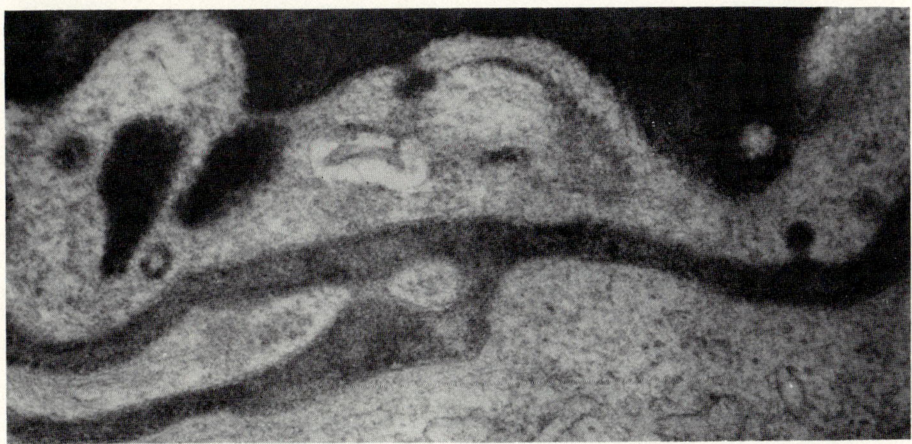

Fig. 287 The lumen and perivascular space of this cerebral vessel in an animal with encephalomyelitis are filled with peroxidase. Pinocytotic vesicles and large pockets also contain peroxidase. (From Hirano, A. et al.: J. Neuropathol. Exp. Neurol., 29: 432, 1970.)

Tubular Bodies and Related Structures (Figs. 288-290)

As pointed out previously, tubular bodies, (Weibel-Palade bodies), characteristic of endothelial cells, are usually confined to the endothelium of large vessels in the normal central nervous system. Under pathological conditions, however, it is not unusual to find large numbers of tubular bodies especially in swollen, reactive or neoplastic endothelial cells (Fig. 288). As described by Kawamura, et al. (1974) tubule-containing vacuoles may be found in such cells as well (Figs. 289, 290). These vacuoles may be bounded by a continuous limiting membrane or may be directly confluent with the lumen or perivascular space. In some cases, typical fenestrae may be seen between the vacuoles and the lumen or between adjacent vacuoles. The tubules within these vacuoles seem to be very similar to those found within tubular bodies.

REFERENCES

Kawamura, J., Kamijyo, Y., Sunaga, T., & Nelson, E.: Tubular bodies in vascular endothelium of a cerebellar neoplasm. Lab. Invest., 30: 358-365, 1974.

Hirano, A.: Further observations of the fine structure of pathological reaction in cerebral blood vessels. *In* The Cerebral Vessel Wall, pp. 41-49, Cervós-Navarro, J., Betz, B., Willenweber, R. & Matakas, F., (eds.), Raven Press, New York, 1976.

Matsumura, H., & Hirano, A.: Further observations of endothelial changes accompanying delayed radiation necrosis in the human brain. J. Clin. Electron Microscopy, 9: 37-43, 1976.

Ohsugi, T., & Hirano, A.: Tubular bodies in endothelial cells in meningiomas. Neuropathol. Appl. Neurol., 3: 1-8, 1977.

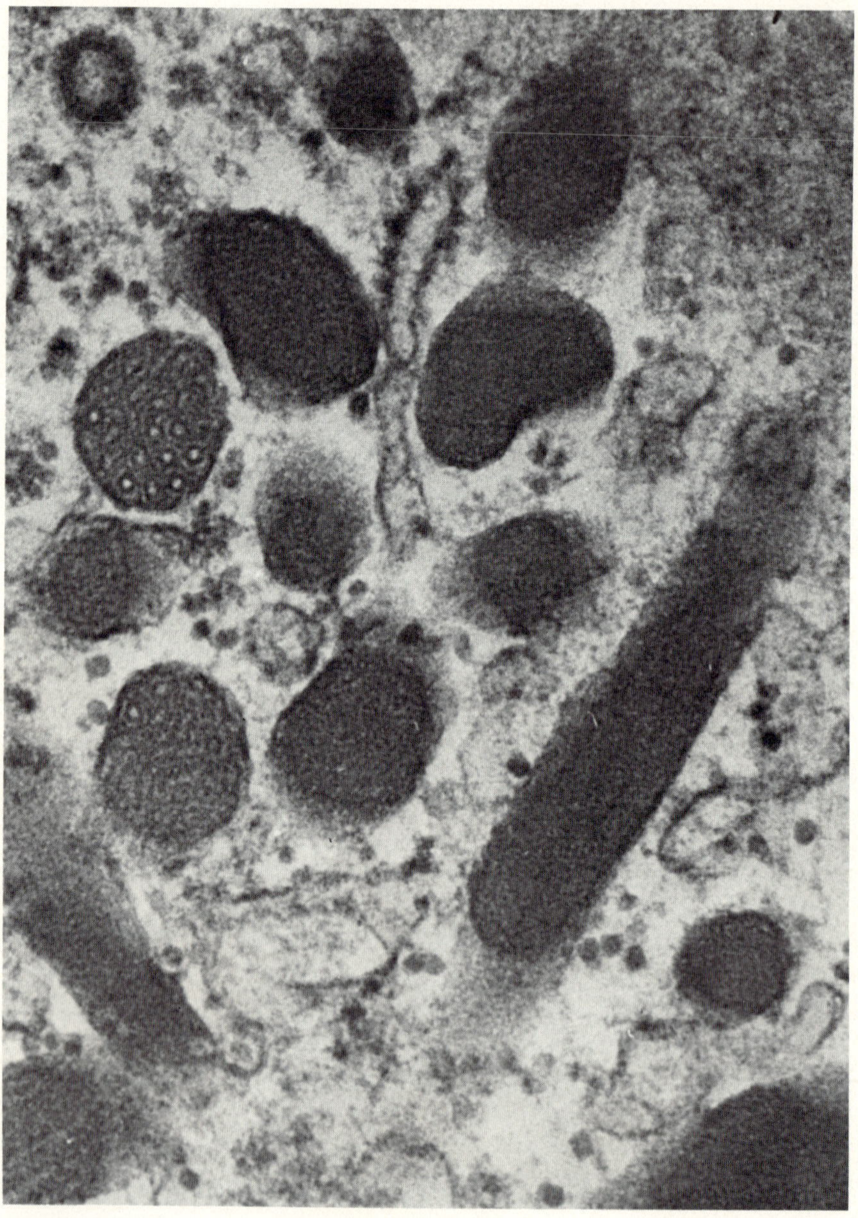

Fig. 288 Cross and longitudinal sections of tubular bodies in an endothelial cell of a capillary in a chromophobe adenoma. × 29,000. (From Hirano, A.: *In* Pathology of Cerebral Microcirculation. p. 203, Walter de Gruyter, Berlin, 1974.)

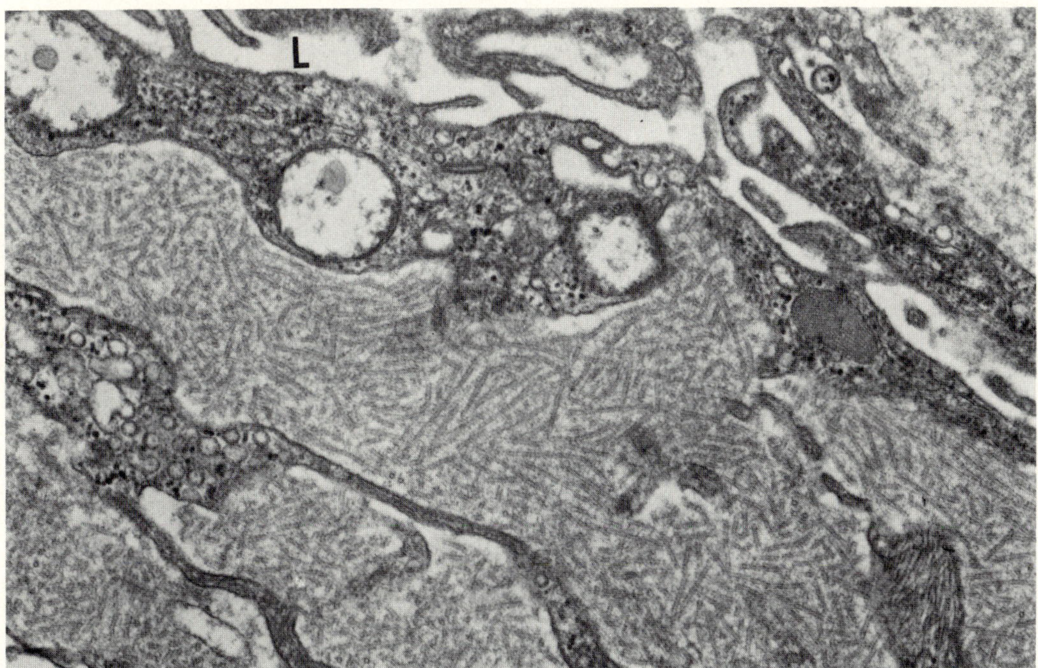

Fig. 289 A vascular wall in a meningioma. The lumen (L) is bordered by a markedly infolded endothelial cell surface. A large tubule-containing vacuole occupies most of the endothelial cell cytoplasm. × 18,000. (From Ohsugi, S. & Hirano, A.: Neuropathol. Appl. Neurobiol., 3: 1, 1977.)

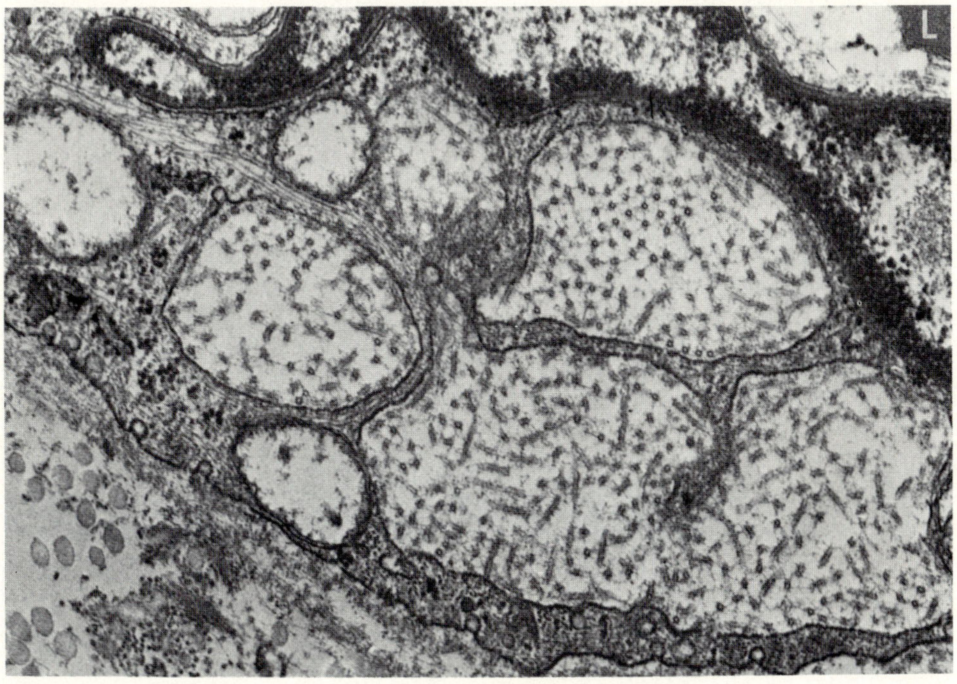

Fig. 290 A vascular wall in a meningioma. The lumen (L) is filled with dense plasma. A large portion of the endothelial cell cytoplasm is occupied by tubule-containing vacuoles. × 31,000. (From Ohsugi, S. & Hirano, A.: Neuropathol. Appl. Neurobiol., 3: 1, 1977.)

Tubular Arrays (Fig. 291)

Tubular arrays consist of finger-like invaginations of the membranes of the rough endoplasmic reticulum into the cisterns. The invaginations are circular in section and roughly equal in diameter so that they frequently appear as tubules within the cisterns of the rough endoplasmic reticulum or between the two membranes surrounding the nuclei.

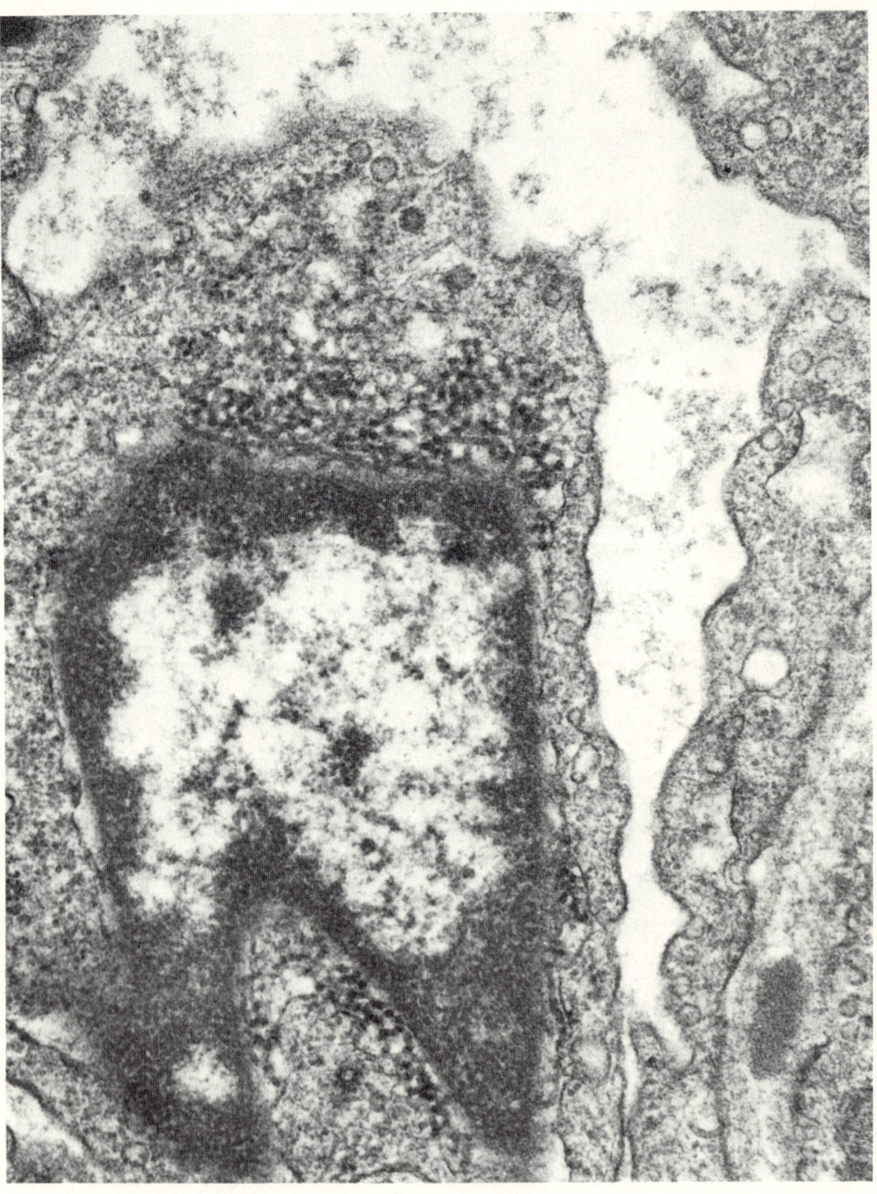

Fig. 291 An endothelial cell with tubular arrays in a dysgerminoma. × 37,000. (From Hirano, A. et al.: Acta Neuropathol., 32: 103, 1975.)

Tubular arrays are not present in the endothelium of the normal nervous system, but they have been observed in the endothelium of a germinoma. They have also been reported in glial cells.

Tubular arrays are also found outside the central nervous system under various pathological conditions including neoplasms and myositis. They have been seen in various cell types but most often in endothelial cells.

REFERENCES

Baringer J.R., & Swoveland, P.: Tubular aggregates in endoplasmic reticulum: Evidence against their viral nature. J. Ultrastruct. Res., 41: 270-276, 1972.

Hirano, A., Llena, J.F., & Chung, H.D.: Some new observations in an intracranial germinoma. Acta Neuropathol., 32: 103-113, 1975.

Hirano, A., Ohsugi, T., & Matsumura, H.: Pores and tubule-containing vacuoles in altered blood vessels of the central nervous system. *In* Advances in Neurology, Vol. 20; Pathology of Cerebrospinal Microcirculation. pp. 461-469, Cervós-Navarro, J., Betz, E., Ebhardt, G., Ferszt, R., & Wullenweber, R., (eds.), Raven Press, New York, 1978.

Endothelial Proliferation

Endothelial proliferation almost always accompanies malignant intracranial neoplasms, especially glioblastoma multiforme. The architecture of the vessels is poorly developed with only a tortuous, often slit-like cavity for a lumen. The cells are plump, closely packed, joined by intercellular junctions and characteristically immature. Mitotic figures are present. Despite a high nucleo-cytoplasmic ratio they may contain large numbers of organelles, especially free ribosomes, and even tubular bodies. In general, the cells resemble normal embryonal endothelium but the number of formed organelles is often greater in the pathological condition.

Other Changes

Depending on the underlying pathology as well as the chronicity of the conditions other changes may also be encountered within the endothelial cells. Abnormal accumulations of filaments may be present and sometimes microtubules may become more obvious. Centrioles become more prominent, especially in proliferating endothelium. Pronounced nuclear deformation may be observed in various pathological conditions, indicating contraction of endothelial cells (Majno et al., 1969).

Dense bodies are sometimes increased in number and in certain lipidoses the endothelium may become filled with lipid inclusions. A peculiar coiled structure has been reported in a case of hemangioblastoma (Cancilla and Zimmerman, 1965).

Another organelle which appears in response to pathological change is the coated vesicle. These have been reported to be quite rare in the adult under normal circumstances but they increase in various pathological conditions.

REFERENCES

Cancilla, P.A. & Zimmerman, H.M.: The fine structure of a cerebellar hemangioblastoma. J. Neuropathol. Exp. Neurol., 24: 621-628, 1965.

Majno, G., Shea, S.M., & Leventhal, M.: Endothelial contraction induced by histamine-type mediators. J. Cell Biol., 42: 647-672, 1969.

4. Brain Edema

Brain edema is a major source of concern in neurological medicine. It is associated with virtually any expanding intracranial lesion and is often the direct cause of the death of the patient. The seriousness of brain edema arises from the presence of a rigid bony case surrounding the brain. This limits its ability to expand and can therefore result in what may be a lethal increase of intracranial pressure. It is not surprising that brain edema has been the focus of many studies.

Light microscopists concluded that brain edema was, for the most part, an extracellular phenomenon such as in other organs (Fig. 292). The advent of the electron microscope, however, produced a puzzling observation. Unlike the image in the light microscope fine structural studies revealed that the normal brain was crowded with cells and processes and there was virtually no extracellular space in the parenchyma. Where, then, was the site of the edema fluid? Initial fine structural studies of edematous brain revealed enormously swollen astrocytes with even smaller extracellular spaces than normal. These observations were seized upon and it was generally concluded that the astrocyte was the site of fluid accumulation and subserved the role played by the extracellular space in other organs (Fig. 293). Soon, however, two facts dawned on the workers in the field. First, their observations had been largely confined to the gray matter, whereas it

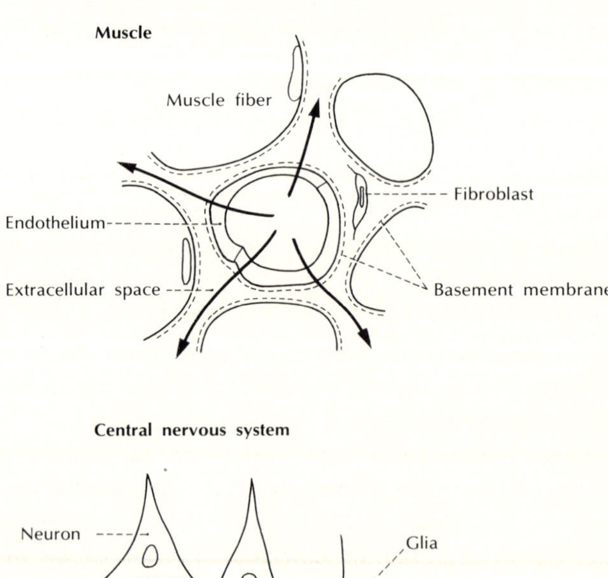

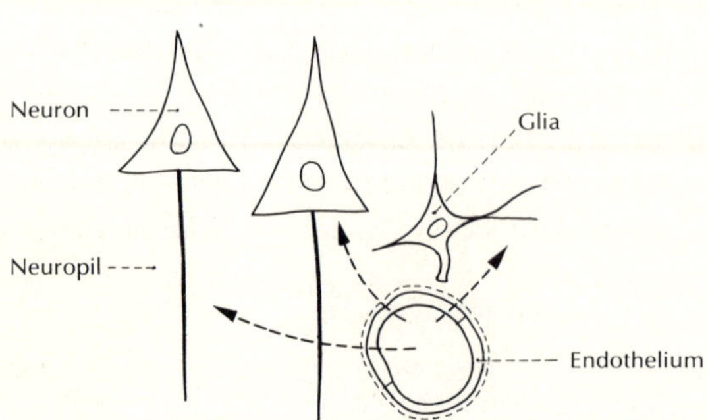

Fig. 292 Route of hematogenous edema fluid. Light microscopic view.

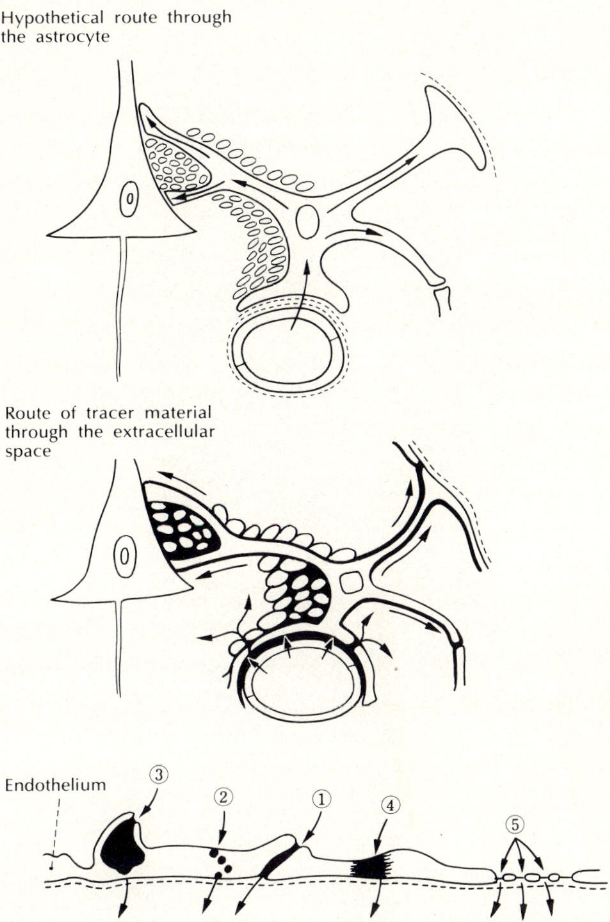

Fig. 293 Route of entry of hematogenous edema fluid.

was well known that edema was, to a great extent, a phenomenon of the white matter. Second, the astrocytes appeared swollen even in presumably non-edematous brain. Both of these facts were due to the relatively poor methods of preservation of the brain. The attendant artifacts affected the white matter even more than the gray and so, led investigators to focus on the gray matter rather than the white matter.

Eventually, the development of the perfusion technique for fixation of the central nervous system and the introduction of better embedding materials permitted improved preservation of intracranial tissue, including the white matter. With these methods it was soon observed that while the extracellular space was narrow under normal conditions brain edema led to the widening of the extracellular space of the white matter (Figs. 294, 295).

A remaining difficulty was that the clear empty spaces seen in edematous brains may have been, at least partly, due to artifact since similar areas could sometimes be seen in poorly preserved areas of normal brains. What was needed was a positive image of edema fluid.

For this purpose tracer substances were selected which were thought to mimic

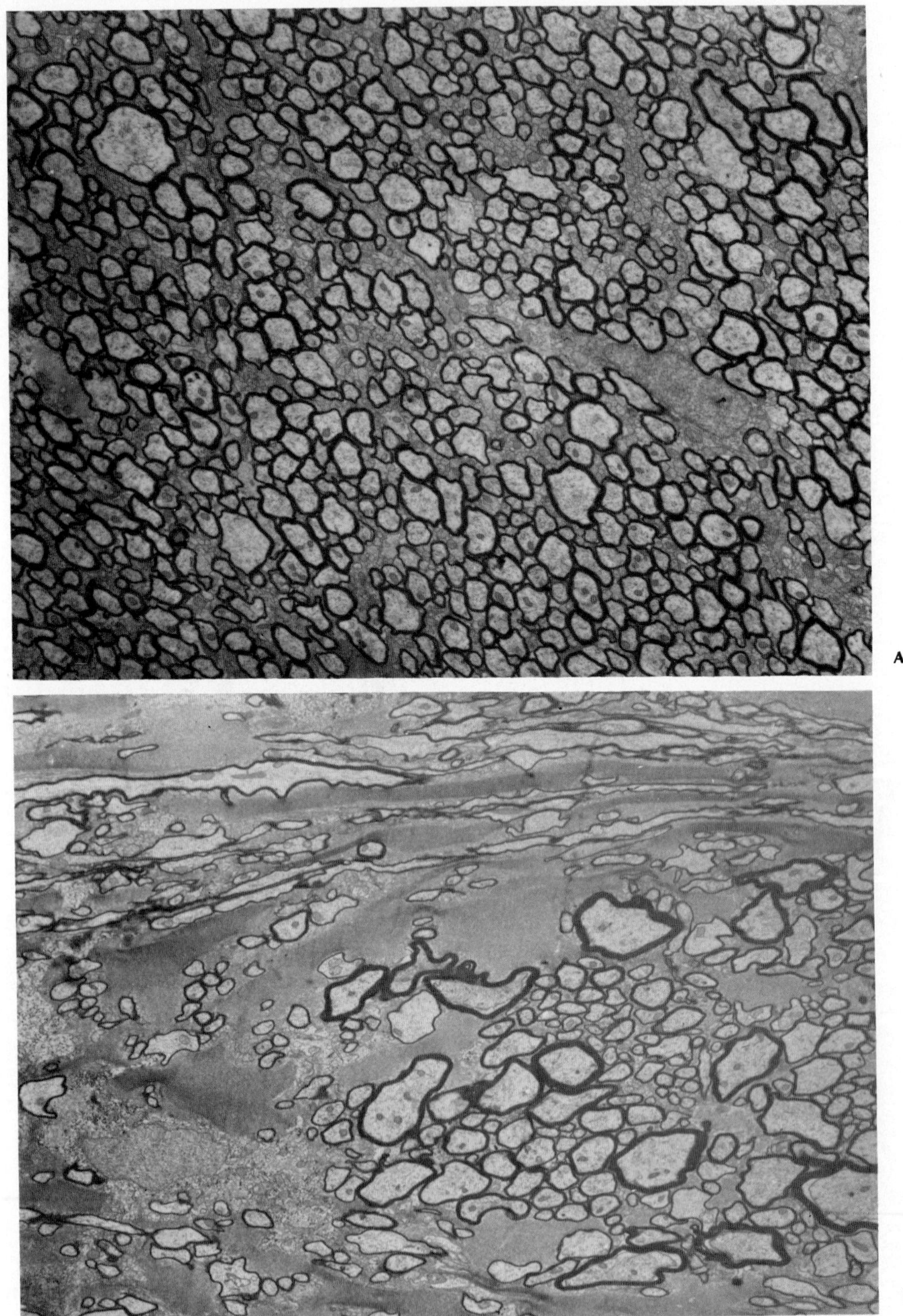

Fig. 294 Cerebral white matter. A. Normal cerebral white matter. × 6,000. (From Hirano, A. et al.: J. Cell Biol., 31: 397, 1966.) B. Edematous cerebral white matter. × 4,000. (From Hirano, A. et al.: Am. J. Path., 45: 1, 1964.)

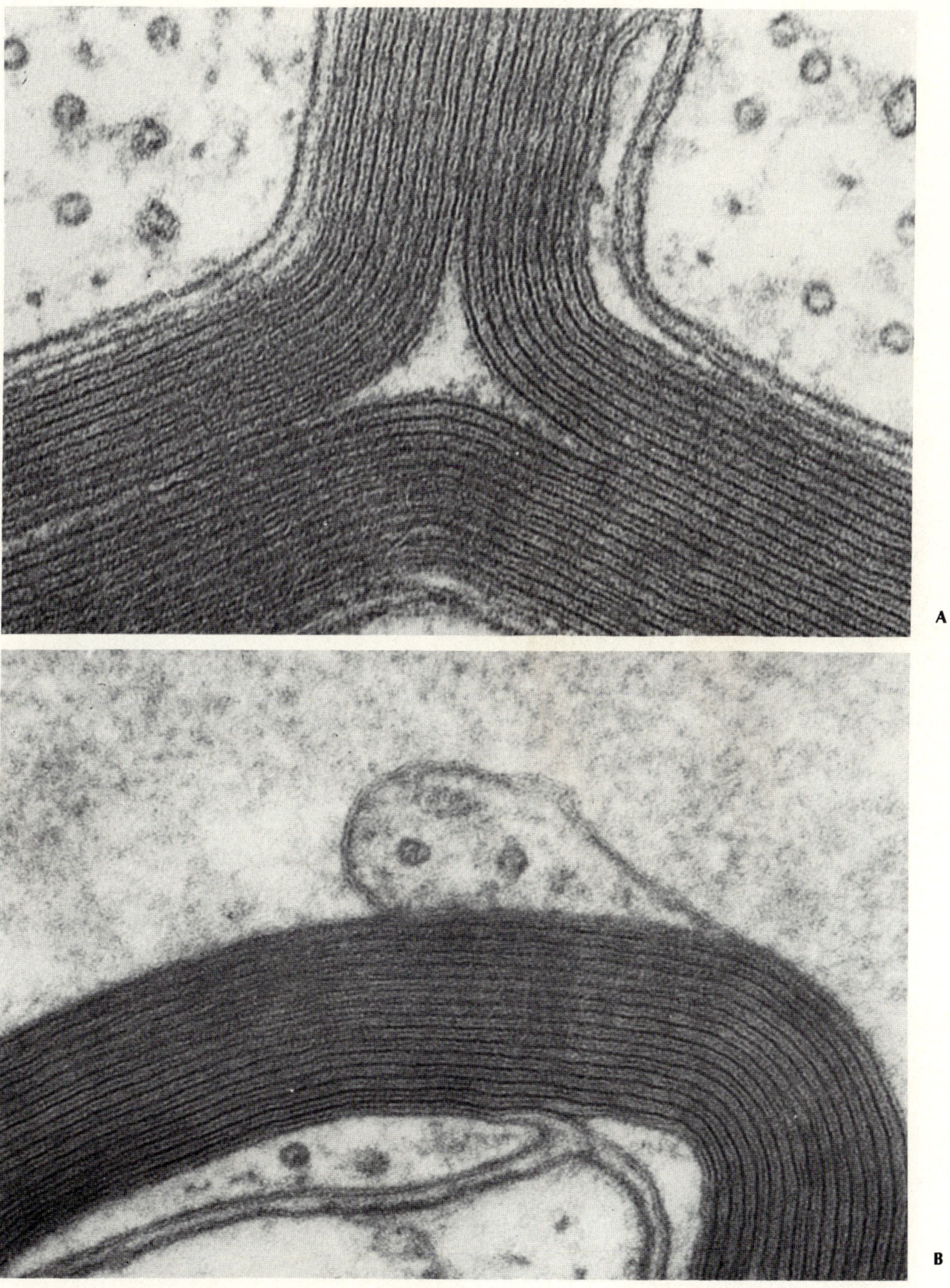

Fig. 295 Cerebral white matter. A. Myelinated axons in normal white matter. × 160,000. B. Myelinated axon in edematous white matter. × 128,000. (From Hirano, A.: Tokyo Igaku, 80: 438, 1973.)

the movement of edema fluid and which, because of their electron density, would allow the tracing of the fluid through the parenchyma. Tracer materials such as cryptococcal polysaccharide, horseradish peroxidase and ferritin were used for this purpose.

It was shown that the endothelium of the normal brain, unlike many other organs, posed a barrier to the movement of tracer substances. When the blood-brain barrier was disrupted by a focal lesion the tracer passed through the endothelium by the various routes described previously and reached the perivascular space (Fig. 296). From there it penetrated between the perivascular astrocytic feet and soon permeated the extracellular space throughout the area of the brain near the lesion, both gray and white matter. With time the tracer moved within the extracellular space, especially that of the white matter (Fig. 297). Depending upon the lesion, after approximately one or two days tracer material could be seen within cells, either normal residents of the brain or more commonly, those derived from the blood stream.

The differences in the extent of involvement between the gray and white matter may be rather easily explained on anatomic grounds. The gray matter is composed of cell bodies and dendrites which are individually oriented in all directions.

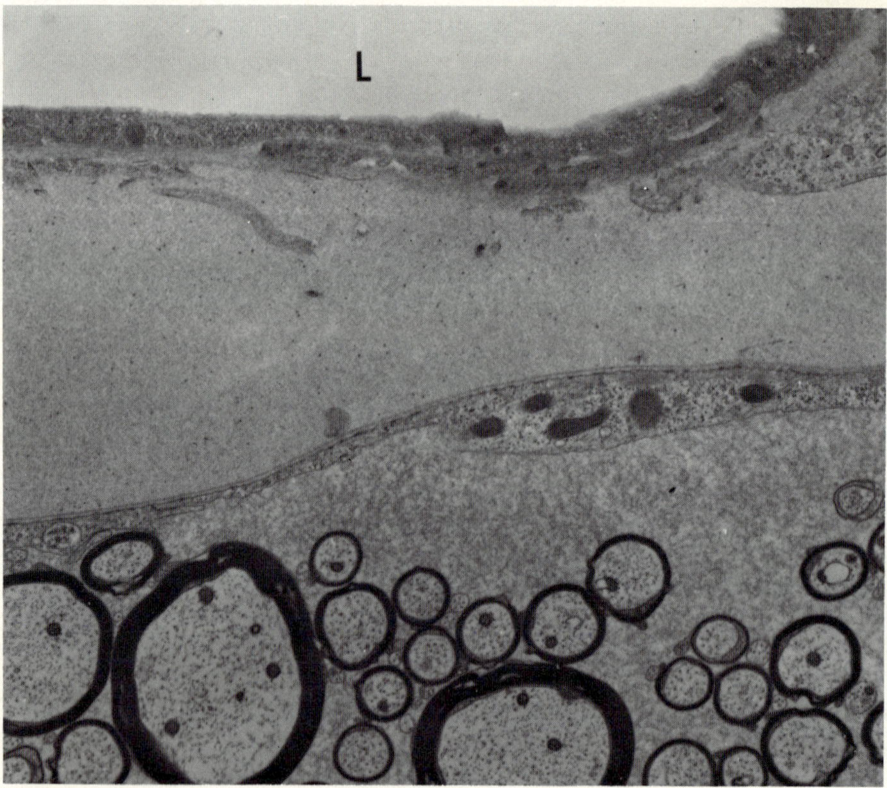

Fig. 296 Edema fluid in the distended perivascular space and intraparenchymal extracellular space of the white matter of edematous brain. The lumen (L) appears empty due to fixation by vascular perfusion. (From Hirano, A. et al.: J. Neuropathol. Exp. Neurol., 27: 571, 1968.)

Furthermore, they are tightly connected to neuronal processes by synaptic junctions (Fig. 298). Astrocytes, too, have sheet-like processes connected by cell junctions which cover various components of the gray matter. All of these elements combine to form a tightly knit tissue with no broad avenues permitting the flow of fluid.

The white matter, on the other hand, is composed of bundles of parallel fibers with very few interconnections. This configuration permits the relatively easy movement of fluid between processes and the possibility of separation of the individual nerve fibers and bundles of fibers.

Thus, edema in the brain is essentially similar to that of any other organ. Its special characteristics arise from the especially lethal effects due to the inability of the brain as a whole to expand and the detailed anatomical differences between the gray and the white matter.

As pointed out above, brain edema is a serious consequence of virtually any insult to the central nervous system by virtue of the attendant increased intracranial pressure and associated cell death. It is conceivable, however, that more subtle effects result from brain edema.

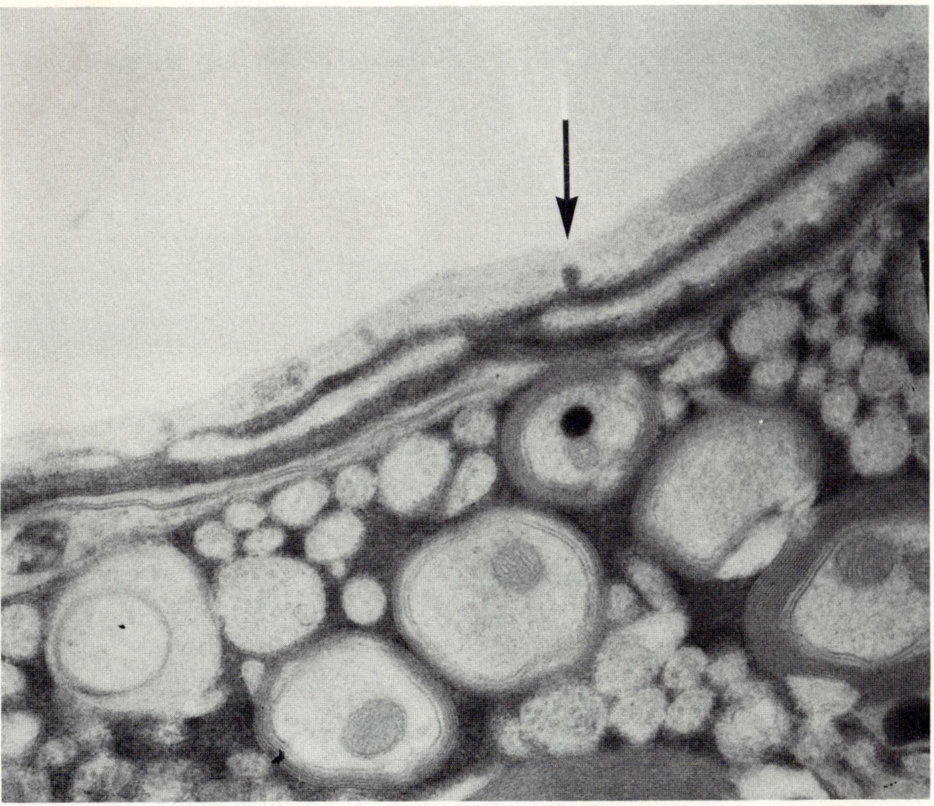

Fig. 297 Penetration of peroxidase is evident in the extracellular space as an electron dense tracer. The arrow indicates pinocytosis in the endothelium of the edematous brain. × 37,000. (From Hirano, A.: The Structure and Function of Nervous Tissue. Vol. 2, p. 69, Academic Press, 1969.)

The large inflow of hematogenous fluid into the parenchymatous spaces conceivably results in an upsetting of the equilibrium of ionic and transmitter substance concentration. Presumably such changes might interfere with neuronal function.

The function of astrocytes, too, is likely to be impaired by the presence of edema fluid. In addition to the swelling of these cells, brain edema also frequently changes the relationship of the astrocytic processes to other intracranial structures. Paramount among these is the surrounding of many synapses by astrocytic processes. The normal intimate relationship between the astrocytic process and the synapse is often destroyed in brain edema.

The function of the myelin sheath may also be interfered with in some forms of brain edema. Under ordinary circumstances the sheath serves to partially isolate the periaxonal space from the general extracellular space. This ability may be impaired in certain pathological conditions by the separation of the outer and inner loops from the myelin lamellae or by the separation of the lateral loops from the axolemma, such changes result in confluency between the periaxonal space and the other extracellular spaces of the central nervous system. In addition, the

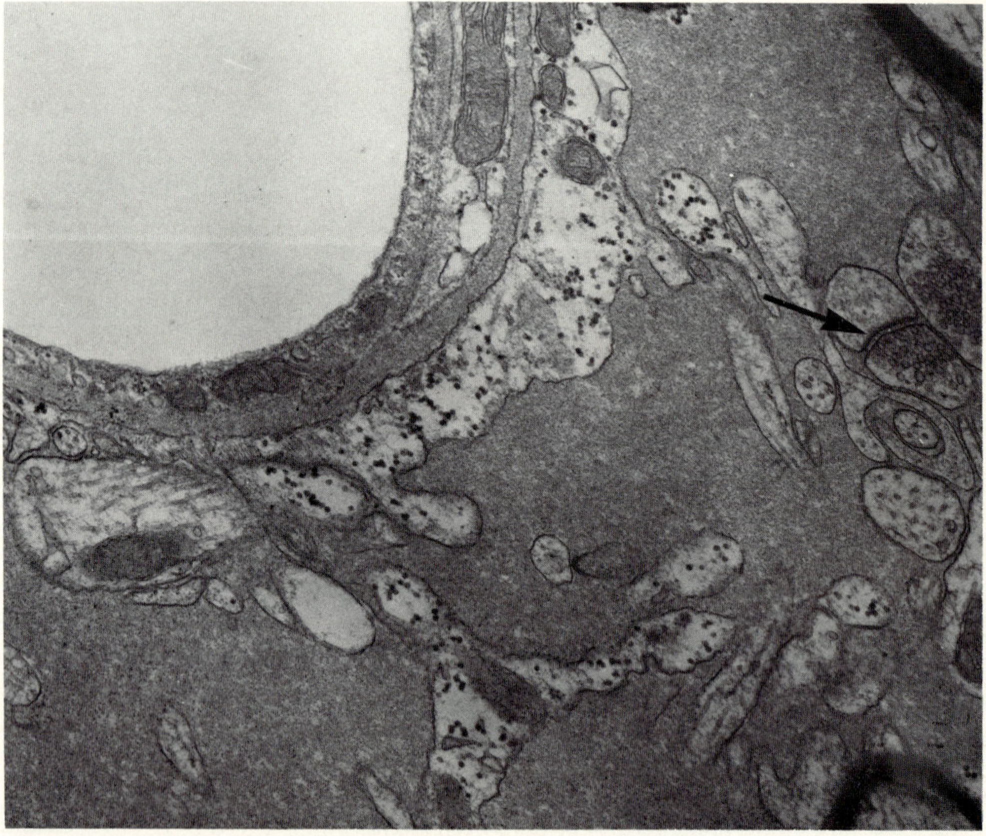

Fig. 298 Electron-dense edema fluid infiltrates the distended extracellular space in the edematous rat brain. Perivascular astrocytes are swollen and contain glycogen granules. A synaptic junction is indicated by the arrow. × 35,000. (From Hirano, A.: The Structure and Function of Nervous Tissue. Vol. 2, p.69, Academic Press, 1969.)

microenvironment of the node of Ranvier may be drastically altered by the intrusion of edema fluid.

REFERENCES

Hirano, A., Zimmerman, H.M., & Levine, S.: The fine structure of cerebral fluid accumulation. III. Extracellular spread of cryptococcal polysaccharide in the acute stage. Am. J. Pathol., 45: 1-19, 1964.

Klatzo, I.: Presidential address. Neuropathological aspects of brain edema. J. Neuropathol. Exp. Neurol., 26: 1-14, 1967.

Klatzo, I., & Seitelberger, F.: Brain Edema. Springer-Verlag, New York, 1967.

Hirano, A.: The fine structure of brain in edema. *In* The Structure and Function of Nervous Tissue. Vol. 2, pp. 69-135, Bourne, G.H. (ed.), Academic Press, New York, 1969.

Hirano, A., Becker, N.H., & Zimmerman, H.M.: The use of peroxidase as a tracer in studies of alterations in the blood-brain barrier. J. Neurol. Sci., 10: 205-213, 1970.

Hirano, A.: Fine structural alterations of small vessels in the nervous system. Pathology of Cerebral Microcirculation. pp. 203-217, Cervós-Navarro, J. (ed.), Walter de Gruyter & Co. Berlin, 1974.

Manz, J.H.: The pathology of cerebral edema. Human Pathol., 5: 291-313, 1974.

Katzman, R., & Pappius, H.M.: Brain Electrolytes and Fluid Metabolism. Williams & Wilkins, Baltimore, 1973.

Hirano, A.: A possible mechanism of dysfunction as the result of brain edema. *In* Advances in Neurology, Vol. 28: Brain Edema, Pathology Diagnosis and Therapy. pp. 83-97, Cervós-Navarro, J. & Ferszt, R. (eds.), Raven Press, New York, 1980.

Spongy States (Figs. 299, 300)

Any lesion which results in clear-appearing vacuolar changes in the central nervous system may be referred to as a "spongy state". In the present section, we shall consider those spongy states in both, the gray and the white matter which are, for the most part, intracellular phenomena and which differ, therefore, from vasogenic edema as described above. It is important to note, however, that the two phenomena, i.e. spongy states and vasogenic edema, are often associated with one another and a clear differentiation is sometimes arbitrary. Furthermore, one must always be aware of the possibility of artifactitious changes especially as the result of inadequate fixation leading to the appearance of spongy states.

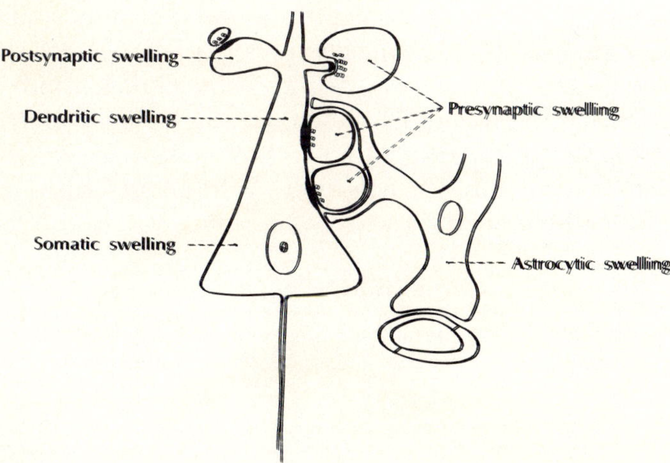

Fig. 299 Sites of swelling found in spongy states in the cerebral cortex.

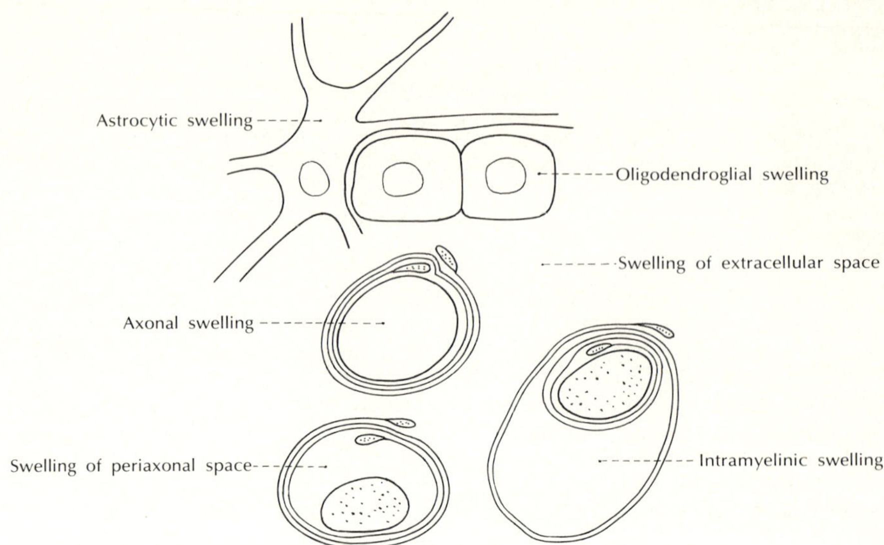

Fig. 300 Sites of swelling found in spongy states of the white matter.

In the gray matter (Fig. 299), astrocytic swelling is common after ischemia or other insults leading to necrosis. These changes are especially visible in perivascular, subpial and perineuronal areas where the astrocytic processes provide a covering function. The perinuclear area of the astrocyte itself is also subject to swelling. In certain conditions, such as Creutzfeldt-Jakob disease parts of the neuron are more selectively involved. These parts include both pre- and postsynaptic terminals in addition to the dendrites and the cell bodies.

The cells of the white matter consist for the most part of oligodendroglia and astrocytes. Both of these are subject to swelling as the result of poor preservation especially in the deeper parts of the white matter (Fig. 300). An example of this phenomenon is the so-called "fried egg" pattern of oligodendroglia. Real spongy changes in the myelinated fibers, however, do occur. During necrosis following, for example, ischemia or cyanide intoxication, the myelinated axon may swell to several times its original width. In some lesions, the periaxonal spaces become abnormally enlarged and sometimes contain extracellular fluid (Hirano and Dembitzer, 1981). Spaces between the myelin lamellae may appear. In triethyltin intoxication, for example, large, clear, intramyelinic splits may be seen. These and other changes of the myelin sheath have already been described in the section dealing with myelin pathology.

REFERENCE

Hirano, A. & Dembitzer, H.M.: The periaxonal space in an experimental model of neuropathy: The mutant Syrian hamster with hind-leg paralysis. J. Neurocytol., in press.

J. NON-NEUROECTODERMAL TISSUES IN THE NEUROAXIS

Structures, not derived from the neuroectoderm, are found in the neuroaxis even under normal circumstances. These include the blood vessels, the meninges and the pituitary gland. Under pathological conditions, other non-neuroectodermal elements can be found within the central nervous system often as the result of an error in development or due to metastatic spread.

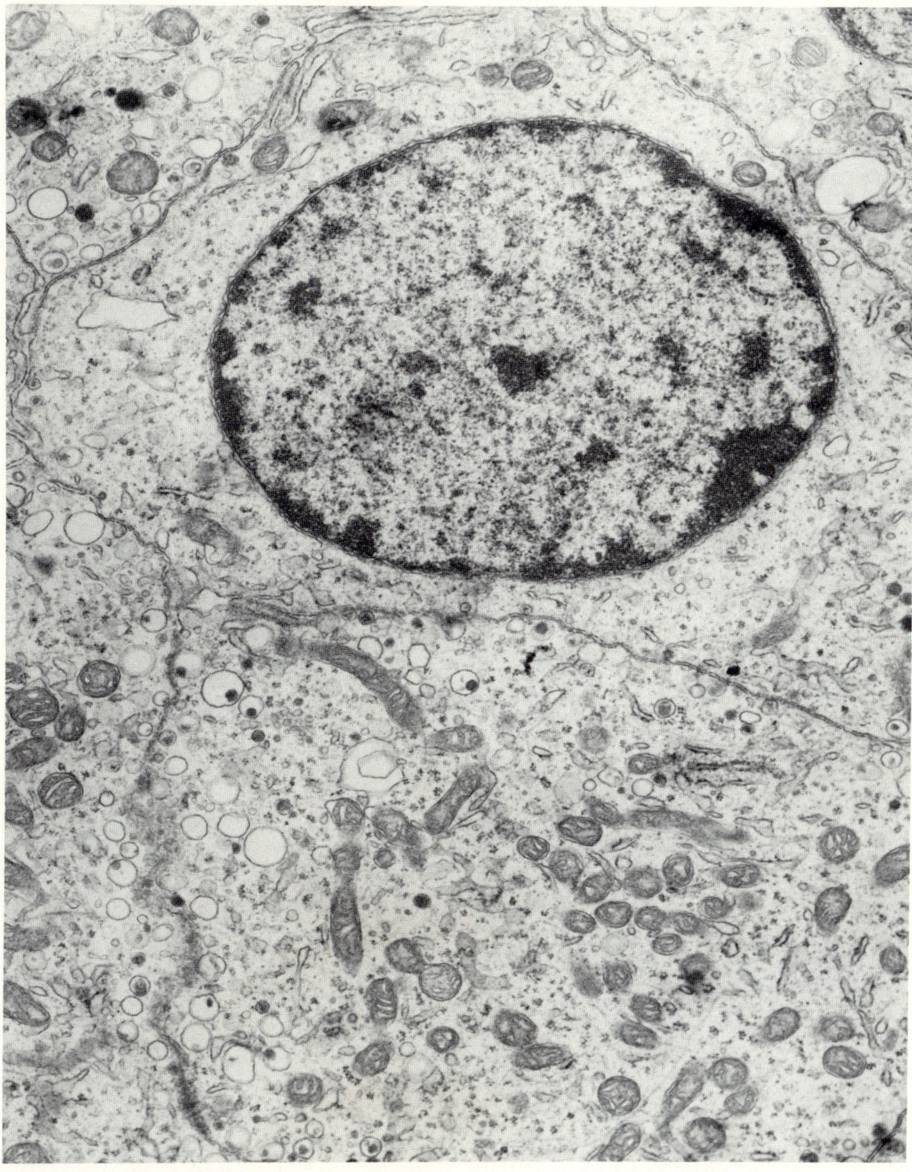

Fig. 301 Pituitary adenoma. Scattered small secretory granules are seen. × 15,000.

1. Pituitary Gland

The normal pituitary (Fig. 280) has been well described in a number of excellent works (Tixier-Vidal and Farquhar, 1975). It is divided into the anterior, endocrine portion and the posterior neural hypophysis. The pituitary gland, as other organs, is subject to various pathological changes including infarcts, hemorrhage (pituitary apoplexy), etc. For the neuropathologist, adenomas of the pituitary constitute the most frequent subject for diagnosis.

In recent times clinicians have differentiated among the pituitary adenomas on the basis of their hormonal secretions. In general, the classification based on secretion correlates with the more traditional morphological classification based on staining reactions.

Adenomas of the pituitary may be divided first into chromophobe or chromophile tumors. Most chromophobes have no apparent specific secretions and present as an expanding mass in the sella turcica and nearby areas (Fig. 88). However, some chromophobe adenomas have been shown to secrete prolactin. Microscopically the tumor appears as a mass of agranular cells forming an "organoid" pattern mimicking an endocrine configuration. Electron microscopic study, however,

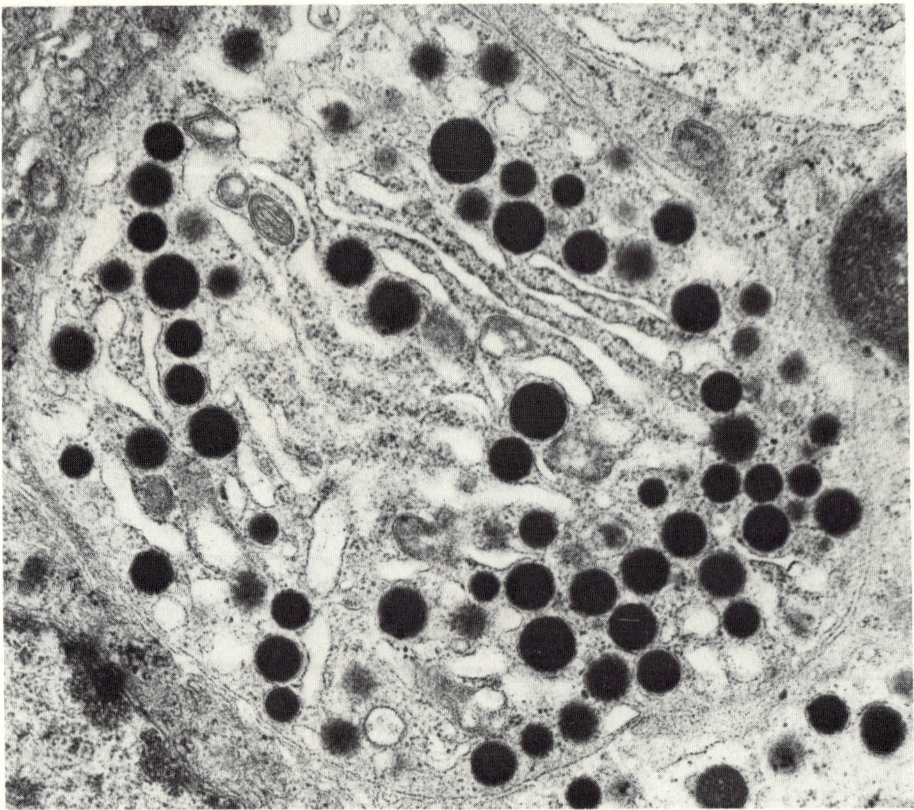

Fig. 302 Pituitary adenoma in a patient with acromegaly. Many large secretory granules are present. × 25,000.

reveals the presence of a few small secretory granules within many of the tumor cells (Fig. 301). Presumably, the secretions found in some chromophobe adenomas may be explained by the presence of these minute granules. The vasculature of chromophobe adenomas is fenestrated as in normal endocrine tissue, but the pores are fewer than ordinarily seen (Hirano et al., 1972).

Chromophile adenomas are classically divided into eosinophilic or basophilic tumors. The eosinophilic adenomas secrete growth hormone and result in acromegaly or gigantism. Fine structural study has revealed that the eosinophilic granules seen in the light microscope consist of large accumulations of membrane-bounded secretory granules (Fig. 302). In some acromegalic patients, however, especially in arrested cases, the eosinophilic granules may not be conspicuous.

Basophilic adenomas may be accompanied by abnormal secretion of ACTH. These tumors are generally small in size and are characterized by the presence of basophilic secretory granules. Certain cases of Cushing's syndrome are associated with a basophilic adenoma.

REFERENCES

Hirano, A., Tomiyasu, U., & Zimmerman, H.M.: The fine structure of blood vessels in chromophobe adenoma. Acta Neuropathol., 22: 200-207, 1972.

Tomiyasu, U., Hirano, A., & Zimmerman, H.M.: Fine structure of human pituitary adenoma. Arch. Pathol., 95: 287-292, 1973.

Tixier-Vidal, A. & Farquhar, M.D. (eds.): The Anterior Pituitary. Academic Press, New York, 1975.

2. Craniopharyngioma (Figs. 69, 89, 303, 304)

Craniopharyngiomas are epidermoid tumors, presumably derived from Rathke's pouch and, while they tend to occur in childhood and adolescence, they may occur at any age. The tumors form masses of stratified epithelium (Fig. 304) and connective tissue in the suprasellar regions which are characterized by cystic spaces

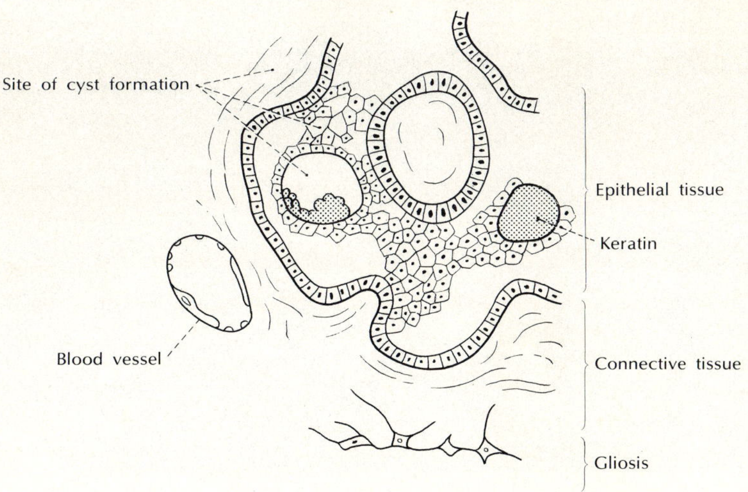

Fig. 303 Craniopharyngioma.

(Fig. 303). The cysts may be widened spaces in the connective tissue, widened extracellular spaces between the epithelial cells forming a honeycomb-like appearance, or they may be keratin-containing spaces lined by squamous cells (Fig. 303) (Ghatak et al., 1971). The blood vessels in the connective tissue are fenestrated (Hirano et al., 1973).

The tumor mass, which may calcify with time, is separated from the parenchyma by a network of glial processes. Rosenthal fibers are commonly found among these processes.

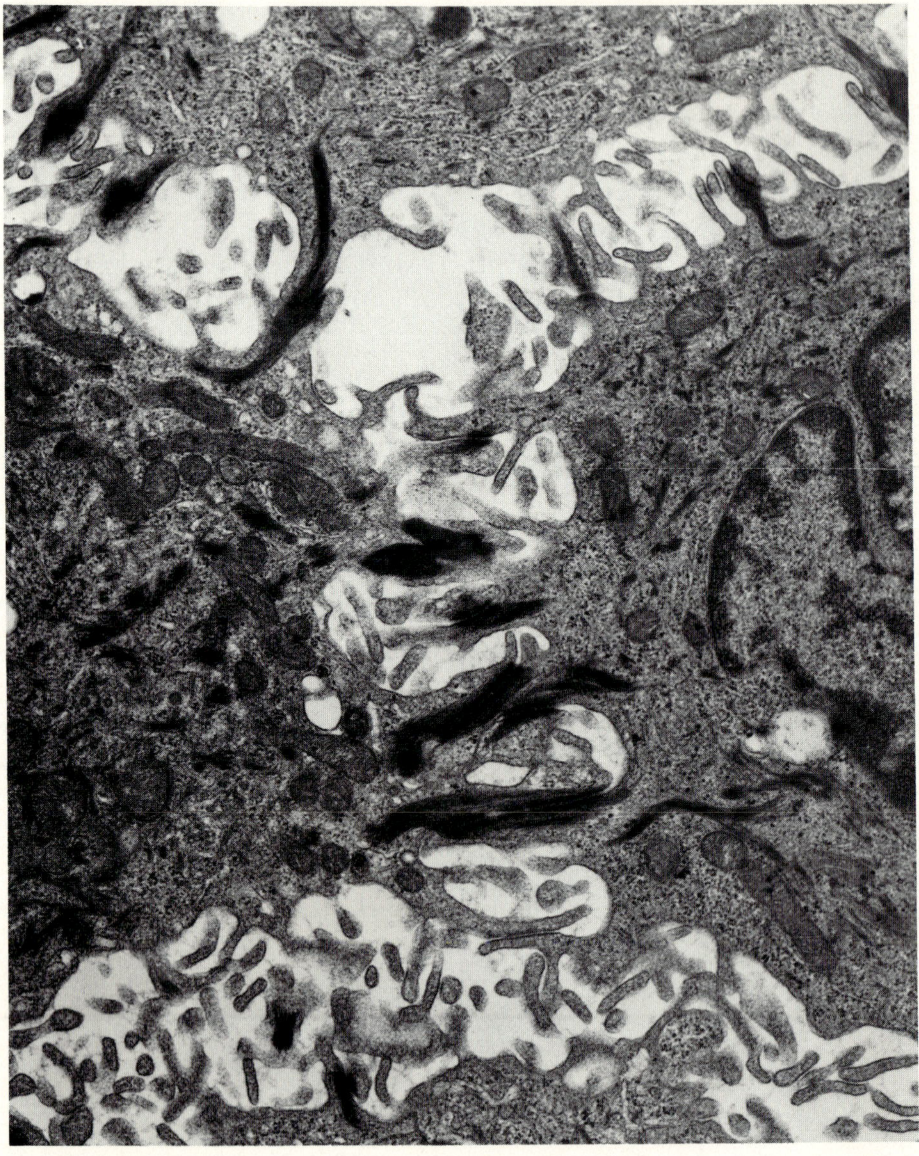

Fig. 304 Craniopharyngioma. There are well developed desmosomes between cells. × 20,000.

REFERENCES

Ghatak, N.R., Hirano, A., & Zimmerman, H.M.: Ultrastructure of a craniopharyngioma. Cancer, 27: 1465-1475, 1971.

Hirano, A., Ghatak, N.R., & Zimmerman, H.M. Fenestrated blood vessels in craniopharyngioma. Acta Neuropathol., 26: 171-177, 1973.

3. Cholesteatoma

Cholesteatomas are also epidermoid in nature. The epithelial-like tumor cells form a cyst around a keratin-containing space. The large amount of keratin is grossly visible and lends the tumor its characteristic "pearly" appearance. Cholesteatomas are most commonly found at the base of the skull, including the cerebello-pontine angle and the suprasellar area, as well as in the lumbosacral region of the spinal cord.

4. Endodermal Cysts (Figs. 305-307)

Endodermal cysts are characterized by a single layer of epithelial cells lining the cystic cavity. They appear at the midline of the neuroaxis and various types of endodermal cysts may be differentiated from one another on the basis of the morphology of the epithelial cells. Cysts with epithelial cells resembling those of the respiratory tract have been seen in the lumbosacral region as well as in the area of the pituitary gland. Other cysts, so-called "enteric" cysts, have epithelial cells with characteristics of the digestive tract. These have been seen in the subarachnoid space of the spinal cord.

Colloid cysts of the third ventricle are benign congenital lesions located at the junction of the lateral and third ventricles. They may be incidental findings at the postmortem examination, but a large cyst may obstruct the foramen of Monro and produce obstructive hydrocephalus.

Histologically, the cyst is surrounded by a single layer of columnar epithelium and contains PAS-positive colloid material within the cavity. Three types of epithelial cells are found. The first is a non-ciliated cell containing secretory vacuoles. The plasma membrane at the apical surface of the cell is covered by a

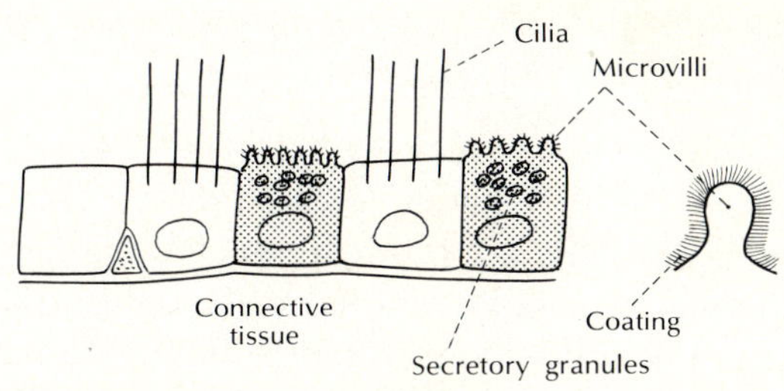

Fig. 305 Wall of an epithelial cyst.

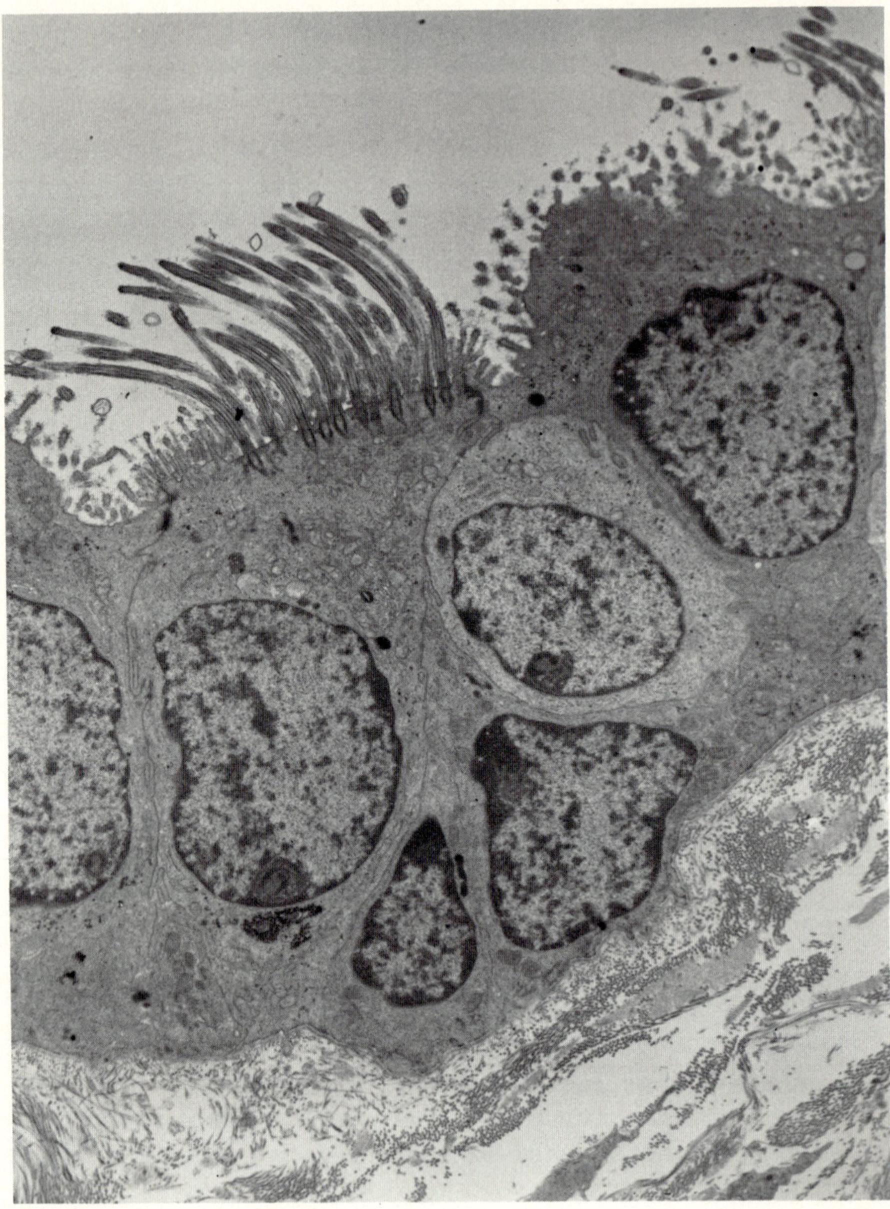

Fig. 306 Wall of an epithelial cyst. Ciliated and non-ciliated cells are present. × 6,000. (From Hirano, A. et al.: Acta Neuropathol., 18: 214, 1971.)

coating material (Hirano and Ghatak, 1977). The secretory cells sometimes resemble goblet cells. These cells are interspersed with ciliated cells devoid of any coating material. In addition, wedge shaped cells are found at the basal region. The third type of epithelial cell is considered to be an immature cell, destined to become either a ciliated or secretory cell (Ghatak et al., 1977). The epithelial cells are separated by a basal lamina from the underlying connective tissue. The cyst

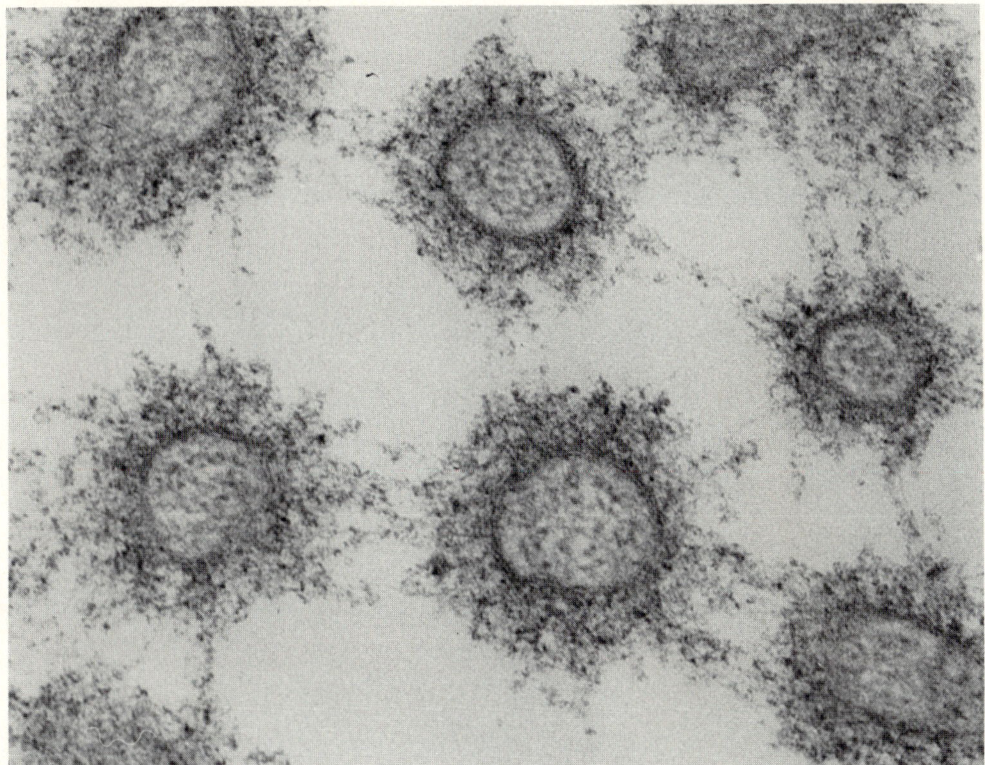

Fig. 307 Cross section of microvilli of non-ciliated cells similar to those illustrated in Fig. 306. Fibrillary and granular material are attached to the surface. Such extensive accumulations of this material are unknown in the normal nervous system. × 128,000. (From Hirano, A., et al.: Acta Neuropathol., 18: 214, 1971.)

cavity contains electron-dense material and floating cellular debris.

Epithelial cysts with essentially the same structure have been seen in the subarachnoid space at the midline of the neuroaxis (Hirano, et al., 1971) and have been regarded by many as neuroepithelial in origin. However, conclusive evidence is still lacking at the present time and the possibility of an endodermal origin must be considered. It should be noted that while the location of colloid cysts is close to the ventricular system they may be regarded as occupying a position in a deeply invaginated portion of the subarachnoid space along the tela choroidea.

REFERENCES

Hirano, A., Ghatak, N.R., Wisoff, H.S., & Zimmerman, H.M.: An epithelial cyst of the spinal cord. An electron microscopic study. Acta Neuropathol., 18: 214-223, 1971.

Hirano, A., & Ghatak, N.R.: The fine structure of colloid cyst of the third ventricle. J. Neuropathol. Exp. Neurol., 33: 333-341, 1974.

Ghatak, N.R., Hirano, A., Kasoff, S.S., & Zimmerman, H.M: Fine structure of an intracerebral epithelial cyst, J. Neurosurg., 41: 75-82, 1974.

Hirano, A. Matsui, T., & Zimmerman, H.M.: The fine structure of epithelial cyst in the central nervous system. Neurol. Surg. (Tokyo), 3: 639-646, 1975.

Ghatak, N.R., Kasoff, I., & Alexander, E., Jr.: Further observation on the fine structure of a colloid cyst of the third ventricle. Acta Neuropathol., 39: 101-107, 1977.

5. Germinoma (Fig. 308)

Germinomas are found in the region of the pineal or suprasellar region. The latter have, in the past, been referred to as "ectopic pinealomas". They usually display a "two cell pattern" containing large epithelial cells and small lymphocyte-like cells. The epithelial cells, which resemble the germ cells of the ovaries or testes, often show annulate lamellae and variable amounts of glycogen. The blood

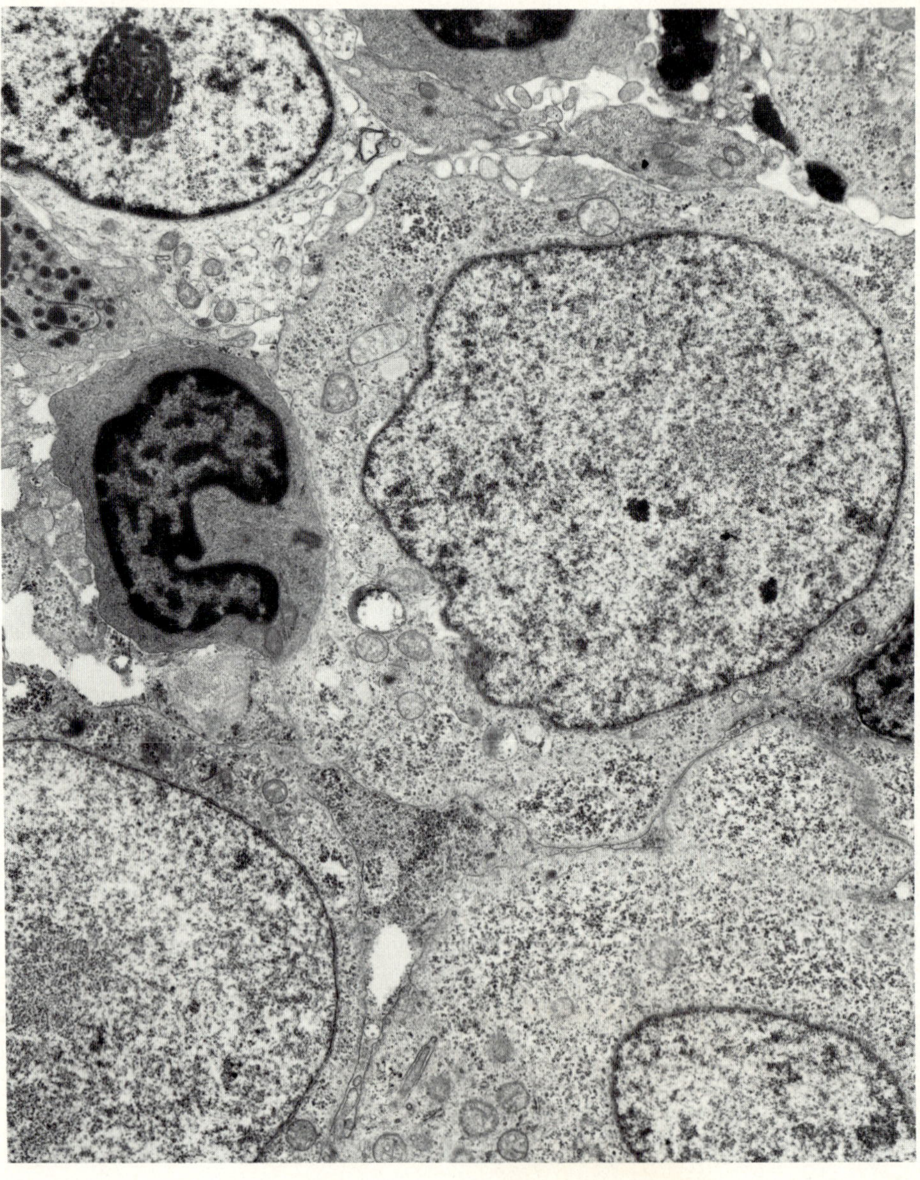

Fig. 308 Germinoma. × 7,000.

vessels are fenestrated. The tumors infiltrate the surrounding neural tissue but are sensitive to radiation.

The region of the pineal gland is also the site of other, rare tumors derived from embryonic tissues. These include teratomas and yolk sac tumors among others.

REFERENCES

Kageyama, N., & Belsky, R.: Ectopic pinealoma in the chiasma region. Neurology, 11: 318-327, 1961.

Ghatak, N.R., Hirano, A., & Zimmerman, H.M.: Intrasellar germinomas: A form of "ectopic pinealoma". J. Neurosurg., 31: 670-675, 1969.

Hirano, A., Llena, J.F., & Chung, H.D.: Some new observations in an intracranial germinoma. Acta Neuropathol., 32: 103-113, 1975.

Matsumura, H., Hirano, A., Zimmerman, H.M. & Ross, E.R.: Fine structure of intracranial germinomas. Report of 3 cases. J. Clin. Electron Microscopy (Tokyo), 9: 195-205, 1976.

6. Teratoma (Fig. 70)

Teratomas are found in the midline of the neuroaxis, especially the pineal region. These benign tumors are not sensitive to radiation and are the subject of surgical removal.

7. Connective Tissue Tumors

As mentioned previously, outside the leptomeninges and the larger blood vessels, connective tissue is not a large component of the normal central nervous system. Nevertheless, these relatively rare components occasionally give rise to neoplastic disease resulting in fibromas or sarcomas. Lipomas, too, while uncommon, have been described in the central nervous system especially along the midline.

REFERENCE

Hirano, A., Llena, J.F., & Chung, H.D.: Fine structure of a cerebellar "fibroma". Acta Neuropathol., 32: 175-186, 1975.

8. Chordoma

Chordomas are derived from the notochord of the embryo and are found along the midline especially the clivus, odontoid process or the vertebral bodies of the sacrococcygeal region. The tumors occupy the epidural space and compress the adjacent tissue including the nerve roots. The cells often contain large amounts of mucopolysaccharide resulting in a "bubble-like" appearance in the light microscope giving rise to their description as "physaliphorous" cells.

REFERENCES

Cancilla, P., Morecki, R., & Hurwitt, E.S.: Fine structure of a recurrent chordoma. Arch. Neurol., 11: 289-295, 1964.

Mair, W.G.P., & Gessaga, E.C.: Ultrastructure of a sacrococcygeal chordoma. Acta Neuropathol., 27: 27-35, 1973.

9. Metastatic Tumors (Figs. 15-17, 95-98, 309-312)

Metastatic tumors to the central nervous system may be derived from a wide variety of primary sites. In men the lung is the most common source and in women most brain metastases arise from carcinoma of the breast. Other common sources are the digestive tract, urinary tract, melanoma, lymphoma, leukemia, sarcoma and others.

Most of these metastases reach the nervous system via the blood stream. Metastatic sites may be either single or, most commonly, multiple. The site of the involvement may be the dura mater, leptomeninges or the parenchyma. Breast carcinoma metastasizes to the dura mater more often than others. Metastatic spread through the subarachnoid space is referred to as leptomeningeal carcinomatosis. In addition to the hematogenous route, metastatic tumors may reach the central nervous system via direct invasion from surrounding structures such as the skull, vertebrae or epidural spaces.

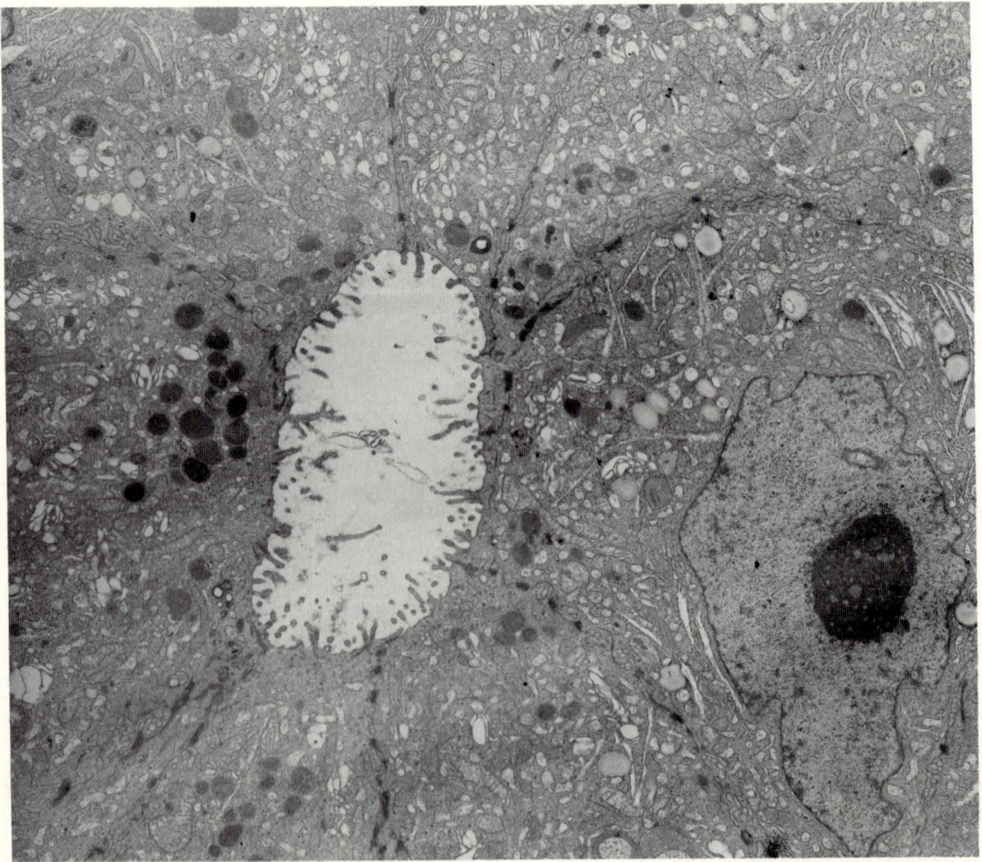

Fig. 309 Metastatic carcinoma. Tumor cells form a lumen into which microvilli protrude. × 4,000. (From Hirano, A.: *In* Progress in Neuropathology. Vol. 1, p. 1, Grune & Stratton, 1971.)

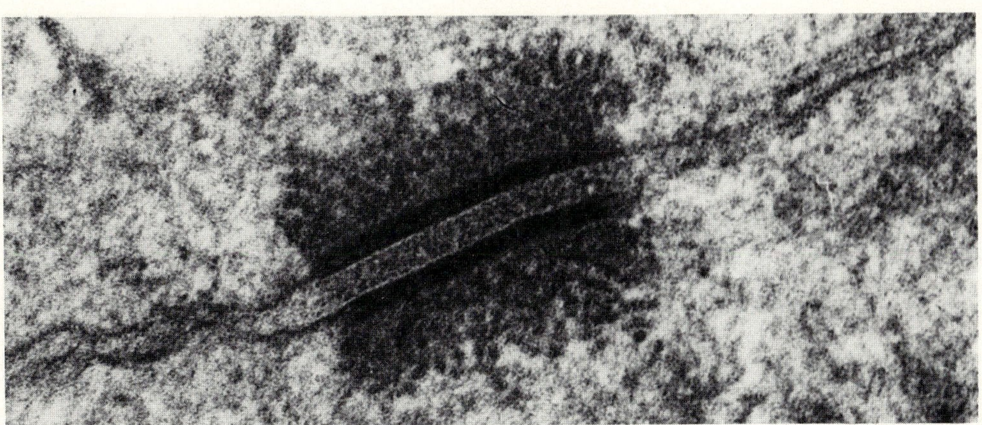

Fig. 310 Metastatic carcinoma. Well developed desmosome. Such well developed structures are unknown in the normal central nervous system. × 160,000. (From Hirano, A.: *In* Progress in Neuropathology. Vol. 1, p. 1, Grune & Stratton, 1971.)

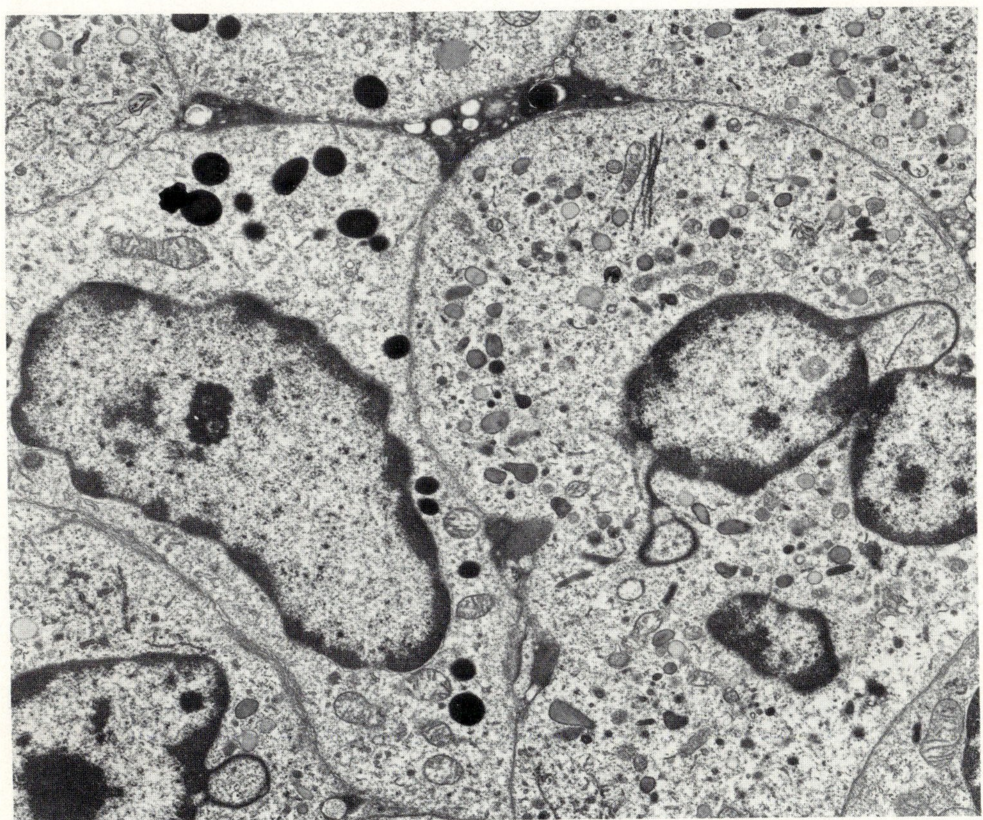

Fig. 311 Tumor cells with variable numbers of granules in an intracranial granulocytic sarcoma. × 3,500. (From Llena, J.F., et al.: Acta Neuropathol., 42: 145, 1978.)

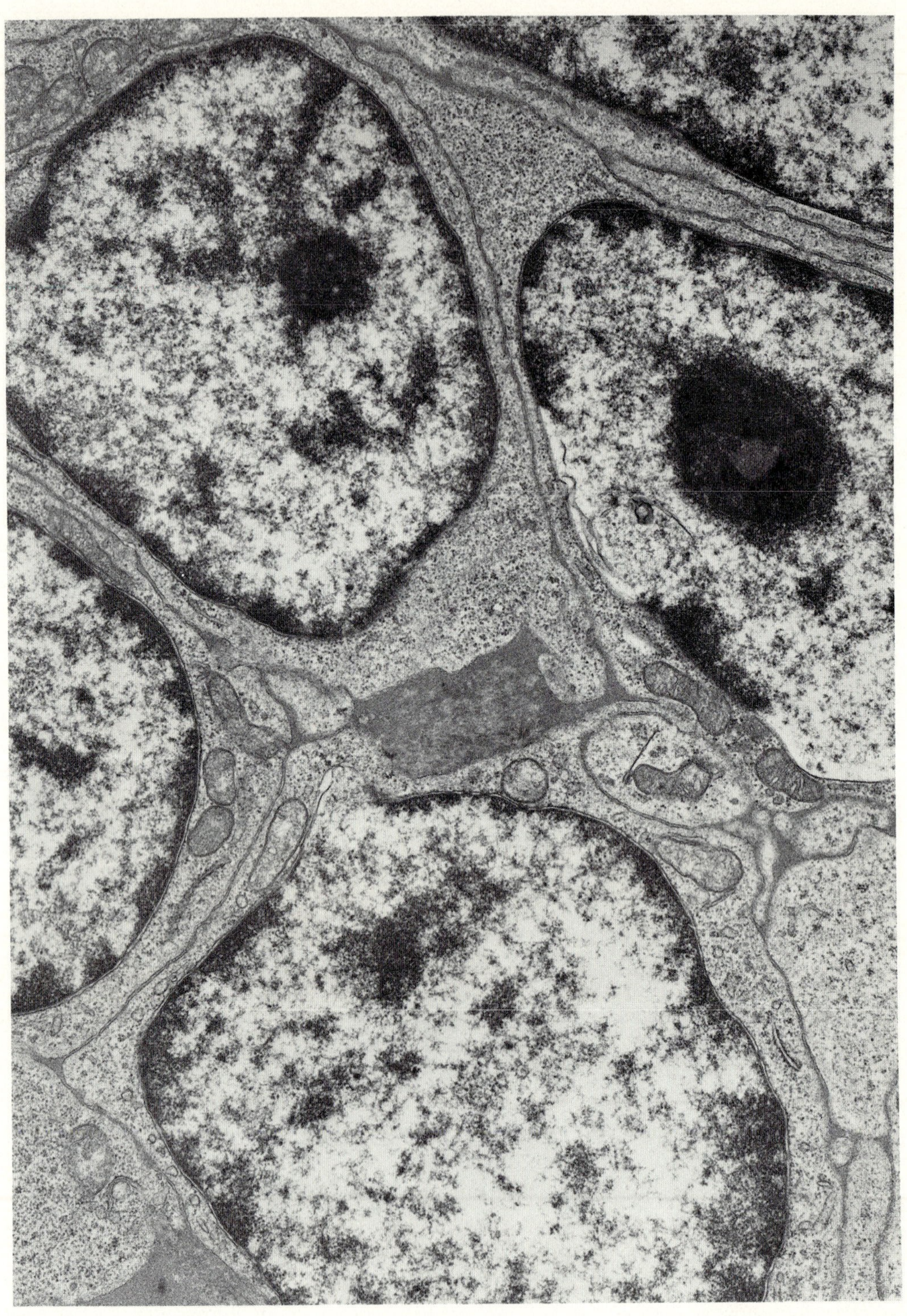

Fig. 312 A primary lymphoma in the central nervous system. The closely packed cells are free of junctional devices. × 15,000. (From Hirano, A.: Acta Neuropathol., 43: 119, 1978.)

Most often, unlike gliomas, metastatic tumors are well circumscribed rather than infiltrative. In many cases, the center becomes necrotic resulting in a cyst-like cavity. Certain tumors such as melanomas, tend to bleed. The reaction of the surrounding brain tissue to the tumor varies a great deal but extensive edema is usually, although not always, present. Final diagnosis of the tumor depends on the histology of the tumor and confirmation of the primary site.

Primary, as well as metastatic lymphomas, of the central nervous system are known. These tumors may be either infiltrative or may form a solid, circumscribed mass. Due to their effect on hematopoietic tissue, lymphomas as well as leukemias may be associated with hemorrhages in the brain even in the absence of any tumor formation in the central nervous system.

The increasing use of chemotherapy and other treatments may be associated with the increased appearance of fungal and viral infections in the central nervous system. Other complications may follow radiotherapy. Delayed radiation necrosis may be observed several months or longer after large doses of radiation. Tissue necrosis associated with vascular alterations, especially fibrinoid necrosis and fibrous sclerosis are seen. These changes may mimic the symptoms of the tumor and be mistaken for its recurrence.

REFERENCES

Barron, K.D., Hirano, A., Araki, S., & Terry, R.D.: Experience with metastatic neoplasms involving the spinal cord. Neurology, 9: 91-106, 1959.

Ghatak, N.R., & White, B.E.: Delayed radiation necrosis of the hypothalmus. Arch. Neurol., 21: 425-430, 1969.

Zimmerman, H.M.: Malignant lymphomas. *In* Pathology of the Nervous System. Vol. 2, 2165-2178, Minckler, J. (ed.), McGraw Hill, New York, 1971.

Hirano, A., & Zimmerman, H.M.: Fenestrated blood vessels in a metastatic renal carcinoma in the brain. Lab. Invest., 26: 465-468, 1972.

Hirano, A., Ghatak, N.R., Becker, N.H., & Zimmerman, H.M.: A comparison of the fine structure of small blood vessels in intracranial and retroperitoneal malignant lymphomas. Acta Neuropathol., 27: 93-104, 1974.

Jellinger, K., & Seitelberger F. (eds.): Lymphomas of the Nervous System. Supplement to Acta Neuropathologica VI, 1975.

Llena, J.F., Cespedes, G., Hirano, A., Zimmerman, H.M., Feiring, E.H., & Fine, D.: Vascular alterations in delayed radiation necrosis of the human brain. An electron microscopic study. Arch. Pathol. Lab. Med., 100: 531-534, 1976.

Llena, J.F., Kawamoto, K., Hirano, A., & Feiring, E.H.: Granulocytic sarcoma of the central nervous system: Initial presentation of leukemia. Acta Neuropathol., 42: 145-147, 1978.

Hirano, A., & Hojo, S.: Metastatic tumors in the central nervous system. The neuropathologial point of view. Neurol. Surg. (Tokyo), 8: 509-518, 599-603, 1980.

III
Selected Textbooks and Journals in Neuropathology

1) Textbooks and Reviews of Neuropathology

Adams, R.D., & Sidman, R.L.: Introduction to Neuropathology. McGraw-Hill Book Co., New York, 1968.

Biggart, J.H.: Pathology of the Nervous System. 3rd Ed., Livingstone, Edinburgh, and London, 1961.

Blackwood, W., & Corsellis, J.A.N. (eds.): Greenfield's Neuropathology. 3rd Ed., Edward Arnold, London, 1976.

Burger, P.C., & Vogel, F.S.: Surgical Pathology of the Nervous System and its Coverings. J. Wiley and Sons, New York, 1976.

Escourolle, R., & Poirier, J.P.: Manual of Basic Neuropathology. 2nd Ed. Translated by L.J. Rubinstein, W.B. Saunders Co., Philadelphia, 1978.

Friede, R.L.: Developmental Neuropathology. Springer-Verlag, New York, 1975.

Haymaker, W.: Bing's Local Diagnosis in Neurological Diseases. C.V. Mosby Co., St. Louis, 1969.

Johannessen, J.V. (ed.): Electron Microscopy in Human Medicine, Vol. 6: Nervous System, Sensory Organs, and Respiratory Tract. McGraw-Hill, New York, 1979.

Lubarsch, O., Henke, F., & Rössle, R.: Handbuch der spezielle pathologischen Anatomie und Histologie Nervensystem. Edited by Scholz, W., Springer-Verlag, Berlin, Part XIII (1-5), 1955-1958.

Minckler, J.: Pathology of the Nervous System. 3 Vols. McGraw-Hill Book Co., New York, 1968-1972.

Peters, G.: Klinische Neuropathologie. 2nd Ed. Georg Thieme Verlag, Stuttgart, 1970.

Robertson, D.M., & Dinsdale, H.B.: The Nervous System. Structure and Function in Disease. Williams & Wilkins, Baltimore, 1972.

Slager, U.T.: Basic Neuropathology. Williams & Wilkins, Baltimore, 1970.

Smith, J.F.: Pediatric Neuropathology. McGraw-Hill Book Co., New York, 1974.

Smith, W.T., & Cavanagh, J.B. (eds.): Recent Advances in Neuropathology. Vol. 1. Churchill Livingstone, Edinburgh, 1979.

Spencer, P., & Schaumburg, H.H. (eds.): Experimental and Clinical Neurotoxicology. Williams & Wilkins, Baltimore, 1980.

Tedeschi, C.G. (ed.): Neuropathology. Methods and Diagnosis. Little, Brown & Co., Boston, 1970.

Vinken, P.J., & Bruyn, G.W. (eds.): Handbook of Clinical Neurology. North Holland Publish., Amsterdam and London. Vol. 1-36, 1968-1979.

Zimmerman, H.M. (ed.): Progress in Neuropathology. Grune & Stratton, New York. Vols. 1, 2 & 3, 1971, 1973 and 1976, Raven Press, New York, Vol. 4, 1979.

2) Atlases of Neuropathology

Blackwood, W., Dodds, T.C., & Sommerville, J.C.: Atlas of Neuropathology. 2nd Edition, E. & S. Livingstone, Ltd. Edinburgh, 1970.

Doerr, W., Schumann, G., & Ule, G.: Atlas of Pathologic Anatomy. Georg Thieme Publishers, Stuttgart, 1978.

Hirano, A., Iwata, M., Llena, J.F., & Matsui, T.: Color Atlas of Pathology of the Nervous System. Igaku-Shoin, Tokyo and New York, 1980.

Malamud, N., & Hirano, A.: Atlas of Neuropathology. 2nd Ed., University of California Press, Berkeley, 1975.

Society of Neuropathology (ed.): Atlas of Neuropathology, Igaku Shoin, 1967.

Treip, C.S.: Color Atlas of Neuropathology. Year Book Medical Publishers, Chicago, 1978.

Zacks, S.I.: Atlas of Neuropathology. Harper & Row, New York, 1971.

3) References on the Pathology of Peripheral Nerve and Muscle

Aguayo, A.J., & Karpati, G. (eds.): Current Topics in Nerve and Muscle Research. Excerpta Medica, Amsterdam, 1979.

Adams, R.D.: Diseases of Muscles. 3rd ed., Hoeber Medical Books, Harper & Row, New York, 1975.

Asbury, A.K., & Johnson, P.C.: Pathology of Peripheral Nerve. W.B. Saunders Co., Philadelphia, 1978.

Bethlem, J.: Muscle Pathology. Introduction and Atlas. North-Holland Publish., Amsterdam and London, 1970.

Coërs, C., & Woolf, A.L.: The Innervation of Muscle. A Biopsy Study. Blackwell Scientific Publications, Oxford, 1959.

Dubowitz, V., & Brooke, M.H. Muscle Biopsy. A Modern Approach. W.B. Saunders Co., Philadelphia, 1973.

Dyck, P.J., Thomas, P.K., & Lambert, E.H.: Peripheral Neuropathy. Vol. I & II. W. B. Saunders Co., Philadelphia, 1975.

Hughes, J.T.: Pathology of Muscle. W.B. Saunders Co., Philadelphia, 1974.

Landon, D.N. (ed.): The Peripheral Nerve. Chapman & Hall, London, 1976.

Walton, J.N.: Disorders of Voluntary Muscles. 3rd Ed. Churchill Livingstone, Edinburgh & London, 1974.

4) Atlases of Peripheral Nerve and Muscle

Babel, J., Bischoff, A., & Spoendlin, H.: Ultrastructure of the Peripheral Nervous System and Sense Organs. Atlas of Normal and Pathological Anatomy. C.V. Mosby Co., St. Louis, 1970.

Mair, W.G.P., & Tome, F.M.S.: Atlas of the Ultrastructure of Diseased Human Muscle. Churchill Livingstone, Edinburgh, 1972.

Uono, M., & Kinoshita, M.: Atlas of Muscle Pathology. Igaku Shoin, Ltd., Tokyo, 1972.

5) Text Books on Tumors

Harkin, J., & Reed, R.J.: Tumors of the Peripheral Nervous System. Armed Forces Institute of Pathology. Washington, D.C., Atlas of Tumor Pathology, Second Series, Fasc.3, 1969.

Rubinstein, L.J. : Tumors of the Central Nervous System. Armed Forces Institute of Pathology. Washington, D.C., Atlas of Tumor Pathology, Second Series, Fasc.6, 1972.

Russell, D.S., & Rubinstein, L.J.: Pathology of Tumours of the Nervous System. 4th ed., Edward Arnold, London, 1977.

Zülch, K.J.: Brain Tumors. Their Biology and Pathology. 2nd ed. Translated by J. Olszewski & A.B. Rothballer, Springer, New York, 1965.

6) Atlases of Tumors

Barnard, R.O., Logue, V., & Reaves, P.S.: An Atlas of Tumours Involving the Central Nervous System. Bailliere-Tindall, London, 1976.

Poon, T.P., Hirano, A., & Zimmerman, H.M.: Electron Microscopic Atlas of Brain Tumors. Grune & Stratton, New York, 1971.

Zimmerman, H.M., Netzky, M.G., & Davidoff, L.M.: Atlas of Tumors of the Nervous System. Lea & Febiger, Philadelphia, 1956.

Zülch, K.J.: Atlas of the Histology of Brain Tumors. Springer-Verlag, New York, 1971.

7) Reference Books on Electron Microscopy of Normal Nervous Tissue

Palay, S.L., & Chan-Palay, V.: Cerebellar Cortex. Cytology and Organization. Springer-Verlag, New York, 1974.

Peters, A., Palay, S.L., & Webster, H. DeF.: The Fine Structure of the Nervous System. The Cells and Their Processes. Harper & Row, New York, 1970.

Sandri, C., Van Buren, J.M. & Akert, K.: Progress in Brain Research, Vol. 46: Membrane Morphology of the Vertebrate Nervous System. A study in Freeze-etch Technique. Elsevier, Amsterdam, 1977.

8) Cytology

Koss, L.G.: Diagnostic Cytology and its Histopathologic Bases. Third Edition. Professional Book Service, New York, 1979.

9) Journals of Neuropathology

Acta Neuropathologica
Journal of Neuropathology and Experimental Neurology
Neuropathology and Applied Neurobiology

10) Neurology Journals

Annals of Neurology
Archives of Neurology
Brain
Clinical Neurology (Tokyo)
Journal of Neurological Science
Journal of Neurology (Berlin)
Journal of Neurology, Neurosurgery and Psychiatry
Muscle and Nerve
Neurology
Neurological Medicine (Tokyo)
Revue Neurologique (Paris)

11) Neurosurgery Journals

Journal of Neurosurgery
Neurologia Medico-Chirurgica (Tokyo)
Neurological Surgery (Tokyo)
Neurosurgery
Surgical Neurology

12) Pathology Journals

American Journal of Pathology
Archives of Pathology and Laboratory Medicine
Human Pathology
Laboratory Investigation

13) Journals of Neuroscience and Related Areas

Advances in Neurological Sciences (Tokyo)
American Journal of Anatomy
Anatomical Record
Brain and Nerve (Tokyo)
Brain Research
Journal of Cell Biology
Journal of Comparative Neurology
Journal of Neurocytology (London)
Journal of Ultrastructural Research
Neurotoxicology
Tissue and Cell (Edinburgh)

INDEX

Page numbers in *italics* indicate illustrations.